Pocket Companion to
Robbins

PATHOLOGIC BASIS OF DISEASE

5th Edition

Stanley L. Robbins, M.D.
Senior Pathologist
Brigham and Women's Hospital
Boston, Massachusetts

Ramzi S. Cotran, M.D.
Frank Burr Mallory Professor of Pathology
Harvard Medical School
Chairman, Departments of Pathology
Brigham and Women's Hospital
The Children's Hospital
Boston, Massachusetts

Vinay Kumar, M.D.
Vernie A. Stembridge Chair in Pathology
University of Texas
Southwestern Medical School
Dallas, Texas

W.B. SAUNDERS COMPANY
A Division of Harcourt Brace & Company
Philadelphia   London   Toronto   Montreal   Sydney   Tokyo

W.B. SAUNDERS COMPANY
A Division of
Harcourt Brace & Company

The Curtis Center
Independence Square West
Philadelphia, Pennsylvania 19106

Library of Congress Cataloging-in-Publication Data

Pocket companion to pathologic basis of disease / [edited by] Stanley L. Robbins, Ramzi S. Cotran, Vinay Kumar. — 2nd ed.

   p.   cm.

   Rev. ed. of: Pocket companion to Robbins pathologic basis of disease / Stanley L. Robbins, Ramzi S. Cotran, Vinay Kumar.

   Includes index.

   ISBN 0–7216–5742–7

   1. Pathology—Handbooks, manuals, etc. I. Robbins, Stanley L. (Stanley Leonard). II. Cotran, Ramzi S. III. Kumar, Vinay. IV. Robbins, Stanley L. (Stanley Leonard). Pocket companion to Robbins pathologic basis of disease. V. Cotran, Ramzi S. Robbins pathologic basis of disease.

   [DNLM: 1. Pathology—handbooks. VERIFIER: 5th ed. for main work not available at CIP stage: related work a.e. for main work made based on 4th ed.; adjust a.e. if necessary.]

RB111.R62   1995 Suppl.

616.07—dc20

DNLM/DLC   95–2348

Pocket Companion to
Robbins Pathologic Basis of Disease   ISBN 0–7216–5742–7
International Edition   ISBN 0–7216–6283–8

Printed in the United States of America.

Last digit is the print number: 9   8   7   6   5   4   3   2

Contributors

Douglas C. Anthony, M.D., Ph.D.
Assistant Professor of Pathology, Harvard Medical School;
Director of Neuropathology, The Children's Hospital;
Neuropathologist, Brigham and Women's Hospital, Boston, MA
Chapter 24: Peripheral Nerve and Skeletal Muscle
Chapter 25: The Central Nervous System

Dennis K. Burns, M.D.
Associate Professor of Pathology, University of Texas
Southwestern Medical School; Pathologist, Parkland Memorial
Hospital and Zale Lipshy University Hospital, Dallas, TX
Chapter 19: Male Genital System
Chapter 21: The Endocrine system

Christopher Corless, M.D.
Pathologist, Veterans Affairs Medical Center; Assistant
Professor of Pathology, Oregon Health Sciences University,
Portland, OR
Chapter 18: Urinary Tract

James M. Crawford, M.D., Ph.D.
Assistant Professor of Pathology, Harvard Medical School;
Associate Pathologist, Brigham and Women's Hospital,
Boston, MA
Chapter 16: The Gastrointestinal Tract
Chapter 17: Liver, Biliary System, and Pancreas

Christopher P. Crum, M.D.
Associate Professor of Pathology, Harvard Medical School;
Director, Division of Women's and Perinatal Pathology,
Brigham and Women's Hospital, Boston, MA
Chapter 20: Female Genital Tract and Breast

Umberto De Girolami, M.D.
Associate Professor of Pathology, Harvard Medical School;
Neuropathologist, Brigham and Women's Hospital and The
Children's Hospital, Boston, MA
Chapter 24: Peripheral Nerve and Skeletal Muscle
Chapter 25: The Central Nervous System

Matthew P. Frosch, M.D., Ph.D.
Instructor in Pathology, Harvard Medical School; Associate
Pathologist, Brigham and Women's Hospital; Consultant in
Pathology, The Children's Hospital, Boston, MA
Chapter 24: Peripheral Nerve and Skeletal Muscle
Chapter 25: The Central Nervous System

Jose Hernandez, M.D.
Associate Professor of Pathology, University of Texas
Southwestern Medical School; Director, Hematology
Laboratory, Parkland Memorial Hospital, Dallas, TX
Chapter 13: Red Cells and Hemostasis
Chapter 14: White Cells, Lymph Nodes, and Spleen

Lester Kobzik, M.D.
Assistant Professor, Department of Pathology, Brigham and
Women's Hospital and Physiology Program, Harvard Medical
School, Boston, MA
Chapter 15: The Respiratory System

Richard N. Mitchell, M.D.
Assistant Professor of Pathology, Harvard Medical School;
Pathologist, Brigham and Women's Hospital, Boston, MA
Chapter 22: The Skin

John Samuelson, M.D., Ph.D.
Associate Professor, Department of Tropical Public Health,
Harvard School of Public Health, Boston, MA
Chapter 8: Infectious Diseases

Frederick J. Schoen, M.D., Ph.D.
Associate Professor of Pathology, Harvard Medical School;
Vice-Chairman, Department of Pathology, Brigham and
Women's Hospital, Boston, MA
Chapter 11: Blood Vessels
Chapter 12: The Heart

Deborah Schofield, M.D.
Assistant Professor of Pathology, Harvard Medical School and
The Children's Hospital, Boston, MA
Chapter 10: Diseases of Infancy and Childhood

Preface

The publication of a new edition of *Robbins Pathologic Basis of Disease (RPBD)* has made necessary a parallel revision of its "Pocket Companion." Despite some hard-gained reduction in the size of the parent text, there continues to be a need for a guide to its use to alleviate the continued pressure of "too much to read and too little time."

More than a topical outline, this small book attempts to distill and extract the essence of the central body of knowledge in *RPBD*. Five new chapters have been added—Cellular Growth and Differentiation: Normal Regulation and Adaptations, Infectious Diseases, Environmental and Nutritional Diseases, Diseases of Infancy and Childhood, and The Skin—to make the two books more completely concordant. Accordingly, the goals of this edition of the Pocket Companion are

- To facilitate the reading and comprehension of the more extended presentations in *RPBD* by providing introductory overviews along with the relevant page numbers to the presentations in the parent book.
- To help students identify the core material requiring their primary attention.
- To provide an "at-a-glance" pocket reference source of the central body of pathologic knowledge.
- To serve as a useful tool for the review of a large body of information.

As before, we must caution against the use of the Pocket Companion as the sole source of information in the study of pathology. Although it contains the salient facts, they are devoid of the discussions and expositions that enrich the fuller presentations. We hope, therefore, that this abbreviated overview of pathology will be used as a companion to the parent book, enhancing the pleasure to be derived from and value of both.

STANLEY L. ROBBINS
RAMZI S. COTRAN
VINAY KUMAR

Contents

Cellular Injury and Cellular Death

INTRODUCTION (p. 1)

Pathology focuses on four aspects of disease:

- Its cause (etiology).
- The mechanisms of its development (pathogenesis).
- The structural alterations induced in cells and tissues (morphology).
- The functional consequences of the morphologic changes, as observed clinically.

DEFINITIONS (p. 2)

All forms of tissue injury start with molecular or structural alterations in cells. Under normal conditions, cells are in a homeostatic "steady state." Cells react to adverse influences by (1) adapting, (2) sustaining reversible injury, or (3) suffering irreversible injury and dying.

Cellular adaptation occurs when excessive physiologic stresses, or some pathologic stimuli, result in a new but altered state that preserves the viability of the cell. Examples are hypertrophy (increase in mass of the cell) or atrophy (decrease in mass of the cell). *Reversible cell injury* denotes pathologic changes that can be reversed when the stimulus is removed, or if the cause of injury is mild. *Irreversible injury* denotes pathologic changes that are permanent and cause cell death.

There are two morphologic patterns of cell death, *necrosis* and *apoptosis*. Necrosis is the more common type after exogenous stimuli and is manifested by swelling, denaturation and coagulation of proteins, breakdown of cellular organelles, and cell rupture. *Apoptosis* is characterized by chromatin condensation and fragmentation, occurs in single or small clusters of cells, and results in the elimination of unwanted cells during embryogenesis and in various physiologic and pathologic states (*see p. 17*).

CAUSES OF CELLULAR INJURY (p. 3)

1. Hypoxia (decrease of oxygen) occurs as a result of (a) ischemia (loss of blood supply), (b) inadequate oxygenation (e.g., cardiorespiratory failure), or (c) loss of oxygen-carrying capacity of the blood (e.g., anemia, carbon monoxide poisoning).

2. Physical agents, including trauma, heat, cold, radiation, and electric shock.
3. Chemical agents and drugs, including:
    a. Therapeutic drugs (e.g., acetaminophen [Tylenol]).
    b. Nontherapeutic agents (e.g., lead, alcohol).
4. Infectious agents, including viruses, rickettsiae, bacteria, fungi, and parasites.
5. Immunologic reactions.
6. Genetic derangements.
7. Nutritional imbalances.

CELL INJURY AND NECROSIS

GENERAL MECHANISMS (p. 4–5)

Certain intracellular systems are particularly vulnerable to cell injury:

- Maintenance of the integrity of cell membranes.
- Aerobic respiration and production of ATP.
- Synthesis of enzymes and structural proteins.
- Preservation of the integrity of the genetic apparatus.

These systems are closely related, and thus injury at one locus leads to wide-ranging secondary effects. The consequences of cell injury depend on the type, duration, and severity of injurious agents, and also the type, state, and adaptability of the responding cell.

The morphologic changes of cell injury become apparent only after some critical biochemical system within the cell has been deranged.

Four biochemical themes are important in mediating cell injury and death.

1. *Oxygen-derived free radicals* are produced in many pathologic conditions and cause deleterious effects on cell structure and function (*see p. 11*).

2. *Loss of calcium homeostasis*, and *increased intracellular calcium*. Ischemia and certain toxins cause net influx of Ca^{++} across the plasma membrane and release of Ca^{++} from mitochondria and endoplasmic reticulum. Increased cytosolic calcium activates *phospholipases* that degrade membrane phospholipids, *proteases* that break down membrane and cytoskeletal proteins, *ATPases* that hasten ATP depletion, and *endonucleases* that are associated with chromatin fragmentation.

3. *ATP depletion,* because it is required for such important processes as membrane transport, protein synthesis, and phospholipid turnover.

4. *Defects in membrane permeability.* Membranes can be damaged directly by toxins, physical and chemical agents, lytic complement components, and perforins, or indirectly as described by the preceding events (*see also p. 10*).

ISCHEMIC AND HYPOXIC INJURY (p. 6)

Reversible Injury

Hypoxia first causes loss of oxidative phosphorylation and ATP generation by mitochondria. Decreased ATP (and an associated increase in AMP) stimulates fructokinase and phosphorylation, resulting in aerobic *glycolysis*. Glycogen is rapidly depleted, and

lactic acid and inorganic phosphate are produced, thus reducing intracellular pH. At this point, there is also clumping of nuclear chromatin (Fig. 1–1).

An early and common manifestation of nonlethal hypoxic injury is *acute cellular swelling*. This is caused by

- Failure of ouabain-sensitive Na^+,K^+-ATPase active membrane transport, causing sodium to enter the cell, potassium to diffuse out of the cell, and an isosmotic gain of water.
- Increased intracellular osmotic load due to the accumulation of inorganic phosphates, lactate, and purine nucleosides.

Other early findings of hypoxic injury include loss of functional polarity in polarized epithelia, detachment of ribosomes from the endoplasmic reticulum, formation of membrane blebs, and myelin figures. *All of the above changes are reversible if oxygenation is restored.*

Irreversible Injury (p. 7)

Irreversible injury is marked by severe mitochondrial vacuolization, extensive damage to plasma membranes, swelling of lysosomes, and the appearance of large, amorphous densities in mitochondria. Injury to lysosomal membranes leads to leakage of the enzymes into the cytoplasm, and by their activation, enzymatic digestion of cell and nuclear components.

Two critical events are involved in irreversible injury: ATP depletion and cell membrane damage.

- *ATP depletion.* An early event in cell injury that contributes to the functional and structural consequences of ischemic hypoxia, and also to cell membrane damage; however, it is controversial whether it is the immediate or primary cause of irreversibility.
- *Cell membrane damage.* The earliest phase of irreversible injury is associated with functional and structural defects of cell membranes. Several mechanisms may contribute to such membrane damage:

  1. *Progressive loss of phospholipids,* due to

     - Activation of membrane phospholipases by the increased cytosolic calcium, leading to phospholipid degradation and phospholipid loss; or
     - Decreased phospholipid reacylation and synthesis, possibly related to loss of ATP.

  2. *Cytoskeletal abnormalities.* Activation of intracellular proteases, induced by increased cytosolic calcium, may cause degradation of intermediate cytoskeletal elements, rendering the cell membrane susceptible to stretching and rupture, particularly in the presence of cell swelling.

  3. *Reactive oxygen species.* These are involved in *reperfusion injury* occurring after restoration of blood flow to the ischemic organ. The toxic oxygen species are produced largely by infiltrating polymorphonuclear leukocytes.

  4. *Lipid breakdown products.* Free fatty acids and lysophospholipids accumulate in ischemic cells as a result of phospholipid degradation and are directly toxic to membranes.

  5. *Loss of intracellular amino acids,* such as glycine and L-alanine, by currently unknown mechanisms.

Loss of membrane integrity causes massive influx of calcium from the extracellular space, resulting in mitochondrial dysfunction, inhibition of cellular enzymes, denaturation of proteins, and

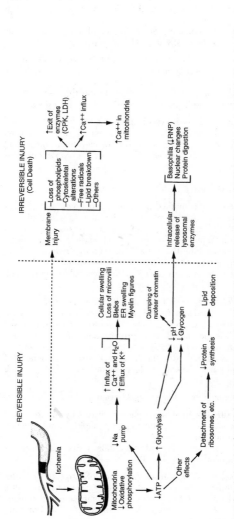

REVERSIBLE INJURY

Ischemia

Mitochondria
↓ Oxidative phosphorylation

↓ATP

↓Na pump → ↑Influx of Ca⁺⁺ and H₂O ↑Efflux of K⁺ → Cellular swelling
Loss of microvilli
Blebs
ER swelling
Myelin figures

↑Glycolysis → ↓pH
↓Glycogen → Clumping of nuclear chromatin

Other effects

Detachment of ribosomes, etc. → ↓Protein synthesis → Lipid deposition

IRREVERSIBLE INJURY (Cell Death)

Membrane Injury
- Loss of phospholipids
- Cytoskeletal alterations
- Free radicals
- Lipid breakdown
- Others

↑Exit of enzymes (CPK, LDH)
↑Ca⁺⁺ influx → ↑Ca⁺⁺ in mitochondria

Intracellular release of lysosomal enzymes → Basophilia (↓RNP)
Nuclear changes
Protein digestion

Figure 1–1. Postulated sequence of events in ischemic injury. Note that although reduced oxidative phosphorylation and ATP levels have a central role, ischemia can cause direct membrane damage. (From Cotran, R.S., Kumar, V., and Robbins, S.L.: Robbins Pathologic Basis of Disease. 5th ed. Philadelphia, W.B. Saunders Co., 1994, p. 6.)

the cytologic alterations characteristic of coagulative necrosis (see below).

In summary, hypoxia affects oxidative phosphorylation and hence the synthesis of vital ATP supplies; membrane damage is critical to the development of lethal cell injury; and calcium is an important mediator of the biochemical and morphologic alterations leading to cell death.

FREE RADICAL-INDUCED CELL INJURY (p. 11)

Free radicals are highly reactive, unstable species that interact with proteins, lipids, and carbohydrates and are involved in cell injury induced by a variety of chemical and biologic events.

Free radical initiation occurs by

- Absorption of radiant energy (UV light, x-rays).
- Oxidative metabolic reactions.
- Enzymatic conversion of exogenous chemicals or drugs (CCl_4 to $\overset{\bullet}{CCl_3}$).
- *Oxygen-Derived Radicals* are a particularly important toxic species (see below).
- *Superoxide* is generated directly during auto-oxidation in mitochondria, or enzymatically by oxidases:

$$O_2 \xrightarrow{\text{oxidase}} O_2^{\bullet-}$$

Superoxide is inactivated by superoxide dismutase (SOD):

$$O_2^{\bullet-} + O_2^{\bullet-} + 2H^+ \xrightarrow{\text{SOD}} H_2O_2 + O_2$$

- *Hydrogen peroxide* is produced

  1. By dismutation of superoxide (as above).
  2. Directly by oxidases present in peroxisomes.

- *Hydroxyl radicals* are formed

  1. By hydrolysis of water caused by ionizing radiation

$$H_2O \rightarrow H^{\bullet} + OH^{\bullet}$$

  2. By interaction with transitional metals in the Fenton reaction

$$Fe^{++} + H_2O_2 \rightarrow Fe^{+++} + OH^{\bullet} + OH^-$$

  3. Through the Haber-Weiss reaction:

$$H_2O_2 + O_2^{\bullet-} \rightarrow OH^{\bullet} + OH^- + O_2$$

- *Nitric oxide* (see Chapter 3) can act as a free radical and can also be converted to highly reactive species ($ONOO^-$), $NO_2^{\bullet}$ and NO_3^- by superoxide ion.

$$NO^{\bullet} + O_2^{\bullet-}H \rightarrow ONOO^- + H^+$$

$$\uparrow \downarrow$$

$$OH^{\bullet} + NO_2^{\bullet} \leftrightarrows ONOOH \rightarrow NO_3^-$$

Free radicals cause cell injury through peroxidation of lipids, cross-linking of proteins by the formation of disulfide bonds, inactivation of sulfhydryl enzymes, and induction of DNA damage that has been implicated both in cell killing and malignant transformation.

Free radical *termination* occurs either by spontaneous decay or by inactivation by several mechanisms:

1. Antioxidants (vitamin E, glutathione, ceruloplasmin, and transferrin). Transferrin in particular binds free iron, which catalyzes free radical formation.
2. Enzymes:

   - Superoxide dismutase (see earlier)
   - Catalase

   $$2H_2O_2 \rightarrow O_2 + 2H_2O$$

   - Glutathione peroxidase

   $$2OH^{\bullet} + 2GSH \rightarrow 2H_2O + GSSG$$

   OR

   $$H_2O_2 + 2GSH \rightarrow 2H_2O + GSSG$$

In many pathologic processes the final outcome of stimulus-induced free radicals depends on the net balance between free radical formation and termination.

CHEMICAL INJURY (p. 13)

Chemicals cause cell injury by two mechanisms:

- Directly; e.g., mercury of mercuric chloride binds to SH groups of cell membrane proteins, causing increased permeability and inhibition of ATPase-dependent transport.
- By conversion to reactive toxic metabolites. Toxic metabolites in turn cause cell injury either by direct covalent binding to membrane protein and lipids, or more commonly by the formation of reactive free radicals, as previously described. For example, *carbon tetrachloride (CCl$_4$)*, widely used in the dry-cleaning industry, is converted to CCl$_3$$^{\bullet}$ in the smooth ER in the liver by P-450. CCl$_3$$^{\bullet}$ initiates lipid peroxidation and autocatalytic reactions that cause swelling and breakdown of the endoplasmic reticulum, dissociation of ribosomes, and decreased hepatic protein synthesis. Loss of lipid acceptor protein leads to lipid accumulation and fatty change in the liver. This is followed by progressive cellular swelling, plasma membrane damage, and cell death.

Acetaminophen (Tylenol) acts by both oxidative damage and covalent binding. The drug is detoxified in the liver through sulfation and glucuronidation and is also converted to a toxic metabolite by cytochrome P-450. When large doses are ingested, the metabolites accumulate in the cell owing to GSH depletion and covalently bind proteins and nucleic acids, thus increasing drug toxicity and resulting in massive liver cell necrosis.

MORPHOLOGY OF REVERSIBLE CELL INJURY AND NECROSIS (p. 14)

The ultrastructural changes were described earlier and are shown in Figure 1–2. *Cellular swelling* is a near-universal manifestation of *reversible* injury by light microscopy. In cells involved in fat metabolism, *fatty change* can also denote *reversible* injury.

Necrosis is the sum of the morphologic changes that follow cell death in living tissue or organs.

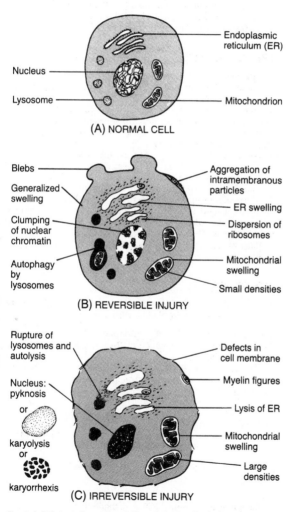

Figure 1-2. Schematic representation of a normal cell (A) and the ultra-structural changes in reversible (B) and irreversible (C) cell injury (see text). (From Cotran, R. S., Kumar, V., and Robbins, S. L.: Robbins Pathologic Basis of Disease. 5th ed. Philadelphia, W. B. Saunders Co., 1994, p. 7.)

Two processes cause the basic morphologic changes of necrosis:

- Denaturation of proteins.
- Enzymatic digestion of organelles and cytosol.

Autolysis indicates enzymatic digestion by lysosomal enzymes of the dead cells themselves. *Heterolysis* is digestion by lysosomal enzymes of immigrant leukocytes.

- The necrotic cell is eosinophilic and glassy and may be vacuolated. The cell membranes are fragmented. Nuclear changes in necrotic cells include *pyknosis* (small, dense nucleus); *karyolysis* (faint, dissolved nucleus); and *karyorrhexis* (nucleus broken up into many clumps).

TYPES OF NECROSIS (p. 16)

- *Coagulation necrosis.* This common pattern of ischemic necrosis, described earlier, occurs in the myocardium, kidney, liver, and other organs.
- *Liquefaction necrosis.* Occurs when autolysis and heterolysis prevail over protein denaturation. The necrotic area is soft and filled with fluid. Most frequently seen in the brain and localized bacterial infections (abscesses).
- *Caseous necrosis.* Characteristic of tuberculous lesions, this appears grossly as soft, friable, cheesy material and microscopically as amorphous eosinophilic material with cell debris.
- *Fat necrosis.* This refers to necrosis in adipose tissue, induced by the action of lipases (derived from injured pancreatic cells or macrophages) that catalyze decomposition of triglycerides to fatty acids, which then complex with calcium to create calcium soaps. Histologically, the necrotic fat shows shadowy outlines of cells and basophilic stippling due to calcium deposition.

APOPTOSIS (p. 17)

This form of cell death differs from necrosis in several respects (Table 1–1) and occurs in the following settings:

- programmed destruction of cells during embryogenesis
- hormone-dependent involution of tissues (e.g., endometrium, prostate) in the adult
- cell deletion in proliferating cell populations (e.g., intestinal crypt epithelium), tumors, and lymphoid organs
- pathologic atrophy in parenchymal organs after duct obstruction
- cell death by cytotoxic T cells
- cell injury in certain viral diseases
- cell death produced by a variety of injurious stimuli when given in low doses (e.g., mild thermal injury)

The *morphologic features* of apoptosis include:

- cell shrinkage
- chromatin condensation and fragmentation
- formation of cytoplasmic blebs and apoptotic bodies
- phagocytosis of apoptotic bodies by adjacent healthy cells or macrophages
- lack of inflammation

Because apoptosis occurs in single or small clusters of cells and

Table 1–1. Features of Necrosis Versus Apoptosis

	Necrosis	**Apoptosis**
Stimuli	Hypoxia, toxins	Physiologic and pathologic
Histology	Cellular swelling	Single cells
	Coagulation necrosis	Chromatin condensation
	Disruption of organelles	Apoptotic bodies
DNA breakdown	Random, diffuse	Internucleosomal
Mechanisms	ATP depletion	Gene activation
	Membrane injury	Endonuclease
	Free radical damage	
Tissue reaction	Inflammation	No inflammation
		Phagocytosis of apoptotic bodies

From Cotran, R. S., Kumar, V., and Robbins, S. L.: Robbins Pathologic Basis of Disease. 5th ed. Philadelphia, W. B. Saunders Co., 1994, p. 18.

does not cause inflammation, it may be difficult to demonstrate histologically.

MECHANISMS. The chromatin condensation and fragmentation are associated with a characteristic *internucleosomal* DNA fragmentation as seen on agar gel electrophoresis. The fragmentation is thought to be mediated by activation of a calcium-sensitive *endonuclease*, due to an increase in free cytosolic calcium that occurs early in apoptosis. Transglutaminase activation partly accounts for the shape and volume changes, and phagocytosis of apoptotic bodies is mediated by receptors on macrophages for surface components on apoptotic cells.

In many instances, apoptosis is dependent on gene activation and new protein synthesis, and it is thought that the process is regulated by a number of apoptosis-associated genes. In humans, these include *bcl-2*, which inhibits apoptosis and therefore extends cell survival; *p-53*, which normally stimulates apoptosis but when mutated or absent favors cell survival; and c-*myc*, whose protein product either stimulates or inhibits apoptosis, depending on the presence of other signals (see also discussion of these genes, and the involvement of apoptosis in tumor growth in Chapter 7).

SUBCELLULAR ALTERATIONS IN CELL INJURY (p. 21)

LYSOSOMES

- *Heterophagy* is the uptake of materials from the external environment by phagocytosis. Examples: phagocytosis and degradation of bacteria by leukocytes, removal of necrotic debris by macrophages, reabsorption of protein by the proximal tubules.
- *Autophagy* is the phagocytosis by lysosomes of deteriorating intracellular organelles, including mitochrondria and endoplas-

mic reticulum. Autophagy is particularly pronounced in cells undergoing atrophy. Lysosomes with undigested debris (autophagic vacuoles) may persist within cells as *residual bodies*, or may be extruded from the cell.

HYPERTROPHY OF SMOOTH ENDOPLASMIC RETICULUM

Certain drugs (e.g., phenobarbital) stimulate hypertrophy of the smooth endoplasmic reticulum, the site of detoxification of these drugs by the mixed-function oxidase electron transport pathway (P-450). This results in increased tolerance to the drug and increased capacity to detoxify other drugs handled by the same system.

INTRACELLULAR ACCUMULATIONS (p. 24)

Proteins, carbohydrates, and lipids can accumulate in cells and sometimes cause cellular injury. They may be

- A *normal* cellular constituent accumulating in excess.
- An *abnormal* substance, usually a product of abnormal metabolism.
- A *pigment*.

Processes that result in abnormal intracellular accumulations include

- *Abnormal* metabolism of a *normal* endogenous substance (e.g., fatty liver).
- *Lack of an enzyme* necessary for the metabolism of a normal or abnormal endogenous substance (e.g., lysosomal storage disease).
- *Deposition of abnormal exogenous substances* (e.g., carbon-laden macrophages).

STEATOSIS (FATTY CHANGE) (p. 25)

This represents a normal constituent (triglycerides) accumulating in excess and leading to an absolute increase in intracellular lipids. It results in the formation of intracellular fat vacuoles. It occurs occasionally in almost all organs but is most common in the liver; when excessive it may lead to cirrhosis.

PATHOGENESIS OF FATTY LIVER. Causes of fatty liver include alcohol abuse, protein malnutrition, diabetes mellitus, obesity, hepatotoxins, and drugs. Fatty livers are enlarged, yellow, and greasy and the fat is seen microscopically as small, fatty, cytoplasmic droplets or as large vacuoles. The condition is caused by one of the following mechanisms, as illustrated in Figure 1–3:

- Excessive entry of free fatty acids into the liver (e.g., starvation, corticosteroid therapy).
- Enhanced fatty acid synthesis.
- Decreased fatty acid oxidation.
- Increased esterification of fatty acids to triglycerides, due to an increase in alpha-glycerophosphate (alcohol).
- Decreased apoprotein synthesis (carbon tetrachloride poisoning).
- Impaired lipoprotein secretion from the liver (alcohol, orotic acid administration).

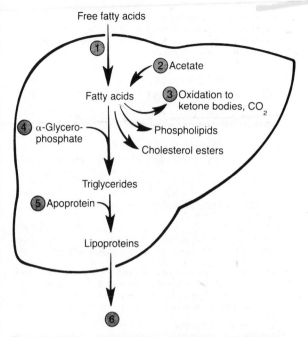

Free fatty acids

Figure 1-3. Possible mechanisms in the pathogenesis of fatty liver. The illustration depicts the uptake and metabolism of fatty acids by the liver, formation of triglycerides, and secretion of lipoproteins. Defects in any of the six numbered steps can lead to accumulation of triglycerides and fatty liver. (From Cotran, R. S., Kumar, V., and Robbins, S. L.: Robbins Pathologic Basis of Disease. 5th ed. Philadelphia, W. B. Saunders Co., 1994, p. 25.)

Acute fatty liver of pregnancy and *Reye's syndrome* are sometimes fatal but rare conditions in which a defect in mitochondrial oxidation is suspected.

CHOLESTEROL AND CHOLESTEROL ESTERS

- In atherosclerosis, these lipids accumulate in smooth muscle cell and macrophages owing to mechanisms discussed on *page 481.* Intracellular cholesterol accumulates in the form of small cytoplasmic vacuoles. Extracellular cholesterol gives characteristic rhomboid cleftlike cavities formed by the dissolved cholesterol crystals.
- In acquired and hereditary hyperlipidemia, lipid accumulates in macrophages and mesenchymal cells.
- In foci of cell injury and inflammation, lipid-laden macrophages result from phagocytosis of membrane lipids derived from injured cells ("foamy macrophages").

OTHER INTRACELLULAR ACCUMULATIONS (p. 27)

- *Proteins.* Example: with proteinuria, reabsorption of protein forms droplets in proximal convoluted tubules. Plasma cells filled with immunoglobulin within distended cisternae of the endoplasmic reticulum (Russell bodies).

- *Glycogen.* Example: genetic storage disease (*see p. 146*).
- *Complex lipids and polysaccharides.* Examples: Gaucher's disease, Niemann-Pick disease.
- *Exogenous pigments:*

  - *Anthracosis.* Accumulation of carbon in the macrophages of the lungs and lymph nodes from air pollution.
  - *Tattooing.* Injected pigment is taken up by macrophages and persists forever in the cells and extracellularly.

- *Endogenous pigments.* These include

  - *Lipofuscin.* The "wear-and-tear" pigment, seen microscopically as yellow-brown, fine, intracytoplasmic granules, usually associated with atrophy ("brown atrophy"). Composed of complex lipids, phospholipids, and protein, suggesting that it is derived from peroxidation of polyunsaturated lipids of cellular membranes.
  - *Melanin.* An endogenous, non–hemoglobin-derived, brown-black pigment formed when the enzyme tyrosinase catalyzes the oxidation of tyrosine to dihydroxyphenylalanine in melanocytes.
  - *Hemosiderin.* A hemoglobin-derived, golden-yellow to brown, granular pigment. Composed of aggregates of ferritin micelles. Intracellular accumulation occurs as a localized process or a systemic derangement.

  Local hemosiderosis results from gross hemorrhage or rupture of small vessels due to vascular congestion. Macrophages take up hemoglobin, and lysosomal enzymes convert it to hemosiderin, a ferritin-containing pigment.

  Systemic hemosiderosis occurs with

- Increased absorption of dietary iron (primary hemochromatosis).
- Impaired utilization of iron (e.g., thalassemia).
- Hemolytic anemias, causing excessive breakdown of red cells.
- Transfusions, increasing the exogenous load of iron.

PATHOLOGIC CALCIFICATION (p. 30)

Pathologic calcification implies the abnormal deposition of calcium salts in soft tissues. *Dystrophic calcification* occurs in nonviable or dying tissues in the presence of normal calcium serum levels. In *metastatic calcification,* deposition of calcium salts is in vital tissues and is always associated with hypercalcemia.

Dystrophic Calcification

This occurs in arteries in atherosclerosis, in damaged heart valves, and in areas of necrosis (coagulative, caseous, and liquefactive). Calcium can be intracellular, extracellular, or in both locations.

Calcification involves two phases:

- *Initiation* occurs *extracellularly* in membrane-bound vesicles derived from dead or dying cells (200 nm) that concentrate calcium by their affinity for acidic phospholipids; phosphates accumulate as a result of the action of membrane-bound phosphatases. Initiation of *intracellular* calcification occurs in mitochondria of dead or dying cells.

- *Propagation* of crystal formation depends on the concentration of calcium and phosphates, the presence of mineral inhibitors, and the presence of collagen.

Metastatic Calcification

This results from hypercalcemia caused by hyperparathyroidism, vitamin D intoxication, systemic sarcoidosis, hyperthyroidism, Addison's disease, bone tumors, metastatic bone cancers, immobilization, and idiopathic hypercalcemia. Calcium deposits occur widely throughout the body, affecting the interstitial tissues of blood vessels, kidneys, lungs, and stomach.

HYALINE CHANGE (p. 31)

Hyalin refers to any alteration within cells or in the extracellular spaces or structures that gives a homogeneous, glassy-pink appearance in routine histologic sections stained with H&E.
    Examples of *intracellular hyalin* include

1. Absorption of protein causing hyaline droplets in proximal epithelial cells of the kidney.
2. Russell bodies in plasma cells.
3. Viral inclusions in the cytoplasm or the nucleus.
4. Masses of altered intermediate filaments (such as alcoholic hyalin, *see p. 858*).

Extracellular hyalin occurs in hyaline arteriolosclerosis, in atherosclerosis, and in damaged glomeruli. *Amyloid* (*see p. 231*) also has a hyaline appearance but is a fibrillar protein with specific biochemical characteristics. Amyloid can be differentiated from hyaline connective tissue by its characteristic staining with *Congo red*, with which it appears red and shows apple-green bipolar refringence.

CELLULAR AGING

With age, there are physiologic and structural alterations in almost all organ systems. Aging is effected in individuals by genetic factors, diet, social conditions, and the occurrence of age-related diseases such as arteriosclerosis, diabetes, and arthritis. In addition, however, age-induced alterations in cells, which could represent the progressive accumulation over the years of sublethal injury or cell death, are thought to be important components of aging.
    A number of functional and morphologic alterations occur in aging cells. These include

- reduced oxidative phosphorylation by mitochondria.
- diminished DNA and RNA synthesis of structural and enzymatic proteins and cell receptors.
- decreased capacity for uptake of nutrients and repair of chromosomal damage.
- irregular and abnormally lobed nuclei.
- pleomorphic mitochondria, decreased ER, and distorted Golgi apparatus.
- a steady accumulation of *lipofuscin* pigment.

The genesis of cell aging is unclear, but it is probably multifactorial. It involves an *endogenous* molecular program of *cellular senescence* as well as continuous *exogenous* influences leading to decreased cell survivability (so-called wear and tear).

Cellular senescence can be inferred from *in vitro* studies showing that normal human diploid fibroblasts in culture have finite life spans and population doublings, which are age dependent. Possible causes of such replicative senescence include the activation of senescence-specific genes; altered or loss of growth regulatory genes; induction of growth inhibitors in senescent cells, and other mechanisms. One hypothesis for these gene defects is chromosomal *"telomeric shortening"* with age, causing loss of DNA from the telomeric ends of the chromosome, leading to the deletion of essential genes and consequent limiting of the lifespan.

Potential mechanisms of the exogenous *wear and tear* defects include:

- *Free radical damage* due to repeated environmental exposure to exogenous agents or progressive reduction of antioxidant defense mechanisms (e.g., vitamin E). Free radicals cause lipofuscin accumulation, nucleic acid damage, mitochondrial DNA mutations, and oxidative modification of enzymes rendering them degradable by proteases, further affecting cell function.
- *Nonenzymatic glycosylation of proteins* leading to the formation of advanced glycosylation end products, which, as we shall see (diabetes discussion) cause cross-linking of adjacent proteins and a number of other potentially damaging biochemical effects.
- *Alterations in the induction of heat-shock proteins.* The heat-shock response is an important defense mechanism against stresses, and its loss with age may decrease cell survival.

CHAPTER TWO

Cellular Growth and Differentiation: Normal Regulation and Adaptations

Replacement of injured or dead cells is critical to survival. Repair of tissues involves two distinct processes: (1) *regeneration,* denoting replacement of dead cells by proliferation of cells of the same type, and (2) *replacement by connective tissue* or fibroplasia. In most cases both contribute to repair. Both regeneration and fibroplasia are determined by largely similar mechanisms involving *cell growth and differentiation* and cell-matrix interactions.

CONTROL OF CELL GROWTH (p. 36)

The most important factors that regulate cell growth are those that recruit quiescent (G_0) cells into the cell cycle.

CELL CYCLE AND TYPES OF CELLS

Cells are divided into three groups based on their proliferative capacity and their relationship to the cell cycle.

- *Continuously dividing cells (labile cells),* such as surface epithelia, and cells of the bone marrow and hematopoietic cells.
- *Quiescent (or stable) cells,* normally with slow turnover but capable of rapid division in response to stimuli—such as liver, kidney, fibroblasts, smooth muscle, and endothelial cells.
- *Nondividing (permanent) cells,* which cannot undergo division in postnatal life—for example, neurons, skeletal and cardiac muscle.

MOLECULAR EVENTS IN CELL GROWTH (p. 37)

Growth is stimulated largely by polypeptide growth factors in serum or produced by cells.

The chain of molecular events induced by growth factors (GF) includes the following:

1. **Binding of GF to Receptors,** most commonly on the plasma membrane but occasionally intracellularly.
2. **GF Receptor Activation.** Most GF receptors have intrin-

sic tyrosine kinase (TK) activity, which is activated (phosphorylated) by ligand binding. Receptors without TK activity recruit intracellular kinases, such as protein kinase-C (PKC), leading, in either case, to a protein phosphorylation cascade (see below).

3. **Signal Transduction and Second Messengers.** The phosphorylated receptors (or PKC) bind to SH2 domain containing proteins, which, through SH3 domains phosphorylate several signaling proteins, including:

- *Phospholipase C-γ*, which degrades PIP_2 (phosphoinositol-4,5-biphosphate) to form IP_3 (inositol triphosphate) and DAG (diacylglycerol), the latter in turn activating PKC.
- *GTP binding proteins,* including G proteins and the *ras* protein family, which are converted from the inactive GDP-binding form to the active GTP-binding form by phosphorylation. *Activated ras* activates *Raf-1,* which in turn activates a cascade of mitogen-activated protein kinases (MAPKs) culminating in the activation of transcription factors important for cell division (Fig. 2–1). *Ras* mutations are extremely common in human cancers.

4. **Transcription.** This includes the activation of *early growth-regulated genes* (such as c-*myc,* c-*fos,* c-*jun*) induced in

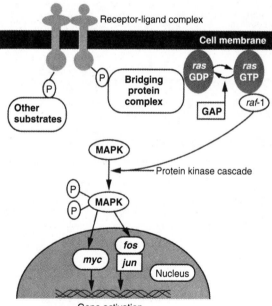

Figure 2–1. The *ras* signal transduction pathway. The phosphorylated receptor tyrosine kinase binds to a bridging protein complex which converts inactive *ras* GDP to active *ras* GTP. The *ras* GTP activates *raf*-1, which in turn phosphorylates a series of other mitogen-induced protein kinases (MAPKs), leading to activation of nuclear transcription factors. GAP, also phosphorylated by receptor-ligand binding, counteracts *ras* activation. (From Cotran, R. S., Kumar, V., and Robbins, S. L.: Robbins Pathologic Basis of Disease. 5th ed. Philadelphia, W. B. Saunders Co., 1994, p. 39.)

the absence of protein synthesis, and *late growth-regulated genes*, some being proto-oncogenes that code for transcription factors and that when mutated, may be associated with malignant transformation (Chapter 7).

5. **Cell Cycle.** The cell cycle itself is controlled by a series of regulatory proteins, called *cyclins*, whose concentrations rise and fall during the cell cycle and which form a complex with constitutively present protein kinases called cdc2. G1 and G2 cyclin-kinase complexes then phosphorylate a number of substrate proteins involved in initiation of DNA replication, formation of mitotic spindles, and other events in the cell cycle. Some of the tumor suppressor genes (Rb gene; p53; see Chapter 7) act in the cyclin pathway to control cell growth.

GROWTH INHIBITION (p. 40)

Growth inhibition, in addition to growth stimulation, regulates cell growth. Inhibitors are also largely polypeptide factors that utilize receptors, signal transduction, second messengers, and transcriptional factors. The best-studied are transforming growth factor-β (TGF-β), tumor necrosis factor (TNF), and β-interferon.

GROWTH FACTORS (p. 40)

These act by endocrine, paracrine, or autocrine signaling and, in addition to their growth effects, influence cell movement, contractibility, and differentiation—all important processes in wound healing (Chapter 3). The major growth factors (Table 2–1) include:

- *Epidermal growth factor (EGF)* and *transforming growth factor-α (TGF-α)*. These two GFs have extensive homology and bind to an identical cell receptor, c-*erb*-B1. They are mitogenic for epithelial cells and fibroblasts.
- *Fibroblast growth factors (FGF)*. Basic FGF is mitogenic for fibroblasts and smooth muscle and also causes endothelial cell migration, proliferation, and differentiation—steps necessary for angiogenesis (Chapter 3). FGF is elaborated by activated macrophages and is strongly heparin binding. Acidic FGF is similar but confined to neural tissue.
- *TGF-β*. Belongs to a family of growth factors with wide-ranging functions. TFG-β is a growth inhibitor to epithelial cells in culture but has variable effects on fibroblast growth, being mitogenic in low doses (due to induction of platelet-derived GF—PDGF) and inhibitory in large ones. Most importantly, it induces deposition of extracellular matrix (ECM) and fibrosis by (1) stimulating fibroblast chemotaxis, (2) stimulating collagen and fibronectin synthesis, and (3) inhibiting collagen degradation (*see p. 87*, Chapter 3). It is produced by platelets, endothelial cells, T cells, and macrophages.
- *Cytokines*. IL1 and TNF are mitogenic and chemotactic for fibroblasts and induce collagen synthesis (fibrogenic cytokines). β- and γ-interferons inhibit cell growth.

EXTRACELLULAR MATRIX AND CELL-MATRIX INTERACTIONS (p. 41)

The ECM markedly influences cell growth and function. The ECM consists of *fibrous structural proteins* and an interstitial

Table 2-1. Growth Factors

EPIDERMAL GROWTH FACTOR FAMILY (EGF)
  EGF
  Transforming growth factor-α
PLATELET-DERIVED GROWTH FACTOR (PDGF)
FIBROBLAST GROWTH FACTOR
  Basic
  Acidic
TRANSFORMING GROWTH FACTOR-β (TGF) FAMILY
  TGF isoforms
INSULIN-LIKE GROWTH FACTORS (IGF)
  IGF-1
  IGF-2
VASOPERMEABILITY FACTOR (VPF)
  (Endothelial cell–derived growth factor [ECGF])
HEPATIC GROWTH FACTOR
  (Scatter factor)
MYELOID COLONY-STIMULATING FACTORS (CSFs)
  Granulocyte-macrophage CSF (GM-CSF)
  Granulocyte CSF (G-CSF)
  Macrophage CSF (M-CSF)
ERYTHROPOIETIN
CYTOKINES
  Interleukins
  Tumor necrosis factor (TNF)
  Interferons
NERVE GROWTH FACTOR (NGF)

From Cotran, R. S., Kumar, V., and Robbins, S. L.: Robbins Pathologic Basis of Disease. 5th ed. Philadelphia, W. B. Saunders Co., 1994, p. 40.

matrix composed of *adhesive glycoproteins* embedded in a gel of *proteoglycans.*

- **Collagens,** consisting of different α chains making up 15 types of collagen, can be fibrillar (or interstitial), such as types I, III, V; or nonfibrillar (such as type IV), forming components of the basement membrane (BM) (see Chapter 3).
- **Fibronectin,** a 400-kD adhesion glycoprotein, binds to several ECM components (collagen, heparin, fibrin, proteoglycans) on the one hand and to cell membranes on the other. Binding to ECM is mediated by recognition of a specific triamino acid sequence, RGD (arginine, glycine, aspartic acid), on the ECM. Binding to cells is via *integrins,* cell receptors that span the membrane and interact with the cytoskeleton at points of *focal adhesion,* thus signaling locomotion and differentiation. Thus fibronectin is directly involved in cell attachment, spreading, and locomotion and interacts with growth factors to affect growth and differentiation.
- **Laminin,** a cross-shaped glycoprotein spanning BM, also binds to cells through specific receptors and to collagen type IV and heparin and is involved in cell attachment, locomotion, and growth.
- **Proteoglycans,** consisting of glycosaminoglycans (GAGs) linked to protein (heparin and dermatan sulfate) and nonlinked GAGs (hyaluronic acid), regulate connective tissue structure and permeability and modulate cell growth and differentiation. *Syndecan,* an integral membrane proteoglycan, maintains the

morphology of epithelial cell sheets. A schema by which ECM and growth factors interact in influencing cell shape, motility, and growth is shown in Figure 2–2.

CELLULAR ADAPTATIONS OF GROWTH AND DIFFERENTIATION (p. 44)

Hyperplasia

Hyperplasia constitutes an increase in the number of cells in an organ or tissue. It is usually accompanied by hypertrophy. Hyperplasia can occur only with cells capable of synthesizing DNA (such as epithelial, hematopoietic, and connective tissue cells). Nerve, cardiac, and skeletal muscle cells have little or no capacity for hyperplastic growth, and so muscle cells undergo almost pure hypertrophy when stimulated by increased functional load or hormones.

Hyperplasia can be physiologic or pathologic.

1. *Physiologic hyperplasia:*

   • Hormonal hyperplasia (e.g., endometrial proliferation after estrogen stimulation).
   • Compensatory hyperplasia (e.g., hyperplasia of the liver after partial hepatectomy).

After partial hepatectomy, the hepatic cell mitotic index increases markedly, eventually restoring the liver to normal weight (12 days after hepatectomy). This liver regeneration is caused by growth factors: *transforming growth factor-α* produced by the

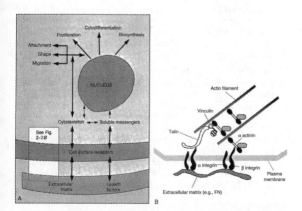

Figure 2–2. *A,* Schema of possible mechanisms by which extracellular matrix (ECM) and growth factors influence cell shape, motility, and growth. Receptors for ECM, such as the integrins—which recognize the RGD sequence—interact with various proteins of the cytoskeleton at focal adhesions and initiate the production of diffusible second messengers, which act on both nucleus and cytoplasm to cause the cell responses, as illustrated. Cell surface receptors to growth factors also initiate second messengers, which modulate cell growth, locomotion, and differentiation. (Redrawn from Madri, J., et al.: *In* Simionescu, N., and Simionescu, M. (eds.): Endothelial Cell Biology. New York, Plenum Publishing, 1988.) *B,* One scenario for the molecular interactions in a focal adhesion complex. Note that integrins join the ECM to contractile elements (actin) via a variety of cytoskeletal proteins. (Courtesy of Dr. Donald Ingber, Harvard Medical School.)

residual liver cells, and *hepatocyte growth factor* (HGF), produced by nonparenchymal cells in the liver and other organs. It is thought that liver cells are "primed" for the action of growth factors by metabolic overload, cytokines, and other factors and that adjuvant hormones such as glucagon and epinephrine potentiate the growth factor effects. Eventual cessation of cell growth is caused by growth inhibitors (e.g., transforming growth factor-β), produced by nonparenchymal liver cells.

2. *Pathologic hyperplasia:*

- Excessive hormonal stimulation (e.g., hyperestrinism and atypical endometrial hyperplasia).
- Effects of locally produced growth factors on target cells (e.g., proliferation of connective tissue cells in wound healing, or squamous epithelium induced by viruses).

In pathologic hyperplasia, if the stimulus abates, the hyperplasia disappears. Thus, cells respond to regular growth control, differentiating the process from neoplasia. However, pathologic hyperplasia constitutes a fertile soil in which cancerous proliferation may eventually arise. Examples are endometrial and cervical hyperplasia (Chapter 23), which are precursors of cancers of the endometrium and cervix, respectively.

Hypertrophy (p. 45)

Hypertrophy is an increase in the number of organelles (e.g., myofilaments) and size of cells and, with such change, an increase in the size of the organ. Hypertrophy can be *physiologic or pathologic* and is caused by

1. Increased functional demand, e.g., hypertrophy of striated muscles in muscle builders (physiologic) or of cardiac muscle in cardiac disease (pathologic).
2. Specific hormonal stimulation, e.g., uterine hypertrophy during pregnancy.

Hypertrophy is triggered by cell membrane interactions, which in the myocardium include *mechanical* factors (stretch) and *trophic* chemicals (GFs and vasoactive agents). These lead to intracellular gene-regulated events that include not only an increase in cell organelles but also phenotypic alterations of the hypertrophied cell. In the heart, for example, there are isoform switches of the myosin to the β heavy chain and the actin to α skeletal forms—both resulting in a salutary slowing of the velocity of contraction of hypertrophied muscle fibers. Hypertrophy eventually reaches a limit, at which time degenerative changes occur in cells and in the heart, and cardiac failure ensues.

Atrophy (p. 47)

Atrophy is shrinkage in the size of the cell due to loss of cell substance. Causes of atrophy are

- decreased workload
- loss of innervation
- diminished blood supply
- inadequate nutrition
- loss of endocrine stimulation
- aging

Atrophic cells have diminished function but are not dead. They exhibit autophagy with a reduction in the number of cell organelles, and often a marked increase in the number of *autophagic vacuoles*. Components resisting digestion are converted to lipofuscin granules, which, in sufficient numbers, make the organ brown ("brown atrophy").

Metaplasia (p. 48)

Metaplasia is a reversible change in which one adult cell type is replaced by another (epithelial or mesenchymal). The most common example is a change from *columnar* to *squamous* epithelium, as occurs in the squamous metaplasia of respiratory epithelium in response to chronic irritation. Although metaplastic epithelium is benign, the influences that predispose to such metaplasia, if persistent, may induce atypical metaplasia, which may progress to cancer transformation. Metaplasia can also occur in mesenchymal cells by which fibroblasts may become transformed to osteoblasts or chondroblasts to produce bone or cartilage.

Metaplasia is thought to occur from genetic reprogramming of stem cells that are known to exist in most epithelia or of undifferentiated mesenchymal cells. Certain chemicals (cytostatic drugs), vitamins (retinoids, vitamin A), and growth factors (TGF-β) play a role in metaplasia.

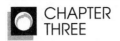

CHAPTER
THREE

Inflammation
and Repair

Inflammation is the reaction of vascularized living tissue to local injury. It is caused by microbial infections, physical agents, chemicals, necrotic tissue, and immunologic reactions. The role of inflammation is to contain and isolate injury, to destroy invading microorganisms and inactivate toxins, and to achieve healing and repair. However, inflammation and repair may be potentially harmful, causing life-threatening hypersensitivity reactions, progressive organ damage, and scarring.

ACUTE INFLAMMATION (p. 53)

CLASSIC SIGNS

Heat (calor); redness (rubor); edema (tumor); pain (dolor); loss of function (functio laesa).

DEFINITION OF TERMS

Exudation The escape of fluid, proteins, and blood cells from the vascular system into the interstitial tissue or body cavities.

Exudate An inflammatory extravascular fluid that has a high protein concentration, much cellular debris, and a specific gravity above 1.020.

Transudate A fluid with low protein content and a specific gravity of less than 1.012. It is essentially an ultrafiltrate of blood plasma and results from hydrostatic imbalance across the vascular endothelium.

Edema Denotes an excess of fluid in the interstitial tissue or serous cavities; it can be either an exudate or a transudate.

Pus A purulent inflammatory exudate rich in leukocytes and parenchymal cell debris.

MAJOR EVENTS IN INFLAMMATION

Changes in Vascular Flow and Caliber (p. 53)

- Initial transient vasoconstriction of arterioles.
- Vasodilatation follows, causing increased flow; it accounts for the heat and redness.
- Slowing of the circulation, eventually, due to increased vascular permeability (see below), leading to *stasis*. The increased permeability is the cause of edema.
- With slowing, leukocytic margination appears, a prelude to the cellular events (see below).

Increased Vascular Permeability (p. 54)

- Normal fluid exchange is dependent on Starling's law and an intact endothelium. Starling's law maintains that normal fluid balance is modulated mainly by two opposing forces: hydrostatic pressure causing fluid to move out of the circulation, and plasma colloid osmotic pressure causing fluid to move into the capillaries (Fig. 3–1A).
- In inflammation, there is increased hydrostatic pressure, caused by the vasodilatation, and decreased osmotic pressure, due to leakage of high-protein fluid across a hyperpermeable endothelium—resulting in marked net outflow of fluid and edema formation (Fig. 3–1B).

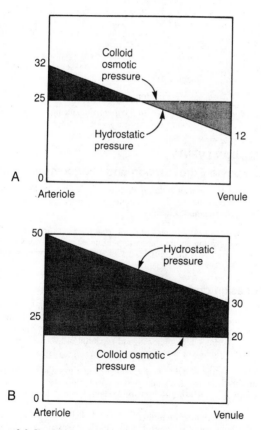

Figure 3–1. Blood pressure and plasma colloid osmotic forces in normal and inflamed microcirculation. *A,* Normal hydrostatic pressure of about 32 mm Hg at the arterial end of the capillary and 12 mm Hg at the venous end. Mean capillary pressure equals colloid osmotic pressure (horizontal line). *B,* Acute inflammation. Mean capillary pressure is increased because of arteriolar dilatation, while osmotic pressure is reduced because of protein leakage across the venule. The result is a net excess of extravasated fluid. (Redrawn from Wright, G. P.: An Introduction to Pathology. 3rd ed. London, Longmans, Green and Co., 1958.)

There are five possible mechanisms of increased endothelial permeability:

1. *Endothelial cell contraction,* leading to the formation of widened intercellular junctions, or intercellular gaps. This is the most common form elicited by chemical mediators (e.g., histamine); occurs immediately after injection of the mediator; is short lived (*immediate-transient response*); and classically involves only venules 20 to 60 μM in diameter, leaving capillaries and arterioles unaffected.

2. *Endothelial retraction* due to cytoskeletal and junction reorganization, and also resulting in widened interendothelial junctions. This effect is somewhat delayed, can be long lived, and is induced by cytokine mediators, such as interleukin-1 (IL-1) and tumor necrosis factor (TNF).

3. *Direct endothelial injury,* resulting in endothelial cell necrosis and detachment. This is caused by severe necrotizing injuries and affects venules, capillaries, and arterioles. The damage is usually *immediate* and *sustained.*

4. *Leukocyte-mediated endothelial injury* resulting from leukocyte aggregation, adhesion, and emigration across the endothelium. These leukocytes release toxic oxygen species and proteolytic enzymes, which cause endothelial injury or detachment, resulting in increased permeability.

5. *Leakage from regenerating capillaries,* during wound healing, when new capillary sprouts are leaky.

CELLULAR EVENTS

Leukocyte Extravasation and Phagocytosis (p. 57)

A critical function of inflammation is the delivery of leukocytes to the site of injury. The sequence of events in this journey, called *extravasation,* includes:

- In the vessel lumen: *margination, rolling,* and *adhesion*
- *Transmigration* across the endothelium (also called diapedesis)
- *Migration* in the interstitial tissues toward a chemotactic stimulus (Fig. 3–2)

Adhesion and Transmigration

These occur largely due to interactions between complementary adhesion molecules on the leukocytes and on the endothelium. Chemical mediators produced during inflammation modulate such adhesion. The major ligand-receptor adhesion pairs are shown in Table 3–1 and include

- *The selectins (E, P, and L),* which bind through their sugar-binding (lectin) domains to oligosaccharides (e.g., sialylated Lewis X), which themselves are covalently bound to cell surface glycoproteins.
- *Immunoglobulins,* including the endothelial *ICAM-1* (intercellular adhesion molecular 1) and *VCAM-1* (vascular cell adhesion molecular 1). ICAM-1 binds to the β_2 *integrins* LFA-1 and MAC-1, and VCAM-1 binds to the β_1 *integrin* VLA-4.

Chemical mediators stimulate adhesion by three mechanisms:

1. *Redistribution of preformed adhesion molecules to the cell surface.* For example, after exposure to histamine or thrombin, P-selectin is rapidly translocated from the endothelial Weibel

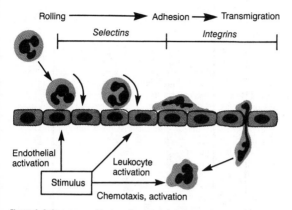

Figure 3–2. Sequence of leukocytic events in inflammation. The leukocytes first *roll*, then arrest and adhere to endothelium, then transmigrate through an intercellular junction, pierce the basement membrane, and migrate toward chemoattractants emanating from the source of injury. The roles of selectins, activating agents, and integrins are also shown. (Modified and redrawn from Travis, J. T.: Biotech gets a grip on cell adhesion. Science 26:906, 1993.)

Palade body membranes to the cell surface, where it can bind leukocytes.

2. *Induction of adhesion molecules on endothelium.* For example, IL-1 and TNF induce the synthesis and surface expression of E-selectin and increase expression of ICAM-1 and VCAM-1, rendering such "activated" endothelial cells more adherent to leukocytes.

3. *Increased avidity of binding.* This is most relevant to the binding of *integrins* (LFA-1 and MAC-1), which are normally present on leukocytes but can be converted from a state of low to high affinity binding toward their ligand ICAM-1 by chemical mediators. Such activation causes firm adhesion of the leukocytes to the endothelium and is also necessary for subsequent transmigration across endothelial cells.

It is now thought that neutrophil adhesion and transmigration in acute inflammation occur by three sometimes overlapping steps:

- Initial rapid and relatively loose adhesion that accounts for rolling, involving the *selectins.*
- Activation of the leukocytes by chemical mediators made by endothelium or other cells, resulting in an increased avidity of integrins to bind to their ligands.
- *Stable binding* of integrins on activated leukocytes (LFA-1; MAC-1; VLA-4) to endothelial immunoglobulins (ICAM-1; VCAM-1), followed by transmigration.

The importance of adhesion molecules is emphasized by the clinical genetic deficiencies in adhesion molecules: In *leukocyte adhesion deficiency type I,* there is a defect in synthesis of β_2 integrins. In *leukocyte adhesion deficiency type II,* a defect in fucose metabolism results in the absence of sialyl Lewis X, the ligand for E- and P-selectin. Both deficiencies result in impaired leukocyte adhesion and recurrent bacterial infections.

Table 3-1. Leukocyte–Endothelial Adhesion Molecules

Endothelial Molecule	Family	Leukocyte Receptor	Family	Distribution
E-selectin (ELAM-1)	Selectin	Sialyl-Le^x glycoprotein	Oligosaccharides	Neutrophils T cells Monocytes
P-selectin (GMP-140)	Selectin	Sialyl-Le^x glycoprotein	Oligosaccharides	Neutrophils Monocytes
ICAM-1	Immunoglobulin	LFA-1 Mac-1	β_2 integrin	All leukocytes
VCAM-1	Immunoglobulin	VLA-4	β_1 integrin	Lymphocytes Monocytes Basophils Eosinophils
LAM-1-ligand(s) (GlyCam-1; CD34)	Mucin-like glycoproteins	L-selectin (LAM-1)	Selectin	Neutrophils Lymphocytes Monocytes

Modified and used with permission from Briscoe, D. M. and Cotran, R. S.: Role of leukocyte–endothelial cell adhesion molecules in renal inflammation: In vitro and in vivo studies. Kidney Int. 42:S-28, 1993.

CHEMOTAXIS AND LEUKOCYTE ACTIVATION (p. 59)

Adherent leukocytes emigrate through interendothelial junctions, traverse the basement membrane, and move toward the site of injury along a gradient of chemotactic agents. Neutrophils emigrate first and monocytes follow. Chemotactic agents for neutrophils include bacterial products, complement fragments, arachidonic acid metabolites (e.g., leukotriene B_4), and certain cytokines.

Chemotaxis involves binding of chemotactic agents to receptors on leukocytes, phospholipase C activation, increased intracellular calcium, activation of protein kinase-C, protein phosphorylation leading to activation of intracellular contractile proteins. Locomotion is controlled by the effects of *calcium* ions and *phosphoinositols* on *actin regulatory proteins* such as *gelsolin* and *filamin*.

Chemotactic agents also cause *leukocyte activation*, characterized by:

• Production of arachidonic acid metabolites
• Degranulation and secretion of enzymes
• Activation of an oxidative burst
• Modulation of leukocyte adhesion molecules

PHAGOCYTOSIS (p. 60). Phagocytosis involves

• *Attachment* of opsonized particles to Fc and C3b receptors on the surface of leukocytes.
• *Engulfment* by pseudopods encircling the phagocytosed particle, creating a *phagosome.*
• *Fusion* of lysosomal granules with the phagosome, leading to degranulation.
• *Killing and degradation of bacteria.*

There are two types of bactericidal mechanisms:

1. *Oxygen-dependent mechanisms.* This is triggered by activation of NADPH oxidase, in the process reducing O_2 to superoxide ($O_2^{\cdot-}$) and hence to H_2O_2 (Fig. 3–3). Myeloperoxidase from specific granules (MPO) then converts H_2O_2, in the presence of Cl^- to the highly bactericidal $HOCl^{\cdot}$.

2. *Oxygen-independent mechanisms* include bactericidal permeability increasing protein (BPIP), lysozyme, lactoferrin, major basic protein (MPB) of eosinophils, and arginine-rich *defensins.* Killed organisms are then degraded by hydrolase and other enzymes in lysosomes.

EXTRACELLULAR RELEASE (p. 63). During phagocytosis, leukocytes release

• Lysosomal enzymes by regurgitation during feeding, reverse endocytosis, and cytotoxic release.
• Oxygen-derived active metabolites.
• Products of arachidonic acid metabolism.

DEFECTS IN LEUKOCYTE FUNCTION (p. 64)

These interfere with inflammation and increase susceptibility to infections. They include both genetic and acquired defects.

1. Deficiency in the number of circulating cells (neutropenia).
2. Defects in adherence (e.g., leukocyte adhesion deficiency)—type I and type II.

CYTOPLASM   PHAGOCYTIC VACUOLE

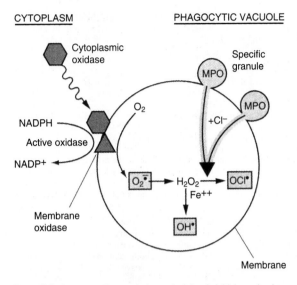

Figure 3-3. Summary of oxygen-dependent bactericidal mechanisms within phagocytic vacuole, as described in text. (From Cotran, R. S., Kumar, V., Robbins, S. L.: Robbins Pathologic Basis of Disease. 5th ed. Philadelphia, W. B. Saunders Co., 1994, p. 62.)

3. Defects in migration and chemotaxis (e.g., *Chédiak-Higashi syndrome*, a genetic disease in which there are several defects in leukocyte function).

4. Defects in phagocytosis (e.g., diabetes mellitus).

5. Defects in microbicidal activity. In *chronic granulomatous disease* there are inherited defects in NADPH oxidase leading to a defect in the respiratory burst, H_2O_2 production, and the MPO-H_2O_2 halide bactericidal mechanism.

6. Mixed defects (e.g., *Chédiak-Higashi syndrome*).

CHEMICAL MEDIATORS (p. 64)

The vascular and white cell events described above are brought about by a variety of chemical mediators, derived either from plasma or from cells. Most perform their biologic activity by binding initially to specific receptors on target cells, although some have direct enzymatic activity (e.g., proteases) and others mediate oxidative damage (e.g., oxygen metabolites). One mediator can stimulate the release of other mediators by the target cells themselves, providing a mechanism for amplification, or in certain instances counteracting the initial mediator action. Once activated and released, most mediators are short lived, either quickly decaying or becoming inactivated by enzymes or inhibited by inhibitors. There is thus a system of check and balances in the regulation of mediator action, because most mediators also have potentially harmful effects.

VASOACTIVE AMINES. Histamine and serotonin, found in mast cells, basophils, and platelets, cause vasodilatation and increased vascular permeability. Release from mast cells is caused by (1) physical agents, (2) immunologic IgE reactions, (3) C3a and

C5a (anaphylatoxins), (4) interleukin-1, and (5) other histamine releasing factors. Release from platelets is stimulated by contact with collagen, thrombin, ADP, and antigen-antibody complexes and by platelet activating factor (PAF). Histamine is important in early inflammation.

COMPLEMENT SYSTEM (p. 66). Activation of complement (Fig. 3–4) occurs via

- The classic pathway, initiated by antigen-antibody complexes.
- The alternate complement pathway, activated by endotoxin, complex polysaccharides, and aggregated globulins.

Complement components with inflammatory activity include

- C3a, which increases vascular permeability.
- C5a, which increases vascular permeability and is highly chemotactic to most leukocytes.
- C3b and C3bi—the opsonins, important in phagocytosis.
- C5b–9, the membrane attack complex that lyses cells and stimulates arachidonic acid metabolism and production of reactive oxygen metabolites by leukocytes.

KININ SYSTEM (p. 67). Surface activation of Hageman factor produces clotting factor XIIa, which converts plasma prekallikrein into kallikrein; the latter cleaves high-molecular-weight kininogen (HMWK) to produce bradykinin, a potent stimulator of increased vascular permeability. Kallikrein in an autocatalytic loop is a potent activator of Hageman factor, has chemotactic activity, and causes neutrophil aggregation.

CLOTTING SYSTEM (p. 68). Also activated by Hageman factor, culminates in the conversion of fibrinogen to fibrin by thrombin

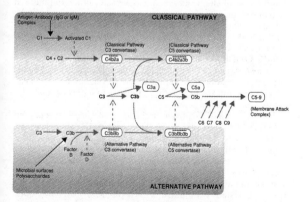

Figure 3–4. Overview of complement activation pathways. The classic pathway is initiated by C1 binding to antigen-antibody complexes, and the alternative pathway is initiated by C3b binding to various activating surfaces, such as microbial cell walls. The C3b involved in alternative pathway initiation may be generated in several ways, including spontaneously, by the classic pathway, or by the alternative pathway itself (see text). Both pathways converge and lead to the formation of inflammatory complement mediators (C3a and C5a) and the membrane attack complex. In this figure, bars over the letter designations of complement components indicate enzymatically active forms, and dashed lines indicate proteolytic activities of various components. (Modified from Abbas, A. K., et al.: Cellular and Molecular Immunology, 2nd ed. Philadelphia, W. B. Saunders Co., 1994.)

and the release of fibrinopeptides, which increase vascular permeability and are chemotactic.

ARACHIDONIC ACID METABOLITES (Fig. 3–5) (p. 69). The inflammatory prostaglandins and leukotrienes include

- PGI_2 (prostacyclin) and PGE_2, which cause vasodilatation.
- Thromboxane A_2, which causes vasoconstriction.
- Leukotrienes C_4, D_4, and E_4, which increase vascular permeability and cause vasoconstriction.
- Leukotriene B_4, which is a powerful chemotactic agent.

PLATELET ACTIVATING FACTOR (p. 70). Produced by mast cells and other leukocytes following a number of stimuli, including IgE reactions. PAF causes platelet aggregation and release, bronchoconstriction, vasodilatation, increased vascular permeability, increased leukocyte adhesion, and leukocyte chemotaxis.

CYTOKINES (p. 70). Cytokines are polypeptide factors produced by activated macrophages, lymphocytes, and other cell types. IL-1 and TNF in particular have the following shared inflammatory effects (Fig. 3–6):

- On the *endothelium,* they increase leukocyte adhesion, stimulate the synthesis of PGI_2 and PAF, increase surface thrombogenicity, and induce the production of other cytokines and growth factors (e.g., IL-8, IL-6); these endothelial effects are referred to as "endothelial activation."
- They induce systemic *acute phase responses,* including fever, neutrophilia, hemodynamic effects, and slow-wave sleep.
- On *fibroblasts,* they induce proliferation, increased collagen formation, and increased collagenase synthesis.

IL-8 belongs to a family of small proteins, called *chemokines,* characterized by four cysteine residues at identical positions. IL-8 is a powerful chemoattractant and activator of neutrophils and is induced in activated macrophages and endothelial cells by other cytokines (IL-1 and TNF). *Monocyte chemoattractant protein* (MCP-1) is chemotactic for monocytes and *RANTES* is chemotactic for lymphocytes.

NITRIC OXIDE (p. 71). Also known as *endothelium-derived relaxation factor* (EDRF), this molecule causes vasodilation, inhibits platelet aggregation and adhesion, and may act as a free radical, becoming cytotoxic to certain microbes, tumor cells, and also possibly other tissue cells.

NO is synthesized from arginine, molecular oxygen, and NADPH by the enzyme nitric oxide synthase (NOS). There are two types of NOS: the endothelial type (also present in neurons) is present constitutively and is rapidly activated by an increase in cytoplasmic calcium. Macrophage type NOS is *induced* when macrophages are activated by cytokines such as γ-interferon without an increase in intracellular calcium. NO has been implicated in a variety of inflammatory diseases, including septic shock.

LYSOSOMAL CONSTITUENTS OF LEUKOCYTES (p. 72). Neutrophils exhibit two major types of granules: *specific,* containing lactoferrin, lysozyme, alkaline phosphatase, and collagenase; and *azurophilic,* containing myeloperoxidase, cationic proteins, acid hydrolases, and neutral proteases. Monocyte granules contain acid hydrolases, elastase, collagenase, and plasminogen activator.

Cationic proteins increase vascular permeability and cause chemotaxis. *Neutral proteases* degrade extracellular matrices. Proteases are checked by antiproteases, which include alpha$_1$-antitrypsin and α_2-macroglobulin.

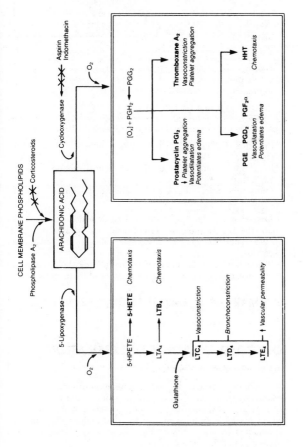

Figure 3-5. Arachidonic acid metabolites in inflammation. (From Cotran, R. S., Kumar, V., and Robbins, S. L.: Robbins Pathologic Basis of Disease. 4th ed. Philadelphia, W. B. Saunders Co., 1989, p. 56.)

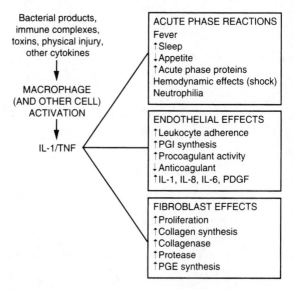

Figure 3–6. Major effects of interleukin-1 (IL-1) and tumor necrosis factor (TNF) in inflammation. (From Cotran, R. S., Kumar, V., and Robbins, S. L.: Robbins Pathologic Basis of Disease. 5th ed. Philadelphia, W. B. Saunders Co., 1994, p. 70.)

OXYGEN-DERIVED FREE RADICALS (p. 73). These include H_2O_2, superoxide (O_2^-), and hydroxyl radicals ($OH^·$), which cause

- Endothelial cell damage with resultant increased vascular permeability.
- Inactivation of antiproteases, thus leading to unopposed protease activity.
- Injury to a variety of cell types (tumor cells, red cells, parenchymal cells).

Oxygen metabolites are detoxified by antioxidants, which include the serum proteins ceruloplasmin and transferrin, and enzymes such as superoxide dismutase, catalase, and glutathione peroxidase.

The net effects on tissue injury of oxygen metabolites depend on the balance between their production and inactivation.

SUMMARY OF CHEMICAL MEDIATORS (Table 3–2) (p. 73)

OUTCOME OF ACUTE INFLAMMATION (p. 74)

Acute inflammation may result in

1. Complete resolution, with regeneration of native cells and restoration of the site of acute inflammation to normal.

2. Healing by connective tissue replacement and scarring, which occurs after substantial tissue destruction, when the inflammation occurs in tissues that do not regenerate, or when there is abundant fibrin exudation.

Table 3-2. Summary of Mediators of Acute Inflammation

Mediator	Source	Vascular Leakage	Chemotaxis	Other
			Action	
Histamine and serotonin	Mast cells, platelets	+	—	
Bradykinin	Plasma substrate	+	—	Pain
C3a	Plasma protein via liver; macrophages	+	—	Opsonic fragment (C3b)
C5a		+	+	Leukocyte adhesion, activation
Prostaglandins	Mast cells, from membrane phospholipids	Potentiate other mediators	—	Vasodilation, pain fever
Leukotriene B$_4$	Leukocytes	—	+	Leukocyte adhesion, activation
Leukotriene C$_4$, D$_4$, E$_4$	Leukocytes, mast cells	+	—	Bronchoconstriction, vasoconstriction
Oxygen metabolites	Leukocytes	+	+±	Endothelial damage, tissue damage
PAF	Leukocytes; mast cells	+	+	Bronchoconstriction Leukocyte priming
IL-1 and TNF	Macrophages; other	—	+	Acute phase reactions Endothelial activation
IL-8	Macrophages, Endothelium	—	+	Leukocyte activation
Nitric oxide	Macrophages, Endothelium			Vasodilation Cytotoxicity

From Cotran, R. S., Kumar, V., and Robbins, S. L.: Robbins Pathologic Basis of Disease. 5th ed. Philadelphia, W. B. Saunders Co., 1994, p. 73.

3. Abscess formation.
4. Progression to chronic inflammation.

CHRONIC INFLAMMATION (CI) (p. 75)

This is defined as inflammation of prolonged duration in which *active inflammation, tissue destruction,* and *attempts at healing* are proceeding simultaneously.

CI arises in several ways:

- It may follow acute inflammation, either because of the persistence of the inciting stimulus, or because of some interference in the normal process of healing.
- It may result from repeated bouts of acute inflammation.
- Most commonly, it begins insidiously as a low-grade, smoldering response that does not follow classic acute inflammation, in one of the following settings:

  - Persistent infection by intracellular microbes (e.g., tubercle bacilli, viral infection), which are of low toxicity but evoke an immunologic reaction.
  - Prolonged exposure to nondegradable but potentially toxic substances (e.g., silicosis and asbestosis in the lung).
  - Immune reactions, particularly those perpetuated against the individual's own tissues (e.g., autoimmune diseases).

The histologic features of CI include (1) infiltration by mononuclear cells, principally macrophages, lymphocytes, and plasma cells; (2) tissue destruction; and (3) connective tissue replacement of injured tissue by a process involving proliferation of blood vessels (angiogenesis) and fibrosis.

Mononuclear Infiltration (p. 76)

Macrophages

- These are central figures in chronic inflammation because of the great number of biologically active products they can secrete (Fig. 3–7).
- They are derived from peripheral blood monocytes that have been induced to emigrate across the endothelium by chemotactic agents. The latter include C5a, fibrinopeptides, cytokines (MCP-1), platelet-derived growth factor (PDGF), and collagen and fibronectin fragments.
- Macrophages can be *activated* to secrete numerous factors, including (1) neutral proteases, (2) chemotactic factors, (3) arachidonic acid metabolites, (4) reactive oxygen species, (5) complement components, (6) coagulation factors, (7) growth factors, (8) cytokines (such as IL-1 and TNF), and (9) other factors (e.g., PAF and α-interferon).
- Macrophage activation in inflammation is triggered by lymphokines (γ-interferon) produced by immune activated T cells, or by nonimmune factors (e.g., endotoxin).
- The secretory products of macrophages induce the changes characteristic of chronic inflammation, tissue destruction (proteases and oxygen-derived free radicals), neovascularization, fibroblast proliferation (growth factors), connective tissue accumulation (cytokines and growth factors), and remodeling (collagenases).

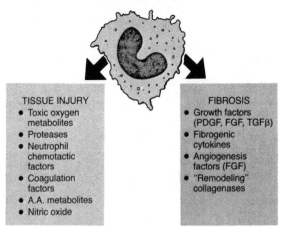

Activated macrophage

TISSUE INJURY	FIBROSIS
• Toxic oxygen metabolites	• Growth factors (PDGF, FGF, TGFβ)
• Proteases	• Fibrogenic cytokines
• Neutrophil chemotactic factors	• Angiogenesis factors (FGF)
• Coagulation factors	• "Remodeling" collagenases
• A.A. metabolites	
• Nitric oxide	

Figure 3–7. Macrophage products involved in tissue destruction and fibrosis. (From Cotran, R. S., Kumar, V., and Robbins, S. L.: Robbins Pathologic Basis of Disease. 5th ed. Philadelphia, W. B. Saunders Co., 1994, p. 77.)

Other Cells in CI (p. 78)

- *Lymphocytes* are mobilized by antibody and cell-mediated immune reactions and also for unknown reasons by nonimmunologic reactions. They have a unique reciprocal relationship to macrophages in CI (Fig. 3–8). They can be activated by contact with antigen and nonspecifically by bacterial endotoxin. Activated lymphocytes produce lymphokines, and these (particularly γ-interferon) are major stimulators of monocytes and macrophages. Activated macrophages produce monokines, which in turn influence B- and T-cell function.
- *Plasma cells* produce antibodies directed against either foreign antigen or altered tissue components.
- *Eosinophils* are common in immunologic reactions and their granules contain major basic protein (MBP), which is highly toxic to parasites and also causes lysis of host cells.

Repair by Connective Tissue (Fibrosis) (p. 79)

Because tissue destruction in chronic inflammation involves both parenchymal cells and the stromal framework, repair cannot be accomplished solely by regeneration of parenchymal cells, and repair thus involves replacement by connective tissue, which in time produces *fibrosis* and *scarring*. There are four components to this process:

- Formation of new blood vessels (angiogenesis)
- Migration and proliferation of fibroblasts
- Deposition of extracellular matrix
- Maturation and reorganization of the fibrous tissue, also known as *remodeling*

Four steps underlie *angiogenesis:* enzymatic degradation of the basement membrane of the parent vessel; migration of endothelial cells; proliferation of endothelial cells; maturation and

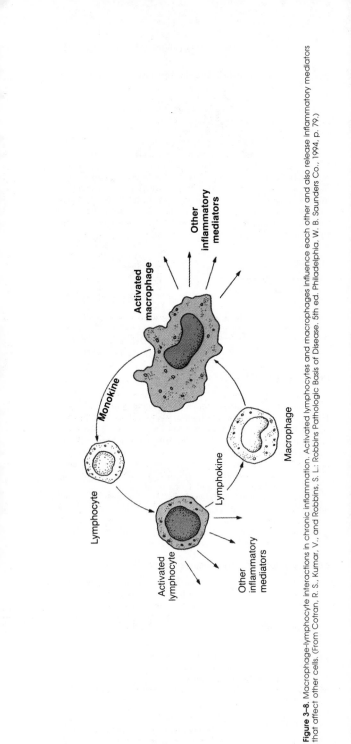

Figure 3–8. Macrophage-lymphocyte interactions in chronic inflammation. Activated lymphocytes and macrophages influence each other and also release inflammatory mediators that affect other cells. (From Cotran, R. S., Kumar, V., and Robbins, S. L.: Robbins Pathologic Basis of Disease. 5th ed. Philadelphia. W. B. Saunders Co., 1994, p. 79.)

organization into capillary tubes. At least two growth factors are important in inducing angiogenesis: *basic fibroblast growth factor (bFGF)*, which can mediate all the steps in angiogenesis; and *vascular permeability* or *vascular endothelial growth factor (VPF, VEGF)*, which causes both angiogenesis and increased permeability.

Migration of fibroblasts and their subsequent proliferation are also mediated by growth factors such as PDGF, EGF, FGF, and TGF-β. TGF-β is particularly critical in favoring fibrous tissue deposition (Table 3–3). It induces fibroblast migration and proliferation as well as increased collagen synthesis and decreased collagen degradation of excess cellular matrix biometalloproteinases. TG-β is thus thought to play an important role in chronic inflammatory fibrosis (see also later under Wound Healing).

GRANULOMATOUS INFLAMMATION

(p. 80)

- A form of CI is characterized by *granulomas*—small nodular collections of modified macrophages. The latter when modified acquire abundant pink cytoplasm and are called *epithelioid cells* (see below). Epithelioid cells may coalesce to form multinucleate giant cells. Lymphocytes, plasma cells, neutrophils, and central necrosis may also be present in a granuloma.
- There are two types of granulomas:

  1. Foreign body granulomas, incited by relatively inert foreign bodies.
  2. Immune granulomas, formed by immune T cell–mediated reactions to poorly degradable antigens. *Lymphokines*, principally γ-interferon from activated T cells, cause transformation of macrophages to epithelioid cells and multinucleate giant cells.

- Granulomas are characteristic of certain diseases caused by particular infectious agents (e.g., tuberculosis), mineral dusts (e.g., silicosis), or other unknown conditions (e.g., sarcoidosis).
- Table 3–4 lists characteristics of the major immune granulomatous diseases.

Table 3–3. Transforming Growth Factor-β (TGF-β)

Produced by:
Platelets, macrophages, other cells
Released in inactive form
Actions
Monocyte chemotaxis
Fibroblast migration
Fibroblast proliferation
Collagen and ECM
Increased synthesis
Decreased degradation

From Cotran, R. S., Kumar, V., and Robbins, S. L.: Robbins Pathologic Basis of Disease. 5th ed. Philadelphia, W.B. Saunders Co., 1994, p. 81.

AMBROSIA

Table 3–4. Examples of Granulomatous Inflammations

Disease	Cause	Tissue Reaction
Bacterial		
Tuberculosis	*Mycobacterium tuberculosis*	*Noncaseating tubercle (granuloma prototype):* a focus of epithelioid cells, rimmed by fibroblasts, lymphocytes, histiocytes, occasional Langhans' giant cell; *caseating tubercle:* central amorphous granular debris, loss of all cellular detail, acid-fast bacilli
Leprosy	*Mycobacterium leprae*	Acid-fast bacilli in macrophages; granulomas and epithelioid types
Syphilis	*Treponema pallidum*	*Gumma:* Microscopic to grossly visible lesion, enclosing wall of histiocytes; plasma cell infiltrate; center cells are necrotic without loss of cellular outline
Cat-scratch disease	Gram-negative bacilli	Rounded or stellate granuloma containing central granular debris and recognizable neutrophils; giant cells uncommon
Parasitic		
Schistosomiasis	*Schistosoma mansoni, S. haematobium, S. japonicum*	Egg emboli; eosinophils
Fungal		
	Cryptococcus neoformans	*Organism is yeastlike, sometimes budding; 5 to 10 μm; large, clear capsule*
	Coccidioides immitis	Organism appears as spherical (30–80 μm) cyst containing endospores of 3 to 5 μm each
Inorganic Metals and Dusts		
Silicosis, berylliosis		Lung involvement; fibrosis
Unknown		
Sarcoidosis		*Noncaseating granuloma:* giant cells (Langhans' and foreign-body types); asteroids in giant cells; occasional Schaumann's body (concentric calcific concretion); no organisms

From Cotran, R. S., Kumar, V., and Robbins, S. L.: Robbins Pathologic Basis of Disease. 5th ed. Philadelphia, W. B. Saunders Co., 1994, p. 81.

MORPHOLOGIC PATTERNS
OF INFLAMMATION (p. 82)

Some inflammatory responses have certain features that create distinctive morphologic patterns:

1. *Serous inflammation* (e.g., pleural tuberculous effusion and skin burn blisters).
2. *Fibrinous inflammation* (e.g., fibrinous pericarditis after an acute myocardial infarct).
3. *Suppurative or purulent inflammation* (e.g., pyogenic staphylococcal abscesses).
4. *Ulcer:* a surface inflammation (mucosa, skin) with sloughing of necrotic tissue.

SYSTEMIC EFFECTS (p. 84)

These include

1. *Fever,* caused by the release of IL-1, TNF, and IL-6 activates macrophages and lymphocytes. IL-1 and TNF interact with vascular receptors in the thermoregulatory centers of the hypothalamus, inducing local PGE_2 production and resulting in sympathetic nerve stimulation, vasoconstriction of skin vessels, and fever.
2. *Leukocytosis,* occurring because of (1) accelerated release of bone marrow cells, induced by IL-1 and TNF; and (2) proliferation of precursors in the bone marrow induced by colony-stimulating factors (CSFs).
3. Elaboration of *acute phase proteins* by the liver (e.g., C-reactive protein, amyloid-A) induced by IL-1, TNF, and IL-6 release.
4. *Other* acute phase reactions such as sleepiness, hypotension, and lipolysis.

WOUND HEALING (p. 85)

Healing of a clean surgical approximated incision (first intention) involves an orchestrated sequence of events, as follows:

- *0 hours.* The incision is filled with clot.
- *3 to 24 hours.* Neutrophils from the margins infiltrate the clot. Mitoses begin to appear in epithelial basal cells; epithelial closure takes place by 24 to 48 hours.
- *Day 3.* Neutrophils are replaced by macrophages. Granulation tissue begins to appear.
- *Day 5.* The incision space is filled with granulation tissue, neovascularization is maximal, collagen fibrils begin to appear, and epithelial proliferation is now maximal.
- *Week 2.* There is proliferation of fibroblasts and continued collagen accumulation. Inflammation and newly formed vessels have largely disappeared.
- *Month 2.* Scar now consists of connective tissue devoid of inflammation covered by intact epidermis.

Healing with second intention occurs when there is more extensive loss of tissue, such as infarction, ulceration, abscess formation, and large wounds. Abundant granulation tissue grows in from the margins to fill the defect, but at the same time the wound *contracts;* i.e., the defect is markedly reduced from its original size. *Myofibroblasts* contribute to wound contraction.

MECHANISMS OF WOUND HEALING (p. 87)

Three influences are important in wound repair:

- Growth factors.
- Cell-cell and cell-matrix interactions.
- ECM (collagen) synthesis, degradation, remodeling.

The first two were discussed in Chapter 2. The major growth factors and their role in wound healing are summarized in Table 3–5.

Collagen Synthesis and Degradation and Wound Strength

- Collagen fibers account in large part for wound strength. The collagens are divided into 15 types: types I, II, and III are the interstitial or fibril collagens, and types IV, V, and VI are amorphous and present in interstitial tissue and basement membranes. Adult skin collagen is mostly type I, but collagen deposited early in granulation tissue is type III, which is then replaced by adult type I collagen.
- Collagen synthesis involves first synthesis of alpha chains on ribosomes, followed by a number of enzymatic hydroxylations, which are necessary to hold the three alpha chains together. Clipping of a C terminal fragment of the procollagen molecule during or shortly after excretion from the cell results in the formation of fibrils, and extracellular lysyl hydroxylysyl oxidation results in cross-linkages between alpha chains of adjacent molecules, which contribute to the tensile strength of collagen (dependent on vitamin C).
- Collagen synthesis is stimulated by growth factors and cytokines secreted by leukocytes and fibroblasts in healing wounds (Table 3–5).
- Net collagen accumulation depends not only on collagen synthesis but also on *degradation*, which is achieved by a family of *metalloproteinases* dependent on zinc for their activity. These include *interstitial collagenases*, which cleave fibrillar collagen; *gelatinases*, which degrade type IV collagen; and *stromelysins*, which degrade other ECM components (proteoglycans, fibronectin). Secretion of metalloproteinases by fibroblasts and leukocytes is induced by growth factors and cytokines and inhibited by TGF-β. They are secreted as proenzymes, which are activated by *plasmin* extracellularly. Once formed, activated collagenases can be rapidly inhibited by a family of specific tissue inhibitors of metalloproteinase (TIMP) produced by

Table 3–5. Growth Factors In Wound Healing

Monocyte chemotaxis	PDGF, FGF, TGF-β
Fibroblast migration	PDGF, EGF, FGF, TGF-β, TNF
Fibroblast proliferation	PDGF, EGF, FGF, TNF
Angiogenesis	VEGF, FGF
Collagen synthesis	TGF-β, PDGF, TNF
Collagenase secretion	PDGF, FGF, EGF, TNF, TGF-β inhibits

From Cotran, R. S., Kumar, V., and Robbins, S. L.: Robbins Pathologic Basis of Disease. 5th ed. Philadelphia, W. B. Saunders, 1994, p. 88.

most mesenchymal cells. These mechanisms provide multiple checks against the uncontrolled actions of collagenases, and aid in the debridement of injured sites and in the remodeling of connective tissue, necessary to repair the defects in wound healing.

- Wound strength at the end of the first week is approximately 10% of normal; it is largely dependent on surgical suturing/tissue adhesion. The progressive recovery of tensile strength to 70 to 80% of normal by the third month (which may persist for life) is associated first with increased collagen synthesis exceeding collagen degradation, and subsequently from the cross-linking and increased fiber size of collagen fibers.

Thus wound healing involves orchestrated events of *early inflammation,* followed by a stage of *fibroplasia* characterized by *granulation tissue,* followed by *extracellular matrix deposition,* tissue *remodeling,* and *scarring.*

FACTORS MODIFYING QUALITY OF INFLAMMATORY-REPARATIVE RESPONSE

A number of systemic and local factors modify the severity of the inflammatory response and the quality of repair.
  The major influences are

- The adequacy of the blood supply.
- The nutritional status of the host, e.g., protein nutrition and vitamin C intake.
- The presence or absence of infection.
- The presence or absence of diabetes mellitus.
- Intercurrent glucocorticosteroid therapy, which hinders the inflammatory-reparative process.
- Adequate levels of circulating white cells.

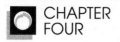

CHAPTER
FOUR

Hemodynamic Disorders, Thrombosis, and Shock

EDEMA (p. 93)

An abnormal accumulation of fluid within interstitial spaces or body cavities, e.g., pericardial, pleural, peritoneal (ascites).
May be

- *Inflammatory* related to increased vascular permeability with escape of protein-rich *exudate* (discussed previously).
- *Non-inflammatory or hemodynamic,* related to imbalance in Starling's forces with seepage of protein-poor *transudate.*
- *Lymphedema,* secondary to reduced lymph drainage.

Edema may be localized, as in obstruction of venous return in an extremity or blockage of a regional group of lymph nodes or lymphatics, or *systemic,* called *anasarca* when severe. Edematous collections in the body cavities are called *hydrothorax, hydropericardium* and *hydroperitoneum* (more commonly *ascites*).

MAJOR CAUSES OF NONINFLAMMATORY EDEMA

Will appear whenever there is:

- An increase in intravascular hydrostatic pressure
- A fall in colloid osmotic pressure
- An impairment to the flow of lymph
- Renal retention of salt and water when there is an underlying kidney disease. May also contribute to edema of other causes. Various physiologic categories of noninflammatory edema are listed in Table 4–1.

CLINICAL SETTINGS WITH SYSTEMIC EDEMA

Congestive heart failure is the most common cause of systemic edema. Although increased hydrostatic pressure is the major factor, the reduced cardiac output and reduced renal flow lead to activation of the renin-angiotensin-aldosterone axis, resulting in renal retention of sodium and water, which in turn expands the fluid volume and the workload of the heart, resulting in further cardiac failure and further increase in hydrostatic pressure.

Table 4–1. Pathophysiologic Categories of Edema

I. Increased hydrostatic pressure
   A. Impaired venous return
      1. Congestive heart failure
      2. Constrictive pericarditis
      3. Cirrhosis of liver (ascites)
      4. Obstruction or narrowing of veins
         a. Thrombosis
         b. External pressure
         c. Inactivity of the lower extremities with long periods of dependency
   B. Arteriolar dilation
      1. Heat
      2. Neurohumoral excess or deficit
II. Reduced oncotic pressure of plasma—hypoproteinemia
   A. Protein-losing glomerulopathies—nephrotic syndrome
   B. Cirrhosis of liver (ascites)
   C. Malnutrition
   D. Protein-losing gastroenteropathy
III. Sodium retention
   A. Excessive salt intake with reduced renal function
   B. Increased tubular reabsorption of sodium
      1. Reduced renal perfusion
      2. Increased renin-angiotensin-aldosterone secretion
IV. Lymphatic obstruction
   A. Inflammatory
   B. Neoplastic
   C. Postsurgical
   D. Postirradiation

Modified from Leaf, A., and Cotran, R. S.: Renal Pathophysiology. 3rd ed. New York, Oxford University Press, 1985, p. 146.

Reduced oncotic pressure of plasma occurs in several states, but the most important is the proteinuria of the nephrotic syndrome (p. 948). Impaired synthesis of plasma proteins in cirrhosis of the liver is another important cause of reduced oncotic pressure. The movement of fluid from the intravascular to the interstitial compartment contracts the plasma volume, activating the renin-angiotensin-aldosterone axis with retention of salt and water, but the basic lowered plasma oncotic pressure persists, and so does the movement of water out of the intravascular compartment producing the non-inflammatory edema.

The other two categories require no comment.

CLINICAL SETTINGS WITH LOCALIZED EDEMA

• *Bilateral leg edema.*

   • Obstruction or narrowing of the vena cava by thrombosis or external pressure, e.g., pregnancy, tumor, ascites.

• *Unilateral leg edema.*

   • Obstruction of major outflow veins of one leg, e.g., thrombosis of the femoral or iliac veins.
   • Varicose veins in the legs with impaired venous return.

- *Uncommon causes of localized edema.*

  - Destruction or blockage of inguinal nodes or lymphatics, e.g., filariasis, surgical excision, lymph nodes, radiation, tumor.

Morphology

Subcutaneous Edema. Most evident in the feet, ankles, and lower legs—*dependent edema.* Generalized edema—*anasarca*—is marked by facial, particularly periorbital, edema.
Edema of Solid Organs. Slight increase in size and weight, separation of parenchymal elements, and compression of microcirculation.
Lungs. Heavy, subcrepitant, and wet. Septa widened and protein-poor fluid in the alveolar spaces. Usually congestive changes are also present, as described later, but there may be "pure" edema with hypersensitivity reactions and early in pneumonia.

HYPEREMIA AND CONGESTION (p. 97)

Both terms mean increased volume of blood in the affected tissue or part.

Active *hyperemia* refers to arteriolar dilatation of sympathetic or humoral origin. It is an active physiologic or pathologic response, as in skin and muscle after exercise or in acute inflammation (as discussed in Chapter 3).

Congestion results from impaired venous drainage with passive distention of distal veins, venules, and capillaries. The affected part is red-blue owing to deoxygenation of impounded red cells—*cyanosis.* It may be localized, as with venous obstruction, or systemic, as with heart failure.

In left ventricular failure, the lungs are mainly affected; in right-sided failure, systemic organs are affected, e.g., liver, spleen, sparing the lungs.

Morphology

General features. Often associated with edema. When *acute,* vessels are distended and organs or tissues unusually bloody. When *chronic,* it may lead to hypoxic atrophy or death of parenchymal cells, or microhemorrhages with hemosiderin deposition and fibrous scarring.
ORGANS MOST AFFECTED. **Lungs.** Congestion and edema —seen mainly with left ventricular failure, e.g., myocardial infarction, myocarditis, cardiomyopathy; rheumatic heart disease with mitral stenosis; floppy mitral valve with regurgitation.

- Alveolar capillaries engorged and tortuous
- Intraseptal edema about the alveolar capillaries with widening septa
- Proteinaceous fluid in air spaces
- Rupture of capillaries with hemosiderin-laden, intra-alveolar macrophages ("heart failure" cells)
- In time, edematous, hemosiderin-laden septa become fibrotic—*"brown induration"* of lungs

Liver. Acute and chronic congestion with right-sided heart failure, rarely with obstruction of the hepatic vein or inferior vena cava.
Acute: dusky red, tense, slightly heavy; oozes blood from distended central veins when sectioned.

Chronic: red-blue, congested centers of lobules rimmed by tan-brown, sometimes fatty (hypoxic) parenchyma—"nutmeg liver".

Severe congestive changes, hypoxic necrosis of central hepatocytes—*centrilobular necrosis.* If central sinusoids rupture, *central hemorrhagic necrosis.*

When persistent, fibrous thickening of walls of veins and central sinusoids leads to *cardiac sclerosis* (sometimes called cardiac cirrhosis).

Spleen. Acute congestion with blood-borne infections. Chronic with cirrhosis of liver.

Acute: slightly enlarged, cyanotic; on section exudes blood and collapses.

Chronic: congestive splenomegaly (500 to 700 gm), perisinusoidal fibrosis; organization of microhemorrhages leads to fibrosis.

HEMOSTASIS AND THROMBOSIS (p. 99)

Both processes closely related. *Hemostasis* vital to normal control of bleeding by the formation of a solid clot at site of vessel injury, but *thrombosis* is a pathologic process, with formation of a clotted mass of blood within the uninterrupted vascular system.

Thrombosis has the potential of:

- Diminishing or obstructing vascular flow to critical structures, e.g., heart, brain.
- Being dislodged or fragmented to create obstructive emboli.
- Producing an infarction, as is discussed later.

Three important contributors to hemostasis and thrombosis:

1. The vascular wall with its lining endothelium and underlying subendothelial connective tissues.

2. Platelets, essential for both hemostasis and thrombus formation.

3. Coagulation system.

NORMAL HEMOSTASIS (p. 100)

Essential events in formation of a hemostatic plug are:

- Brief period of neurogenic vasoconstriction, possibly augmented by humoral factors such as endothelin (a potent endothelium-derived vasoconstrictor).
- Injury to endothelial cells exposes thrombogenic subendothelial collagen to which platelets adhere and undergo "activation," with the release of adenosine diphosphate (ADP) thromboxane A_2 and serotonin. Further platelets adhere to form a *temporary plug.*
- Release of tissue factors at site of injury in combination with platelet factors activates coagulation sequence converting fibrinogen to fibrin.
- In this way a *permanent plug* is produced, made up of polymerized fibrin and platelet aggregates.

Now the three major contributors to hemostasis and thrombosis.

Endothelium

Endothelial cells, on the one hand, possess antiplatelet, anticoagulant, and fibrinolytic properties, but on the other hand, when injured or activated they exert procoagulant functions. These schizophrenic functions are listed in Figure 4–1.

Platelets

Play a central role in both hemostasis and thrombosis. With injury to a vessel, platelets are exposed to the subendothelial collagen and other connective tissue glycoproteins. They then undergo (a) adhesion and shape change, (b) secretion (release reaction), and (c) aggregation, collectively referred to as "platelet activation."

- *Adhesion* refers to attachment at the sites of endothelial injury by means of von Willebrand's factor (vWF), molecular bridges, and glycoprotein receptors on collagen and other connective tissue elements (mostly Gp1b). Genetic deficiency of von Willebrand's disease causes bleeding disorder.
- *Secretion or release reaction* liberates contents of platelet *alpha*-granules (coagulation proteins, growth factors, and enzymes) and dense bodies (contain ADP and ionized calcium), resulting in the appearance of a membrane phospholipid complex (platelet factor 3) on the platelet surface to which clotting factors may adhere.
- *Platelet aggregation* implies interadherence, initiated by ADP thromboxane A_2, followed in turn by generation of thrombin and ultimately fibrin.

A platelet deficiency produces serious bleeding disorders, as discussed in Chapter 13 of PBD.

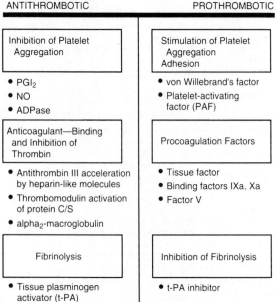

ANTITHROMBOTIC	PROTHROMBOTIC
Inhibition of Platelet Aggregation	Stimulation of Platelet Aggregation Adhesion
• PGI_2 • NO • ADPase	• von Willebrand's factor • Platelet-activating factor (PAF)
Anticoagulant—Binding and Inhibition of Thrombin	Procoagulation Factors
• Antithrombin III acceleration by heparin-like molecules • Thrombomodulin activation of protein C/S • $alpha_2$-macroglobulin	• Tissue factor • Binding factors IXa, Xa • Factor V
Fibrinolysis	Inhibition of Fibrinolysis
• Tissue plasminogen activator (t-PA)	• t-PA inhibitor

Figure 4–1. The endothelial thrombotic-antithrombotic balance. The major factors favoring and inhibiting thrombosis are shown. (From Cotran, R. S., Kumar, V., and Robbins, S. L.: Robbins Pathologic Basis of Disease. 5th ed. Philadelphia, W. B. Saunders Co., 1994, p. 100.)

Coagulation System

Consists in essence of a series of transformations of proenzymes to activated enzymes, culminating in polymerization of fibrinogen into fibrin. It has been customary to divide coagulation into an *extrinsic* and an *intrinsic* pathway, both of which converge on activation of factor X. In theory, the intrinsic pathway is activated by Hageman factor (factor XII) and the extrinsic pathway by tissue factor. Note in Figure 4–2, however, the many links between intrinsic and extrinsic pathways, and so tissue factor also can activate the intrinsic pathway. *In vivo* studies indicate that factor XI activation is not important.

Control Mechanisms

There are checks and balances against uncontrolled spread of the coagulation process:

- Thrombin (in the presence of fibronectin and fibrinogen) induces endothelial cell release of urokinase and tissue-type plasminogen activators (tPA) to convert plasminogen to plasmin.

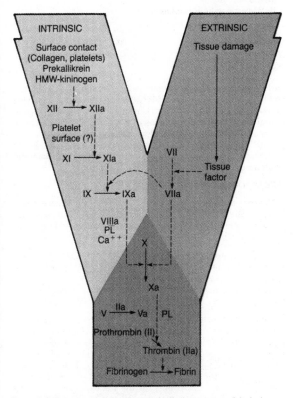

Figure 4–2. The coagulation cascade. Note the common links between the intrinsic and extrinsic coagulation pathways. (From Cotran, R. S., Kumar, V., and Robbins, S. L.: Robbins Pathologic Basis of Disease. 5th ed. Philadelphia, W. B. Saunders Co., 1994, p. 103.)

- Fibrin split products formed by fibrinolysis inhibit clotting.
- Antithrombin III in the presence of heparin-like molecules on endothelial cells inhibits thrombin and down-regulates factors XIIa, XIa, Xa, and IXa.
- Activated clotting factors are depleted by dilution at sites of clot formation.
- Activated factors are cleared by the liver and mononuclear phagocyte system.
- Thrombin unmasks endothelial cell receptors (thrombomodulin) that bind and activate protein C, which in turn inactivates factors Va and VIIIa.

Thus, normal hemostasis constitutes a balanced mechanism involving numerous pro- and anticoagulation reactions.

THROMBOSIS (p. 105)

Represents hemostasis in the intact vascular system. *Three influences are involved (Virchow's triad):*

1. Endothelial injury (most important). Alone can induce thrombosis.
2. Alterations in normal flow.
3. Hypercoagulability.

When the last two are both present, endothelial injury is not requisite.

Endothelial Injury

Particularly important in thrombi in arteries and heart. Exemplified by ulcerative atherosclerosis with almost invariable overlying thrombi. It also occurs with transmural myocardial infarction (mural intraventricular thrombosis), vasculitis, trauma, radiation, and more subtle influences such as bacterial toxins.

With injury, endothelial cells are activated with release of thrombotic (and antithrombotic) factors, collagen is exposed, and the train of platelet and clotting events is initiated.

Alterations in Normal Blood Flow

Turbulence in the arteries or heart or *stasis* in the veins disrupts the laminar stream and the plasmatic sleeve that separates formed elements from the vessel wall. More important in veins than in arteries.

- Platelets activated by contact with endothelium.
- Slowed flow retards dilution of activated clotting factors and hepatic clearance.
- Stasis or turbulence retards the inflow of inhibitors.
- Turbulence may induce endothelial injury.

Stasis is important in myocardial infarcts when damaged myocardium is unable to contract and at the same time endothelial injury also contributes to thrombogenesis. This sequence is also important in dilated cardiac chambers, especially atrial appendages and abnormally dilated (varicose) veins. It is the major determinant of thrombosis in the deep veins of legs devoid of endothelial injury. It accounts for the frequency of thrombosis in hyperviscosity syndromes (polycythemia, macroglobulinemia, cryoglobulinemia), sickle cell anemia, and cavernous hemangiomas.

Hypercoagulability of Blood

An ill-defined phenomenon, not associated with consistent or significant laboratory findings. Invoked to account for the increased tendency to thrombosis with (a) antithrombin III or protein C deficiency; (b) disseminated cancer; (c) in the nephrotic syndrome; (d) following trauma; (e) with the use of oral contraceptives (OCs); and (f) in late pregnancy or postdelivery. The hypercoagulable states can be divided into (1) primary (genetic) or (2) secondary (acquired) categories, as in Table 4–2.

The basis of hypercoagulability is only sometimes clear, e.g., genetic impairment in antithrombin III synthesis, urinary excretion of antithrombin III in the nephrotic syndrome, secretion of procoagulants by cancer cells, or release of tissue factor after trauma, burns, or delivery. In most thrombotic diatheses, no such clear basis for hypercoagulability is present.

Morphology of Thrombi (p. 106)

Thrombi may form anywhere in the cardiovascular system. In the *cardiac chambers* and *aorta,* because of rapid bypassing flow, they are *nonocclusive (mural).* In the remainder of the arterial tree and within veins, thrombi are usually *occlusive.*

At sites of origin, all thrombi generally are firmly attached, but at both upstream and downstream ends they may propagate to produce loosely attached heads or tails that may fragment and embolize.

On the arterial side (including the heart), thrombi tend to be gray-red; pale layers of platelets and fibrin alternate with darker layers containing more red cells (lines of Zahn).

Table 4–2. Hypercoagulable States

Primary (Genetic)
Antithrombin III deficiency
Protein C deficiency
Protein S deficiency
Fibrinolysis defects
? Other combined defects

Secondary (Acquired)	
High Risk	
Prolonged bed rest or immobilization	Acute leukemia
Myocardial infarction	Myeloproliferative disorders
Tissue damage (including surgery, fractures, burns)	Prosthetic cardiac valves
	Disseminated intravascular coagulation
Cardiac failure	Thrombotic thrombocytopenia
Cancer	Homocystinuria
Lower Risk	
Atrial fibrillation	Hyperlipidemia
Cardiomyopathy	Lupus anticoagulant
Nephrotic syndrome	Sickle cell anemia
Late pregnancy/postdelivery	Smoking
Oral contraceptives	Thrombocytosis

From Cotran R. S., Kumar V., and Robbins, S. L: Robbins Pathologic Basis of Disease. 5th ed. Philadelphia, W. B. Saunders Co., 1994, p. 106.

Frequent sites:

- The left ventricle overlying a myocardial infarct.
- Auricular appendages, particularly when flow is sluggish (atrial fibrillation).
- The aorta (mural) overlying ulcerated and fissured atheromata.
- Atherosclerotic arteries, e.g., coronaries, iliacs, carotids (occlusive).
- Aneurysmal sacs.

On the venous side (phlebothrombosis), thrombi tend to be red-blue, resembling clotted blood in a test tube, but thin strands of fibrin are sometimes evident. Only rarely are lines of Zahn well defined.

Attachment to the vessel wall helps differentiate antemortem venous thrombi from "currant jelly" postmortem clots.

Frequent sites:

- Dilated superficial varicose veins of the legs (rarely embolize).
- Deep veins of the calf and thighs and muscular veins in approximately the following order—deep calf, femoral, popliteal, iliac. Account for about 95% of venous thrombi (often clinically silent and frequently embolize to the lungs).
- Less commonly in the periprostatic plexus and ovarian and periuterine veins (rare source of emboli).

Formation of valvular vegetations:

Infective endocarditis constitutes bacteria- or fungus-laden thrombi on valvular leaflets or mural endocardium, complicating blood-borne infections.

Nonbacterial thrombotic endocarditis seen as small vegetations on any valve in patients with systemic lupus erythematosus (lupus endocarditis). Similar small vegetations in disseminated cancer, or other putative hypercoagulability syndromes.

Fate of Thrombus

If the patient survives the immediate ischemic effects of a thrombus, one of the following sequences may ensue:

1. *Propagation* to obstruct a critical vessel or branch.
2. *Embolization* in part or in whole.
3. *Removal by fibrinolytic action.*
4. *Organization* and *recanalization.*

If thrombus persists, it undergoes organization by invading fibroblasts and capillaries. It is sometimes recanalized by through-and-through capillary channels.

CLINICAL SIGNIFICANCE (p. 109)

Arterial thrombi may obstruct critical vessels, e.g., coronary, cerebral. Those in heart chambers may embolize to leg, kidneys, spleen.

Venous thrombi in deep veins of the legs are common problems. They are often silent, may embolize to the lungs, and are prone to occur in certain clinical settings:

- *Advanced age:* associated with atherosclerosis and endothelial damage, hypercoagulability, and reduced physical activity with venous stasis.
- *Bed rest and immobilization,* e.g., of an extremity after a fracture: associated with vascular stasis and possibly hypercoagulation.

- *Heart disease.*
  - *Myocardial infarction.* Dyskinesis of affected ventricular wall with stasis and endocardial cell injury.
  - *Rheumatic mitral stenosis.* Left atrial and auricular enlargement, often with atrial fibrillation, adding elements of stasis and turbulence.
  - *Congestive heart failure.* Slowed venous return, and stasis within peripheral vessels, notably in the legs.
  - *Valvular damage* or *congenital cardiac anomaly.* Induces jet streams, turbulence, and endocardial damage, sometimes leading to bacterial seeding and infective endocarditis.
- *Tissue injury* (fractures, burns, extensive soft tissue damage, labor and delivery, postoperative states). Released tissue factor from endothelial injury, bed rest, and reduced physical activity.
- *Visceral cancer* (usually disseminated). Often complicated by random, asynchronous, venous thrombi (migratory thrombophlebitis, *Trousseau's phenomenon*)—most frequently encountered with pancreatic or gastrointestinal carcinoma. Vital or necrotic cancer cells release procoagulants.
- *Late pregnancy* and *the postdelivery period* are associated with thrombi, usually in leg veins ("milk leg" or "phlegmasia alba dolens"—painful white leg). The gravid uterus compresses the inferior vena cava, causing venous stasis in the legs; there is also hypercoagulability, reduced fibrinolytic activity, and increased distensibility of veins. Delivery involves release of tissue factor and procoagulants.
- *Oral contraceptives* (high-dose estrogen). Responsible for a fivefold increased death rate from circulatory diseases, mainly myocardial infarction, stroke, and pulmonary embolism in women over 35 years of age. Concomitant cigarette smoking is an important cofactor.

DISSEMINATED INTRAVASCULAR COAGULATION (DIC) (p. 110)

Mentioned here because it is characterized by myriad thrombi in the microcirculation, soon followed in many cases by active fibrinolysis and a bleeding disorder. For the latter reason, this condition is discussed with the bleeding diatheses.

EMBOLISM (p. 111)

Constitutes an intravascular solid, liquid, or gaseous mass carried through the blood to a site distant from its origin. Over 98% arise in thrombi. Among other possible types, the most common are debris from atheromatous plaques (atheroemboli) and fat emboli. Unless otherwise qualified, the term *embolism* implies *thromboembolism.*

Emboli arising in veins usually impact in the lungs and may or may not cause infarction (pulmonary embolism).

Emboli arising on the arterial side of the circulation, most often in intracardiac thrombi, usually impact in the legs, brain, and viscera and often cause infarctions (systemic embolism).

PULMONARY EMBOLISM (PE) (p. 111)

Occlusions of pulmonary arteries are almost always embolic; in situ *thromboses are rare,* occurring only with pulmonary hypertension and pulmonary atherosclerosis. However, thrombosis may complete a partial embolic occlusion.

Over 95% of PE arise in deep veins of legs. They tend to occur in hospitalized patients, particularly following hip fractures and surgery, and in elderly patients confined to bed for long periods.

Potential consequences are

- Large emboli (about 5%) impacting in the major pulmonary artery(ies) or astride the bifurcation of the pulmonary artery (saddle embolus).

  - May cause instantaneous death when more than 60% of the total pulmonary vasculature is occluded.
  - May cause cardiovascular collapse, e.g., acute cor pulmonale (right heart failure). A shower of or repeated small emboli may have the same effect.
  - Hemodynamic compromise is secondary not only to vascular obstruction, but also to reflex vasoconstriction caused by such agents as thromboxane A_2.

- Small emboli (60 to 80%).

  - May be clinically silent in patients without cardiovascular failure.
  - In only 10 to 15% of cases in patients with compromised pulmonary circulation (cardiac failure), infarctions result. Such emboli are generally small.

- Between the extremes of large and small emboli are those of middle size (about 10 to 15%) that occlude moderate-sized peripheral pulmonary branches.

  - Usually induce pulmonary hemorrhages.

Uncommonly, multiple overt or covert small emboli produce right heart strain (chronic cor pulmonale) and eventually pulmonary hypertension and vascular sclerosis.

CLINICAL SIGNIFICANCE. Diagnosis of pulmonary emboli is often difficult; almost two thirds of PE, even when fatal, are not diagnosed before death. Many are silent, others are catastrophic, and even when they produce infarction they may not produce recognizable manifestations.

Even without treatment, there is usually improvement in perfusion within the first day owing to fibrinolysis and contraction of the mass. As with a thrombus, the embolus may become organized if it does not resolve and incorporated in the vessel wall as a mural plaque. Occasionally organization creates bridging, fibrous webs.

SYSTEMIC EMBOLISM (p. 112)

Arterial emboli:

- Most (80 to 85%) arise from thrombi within the heart, secondary to myocardial infarction.
- About 5 to 10% arise from auricular thrombi (usually associated with rheumatic heart disease and atrial fibrillation).
- About 5% arise from thrombi in the dilated cardiac chambers of myocarditis/cardiomyopathy.
- Less common sources include debris from ulcerated atheromata or thrombi associated with aortic aneurysms, infective endocarditis, prosthetic valves, and paradoxic emboli.

- Origin of about 15% is unknown.

Sites of Lodgment. Lower extremities (70 to 75%), brain (10%), viscera (10%), upper limbs (about 5%).

Not all emboli inevitably cause infarction (see below), but they are an important cause of morbidity and mortality.

AMNIOTIC FLUID INFUSION (EMBOLISM) (p. 112)

An uncommon (1 in 50,000 deliveries), grave complication of labor and delivery that appears without warning and is marked by respiratory difficulty, cyanosis, and vascular collapse, progressing sometimes to convulsions, coma, and death. Complicating DIC may introduce a bleeding diathesis.

The *pathogenesis* is thought to involve a tear in the placental membranes and in uterine/cervical veins with the infusion of amniotic fluid.

The *pathophysiology of clinical features* is uncertain but may involve

- Embolization to the pulmonary microcirculation of the particulate debris in amniotic fluid, e.g., fetal epithelial squamae, lanugo hair.
- Release of vasoconstrictor agents, e.g., prostaglandins reducing pulmonary blood flow.
- Intercurrence of DIC with blockade of pulmonary circulation by myriad microthrombi.

The *diagnostic morphologic feature is the amniotic debris in pulmonary capillaries.*

AIR EMBOLISM (CAISSON DISEASE) (p. 113)

When bubbles of air or gas within the circulation obstruct vascular flow, the resultant injury is referred to as "barotrauma." Air or gas may gain access to the circulation:

- During delivery or abortion, when it is forced into ruptured uterine venous sinuses by contractions of the uterus.
- During performance of pneumothorax when a large artery or vein is accidentally ruptured or entered.
- When injury to the lung or chest wall opens a large vein and permits entrance of air during the negative pressure phase of inspiration.

In any of the above circumstances, quantities of air, probably 100 ml, are necessary to become clinically significant.

A specialized form of gas embolism known as *caisson disease* or *decompression sickness* occurs with sudden changes in atmospheric pressure, particularly among scuba and deep-sea divers and underwater workers. When oxygen (often mixed with helium or nitrogen) is breathed under increased pressure, the gases dissolve in the blood and tissue fluids. With decompression, they come out of solution as minute bubbles. Oxygen is soluble, nitrogen and helium persist as gaseous emboli.

Acute decompression sickness is marked by "the bends" from acute obstruction of small vessels in and around joints and skeletal muscles or by "the chokes" with bubbles in lungs and respiratory muscles.

Chronic decompression sickness (caisson disease) is marked by foci of ischemic necrosis in the skeletal system, particularly the normally poorly vascularized heads of the femur, tibia, and humerus.

It is necessary at autopsy to open the heart and major pulmonary vessels under water to be able to detect escaping gas.

FAT EMBOLISM (p. 113)

Next to thromboembolism, the most common form of embolism. Intravascular globules of fat may occur:

- Most often in patients sustaining fractures of large bones that have fatty marrows.
- With extensive trauma to fatty tissue.
- Rarely, in nontraumatic diseases, e.g., diabetes mellitus, sickle cell anemia, pancreatitis.

Depending on the number and size of the microglobules of fat, there may be no symptoms or the development of the *fat embolism syndrome—thrombocytopenia, petechiae in the skin and conjunctivae, respiratory difficulty,* and *obtundation, sometimes coma and death.* To be noted: the mere presence of intravascular fat globules is not synonymous with the fat embolism syndrome. Although fat emboli are present in 90% of patients following a large fracture, in only 1 to 2% is it clinically significant.

MORPHOLOGY. *Diagnosis rests on identification of intravascular fat globules in microvessels, especially in the lungs, kidneys, and brain. Requires special fat stains (oil red-O) and avoidance of fat solvent fixatives.*

- *Lungs* may reveal marked edema and hyaline membranes within the alveolar spaces identical to those seen in the adult respiratory distress syndrome.
- *Brain* may contain microemboli of fat, cerebral edema, scattered perivascular microhemorrhages, and occasionally microinfarcts.
- *Kidneys* may also disclose globules in glomeruli.
- *Skin* may have petechiae, which may also occur in conjunctivae and serosal membranes. These reflect thrombocytopenia secondary to adhesion of platelets to microemboli of fat.

PATHOGENESIS. Still uncertain, but both mechanical obstruction and chemical injury probably are involved. The microaggregates of fat may themselves occlude the pulmonary or cerebral microcirculation. In addition, free fatty acids may cause toxic injury to vascular endothelium with the development of thrombi, thus an element of DIC is added.

INFARCTION (p. 114)

An infarct is a localized area of ischemic necrosis in an organ or tissue, resulting most often from sudden occlusion of its arterial supply (97%). It rarely is caused by obstruction of venous drainage, usually in organs having no potential bypass channels, e.g., ovary, testis.

Vascular obstructions:

- Are thrombotic or embolic in origin in the great majority of cases.
- Rarely are caused by expansile tumors, spasm (as in coronary arteries), trapping of a viscus in a hernial sac, twisting of a

mobile viscus (loop of bowel, ovary) with compression of thin-walled veins and sometimes arteries.

Not all vascular occlusions lead to infarction. Factors that modify the outcome include

- General status of the blood and cardiovascular system (anemia and congestive failure increase the likelihood).
- Anatomic pattern of vascular supply—dual blood supply, e.g., liver, lungs, or interconnecting anastomoses, such as in the intestines or circle of Willis, protects against infarction.
- Rate of development of occlusion.
- Vulnerability of tissue to ischemia; neurons and myocardial and renal proximal tubular epithelial cells are especially sensitive to ischemia (hypoxia).

MORPHOLOGY. Infarcts are classified as hemorrhagic (red) or pale (white, anemic), and also septic or bland.

Hemorrhagic infarcts are encountered with venous occlusion (e.g., torsion of ovary) and in tissues that are loose (e.g., lung) or have a double or anastomotic circulation (e.g., small intestine, lung).

White or pale infarcts occur in solid organs with end arteries (having few anastomoses) such as kidneys and spleen.

Whether hemorrhagic or pale, most infarcts are wedge shaped, with their apex at the locus of vascular obstruction and their bases at the external aspect of the organ. Common to all is ischemic coagulative necrosis with eventual replacement of infarct by scar tissue.

*Infarcts in the brain—encephalomalacia—*are an exception. They may be peripheral or central, depending on the affected vessel and collateral flow, and are marked by liquefactive necrosis.

CLINICAL SIGNIFICANCE. Infarction is a dominant cause of morbidity and mortality in developed countries. Collectively, myocardial, cerebral, and pulmonary infarctions are responsible for well over half of all deaths.

SHOCK (p. 117)

At the most basic level, shock constitutes a widespread hypoperfusion of cells and tissues owing to inadequate effective circulating blood volume. The perfusion deficit results in insufficient delivery of oxygen and nutrients to the cells and tissues, inadequate clearance of metabolites, and a hypoxic shift from aerobic to anaerobic metabolism, resulting sometimes in lactic acidosis.

PATHOGENESIS

Basis for the hypoperfusion can be divided into three major categories:

- *Cardiogenic shock,* i.e., "pump failure" owing to myocardial damage (myocardial infarction), arrhythmias, tamponade, or outflow obstruction.
- *Hypovolemic or hemorrhagic shock,* caused by large losses of plasma (severe burns) or whole blood (traumatic injury).
- *Septic shock,* caused by bacteremic infections, most commonly gram-negative organisms (endotoxic shock) but also gram-positives and, rarely, fungi.
- Rare additional types of shock: *neurogenic* and *anaphylactic.*

Cardiogenic shock and hypovolemic shock require no further explanation for the hyperperfusion. The pathophysiology of septic shock is less well understood, but hypoperfusion is attributed to sequestration blood volume in the peripheral capacitance vessels. The basis for dilatation of capacitance vessels is not clear. Release of a bacterial toxin such as the endotoxins (LPS) from gram-negative organisms may directly alter function of vascular wall and parenchymal cells, but, more importantly, it may act by initiating the synthesis, release, and activation of mediators derived from plasma, white cells, endothelial cells, and others. A long list of mediators is implicated, including:

- cytokines (IL-1, TNF, IL-6, IL-8)
- platelet activating factor
- nitric oxide
- complement (C5a and C3a)
- prostaglandins
- leukotrienes
- others

Mediators, in turn, affect many organ systems—

- heart—myocardial dysfunction
- vascular system—dilatation and hypotension
- lungs—causing ARDS (p. 676)
- kidneys—acute renal failure
- liver—hepatic failure
- others

Among the mediators, IL-1 and TNF-α are thought to be key to pathogenesis of septic shock. They cause endothelial activation and leukocyte adhesion and promote intravascular coagulation. In addition, bacterial toxins, as mentioned, may directly injure cells, reducing their capacity effectively to utilize the minimal amounts of oxygen in the reduced blood supply.

MORPHOLOGY. The systemic hypoxia causes organ injury.

Brain may show hypoxic encephalopathy (*see p. 1308*).

Heart shows two types of changes:

1. Subepicardial and subendocardial hemorrhages accompanied by individual myofiber necroses and/or micro- (sometimes macro-) infarcts.

2. Scattered opaque transverse "contraction bands" within myocytes.

Although distinctive, these changes are not pathognomonic of shock.

Lungs usually are not morphologically affected in pure hypovolemic shock, but in cardiogenic and septic shock, severe pulmonary edema may progress to adult respiratory distress syndrome, "shock lung."

Kidneys suffer ischemic injury to tubules at all levels of the nephron—"acute tubular necrosis" (*see p. 964*).

Other organs may be affected: adrenals, pituitary, GI tract, liver.

CLINICAL CORRELATIONS. Three classic stages of shock:

1. *Compensated stage.* Begins with mild hypotension, tachycardia, pallor, and cold, clammy extremities (in septic shock, peripheral dilatation may produce warm, flushed extremities and facies).

2. *Decompensated stage.* If circulatory insufficiency persists, compensatory mechanisms are overwhelmed with a decline in

blood pressure, rapid pulse, respiratory difficulty, metabolic acidosis, and a decline in renal function, principally output.

3. *"Irreversible" shock.* If circulatory and metabolic deficits are not corrected, a stage may develop when all therapeutic efforts are to no avail, leading to coma and death.

If, however, the underlying cause of the shock, e.g., sepsis, can be controlled and the patient's fluid and electrolyte levels appropriately managed, *shock up to the terminal stages is a reversible condition* with improvement in pulmonary, renal, and cerebral function.

Full recovery is possible, but there is high mortality with cardiogenic shock (80 to 90%) because of underlying cardiac disease, and with septic shock (50%) because of difficulty in control of infection.

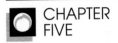

CHAPTER FIVE

Genetic Disorders

CLASSIFICATION

1. Chromosomal (cytogenetic) disorders.
2. Mendelian disorders.
3. Multifactorial disorders.
4. Single gene disorders with nonclassic inheritance.

MENDELIAN DISORDERS (p. 127)

These result from mutations in single genes of large effect.
Some relevant definitions:

Penetrance The percentage of individuals carrying an autosomal dominant gene and expressing the trait.

Variable expressivity Variable expression of autosomal dominant trait in affected individuals.

Codominance Full expression of both alleles of a given gene pair in a heterozygote.

Polymorphism Multiple allelic forms of a single gene.

Pleiotropism Multiple end effects of a single mutant gene.

Genetic heterogeneity Production of a given trait by different mutations at multiple loci.

Autosomal Dominant Disorders (p. 128)

Some general features are

- Mutations affecting structural (e.g., collagen) or regulatory (e.g., receptor) proteins. In some instances, e.g., collagen, the product of the mutant allele interferes with the function of the normal protein. Such mutant alleles, called "dominant negative," can produce severe deficiency of protein, as in osteogenesis imperfecta (Chapter 23).
- Reduced penetrance and variable expressivity.
- Onset of clinical features that may be later than in autosomal recessive disorders.

Autosomal Recessive Disorders (p. 129)

These include most inborn errors of metabolism. In contrast to autosomal dominant disorders, the following features generally apply to most disorders in this category:

- Age of onset is frequently in early life.
- Clinical features tend to be more uniform.
- In many patients enzyme proteins, rather than structural proteins, are affected.

Sex-Linked (X-Linked) Disorders (p. 129)

All sex-linked disorders are X-linked, and almost all are X-linked recessive. They are fully expressed in males because mutant genes on the X chromosome are not paired with alleles on the Y. In contrast, heterozygous females usually express the disease partially because the paired normal allele is randomly inactivated in some, but not all, cells (e.g., G6PD deficiency). Fragile X syndrome is discussed later.

BIOCHEMICAL AND MOLECULAR BASIS OF MENDELIAN DISORDERS (p. 130)

Virtually any type of protein may be affected. Some examples are provided in Table 5–1.

DISORDERS ASSOCIATED WITH DEFECTS IN STRUCTURAL PROTEINS (p. 132)

Marfan Syndrome (p. 132)

A disorder of connective tissues affecting predominantly the skeletal, ocular, and cardiovascular systems.

SKELETAL CHANGES

- Tall stature with exceptionally long extremities.
- Long, tapering fingers and toes (arachnodactyly).
- Laxity of joint ligaments, producing hyperextensibility.
- Spinal deformities (e.g., kyphosis and scoliosis).

OCULAR CHANGES

- Bilateral dislocation of lenses (ectopia lentis).
- Increased axial length of the globe, giving rise to retinal detachments.

CARDIOVASCULAR LESIONS

- Mitral valve prolapse is most common, although not life threatening; affected valves are soft and billowy, producing a floppy valve associated with mitral regurgitation.
- Cystic medionecrosis of the aorta is less common than mitral valve lesions but clinically more important. Histologically, the media undergoes softening with formation of cystlike spaces, giving rise to dilatation of the aortic valve ring and aortic incompetence. More important, the cystic medionecrosis predisposes to an intimal tear through which the blood dissects into the media (a dissecting aneurysm); cleavage of the aortic wall may extend proximally or distally, often resulting in rupture of the aorta.

Death is usually caused by rupture of a dissecting aneurysm, followed in importance by cardiac failure.

Marfan syndrome results from mutations in the *fibrillin* gene. Fibrillin, a glycoprotein secreted by fibroblasts, provides a scaffolding for the deposition of elastin. Abnormal fibrillin leads to defects in the elastic tissue, particularly in the aorta, mitral valve, and ciliary zonules. The fibrillin gene (Marfan locus) has been mapped to 15q21.1.

Ehlers-Danlos Syndromes (EDS) (p. 133)

This clinically and genetically heterogeneous group of disorders results from some *defect in collagen*. They are divided into twelve

Table 5-1. Biochemical and Molecular Basis of Some Mendelian Disorders

Protein Type/ Function	Example	Molecular Lesion	Disease
Enzyme	Phenylalanine hydroxylase	Splice site mutation: reduced amount	Phenylketonuria
	Hexosaminidase	Splice site mutation or frame-shift mutation with stop codon: reduced amount	Tay-Sachs disease
Receptor	Low-density lipoprotein receptor	Deletions, point mutations: reduction of synthesis, transport to cell surface, or binding to low-density lipoprotein	Familial hypercholesterolemia
Transport			
Oxygen	Hemoglobin	Deletions: reduced amount	α Thalassemia
		Defective mRNA processing; reduced amount	β Thalassemia
		Point mutations: abnormal structure	Sickle cell anemia
Ions	Cystic fibrosis transmembrane conductance regulator	Deletions and other mutations	Cystic fibrosis
Structural			
Extracellular	Collagen	Deletions or point mutations cause reduced amount of normal collagen or normal amounts of mutant collagen	Osteogenesis imperfecta; Ehlers-Danlos syndromes
	Fibrillin	Point mutations	Marfan syndrome
Cell membrane	Dystrophin	Deletion with reduced synthesis	Duchenne/Becker muscular dystrophy
Enzyme Inhibitor	α₁-Antitrypsin	Missense mutations—impair secretion from liver to serum	Emphysema and liver disease
Hemostasis	Factor VIII	Deletions, insertions, nonsense mutations, and others: reduced synthesis or abnormal factor VIII	Hemophilia A

From Cotran, R. S., Kumar, V., and Robbins, S. L.: Robbins Pathologic Basis of Disease. 5th ed. Philadelphia, W. B. Saunders Co., 1994, p. 131.

variants on the basis of predominant clinical manifestations and pattern of inheritance. The features listed below are common to most variants:

- *Skin.* Hyperextensible, extremely fragile, and vulnerable to trauma; surgical repair of wounds is markedly impaired owing to defective collagen.
- *Joints.* Hypermobile and prone to dislocation.
- *Internal complications.* These affect several organs rich in collagen; manifestations include rupture of the colon and large arteries, ocular fragility with corneal rupture and retinal detachment, and diaphragmatic hernias.

The biochemical bases of abnormalities in collagen are extremely varied. Some of the better characterized defects are as follows:

- Reduced activity of lysyl hydroxylase, an enzyme essential for cross linking of collagen fibers, is noted in type VI EDS, the most common autosomal recessive form. Collagens (types I and III) lack structural stability.
- Abnormalities of type III collagen, resulting from several distinct mutations in the structural gene, characterize type IV EDS. Because a structural rather than an enzyme protein is affected, the pattern of inheritance is autosomal dominant. Blood vessels and intestines known to be rich in type III collagen are prone to spontaneous rupture.
- Defective conversion of type I procollagen to collagen characterizes type VII EDS. It is caused by mutations affecting type I collagen genes. The mutant procollagen chains resist cleavage of N-terminal peptides, essential for the formation of normal collagen. Even if only one of the two alleles is mutant, their abnormal products interfere with the formation of normal collagen helices, and hence heterozygotes have severe disease.
- Defective copper metabolism is the basis of EDS type IX. Intracellular copper levels are high but serum copper is low. Abnormality of copper metabolism secondarily reduces the activity of the enzyme lysyl oxidase, essential for cross linking of collagen and elastin. It is inherited as an X-linked recessive trait.

DISORDERS ASSOCIATED WITH DEFECTS IN RECEPTOR PROTEINS

Familial Hypercholesterolemia (FH) (p. 135)

This results from a mutation in the gene encoding the receptor for low-density lipoprotein (LDL). At least 35 mutations that can be classified into four groups have been discovered.

- Class I mutations are the most common, and they impair transcription, resulting in failure of synthesis of receptor proteins.
- Class II mutations prevent transport of the receptors from the endoplasmic reticulum to the Golgi complex.
- Class III mutations are associated with production of a receptor protein that has reduced binding capacity.
- Class IV mutations give rise to proteins that can bind LDL but cannot internalize the bound LDL.

NORMAL CHOLESTEROL TRANSPORT AND METABOLISM.

Review Figure 5–1. Only a few salient features will be emphasized:

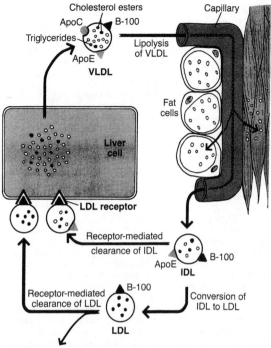

Figure 5–1. Schematic illustration of LDL metabolism and the role of liver in its synthesis and clearance. Lipolysis of VLDL by lipoprotein lipase in the capillaries releases triglycerides that are then stored in fat cells and used as a source of energy in skeletal muscles. (From Cotran, R. S., Kumar, V., and Robbins, S. L.: Robbins Pathologic Basis of Disease. 5th ed. Philadelphia, W. B. Saunders Co., 1994, p. 135.)

- LDL is the major transport form of cholesterol in plasma.
- Although many cells in the body possess high-affinity receptors that recognize apoprotein B-100 of the LDL molecule, about 70% of plasma LDL is cleared by liver. The remaining 30% is transported into other cells, especially mononuclear phagocytes, by binding to distinct receptors for chemically altered (e.g., acetylated) form of LDL.
- The transport of and metabolism of LDL into the liver can be resolved into several steps: (1) binding to surface receptors; (2) internalization, followed by transport to and fusion with lysosomes; (3) lysosomal processing, leading to release of free cholesterol into cytoplasm. Free cholesterol affects three processes:

  1. It suppresses cholesterol synthesis by inhibiting the enzyme (3HMG) CoA reductase.
  2. It activates enzymes that favor esterification of cholesterol.
  3. It suppresses synthesis of LDL receptors, thereby preventing excessive transport of cholesterol into cells.

CLINICAL FEATURES. FH is an extremely common disorder with a gene frequency of one in 500.

Heterozygotes have the following features:

- Cells possess 50% of the normal number of high-affinity LDL receptors. A plasma LDL cholesterol level two to three times higher than normal, resulting from both impaired clearance of plasma LDL and increased synthesis. The latter is secondary to decreased hepatic uptake of IDL, the immediate precursor of plasma LDL.
- Hypercholesterolemia, leading to premature atherosclerosis and accumulation of cholesterol in soft tissues and skin, producing xanthomas.

Homozygotes have much greater elevations of plasma LDL cholesterol and are at much greater risk of developing widespread atherosclerosis; ischemic heart disease often develops before the age of 20. Xanthomas of the skin are also more prominent in homozygotes.

DISORDERS ASSOCIATED WITH DEFECTS IN ENZYMES (p. 138)

Lysosomal Storage Diseases (pp. 138–145)

The synthesis, transport, and functions of lysosomal enzymes (discussed on p. 138 and illustrated in Fig. 5–11 of *Robbins Pathologic Basis of Disease*) should be reviewed.

Lysosomal storage disorders result from inherited lack of functional lysosomal enzymes or other proteins essential for their function. In the absence of normal lysosomal processing, catabolism of complex substrates is impaired, leading to accumulation of partially degraded insoluble metabolites within lysosomes. The lysosomes, packed with undigested macromolecules, are enlarged and interfere with normal cell function.

Lysosomal storage diseases are classified on the basis of the biochemical nature of the accumulated metabolite (Table 5–2). Distribution of the stored material and resultant clinical features depend on

- The site where most of the material to be degraded is normally found.
- The site where most of the degradation normally occurs.

Because cells of the mononuclear phagocytic system are particularly rich in lysosomes and are responsible for degradation of several substrates, organs rich in phagocytic cells, such as liver and spleen, are often enlarged. Some of the more common disorders are described next.

Tay-Sachs Disease (Gm₂-Gangliosidosis: Hexosaminidase α-Subunit Deficiency)

This results from mutations that affect the α-subunit of the hexosaminidase enzyme complex. The resultant deficiency of hexosaminidase A prevents degradation of GM_2-ganglioside. It is most common in Jews of Eastern European origin. The clinical features, derived primarily from accumulation of GM_2-ganglioside in neurons of the central and autonomic nervous systems and retina, include

- Motor and mental deterioration commencing at about 6 months of age.
- Blindness.

Table 5-2. Lysosomal Storage Diseases

Disease	Enzyme Deficiency	Major Accumulating Metabolites
Glycogenosis		
Type 2—Pompe's disease	α-1,4-Glucosidase (lysosomal glucosidase)	Glycogen
Sphingolipidoses		
Tay-Sachs disease	Hexosaminidase-α subunit	G_{M2}-ganglioside
Sandhoff's disease	Hexosaminidase-β subunit	G_{M2}-ganglioside, globoside
Sulfatidoses		
Gaucher's disease	Glucocerebrosidase	Glucocerebroside
Niemann-Pick disease, types A and B	Sphingomyelinase	Sphingomyelin
Mucopolysaccharidoses		
MPS I (Hurler)	α-L-Iduronidase	Dermatan sulfate, heparan sulfate
MPS II (Hunter)	L-Iduronosulfate sulfatase	
Mucolipidoses (ML)		
I-cell disease (MLII) and pseudo-Hurler polydystrophy	Deficiency of phosphorylating enzymes essential for formation of mannose-6-phosphate recognition marker; acid hydrolases lacking recognition marker cannot be targeted to lysosomes but are secreted extracellularly	Mucopolysaccharide, glycolipid

Modified from Cotran, R. S., Kumar, V., and Robbins, S. L.: Pathologic Basis of Disease. 5th ed. Philadelphia, W. B. Saunders Co., 1994, p. 139.

- A cherry-red spot in the retina.
- Death by 2 to 3 years of age.

MORPHOLOGIC FEATURES

- Ballooning of neurons with cytoplasmic vacuoles that stain positive for lipids.
- Whorled configurations in the cytoplasmic vacuoles, revealed by electron microscopy.
- Progressive destruction of neurons with proliferation of microglia.
- Accumulation of lipids in retinal ganglion cells, rendering them pale in color, thus accentuating the normal red color of the macular choroid (cherry-red spot).

Antenatal diagnosis and carrier detection are possible by DNA probe analysis and enzyme assays on cells obtained from amniocentesis.

Niemann-Pick Disease

This is a heterogeneous disorder associated with accumulation of sphingomyelin and cholesterol in mononuclear phagocytic and many other cell types.

Biochemically, two groups can be distinguished:

1. With a deficiency of sphingomyelinase (Types A and B)
2. With normal levels of sphingomyelinase, but possibly defects in intracellular esterification of cholesterol (Type C).

Sphingomyelinase-deficient type A variant is the most common form and is associated with

- Diffuse neuronal involvement, leading eventually to cell death and shrinkage of the brain; there is a retinal cherry-red spot similar to that in Tay-Sachs disease.
- Massive accumulation of lipids in cells of the mononuclear phagocytic system, giving rise to massive splenomegaly, enlargement of liver and lymph nodes, and infiltration of bone marrow.
- Visceral involvement affecting the GI tract and lungs.

Affected cells everywhere are enlarged and filled with numerous small vacuoles that impart foaminess to the cytoplasm.

Clinical manifestations appear soon after birth and consist of hepatosplenomegaly, failure to thrive, and deterioration of psychomotor functions. Survival is limited to 1 or 2 years.

Gaucher's Disease

This refers to a cluster of autosomal recessive disorders in which mutations affecting the glucocerebrosidase locus reduce the levels of this enzyme. Consequently, cleavage of ceramide derived from cell membranes of senescent leukocytes and red cells, as well as from turnover of gangliosides in the brains of neonates is impaired. Accumulation of glucocerebrosides occurs in the mononuclear phagocytic system and, in some forms, in the central nervous system. Two important variants of Gaucher disease can be distinguished:

1. *Type I,* the most common form, occurs in adults. This chronic, non-neuronopathic form is associated with storage of glucocerebrosides in the mononuclear phagocytic system; there is no brain involvement, but massive splenomegaly; involvement of bone marrow produces small or large areas of bone erosions

that can cause pathologic fractures; pancytopenia or thrombocytopenia results from hypersplenism; life span is not affected.

2. *Type II,* also known as the acute neuronopathic form, is associated with hepatosplenomegaly as well as CNS involvement; symptoms such as convulsions and mental deterioration dominate the clinical picture; death occurs at a young age.

These patterns, resulting from different allelic mutations in the structural gene for the enzyme, run within families. Prenatal diagnosis is possible by assay of enzymes in amniotic fluid cells and by DNA probe analysis.

Histologically, affected cells (Gaucher's cells) are distended with PAS-positive material that has a fibrillary appearance resembling crumpled tissue paper.

Mucopolysaccharidoses (MPS)

A group of disorders resulting from inherited deficiencies of enzymes involved in the degradation of MPS. The MPS that accumulate in the cells include heparan sulfate, dermatan sulfate, keratan sulfate, and chondroitin sulfate. Histologically, affected cells are distended with clear cytoplasm (balloon cells) that contains PAS-positive material. Accumulated MPS are found in many cell types, including mononuclear phagocytic cells (giving rise to hepatosplenomegaly); fibroblasts throughout the body; endothelial cells and intimal smooth muscle cells (giving rise to narrowing of coronary arteries); and neurons.

Several clinical variants of MPS classified as MPS I to VII have been described, each resulting from the deficiency of one specific enzyme. Some better known examples are the autosomal recessive Hurler's disease (MPS I) and the X-linked recessive Hunter's disease (MPS II). In general, all forms are progressive disorders characterized by one or more of the following:

- Coarse facial features.
- Hepatosplenomegaly.
- Corneal clouding.
- Lesions of cardiac valves.
- Narrowing of coronary arteries.
- Joint stiffness.
- Mental retardation.

Glycogen Storage Diseases (pp. 146–147)

A group of autosomal recessive disorders resulting from defects in the synthesis or catabolism of glycogen. On the basis of specific enzyme deficiencies and resultant clinical pictures, glycogen storage diseases have been divided into three major groups (Table 5–3):

HEPATIC FORMS. The prototype is von Gierke's disease (type I glycogenosis). This results from deficiency of the hepatic enzyme glucose-6-phosphatase, which is essential for conversion of G6P to glucose. The major effects of this enzyme deficiency are (1) accumulation of glycogen, because it cannot be broken down to free glucose; and (2) low blood glucose (hypoglycemia).

MYOPATHIC FORMS. These result from deficiencies of enzymes that fuel glycolysis in striated muscles. McArdle's disease (type V glycogenosis), the most important example, is caused by lack of muscle phosphorylase. Deficiency of this enzyme leads to (1) storage of glycogen in skeletal muscles, (2) muscle weakness, (3) muscle cramps after exercise, and (4) failure of exercise-induced rise in blood lactate.

Table 5-3. Principal Subgroups of Glycogenoses

Clinicopathologic Category	Specific Type	Enzyme Deficiency	Morphologic Changes	Clinical Features
Hepatic Type	Hepatorenal—von Gierke's disease (type I)	Glucose-6-phosphatase	Hepatomegaly—intracytoplasmic accumulations of glycogen and small amounts of lipid; intranuclear glycogen Renomegaly—intracytoplasmic accumulations of glycogen in cortical tubular epithelial cells	Failure to thrive, stunted growth, hepatomegaly, and renomegaly. Hypoglycemia due to failure of glucose mobilization, often leading to convulsions. Hyperlipidemia and hyperuricemia resulting from deranged glucose metabolism; many patients develop gout and skin xanthomas. Bleeding tendency due to platelet dysfunction. Mortality approximately 50%.
Myopathic Type	McArdle's syndrome (type V)	Muscle phosphorylase	Skeletal muscle only—accumulations of glycogen predominantly in subsarcolemmal location	Painful cramps associated with strenuous exercise. Myoglobinuria occurs in 50% of cases. Onset in adulthood (>20 years). Muscular exercise fails to raise lactate level in venous blood. Compatible with normal longevity.
Miscellaneous Types	Generalized glycogenosis—Pompe's disease (type II)	Lysosomal glucosidase (acid maltase)	Mild hepatomegaly—ballooning of lysosomes with glycogen creating lacy cytoplasmic pattern Cardiomegaly—glycogen within sarcoplasm as well as membrane-bound Skeletal muscle—similar to heart	Massive cardiomegaly, muscle hypotonia, and cardiorespiratory failure within two years. A milder adult form with only skeletal muscle involvement presenting with chronic myopathy.

From Cotran, R. S., Kumar, V., and Robbins, S. L.: Robbins Pathologic Basis of Disease. 5th ed. Philadelphia, W. B. Saunders Co., 1994, p. 147.

MISCELLANEOUS FORMS. There are several of these, the most important being type II glycogenosis, or Pompe's disease, which results from deficiency of the lysosomal enzyme acid maltase (α-glucosidase). As in other lysosomal storage diseases, many organs are involved, but storage of glycogen is most prominent in the heart. Affected neonates have massive cardiomegaly, and death results from cardiac failure by 2 years of age.

Alkaptonuria

In this disorder the lack of homogentisic oxidase blocks the metabolism of phenylalanine and leads to accumulation of homogentisic acid. Excessive homogentisic acid is associated with the following:

- Excretion in urine, imparting to it a black color if allowed to stand.
- Ochronosis—a blue-black pigmentation of the ears, nose, and cheeks resulting from binding of homogentisic acid to connective tissue and cartilage.
- Arthropathy associated with deposition in articular cartilage; the pigmented cartilage loses resilience and is readily eroded; the vertebral column, knee, shoulders, and hips are usually affected.

DISORDERS ASSOCIATED WITH DEFECTS IN PROTEINS THAT REGULATE CELL GROWTH (p. 148)

Neurofibromatosis: Types 1 and 2 (p. 148)

These are two genetically distinct autosomal dominant disorders, both characterized by the presence of tumors of the nerves.

Neurofibromatosis type 1 (also called von Recklinghausen's disease) is characterized by three main features:

1. *Multiple neural tumors* involving nerve trunks in skin as well as internal organs. Skin lesions are usually widespread and vary in size from 1 to 20 cm. The large lesions are multilobed and pendulous and contain multiple, tortuous, and thickened nerves (plexiform neurofibromas), sometimes causing massive enlargement of a limb or other body parts. Histologically, neurofibromas reveal proliferation of neurites, Schwann cells, and fibroblasts, all embedded in loose myxoid stroma.

2. *Cutaneous pigmentations,* present in over 90% of patients, take the form of light brown macules located over nerve trunks (*café au lait* spots).

3. *Lisch nodules* or pigmented iris hamartomas are present in almost all cases.

Several associated abnormalities are present: the important ones are listed below:

- There are skeletal lesions (bone cysts, scoliosis, and erosion of the bone surface) in 30 to 50% of patients.
- There is an increased risk of the development of other tumors, especially meningiomas, optic gliomas, and pheochromocytomas.
- There is a tendency toward reduced intelligence.

The NF-1 locus on chromosome 17 encodes neurofibromin, a protein that regulates the function of the p21 *ras* oncoprotein. NF-1 is a tumor suppressor gene.

The NF-2 locus on chromosome 22 also encodes a tumor

suppressor gene, of unknown function. These patients have the following features:

- Bilateral acoustic nerve tumors in all cases.
- Skin tumors in some but not all patients.
- Café au lait spots.
- Absence of Lisch nodules.

DISORDERS WITH MULTIFACTORIAL INHERITANCE (p. 149)

These result from the combined effects of two or more mutant genes and environmental factors and exhibit the following characteristics:

- The risk of expression is conditioned by the number of mutant genes inherited.
- Environmental influences significantly modify the risk of expression; hence, the concordance rate in identical twins is 20 to 40%.
- The risk of recurrence of the disorder in first-degree relatives is 2 to 7%.
- The risk of recurrence in subsequent pregnancies increases with the birth of each affected child.

Multifactorial inheritance underlies many congenital malformations and common disorders such as diabetes mellitus, gout, hypertension, and coronary heart disease.

CYTOGENETIC DISORDERS (p. 152)

These may be due to

- Alterations in the number of chromosomes.
- Alterations in the structure of chromosomes.

COMMON TYPES OF NUMERICAL DISORDERS

- Monosomy, associated with one less normal chromosome $(2n - 1)$
- Trisomy, associated with one extra chromosome $(2n + 1)$.
- Mosaicism, associated with one or more populations of cells, some with normal chromosomal complement, others with extra or missing chromosomes.

Numerical disorders of chromosomes result from errors during cell division. Monosomy and trisomy usually result from nondisjunction of chromosomes during gametogenesis (the first meiotic division), whereas mosaics are produced when mitotic errors occur in the zygote. Monosomy or trisomy of autosomes usually results in early fetal death and spontaneous abortion, whereas similar imbalances in sex chromosomes are much better tolerated.

STRUCTURAL ABERRATIONS OF CHROMOSOMES (Fig. 5–2)

- *Deletion.* Loss of a terminal or interstitial segment of a chromosome.
- *Translocation* involves transfer of a segment of one chromosome to another, as follows:

  - Balanced reciprocal, involving exchange of chromosomal material between two chromosomes with no net gain or loss of genetic material.

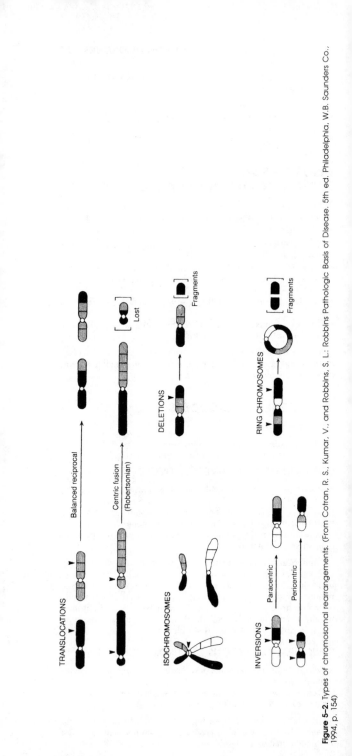

Figure 5–2. Types of chromosomal rearrangements. (From Cotran, R. S., Kumar, V., and Robbins, S. L.: Robbins Pathologic Basis of Disease. 5th ed. Philadelphia, W.B. Saunders Co., 1994, p. 154)

- Robertsonian (centric) fusion, being reciprocal translocation between two acrocentric chromosomes involving the short arm of one and the long arm of the other; transfer of segments leads to formation of one abnormally large chromosome and one extremely small. The latter is usually lost. This translocation predisposes to the formation of abnormal (unbalanced) gametes.
- *Isochromosome.* Formed when one arm (short or long) is lost and the remaining arm is duplicated, resulting in a chromosome of two short arms only or of two long arms. In live births, the most common isochromosome is i(Xq) with duplication of long arm and deletion of short arm.
- *Inversion.* Rearrangement associated with two breaks in a chromosome, followed by inversion and reincorporation of the broken segment.
- *Ring chromosome.* Deletion affecting both ends, followed by fusion of the damaged ends.

CYTOGENETIC DISORDERS INVOLVING AUTOSOMES (p. 154)

Trisomy 21 (Down's Syndrome) (p. 154)

The most common chromosomal disorder (one in 800 births).
KARYOTYPIC FEATURES

- About 95% have a complete extra chromosome 21 (47,XY, + 21). The incidence of this form is strongly influenced by maternal age (one in 1550 births in women under 20 years, increasing to one in 25 in women over 45 years). In 95% of these cases the extra chromosome is maternal in origin.
- Translocation variant making up 4% of all cases; has extra chromosomal material derived from inheritance of a parental chromosome bearing a translocation of the long arm of chromosome 21 to chromosome 22 or 14 (e.g., 46,XX, − 14, + t(14q21q). Because the fertilized ovum already possesses two normal autosomes 21, the translocated chromosomal fragment provides the same triple gene dosage as trisomy 21. Such cases are frequently (but not always) familial because the parent is a carrier of a robertsonian translocation. Such a rearrangement may also occur during gametogenesis.
- Mosaic variants make up about 1% of all cases; they have a mixture of cells with normal chromosome numbers and extra chromosome 21.

CLINICAL FEATURES

- Facial profile: flat with oblique palpebral fissures and epicanthic folds.
- Severe mental retardation.
- Congenital heart disease, especially septal defects, responsible for the majority of deaths in infancy and childhood.
- Ten- to twenty-fold increased risk of developing acute leukemia.
- Serious infections resulting from abnormal immune responses.
- Premature Alzheimer's disease in those who survive after 35 years of age.

Other Trisomies (p. 156)

Trisomy 18 (Edwards' syndrome) and trisomy 13 (Patau's syndrome) occur much less commonly than trisomy 21; affected infants have severe malformations and usually die within the first year of life.

Cri-du-Chat Syndrome (p. 156)

KARYOTYPE. Deletion of short arm of chromosome 5 (5p−).
CLINICAL FEATURES

- A mewing, catlike cry
- Severe mental retardation
- Congenital heart disease
- Survival of some into adult life

CYTOGENETIC DISORDERS INVOLVING SEX CHROMOSOMES (p. 158)

Imbalances of sex chromosomes are better tolerated than similar imbalances of autosomes, and hence sex chromosome disorders are more common than autosomal disorders. The milder nature of X-chromosome aberrations is in part related to the inactivation of X chromosome, explained by the Lyon hypothesis:

- All but one X chromosome is genetically inactive.
- Random inactivation of either paternal or maternal X chromosome occurs early in embryogenesis and leads to the formation of a Barr body. X-inactivation is regulated by the X-inactive-specific transcript gene (XIST), which maps to Xq13.
- Normal females are mosaics, having two cell populations, one with inactivated paternal X and the other with inactivated maternal X.

Because numerical aberrations of X chromosomes (extra or missing) are associated with somatic and gonadal abnormalities, Lyon's hypothesis has to be modified as follows:

- Both X chromosomes are required for normal gametogenesis; the inactivated X is selectively reactivated in germ cells during gamete formation.
- X inactivation spares certain regions of the chromosome necessary for normal growth and development.

Klinefelter's Syndrome (p. 159)

Definition. Male hypogonadism associated with two or more X chromosomes and at least one Y chromosome.
KARYOTYPE. 47,XXY is most common (80% of cases); others are mosaics (e.g., 46,XY/47,XXY).

CLINICAL FEATURES

- Leading cause of male infertility.
- Eunuchoid body habitus.
- Minimal or no mental retardation.
- Failure of male secondary sexual characteristics.
- Gynecomastia; female distribution of hair.
- Atrophic testis with hyperplasia of Leydig cells.
- Plasma FSH and estrogen levels elevated; testosterone levels low.

XYY Syndrome (p. 160)

- Usually tall; phenotypically normal.
- Some have behavioral difficulties (aggressive, antisocial, impulsive nature). This, however, is controversial.

Turner's Syndrome (p. 160)

Definition Hypogonadism in phenotypic females resulting from complete or partial monosomy of X chromosome.

KARYOTYPES

- 45,X most common (57% of cases).
- 46,X,i(Xq) (isochromosome of the long arm with deletion of the short arm).
- Mosaics, e.g., 45,X/46,XX.

CLINICAL FEATURES. Wide-ranging degrees of abnormalities, depending on karyotype; 45,X most severely affected. Typical features include

- Lymphedema of neck, hands, and feet
- Webbing of neck
- Short stature
- Broad chest and widely spaced nipples
- Primary amenorrhea
- Failure of development of breasts
- Infantile external genitalia
- Ovaries severely atrophic and fibrous
- Congenital heart disease, particularly aortic coarctation

Hermaphroditism and Pseudohermaphroditism (p. 161)

TRUE HERMAPHRODITES. Extremely rare. These have both ovaries and testes, either combined as an ovotestes or with one gonad on each side. Two thirds have 46,XX karyotype with translocation of the Y chromosome to the X chromosome, or an autosome. The remaining one third are mosaics.

PSEUDOHERMAPHRODITES. These have disparate gonadal and phenotypic sexual characteristics.

FEMALE PSEUDOHERMAPHRODITES. These have 46,XX karyotype. Ovaries and internal genitalia are normal but external genitalia are ambiguous or virilized. The most common cause is inappropriate exposure to androgenic steroids during gestation. The condition may occur in congenital adrenal hyperplasia or in the presence of androgen-secreting maternal tumors.

MALE PSEUDOHERMAPHRODITES. Y chromosome is present, and therefore the gonads are exclusively testes, but external genitalia are either ambiguous or completely female. The condition results from defective virilization of the male embryo due to reduced androgen synthesis or resistance to action of androgens. The most common form is *complete testicular feminization* associated with mutation in the structural gene for androgen receptor located on Xq11-Xq12.

SINGLE GENE DISORDERS WITH NONCLASSIC INHERITANCE (p. 162)

These are classified into three categories:

TRIPLET REPEAT MUTATIONS— FRAGILE X SYNDROME (p. 162)

Several disorders, such as Huntington's disease, myotonic dystrophy, and fragile X syndrome, are characterized by triplet repeat mutations. In these mutations, there is a long repeating sequence of three nucleotides, and all affected sequences share the nucleotides guanine (G) and cytosine (C).

Fragile X syndrome, the prototypic disorder in this category, is a common cause of familial mental retardation. It is characterized cytogenetically by a fragile site on Xq27.3, which is seen as a discontinuity of staining. At this site there are multiple tandem repeats of the nucleotide sequence CGG. In normal individuals, the average number of repeats is 29, whereas affected individuals have 250 to 4000 repeats. In between are those with "premutations" characterized by 50 to 200 CGG repeats. In carrier females, the premutations undergo amplification during oogenesis, resulting in full mutations that are then passed on to their progeny. Because the mutations are carried on the X-chromosome, this is an X-linked recessive disorder. However, because premutations are silent, and they are amplified only during oogenesis in carrier females, the transmission pattern differs from classic X-linked disorders. Thus, carrier males with premutations do not have any symptoms, and approximately 30% of carrier females are affected.

Clinically, the affected males have severe mental retardation, and 80% have an enlarged testis. Other physical features, such as an elongated face and large mandible, are inconsistent. The clinical features of fragile X worsen with each successive generation, due to amplification of nucleotide repeats during oogenesis. This phenomenon is called *anticipation.*

MUTATIONS IN MITOCHONDRIAL GENES— LEBER'S HEREDITARY OPTIC NEUROPATHY (p. 163)

Ova contain mitochondria but spermatozoa contain few, hence the mitochondrial content of zygotes is derived almost entirely from the ovum. Thus, mitochondrial DNA is transmitted entirely by females, and diseases resulting from mutations in mitochondrial genes are *maternally inherited.* Affected females transmit the disease to all their offspring—male and female; however, daughters and not sons pass the disease further to their progeny. When a cell carrying normal and mutant mitochondrial DNA divides, the proportion of normal and mutant DNA in the daughter cells is random and quite variable. Hence, expression of disorders resulting from mutations in mitochondrial genes is quite variable. Genes contained in the mitochondria encode enzymes involved in oxidative phosphorylation, and hence diseases in this category predominantly affect organs heavily dependent on mitochondrial energy metabolism. These include the neuromuscular system, liver, heart, and kidney. As an example, Leber's hereditary optic neuropathy causes blindness, neurologic dysfunction, and cardiac conduction defects.

GENOMIC IMPRINTING—PRADER-WILLI AND ANGELMAN'S SYNDROMES (p. 164)

Genomic imprinting is an epigenetic process that results in differential "function" of genes carried on paternal versus maternal chromosomes. Two syndromes resulting from genomic imprinting are described below. *Prader-Willi* syndrome, characterized by mental retardation, short stature, hypotonia, obesity, and hypogonadism, results from the deletion of genes located at 15q12 in the paternally derived chromosome 15. In some cases, an entire chromosome 15 derived from the father is absent, replaced instead by two maternally derived chromosomes 15 (uniparental disomy). In the latter case, the patients do not exhibit any structural or numerical cytogenetic abnormality. In contrast with the Prader-Willi syndrome, patients with the phenotypically distinct *Angelman's syndrome* are born with deletion of the same chromosomal region derived from their mothers, or uniparental disomy of paternal chromosome 15. These patients, in addition to mental retardation, have ataxia, seizures, and inappropriate laughter. The molecular mechanism of imprinting is not clear, but it is strongly suspected that differential methylation of DNA during gametogenesis results in imprinting of paternal and maternal chromosomes.

MOLECULAR DIAGNOSIS (p. 165)

This can be applied to *genetic* and *acquired* disorders (such as infectious diseases).

GENETIC DISEASES (p. 165)

Detection of an abnormal gene by DNA probe analysis has two distinct advantages over traditional methods that depend on detection of the abnormal gene products and their clinical effects:

- The amount of DNA required for diagnosis is extremely small. It can be readily obtained from 10^5 cells or less and amplified by the polymerase chain reaction.
- The test is not dependent on a gene product that may be expressed only in certain differentiated cells: e.g., because all cells of the body contain the globin gene, mutations of globin genes can be detected in cells obtained from the amniotic fluid.

Two different approaches are applied to the diagnosis of genetic diseases by recombinant DNA technology:

- *Direct gene diagnosis,* involving detection of the mutant gene.
- *Indirect gene diagnosis,* involving detection of linkage of the disease gene with a harmless "marker gene."

Direct Gene Diagnosis (p. 165)

This is based on the identification of a qualitative difference between DNA sequences in the normal and abnormal genes. Two methods are used:

1. One is based on the fact that some mutations alter or destroy certain restriction sites on normal DNA. For example, the normal β-globin gene has three restriction sites for the enzyme Mst II, one of which is lost in the sickle globin gene. This results in the production of different-sized bands when DNA from normal and affected individuals is digested with Mst II and compared by Southern blot analysis.

2. Oligonucleotide probe analysis is used when the point mutation producing the abnormal gene does not alter any known restriction site. Two oligonucleotides 18 to 20 bases long are synthesized, having at their centers the single base by which the normal and mutant genes differ. Each oligonucleotide hybridizes strongly to the corresponding (normal) gene, but weakly to the gene that does not share the exact sequence. Thus, in Southern

blot analysis, the normal and mutant genes can be distinguished on the basis of the "strength" of hybridization with the two oligonucleotide probes.

Indirect Gene Diagnosis: Gene Tracking (p. 166)

In many genetic diseases, the mutant gene and its normal counterpart have not yet been identified or sequenced, and thus direct gene diagnosis cannot be used. It is therefore necessary to employ "gene tracking," which determines whether a given family member or fetus inherited the same relevant chromosomal region(s) as a previously affected family member. This requires that chromosomes carrying the normal and mutant genes in heterozygotes be distinguishable. To accomplish this, advantage is taken of naturally occurring variations in DNA sequences in the vicinity of (and linked to) the mutant gene. Such an analysis, called restriction fragment length polymorphism (RFLP), relies on DNA polymorphisms that give rise to fragments of different lengths in Southern blot analysis. In cystic fibrosis, for example, heterozygous parents and children have two bands derived from the normal and the affected chromosome. In contrast, an affected (homozygous) individual reveals a single band derived from two identical chromosomes carrying the mutant gene. In addition to RFLPs, another type of polymorphism, resulting from a variable number of tandem repeats (VNTRs), can also be used for linkage analysis.

The RFLP technique has proved useful in antenatal detection of several genetic disorders such as cystic fibrosis, Huntington's disease, polycystic kidney disease, fragile X syndrome, and Duchenne's muscular dystrophy. However, it has certain limitations:

- For prenatal diagnosis, several affected and unaffected family members must be available for testing.
- Key family members (e.g., parents, siblings) must be heterozygous for an RFLP (i.e., the normal chromosome and that carrying the mutant gene must be distinguishable in a Southern blot analysis). In other words, informative DNA polymorphisms should be present in linkage with the gene in question.
- Recombination between homologous chromosomes during gametogenesis may lead to loss of linkage between the DNA polymorphism and the mutant gene.

OTHER DIAGNOSTIC APPLICATIONS

In addition to its value in the diagnosis of genetic disorders, DNA probe analysis is useful in the diagnosis of some forms of *cancer*, (2) positive identification of individuals for forensic pathology, and (3) diagnosis of infectious diseases.

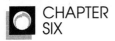

CHAPTER
SIX

Immunity

The immune system protects against exogenous (foreign) substances, microbial invasion, and possibly tumors, but occasionally the immune responses also damage normal host tissues and react to *homologous antigens* (e.g., blood transfusions, transplanted tissues, fetal antigens in pregnancy), and sometimes *endogenous antigens,* the basis of autoimmune disorders.

Pathology related to the immune system falls into three general categories:

1. Hypersensitivity (hyperactive) states (e.g., anaphylaxis).
2. Autoimmunity (e.g., systemic lupus erythematosus [SLE]).
3. Deficiency states, congenital or acquired (e.g., AIDS).

In addition, amyloidosis, in which immunoglobulin fragments are deposited in tissues, is also considered here.

MECHANISMS OF IMMUNE-MEDIATED INJURY (HYPERSENSITIVITY REACTIONS)
(p. 177)

Hypersensitivity reactions are subdivided on the basis of mechanisms of immune injury (Table 6–1).

TYPE I HYPERSENSITIVITY (ANAPHYLACTIC) (p. 178)

Mediated by IgE antibodies bound to mast cells and basophils formed in response to a particular antigen (allergen). Under normal circumstances, IgE probably functions to protect against parasitic infections. On reexposure of sensitized individuals, allergen binds to and cross-links the IgE on mast cells and results in

- Release (*degranulation*) of preformed vesicles containing *primary mediators.*
- De novo synthesis of *secondary mediators.*

Degranulation may also be triggered by a variety of other physical and chemical stimuli, e.g., complement fragments C3a and C5a (*anaphylatoxins*), certain drugs (codeine, morphine), mellitin (in bee venom), sunlight, trauma, heat, or cold.

In many cases of type I hypersensitivity, two phases may be exhibited: the initial (rapid) response, which becomes evident in 5 to 30 minutes after re-exposure, with resolution within 30 minutes; the second (delayed) phase, which sets in 2 to 8 hours later (without additional antigenic challenge), lasts for days, and is characterized by an intense infiltration by inflammatory cells and tissue damage.

Table 6–1. Mechanisms of Immunologically Mediated Disorders

Type	Prototype Disorder	Immune Mechanism
I. Anaphylactic type	Anaphylaxis, some forms of bronchial asthma	Formation of IgE (cytotropic) antibody → release of vasoactive amines and other mediators from basophils and mast cells
II. Cytotoxic type	Autoimmune hemolytic anemia, erythroblastosis fetalis, Goodpasture's syndrome	Formation of IgG, IgM → binds to antigen on target cell surface → phagocytosis of target cell or lysis of target cell by C8,9 fraction of activated complement or antibody-dependent cellular cytotoxicity (ADCC)
III. Immune complex disease	Arthus reaction, serum sickness, systemic lupus erythematosus, certain forms of acute glomerulonephritis	Antigen-antibody complexes → activated complement → attracted neutrophils → release of lysosomal enzymes and other toxic moieties
IV. Cell-mediated (delayed) hypersensitivity	Tuberculosis, contact dermatitis, transplant rejection	Sensitized thymus-derived T lymphocytes → release of lymphokines and T cell-mediated cytotoxicity

From Cotran, R. S., Kumar, V., and Robbins, S. L.: Robbins Pathologic Basis of Disease. 5th ed. Philadelphia, W. B. Saunders Co., 1994, p. 178.

Primary mast cell mediators typically induce the initial rapid response. These mediators include

- *Biogenic amines,* e.g., histamine. Bronchial smooth muscle contraction, increased vascular permeability, and increased mucous gland secretions.
- *Chemotactic mediators,* e.g., eosinophil chemotactic factors and neutrophil chemotactic factors.
- *Enzymes* contained in granule matrix (e.g., chymase, tryptase) lead to generation of kinins and activated complement by acting on their precursor proteins.
- *Proteoglycans,* e.g., heparin.

Secondary mediators include two classes: (1) lipid mediators and (2) cytokines.

The *lipid mediators* are

- *Leukotriene B_4.* Highly chemotactic for neutrophils, monocytes, and eosinophils.
- *Leukotriene C_4, D_4, E_4.* 1000-fold more potent than histamine in increasing vascular permeability and causing bronchial smooth muscle contraction. These also cause marked mucous gland secretion.
- *Prostaglandin D_2* causes intense bronchospasm, vasodilation, and mucous secretion.
- *Platelet activating factor (PAF)* causes platelet aggregation, histamine release, bronchoconstriction, vasodilation, and increased vascular permeability. It also has proinflammatory effects, such as chemoattraction and degranulation of neutrophils.

The *cytokines,* which recruit and activate inflammatory cells, are thought to be produced by mast cells (TNF-α, IL-4, IL-5, IL-6). IL-4 is important for recruitment of eosinophils. TNF-α is a powerful proinflammatory cytokine that recruits and activates many inflammatory cells. Additional cytokines are released by the recruited inflammatory cells. Cytokines and PAF are of particular importance in the late-phase response.

SYSTEMIC ANAPHYLAXIS. Typically follows parenteral or oral administration of allergen. The severity reflects the level of sensitization, and even minuscule doses may induce shock in the appropriate host. Pruritus, urticaria, and erythema occur minutes after exposure, followed by bronchoconstriction and laryngeal edema, escalating into laryngeal obstruction, shock, and death within minutes to hours.

Autopsy findings include pulmonary edema and hemorrhage (reflecting increased vascular permeability), lung hyperdistention, and right ventricular dilatation (reflecting pulmonary vasoconstriction).

LOCAL ANAPHYLAXIS (ATOPIC ALLERGIES). Atopy is a hereditary predisposition to develop local type I responses to inhaled or ingested allergens. It affects 10% of the population and includes urticaria, angioedema, rhinitis, and asthma (all described elsewhere).

TYPE II HYPERSENSITIVITY (CYTOTOXIC)
(p. 182)

Mediated by antibodies against intrinsic antigens or extrinsic antigens adsorbed on the cell surface or on other tissue components. Subsequent injury may occur secondary to

1. *Complement-dependent reactions;* either direct lysis via the C5–9 complement membrane attack complex (MAC) or by *opsonization* (enhanced phagocytosis) due to fixation of C3b fragments. Examples are

- Transfusion reactions. Recipient antibodies against incompatible donor erythrocyte antigens.
- Erythroblastosis fetalis. Maternal IgG antibodies (capable of crossing the placenta) against fetal erythrocyte antigens.
- Autoimmune thrombocytopenia, agranulocytosis, or hemolytic anemia. Autoantibodies against one's own blood cells.
- Certain drug reactions. Antibodies against drugs that have complexed to erythrocyte or other protein antigens.
- Goodpasture's disease. Antibodies against the common basement membrane component of kidneys and lungs.

2. *Antibody-dependent cell-mediated cytotoxicity (ADCC);* targets with low concentrations of bound antibody (IgG or IgE) are lysed (without phagocytosis) by nonsensitized cells with Fc receptors, e.g., monocytes, neutrophils, eosinophils, and natural killer (NK) cells. May be important for parasitic infections or tumors, and may play a major role in graft rejection.

3. *Antibody-mediated cellular dysfunction;* e.g., antiacetylcholine receptor antibodies impair neuromuscular transmission in myasthenia gravis; antithyroid-stimulating-hormone receptor antibodies cause hyperthyroidism in Graves' disease.

TYPE III HYPERSENSITIVITY (IMMUNE COMPLEX-MEDIATED) (p. 184)

Mediated by antigen-antibody complexes—immune complexes (IC)—forming either in the circulation or at extravascular sites of antigen deposition; antigens may be exogenous (e.g., infectious agents) or endogenous. Subsequent injury derives from activation of various serum mediators, particularly complement.

SYSTEMIC IMMUNE COMPLEX DISEASE. Complexes form in the circulation and are systemically deposited.

- *Acute serum sickness* is the prototype caused by administration of large amounts of foreign serum (e.g., horse antithymocyte globulin). About 5 days after serum inoculation, newly synthesized antihorse serum antibodies complex with foreign antigen to form circulating IC. Small IC (formed early in antigen excess) circulate for long periods and bind with low avidity to mononuclear phagocytes. Complexes deposit within a variety of capillary or arteriolar walls (causing vasculitis, see below). This is promoted by increased vascular permeability secondary to an initial *IgE* production, followed by local mast cell-basophil degranulation.

  Affected tissues include renal glomeruli (causing glomerulonephritis), joints (arthritis), skin, heart, and serosal surfaces.

  With continued antibody production, large IC eventually form (i.e., in antibody excess). These are cleared by phagocytes, ending the disease process.

  Deposition of IC activates the complement cascade with

- C3b release, enhancing opsonization.
- C5a (chemotactic factor) release, with secondary neutrophil- and monocyte-mediated injury.

- C3a and C5a release, increasing vascular permeability and causing smooth muscle contraction.
- Cytolysis mediated by the membrane attack complex.
- A decrease in serum complement levels secondary to consumption.

  IC also *aggregate platelets* (with subsequent degranulation) and *activate factor XII* (Hageman factor). The coagulation cascade and kinin systems are thus involved as well.

MORPHOLOGY. Fibrinoid deposits within vessel walls with neutrophil infiltration and surrounding hemorrhage and edema— *acute necrotizing vasculitis (fibrinoid necrosis).* Superimposed thrombosis and downstream tissue necrosis may also be present. The IC and complement may be visualized by immunofluorescence as granular lumpy deposits, or by electron microscopy as electron-dense deposits in the basement membranes.

  With time and clearance (catabolism) of the inciting antigen and IC, the lesions resolve.

- *Chronic serum sickness,* due to recurrent or prolonged antigenemia (e.g., SLE), shows intimal thickening and vascular (and/ or parenchymal) scarring.

LOCAL IMMUNE COMPLEX DISEASE (ARTHUS REACTION).
Localized tissue vasculitis and necrosis due to

- Focal formation or deposition of IC.
- "Planting" of antigen within a particular tissue (e.g., the renal glomerulus) with subsequent in situ formation of IC.

  This may be produced experimentally by *intracutaneous* antigen injection in previously sensitized hosts carrying the appropriate circulating antibody. Antigen seeps into vascular walls where *large* IC precipitate in situ (antibody excess). Complement and coagulation cascade activation and platelet aggregation lead to fibrinoid necrosis. Superimposed thrombosis may cause tissue necrosis.

TYPE IV HYPERSENSITIVITY (CELL-MEDIATED) (p. 187)

Initiated by specifically sensitized T lymphocytes and includes **DELAYED-TYPE HYPERSENSITIVITY (DTH).** Principal pattern of response to *Mycobacterium tuberculosis,* fungi, protozoa, and parasites, as well as contact skin sensitivity. DTH also contributes to graft rejection.

  Mediated by CD4-positive (CD4+) T-helper-1 (T_H1) cells that secrete specific cytokines after encounter with processed antigen in association with class II major histocompatibility complex (MHC). The cytokines such as IFN-γ, IL-2, TNF-α, mediate injury primarily by recruiting and activating antigen-nonspecific monocytes and macrophages; substantial "bystander" injury typically ensues. The mechanisms of macrophage-mediated injury are discussed in *Chapter 3.*

  With persistent or nondegradable antigens, the initial nonspecific infiltrate of T cells and macrophages is replaced by a collection of macrophages that transform into epithelioid cells, thus forming a focal granuloma.

T CELL-MEDIATED CYTOTOXICITY. Generation of CD8+ cytotoxic T lymphocytes (CTL) is the principal pattern of response to many viral infections and to tumor cells. CTL also contribute to graft rejection.

CTL recognize processed antigen in association with class I MHC. CTL-induced injury is thus highly specific with minimal "bystander" injury.

TISSUE TRANSPLANTATION

To understand transplant rejection, a brief review of histocompatibility antigens is desirable.

HISTOCOMPATIBILITY ANTIGENS (p. 175)

The most important are grouped in the MHC (also known as human leukocyte antigen or HLA cluster) on chromosome 6; they are highly polymorphic, i.e., with several alternative genes (alleles) for each locus. Moreover, heterozygotes may express up to 16 *unique* MHC antigens, a formidable barrier to transplantation.

CLASS I ANTIGENS. Present on virtually all nucleated cells and platelets, these are polymorphic heavy-chain glycoproteins (coded on three closely linked loci: HLA-A, -B, and -C) and a nonpolymorphic β-2-microglobulin (coded by a gene on chromosome 15); they elicit antibodies in nonidentical individuals and are typed by conventional serologic techniques.

- These antigens typically bind only those processed antigens that are initially synthesized *endogenously,* e.g., viral products in a virally infected cell. The peptides derived from the processing of antigens bind to the "peptide-binding groove," which faces outward from the cell membrane and is composed of the α_1 and α_2 domains of the class I heavy chain.
- MHC-I antigens "present" processed antigens to CD8+ *cytotoxic T cells* (with the appropriate receptor specificity), resulting in T-cell activation.
- Because T-cell receptors recognize only *antigen-MHC complexes,* CD8+ T cells bind and kill only infected cells that bear self class I antigens; this is called *MHC restriction.*

CLASS II ANTIGENS. Characteristically confined to "antigen-presenting cells" (APC), including dendritic cells, macrophages, B cells, and activated T cells.

- MHC-II antigens are coded in the HLA-D region with three serologically defined subloci (DP, DQ, and DR). Each class II molecule is a heterodimer of noncovalently associated α and β chains.
- Class II MHC antigens typically bind and present *exogenous* (then internalized and processed) antigens to CD4+ T cells. *CD4+ helper T lymphocytes* also exhibit MHC restriction, recognizing processed antigen only in the context of self–class II MHC.

CLASS III PROTEINS. Some components of the complement system (C2, C4, Bf), and some cytokines (TNF-α and TNF-β) are encoded within the MHC cluster. Although linked to class I and II antigens, these are not histocompatibility antigens.

TRANSPLANT REJECTION (p. 190)

Renal transplant rejection will be described in some detail, followed by a brief comment on bone marrow transplantation.

However, with minor variations, the same concepts are true for other tissues and organs, e.g., liver and heart.

CD8+ and CD4+ T cells react to processed MHC antigens in grafts. Consequences include direct CTL-mediated cytolysis, as well as microvascular injury, tissue ischemia, and macrophage-mediated destruction.

Antibody-mediated responses may also be important in some circumstances. They involve initial endothelial cell injury and subsequent vasculitis. This pattern of rejection, in general, responds poorly to immunosuppressive drugs.

HYPERACUTE REJECTION (p. 192)

When the recipient has been previously sensitized to antigens in graft (e.g., by blood transfusion, previous pregnancy, infections with HLA cross-reactive microorganisms), there is an immediate "hyperacute rejection" (minutes to 1 to 2 days) in which preformed circulating antibody fixes to antigens in the graft vascular bed and induces complement- and ADCC-mediated injury.

The gross image is reflected in a cyanotic, mottled, flaccid organ. Microscopically, the lesions resemble an Arthus reaction (described earlier). Ig and complement are deposited in the vessel walls with endothelial injury, fibrin-platelet microthombi, neutrophil infiltrates, and arteriolar fibrinoid necrosis followed by distal parenchymal infarction.

Some time after transplantation, donor class I or II MHC antigens may induce *recipient antibody formation,* with subsequent complement-, ADCC-, or IC-mediated injury (*acute vasculitis*).

ACUTE REJECTION (p. 192)

Typically occurs within a few days of transplantation or after cessation of immunosuppressive therapy. Both cellular and humoral mechanisms contribute to variable degrees.

Acute cellular rejection is characterized by an interstitial mononuclear cell infiltrate (macrophages, plasma cells, and both CD4+ and CD8+ T cells). Cellular rejection typically responds promptly to immunosuppressive drugs.

Subacute vasculitis typically occurs in the first few months after transplantation, is more common than acute rejection vasculitis, and produces repeated bouts of clinical rejection (e.g., altered renal function in a kidney transplant).

Microscopic correlate is markedly thickened arteriolar intima containing Ig and complement deposits, fibroblasts, smooth muscle cells, and foamy macrophages; seen as concentric luminal narrowing or obliteration of lumen with distal parenchymal ischemic effects.

CHRONIC REJECTION (p. 193)

Occurs over months to years and is characterized by progressive organ dysfunction (i.e., rising serum creatinine).

Morphologically, the arteries show dense intimal fibrosis, probably the end stage of recurrent episodes of acute and subacute rejection with parenchymal ischemic injury. Frequently, there is a mononuclear interstitial infiltrate with numerous plasma cells and eosinophils, as well as an occasional superimposed acute arteritis.

BONE MARROW TRANSPLANTATION (p. 194)

Presents special problems. Used for hematologic malignancies (e.g., leukemia), aplastic anemia, or immunodeficiency states. The recipient receives lethal levels of irradiation (and/or chemotherapy) to eradicate malignant cells, create a satisfactory graft bed, and/or minimize host rejection of the grafted marrow. However, recipient NK cells or radiation-resistant T cells may mediate significant transplant rejection.

The unique problem with marrow transplantation is *graft-versus-host disease (GVHD)*, in which donor immunocompetent cells or precursors are introduced into MHC-nonidentical, immunocompromised recipients. The host cells are recognized by the transplanted cells as being foreign. CD8+ and CD4+ T cell-mediated injury ensues. Liver, skin, and GI mucosa are most typically affected.

GVHD and complications (e.g., infections) are often lethal. Aside from close MHC matching, selective T-cell depletion from donor marrow is attempted to reduce the severity of GVHD.

AUTOIMMUNE DISEASES (p. 195)

These disorders result from some breakdown in *self-tolerance*, which is the lack of responsiveness to one's own antigens. Tolerance is achieved by some combination of the following:

- *Clonal deletion.* Immature T-cell clones with T-cell receptors (TCR) that have high affinity for self-antigens are deleted in the thymus during development. A similar negative selection also occurs during B-cell development. However, clonal deletion is not perfect, and normal B cells can be found with surface Ig against self-antigens (e.g., DNA, myelin, collagen, and thyroglobulin).
- *Clonal anergy.* This refers to irreversible functional inactivation of developing T and B cells. One mechanism of clonal anergy is recognition of antigen in the absence of costimulatory signals from the antigen-presenting cell.
- *Suppression of autoreactive lymphocytes.* Components that actively suppress immune responses to self include *suppressor T cells* and their products, such as TGF-β_1 and IL-10.

Tolerance may be maintained if either helper T cells or B cells (or both) are rendered inactive. Because helper T cells control both cellular and humoral immunity, tolerance of T-helper cells is considered critical for prevention of autoimmune diseases.

Autoimmune reactions may result from

1. *Bypass of helper T-cell tolerance* with activation of nontolerant B cells:

- Autoantigenic determinants (haptens) complexed to an immunogenic carrier moiety (e.g., self-antigens modified by drugs or microorganisms).
- Organisms eliciting antibodies that cross-react with host antigen (molecular mimicry).
- Direct (T-cell independent) polyclonal B-cell activation (e.g., bacterial lipopolysaccharide or Epstein-Barr virus infection).

2. *Imbalance of suppressor-helper T-cell function:* Loss of suppressor T cells has been implicated in the development of auto-

immunity in several animal models and is suspected in human autoimmune diseases.

3. *Emergence of previously sequestered antigens* (e.g., sperm, myelin basic protein, and lens crystallin), which therefore did not induce tolerance during development.

HLA linkage (especially to the DR antigens) and familial clustering in some autoimmune diseases suggest a genetic component. Exogenous infection with bacteria, mycoplasmas, or especially viruses may also trigger autoimmunity, suggesting an exogenous component as well.

Autoimmunity may be tissue specific (e.g., autoimmune thyroiditis) or systemic (e.g., SLE). The following are systemic diseases (the single tissue diseases are discussed in their own chapters).

SYSTEMIC LUPUS ERYTHEMATOSUS (SLE)
(p. 199)

The prototypical systemic autoimmune disorder, characterized by numerous autoantibodies, especially *antinuclear antibodies (ANAs)*.

Incidence approaches one in 2500 in some general populations; female:male, 9:1.

ANAs are commonly detected by indirect immunofluorescence. The patterns of immunofluorescence (e.g., homogeneous, peripheral, speckled, nucleolar), although nonspecific, suggest the type of circulating antibody.

However, ANAs occur in other autoimmune disorders and in up to 10% of normal individuals (Table 6–2), but *anti–double-stranded (native) DNA and anti-Smith antigen antibodies strongly suggest SLE*.

ANA cannot penetrate intact cells. However, nuclei of damaged cells react with ANA, lose their chromatin patterns, and become homogeneous *LE bodies* (hematoxylin bodies). Phagocytosis of LE bodies by neutrophils or macrophages in vitro forms *LE cells* in up to 70% of patients with SLE.

In addition to ANAs, lupus patients have many other autoantibodies, some directed against blood elements (red cells, platelets, leukocytes). In addition, up to 20% to 40% of patients have antiphospholipid antibodies. Some bind to cardiolipin antigen, giving rise to false-positive VDRL tests. Others interfere with (prolong) *in vitro* tests for clotting. These so-called lupus anticoagulants actually exert a procoagulant effect *in vivo,* causing recurrent vascular thromboses, miscarriages, and cerebral ischemia. Their mechanism of action *in vivo* is unknown.

ETIOLOGY AND PATHOGENESIS. Monozygotic twin concordance (50 to 60%) and familial and HLA clustering suggest a *genetic predisposition.* In addition, *exogenous factors* such as drug exposure (see later), ultraviolet (UV) irradiation, virus infections, and estrogens are also involved.

Although the etiology is unknown, the pathogenesis is thought to involve some basic defect in the maintenance of self-tolerance with activation of B cells. This may occur secondary to some combination of

• Heritable defects in the regulation of B-cell proliferation.
• Helper T-cell hyperactivity.
• Defects in suppressor T-cell function.

MORPHOLOGY. *Typical in all tissues is an acute necrotizing*

Table 6–2. ANTINUCLEAR ANTIBODIES IN VARIOUS AUTOIMMUNE DISEASES

		Disease, % Positive					
Nature of Antigen	Antibody System	SLE	Drug-Induced LE	Systemic Sclerosis—Diffuse	Limited Scleroderma—CREST	Sjögren's Syndrome	Inflammatory Myopathies
Many nuclear antigens (DNA, RNA, proteins)	Generic ANA (indirect IF)	>95	>95	70–90	70–90	50–80	40–60
Native DNA	Anti–double-stranded DNA	40–60	<5	<5	<5	<5	<5
Histones	Anti-histone	70	>95	<5	<5	<5	<5
Ribonucleoprotein (Smith antigen)	Anti-Sm	20–30	<5	<5	<5	<5	<5
Ribonucleoprotein (U1RNP)	Nuclear RNP	30–40	<5	15	10	<5	<5
Ribonucleoprotein	SS-A(Ro)	30–50	<5	<5	<5	70–95	10
Ribonucleoprotein	SS-B(La)	10–15	<5	<5	<5	60–90	<5
DNA topoisomerase I	Scl-70	<5	<5	40–70	10	<5	<5
Centromeric proteins	Anticentromere	<5	<5	22–36	90	<5	<5
Histidyl-tRNA synthetase	Jo-1	<5	<5	<5	<5	<5	25

Boxed entries indicate high correlation. ANA = antinuclear antibodies; RNP = ribonucleoprotein.

Data from Tan, E. M., et al.: Antinuclear antibodies (ANAs): Diagnostically specific immune markers and clues towards understanding systemic autoimmunity. Clin. Immunol. Immunopathol. 47:121, 1988; McCarty, G. A.: Autoantibodies and their relation to rheumatic diseases. Med. Clin. North Am. 70:237, 1986; and Bernstein, R. M., and Mathews, M. B.: Autoantibodies to intracellular antigens, with particular reference to t-RNA and related proteins in myositis. J. Rheumatol. 14(Suppl. 13):83, 1987.

vasculitis with fibrinoid deposits, involving small arteries and arterioles. Ig, DNA, and C3 may be found within vessel walls. Skin and muscle are most commonly involved. A perivascular lymphocytic infiltrate is frequently present.

In chronic cases, vessels show a fibrous thickening and luminal narrowing.

KIDNEY. Involved in virtually all cases of SLE. There are five patterns of *lupus nephritis:*

- Class I. Normal by light, EM, and fluorescence microscopy; rare.
- Class II. Mesangial lupus glomerulonephritis (GN), present in about 25% of patients; associated with minimal hematuria or proteinuria. Slight increase in mesangial matrix and cells with granular mesangial Ig and complement deposits.
- Class III. Focal proliferative GN; 20% of patients. Associated with recurrent hematuria, moderate proteinuria, and occasional mild renal insufficiency. Focal and segmental glomerular swelling with endothelial and mesangial proliferation, neutrophil infiltration, and sometimes fibrinoid deposits and capillary thrombi.
- Class IV. Diffuse proliferative GN; 35% to 40% of patients, many of whom are overtly symptomatic, with microscopic to gross hematuria, proteinuria (sometimes nephrotic range), hypertension, and diminished glomerular filtration rate. Most glomeruli show endothelial, mesangial, and occasionally epithelial proliferation. IC deposits are typically *subendothelial,* and when extensive form "wire loops." Frequently, there are also tubular changes with granular IC deposits in basement membranes and interstitial changes. Most severe form of lupus nephritis, carrying the worst prognosis.
- Class V. Membranous GN; 15% of patients; induces severe proteinuria or nephrotic syndrome. Diffusely thickened capillary walls similar to idiopathic membranous GN, and characterized by *subepithelial* IC deposits.

SKIN. Classically, malar erythema, including bridge of nose ("butterfly rash").

Also, variable cutaneous lesions from erythema to bullae elsewhere. Sunlight exacerbates the lesions. Microscopically, there is basal layer degeneration with dermal-epidermal junction Ig and complement deposits. The dermis shows variable fibrosis, perivascular mononuclear cell infiltrates, and vascular fibrinoid change.

JOINTS. *Typically a nonspecific, nonerosive synovitis.* Minimal joint deformity in contrast to rheumatoid arthritis.

CENTRAL NERVOUS SYSTEM (CNS). Neuropsychiatric manifestations probably secondary to endothelial injury and occlusion (antiphospholipid antibodies) or impaired neuronal function.

SEROSITIS. Initially fibrinous with focal vasculitis, fibrinoid necrosis, and edema, progressing to adhesions, possibly obliterating serosal cavities (i.e., the pericardial sac).

HEART. Characteristic *nonbacterial verrucous (Libman-Sacks) endocarditis,* much less frequent with the use of steroids. Typically, numerous small, warty vegetations (0.5 to 4 mm) occur on the inflow and/or outflow surfaces of the mitral and tricuspid valves. Microscopically, they are composed of necrotic debris, degenerating fibroblasts, inflammatory cells, and fibrinoid material.

An increasing number of younger patients, especially those treated with corticosteroids, have clinical evidence of coronary

artery disease. The pathogenesis of the coronary atherosclerosis is not clear.

SPLEEN. Moderate splenomegaly with capsular thickening and follicular hyperplasia. Marked perivascular fibrosis around penicilliary arteries is characteristic, producing an *onion-skin* appearance. Ig, C3, and DNA are found within these vessels.

LUNGS. Pleuritis with pleural effusions, interstitial pneumonitis, and diffuse fibrosing alveolitis, all probably related to IC deposition.

CLINICAL COURSE. SLE presents insidiously as a systemic, chronic, recurrent, febrile illness with symptoms referable to virtually any tissue, but especially joints, skin, kidneys, and serosal membranes.

Autoantibodies to hematologic components may induce thrombocytopenia, leukopenia, and anemia. The clinical manifestations are protean (Table 6–3).

The course of the disease is highly variable; rarely, it is fulminant with death in weeks to months.

- Sometimes, the disease may cause minimal symptoms (hematuria, rash) and remit even without treatment.
- More often, the disease is characterized by recurrent flares and remissions over many years, and is held in check by immunosuppressive regimens.
- Ten-year survival is approximately 70%; death is most commonly caused by renal failure or intercurrent infections.

DISCOID LE (DLE). A disease limited to cutaneous lesions that grossly and microscopically mimic SLE. Only 35% of patients have a positive ANA.

- In contrast to SLE, *only lesional skin has deposits of Ig-complement in the basement membrane.*

Table 6–3. Manifestations of Systemic Lupus Erythematosus

Clinical Manifestation	Prevalence in Patients (%)
Hematologic	100
Arthritis	90
Skin	85
Fever	83
Fatigue	81
Weight loss	63
Renal	50
Pleurisy	46
Myalgia	33
Pericarditis	25
Gastrointestinal	21
Raynaud's phenomenon	20
Central nervous system	20
Ocular	15
Peripheral neuropathy	14
Pneumonitis	11
Parotid gland enlargement	8
Liver disease	2

From Condemi, J. J.: The autoimmune diseases. J.A.M.A. 258:2920–2929, 1987. Copyright 1987, American Medical Association.

- After many years, 5 to 10% of affected individuals develop systemic manifestations.

DRUG-INDUCED LE. Drugs such as hydralazine, procainamide, isoniazid, and D-penicillamine frequently induce a positive ANA, less often an LE-like syndrome. With the latter, although there is multiorgan involvement, renal and CNS disease is uncommon. Antidouble-stranded DNA antibodies are rare, but antihistone antibodies are common. There is linkage with HLA-DR4.

Drug-related LE usually remits after cessation of the offending agent.

SJÖGREN'S SYNDROME (p. 208)

Characterized by dry eyes (*keratoconjunctivitis sicca*) and dry mouth (*xerostomia*), resulting from immune-mediated lacrimal and salivary gland destruction. Forty per cent occur in isolation (the primary form or *sicca syndrome*), and the remaining 60% in association with other autoimmune diseases such as rheumatoid arthritis (most common), SLE, or scleroderma.

- Ninety per cent of patients are women between 40 and 60 years of age.
- Most patients have rheumatoid factor in the absence of rheumatoid arthritis, and ANAs especially against ribonucleoproteins SS-A and -B (see Table 6–2).
- Injury is probably a consequence of both cellular and humoral mechanisms.

Morphologically, the lacrimal and salivary glands (other exocrine glands may also be involved) initially show a periductal lymphocytic infiltrate (predominantly CD4+ T cells with some B cells) with ductal epithelial hyperplasia and luminal obstruction. This is followed by acinar atrophy, fibrosis, and eventual fatty replacement.

Secondary changes include

- Corneal inflammation, erosion, and ulceration.
- Atrophy of oral mucosa with inflammatory fissuring and ulceration.
- Difficulty in swallowing solid foods.
- Nasal drying and crusting with ulceration. Rarely, septal perforation.
- Laryngitis, bronchitis, or pneumonitis due to respiratory involvement.

To distinguish lacrimal and salivary gland enlargement (called *Mikulicz's syndrome*) caused by Sjögren's syndrome from other causes (sarcoidosis, leukemia, lymphoma), lip biopsy (to examine minor salivary glands) is helpful.

Some cases of Sjögren's syndrome have extraglandular involvement:

- Commonly a tubulointerstitial nephritis with tubular atrophy causing renal tubular acidosis with excess urate and phosphate excretion.
- Possibly adenopathy with pleomorphic lymph node infiltrates.

There is a 40-fold increased risk of developing lymphoma in involved glands.

SYSTEMIC SCLEROSIS (SCLERODERMA) (p. 210)

Excessive systemic fibrosis, most commonly in the skin (where it may be confined for years), but also eventually in the GI tract, kidneys, heart, muscles, and lung in most patients.

The female:male ratio is 3:1, with mean onset at age 40; it tends to be more severe in blacks.

The disease initially presents with symmetric edema and thickening skin of hands and fingers, or with Raynaud's phenomenon. This is followed by

- Articular symptoms that may mimic rheumatoid arthritis.
- Dysphagia from esophageal fibrosis (up to 50% of patients).
- Malabsorption or intestinal pain or obstruction.
- Pulmonary fibrosis, which may cause respiratory and/or right heart dysfunction.
- Direct cardiac involvement, which may induce arrhythmias or heart failure.
- Development of malignant hypertension, which may result in fatal renal failure.

Systemic sclerosis is subclassified into

- *Diffuse scleroderma.* Widespread cutaneous and early visceral involvement with rapid progression. Associated more or less with specific ANA (see Table 6–2).
- *Localized scleroderma (CREST syndrome).* Acronym for calcinosis, *R*aynaud's phenomenon, *e*sophageal dysmotility, *s*clerodactyly, and *t*elangiectasia. Minimal cutaneous involvement (typically fingers and face) with late visceral involvement and a relatively benign course. Associated with anticentromere antibodies.

PATHOGENESIS. Although the genesis is unknown (and may be multifactorial), the final common pathway involves fibroblast activation with exaggerated synthesis of normal collagen.

Possibilities include

- A delayed hypersensitivity reaction to collagen or other connective tissue components with production of cytokines (TNF-α, IL-1, PDGF, or TGF-β), which promote collagen synthesis.
- Recurrent endothelial injury (due to IC or antibodies) causing platelet aggregation and subsequent release of activating factors that alter vascular permeability and stimulate fibroblasts.

In addition, a host of autoantibodies, reflecting deranged humoral immunity, is also present. Of importance are (1) antibodies to DNA topoisomerase I (anti-Scl 70), which is highly specific for diffuse scleroderma, and (2) anticentromere antibody, characteristic of the CREST syndrome. Whether these antibodies cause tissue injury is not established.

MORPHOLOGY. Skin. Grossly, there is diffuse sclerosis with atrophy. Initially, affected areas are edematous with a doughy consistency. Eventually, fibrotic fingers become tapered and clawlike with diminished mobility, and the face becomes a drawn mask.

- Focal obliteration of the vascular supply causes ulceration. Occasionally, fingertips undergo autoamputation.
- Microscopically, there are perivascular lymphocytic infiltrates with early capillary and arteriolar injury and partial occlusion; edema and collagen fiber degeneration are followed by progressive dermal fibrosis and vascular hyaline thickening.

GI Tract. Progressive atrophy and collagenization of muscularis, mostly in the esophagus; the lower two thirds may develop rubber-hose inflexibility.

- Throughout the alimentary tract, mucosa may be thinned and ulcerated with mural collagenization.
- Vascular changes are as described for skin.

Musculoskeletal System. Typically an inflammatory synovitis progressing to fibrosis; joint destruction is uncommon.

- Muscle involvement begins proximally with edema and mononuclear-perivascular infiltrates, progressing to interstitial fibrosis with myofiber degeneration.
- Vessels show basement membrane thickening.

Kidneys. Affected in two thirds of patients with systemic sclerosis.

- *Renal failure accounts for 50% of deaths in systemic sclerosis.*
- The most prominent changes are in vessel walls (especially interlobular arteries) with intimal proliferation and deposition of mucinous or collagenous material.
- Hypertension in 30% of cases, 10% of which have a malignant course. Hypertension further accentuates the vascular changes, often resulting in fibrinoid necrosis with thrombosis and necrosis.

Lungs. Variable fibrosis of small pulmonary vessels with diffuse interstitial and alveolar fibrosis, progressing in some cases to honeycombing.

Heart. Perivascular infiltrates with interstitial fibrosis, occasionally evolving into a restrictive cardiomyopathy. There may also be conduction system involvement with resultant arrhythmias.

Nervous System. The CNS may have arterial lesions similar to those in the kidney with distal ischemic changes. Peripheral neuropathy may occur owing to perineural vascular sclerosis.

INFLAMMATORY MYOPATHIES (p. 213)

This is an uncommon group of immunologically mediated inflammatory disorders that injure skeletal muscles. Included are *dermatomyositis, polymyositis,* and *inclusion body myositis.*

Dermatomyositis is characterized by involvement of skin and skeletal muscles, and affects children as well as adults.

- Classic skin rash is seen as lilac or heliotrope discoloration of upper eyelids with periorbital edema. Scaling red eruptions (Grotton's lesions) are often present on knuckles, elbows, and knees.
- Muscle weakness is gradual and bilaterally symmetric and typically affects proximal muscles first.
- Adult women have a slightly higher risk of developing visceral cancers—lung, ovary, stomach.
- Caused most likely by antibody-mediated injury to the microvasculature in the perimyseal connective tissue. The resultant perifascicular atrophy of myofibers is characteristic.

Polymyositis. Muscle involvement resembles dermatomyositis, but skin involvement and association with cancers are lacking. Caused by damage to muscle fibers by CD8+ cytotoxic T cells, which can be seen to invade and surround muscle fibers. Both necrotic and regenerating fibers are present.

Inclusion body myositis. Unlike the two other forms, the muscle involvement is asymmetric and involves distal muscles (extensors of foot and flexors of fingers) first. Damage mediated by CD8+ T cells. Histologically characterized by the presence of vacuoles in affected myocytes, which are rimmed by basophilic granules.

The diagnosis of these disorders is based on clinical features, electromyography, increase in serum creatinine kinase, and biopsy.

MIXED CONNECTIVE TISSUE DISEASE (MCTD) (p. 214)

It is controversial whether this condition represents a heterogeneous subgroup of other autoimmune disorders or is a separate clinical entity. It is characterized by

- Features suggestive of SLE, polymyositis, and systemic sclerosis (e.g., Raynaud's phenomenon, esophageal dysmotility, myositis, leukopenia-anemia, fever, lymphadenopathy, and hypergammaglobulinemia).
- High ANA titers to ribonucleoproteins (and unlike SLE *no* antibodies to native DNA or Smith antigens).
- Infrequency of renal disease.
- Excellent response to steroids.
- Eighty percent of patients being female, typically in the 30- to 60-year age range.

POLYARTERITIS NODOSA AND OTHER VASCULITIDES (p. 215)

A group of noninfectious necrotizing vasculitides detailed in Chapter 11.

IMMUNOLOGIC DEFICIENCY SYNDROMES (p. 216)

May be subdivided into primary and secondary forms. *Primary immunodeficiency disorders* are usually hereditary, typically manifesting between 6 months and 2 years of life as maternal antibody protection is lost. *Secondary immunodeficiencies* result from altered immune function due to infections, malnutrition, aging, immunosuppression, irradiation, chemotherapy, or autoimmunity.

X-LINKED AGAMMAGLOBULINEMIA OF BRUTON (p. 216)

One of the most common primary immunodeficiency syndromes. An X-linked disorder. Presents as *recurrent bacterial infections* (e.g., *Staphylococcus, Haemophilus influenzae*) beginning at 8 to 9 months of age. There is virtually no serum Ig, but cell-mediated immune function is normal; consequently, most viral and fungal infections are handled appropriately. Exceptions (for unclear reasons) include enterovirus, echovirus (causing a fatal encephalitis), and vaccine-associated poliovirus (causing paralysis).

- The basic defect is lack of *mature* B cells due to mutations in

a tyrosine-kinase gene expressed in early B cells. Pre-B cells are present in normal numbers in marrow, but lymph nodes and spleen lack germinal centers, and plasma cells are absent from all tissues.
- T-cell numbers and function are entirely normal.
- For unknown reasons, these patients have an increased frequency (up to 20%) of autoimmune connective tissue diseases, including a rheumatoid-like arthritis that responds to gamma-globulin therapy.

COMMON VARIABLE IMMUNODEFICIENCY
(p. 216)

A heterogeneous group of disorders, congenital or acquired, sporadic or familial. *The common feature is hypogammaglobulinemia, generally affecting all Ig classes, but occasionally only IgG.*

Typically, there are recurrent bacterial infections, and patients are also prone to autoimmune diseases and lymphoid malignancies. There are several subvarieties:

- *Intrinsic B-cell defect* in most cases. B cells are present in normal numbers and proliferate in response to antigen, but do not differentiate into plasma cells. Lymphoid follicles are hyperplastic.
- For unclear reasons, there is also frequent multiorgan involvement with noncaseating granulomas.
- *Regulatory T-cell defect* in some cases: either a T-helper deficiency or a T-suppressor hyperactivity.
- Some patients show linkage with the complement genes within HLA complex, as do certain patients with selective IgA deficiency, suggesting some genetically determined defect in B-cell differentiation.

ISOLATED IGA DEFICIENCY (p. 217)

Very common immunodeficiency (one in 600 people) with *virtual absence of serum and secretory IgA, and occasionally of IgG$_2$ and IgG$_4$ subclasses.* May be familial or acquired following toxoplasmosis, measles, or other viral infection.

- Although usually asymptomatic, patients may have recurrent sinopulmonary and GI infections and are prone to respiratory tract allergies and autoimmune diseases (SLE, rheumatoid arthritis).
- The basic defect is failure of maturation of IgA-positive B cells. Immature forms are present in normal numbers.
- Forty per cent of patients have antibodies to IgA. Transfusion of IgA-containing blood products may induce anaphylaxis.

DIGEORGE'S SYNDROME
(THYMIC HYPOPLASIA) (p. 217)

A multiorgan congenital disorder resulting from fetal damage to the third and fourth pharyngeal pouches before the eighth week of gestation.

Characteristic are

- *Thymic hypoplasia or aplasia.* T-cell deficiency with lack of cell-mediated responses (especially to fungi and viruses). B cells and Ig levels are usually normal.

- *Parathyroid hypoplasia.* Abnormal calcium regulation with hypocalcemic tetany.
- *Congenital defects of heart and great vessels.*
- *Dysmorphic facies.*

Patients may be treated with fetal thymus or thymic epithelium transplants. If children survive into their fifth year, T-cell function tends to normalize even with thymic aplasia.

SEVERE COMBINED IMMUNODEFICIENCY DISEASE (SCID) (p. 218)

Heterogeneous group of autosomal or X-linked recessive disorders *characterized by lymphopenia and defects in T- and B-cell function,* more often in the former.

Pathogenetic mechanisms fall into two general categories:

- T- and/or B-cell stem cell defects in a small minority of cases.
- Defects in normal T-cell maturation/differentiation, with secondary deficiencies of B-cell function. Defects in T-cell differentiation are heterogeneous. In the X-linked recessive forms, there is a mutation in the cytokine receptor gene shared by IL-2, IL-4, and IL-7.

Fifty per cent of patients with the autosomal recessive form of SCID lack the enzyme adenosine deaminase (ADA) in their lymphocytes and erythrocytes, leading to the accumulation of metabolites such as deoxyadenosine and deoxy-ATP, which are toxic to lymphocytes.

In X-linked SCID and ADA-deficient patients, the thymus is typically arrested at an early fetal stage, and lymph nodes, spleen, tonsils, and appendix show virtually no lymphoid tissue. Affected infants do not synthesize antibodies and fail to reject skin grafts or mount a delayed-type hypersensitivity response. Death usually occurs within 1 year from opportunistic infections.

GVHD may occur owing to transplacental transfer of maternal T cells.

Bone marrow transplant from matched donors may yield full immunologic reconstitution.

IMMUNODEFICIENCY WITH THROMBOCYTOPENIA AND ECZEMA (WISKOTT-ALDRICH SYNDROME) (p. 218)

X-linked recessive disease characterized by thrombocytopenia, eczema, and recurrent infections with a predilection for the development of lymphomas.

- The thymus is morphologically normal, but there is peripheral T-cell depletion in lymphoid tissues with an associated defect in cellular immunity.
- Antibody responses are variable but are characteristically poor to polysaccharide antigens.
- The pathogenesis is unknown; bone marrow transplantation has occasionally been curative.

GENETIC DEFICIENCIES OF THE COMPLEMENT SYSTEM (p. 219)

These have been described for virtually all complement components and for two inhibitors. Deficiency of C3 leads to increased susceptibility to bacterial infections. Inherited deficiencies of C1q, C2, and C4 impair clearance of immune complexes and hence increase the risk of immune complex–mediated diseases (e.g., SLE). An absence of C1 esterase inhibitor is associated with *hereditary angioedema* due to uncontrolled generation of vasoactive C2 kinin. Defects in later-acting components (C5–C8) result in recurrent neisserial infections.

ACQUIRED IMMUNODEFICIENCY SYNDROME (AIDS) (p. 219)

An infectious secondary form of immunodeficiency caused by the human immunodeficiency virus (HIV-I). It is characterized by profound suppression of T-cell mediated immunity, opportunistic infections, secondary neoplasms, and neurologic disease.

EPIDEMIOLOGY AND MODES OF TRANSMISSION. Transmission of the HIV occurs through (1) sexual contact, (2) parenteral inoculation, or (3) passage from infected mothers to fetuses or newborns.

In the United States, there are five major risk groups:

1. *Homosexual/bisexual males.* Approximately 60% of reported cases of AIDS (in homosexual males the virus enters via lymphocytes in semen through traumatized rectal mucosa).

2. *Intravenous drug users* (without a history of homosexual contact). Approximately 23% of all patients. Caused by sharing of contaminated needles and paraphernalia.

3. *Hemophiliacs.* Especially those receiving large amounts of pooled factor VIII concentrate before 1985; 1% of cases.

4. *Blood/component recipients (excluding hemophiliacs);* 2% of all patients. Transmission by this route has been virtually eliminated in the U.S. However, because recently infected individuals may be seronegative, a small but definite risk of acquiring AIDS through blood transfusion persists.

5. *Other high-risk groups.* Six per cent of patients acquire disease through heterosexual contacts with members of other high-risk groups. Eighty per cent of children with AIDS have an HIV-infected parent and suffer transplacental or perinatal transmission.

- The risk of seroconversion after an accidental needle stick with infected blood is approximately 0.5%.
- In about 6% of patients the mode of transmission is unknown.
- HIV is *not* transmitted by casual (nonsexual) contact.
- Outside the United States and Europe, male-to-female transmission (most with vaginal intercourse) is the most common mode of spread.
- Increased heterosexual transmission is beginning to outpace other modes in the United States.
- Although HIV has been found in vaginal and cervical secretions, monocytes, and endothelium, female-to-male transmission is not common in the U.S.

BIOLOGY OF HIV-I. A human type C retrovirus in the same family as the animal lentivirus family. Also closely related to HIV-II, which causes a similar disease, primarily in West Africa.

- HIV is a *nontransforming cytopathic retrovirus* inducing immunodeficiency by destruction of target T cells.
- The HIV-I lipid envelope, derived from the infected host membrane during budding, is studded with two viral glycopro-

teins, gp120 and gp41, the former important in binding to host CD4 molecules to initiate viral infection.

- It has several genes not present in the other retroviruses. These include *tat, vpu, vif, nef,* and *rev.* Many, such as *tat* and *rev,* regulate HIV transcription and hence may be targeted for therapy.
- *The virus has been isolated from lymphoid cells, serum, cerebrospinal fluid, and all secretions of infected patients.*

HIV INFECTION OF LYMPHOCYTES AND MONOCYTES. Central to the pathogenesis of AIDS is depletion of CD4 + helper T cells. The CD4 antigen (also present at lower levels on monocytes and macrophages) is the high-affinity receptor for the gp120 protein on HIV-I.

- After binding the virus is internalized; the genome undergoes reverse transcription; the proviral DNA is then integrated into the host genome.
- *Transcription/translation and viral propagation may subsequently occur only with T-cell activation (e.g., antigenic stimulation). In the absence of T-cell activation, the infection enters a latent phase.*
- Perhaps 0.1% to 13% of circulating T cells express viral mRNA. However, a much greater proportion of CD4 + T cells in lymph nodes (20% to 30%) contain HIV DNA, most of which is in latent form.
- Infected monocytes and macrophages refractory to HIV cytopathic effects act (1) as reservoirs for HIV (perhaps transferring virus to T cells during antigen presentation) and (2) as vehicles for viral transport, especially to the CNS.
- In addition to macrophages, the follicular dendritic cells (FDCs) in the germinal center of lymph nodes are also important reservoirs of HIV. The viral particles coated with anti-HIV antibodies are found attached to the Fc receptor for Ig on the surface of FDCs. These HIV virions continually infect T cells as they come in close contact with the FDCs during passage through lymph nodes.
- The consequences of CD4 + cell depletion on immune function are listed in Table 6–4.
- In addition to T-cell depletion, there are also qualitative defects in T-cell function, with a selective loss of T-cell memory early in the course of disease.
- There is paradoxic B-cell activation, but nonetheless patients with AIDS are unable to mount appreciable antibody responses to new antigens, probably owing to CD4 + T cell depletion and/or intrinsic B cell defects.

CENTRAL NERVOUS SYSTEM INVOLVEMENT BY HIV. The CNS is a major target in HIV infection. This occurs predominantly, if not exclusively, via monocytes. Infected monocytes circulate to the brain and are somehow activated either to release toxic cytokines directly or to recruit other neuron-damaging inflammatory cells.

NATURAL HISTORY OF HIV INFECTION. On the basis of interactions of HIV with the host immune system, it can be divided into three phases (Fig. 6–1).

1. The *early, acute phase,* characterized by transient viremia, seeding of lymphoid tissue, a temporary fall in CD4 + T cells, followed by seroconversion and control of viral replication by generation of CD8 + antiviral T cells. Clinically, a self-limited acute illness with sore throat, nonspecific myalgias, and aseptic

Table 6-4. Major Abnormalities of Immune Function in AIDS

Lymphopenia
   Predominantly due to selective loss of the CD4+ helper-inducer T-cell subset; inversion of CD4-CD8 ratio

Decreased T-Cell Function *in Vivo*
   Preferential loss of memory T cells
   Susceptibility to opportunistic infections
   Susceptibility to neoplasms
   Decreased delayed-type hypersensitivity

Altered T-Cell Function *in Vitro*
   Decreased proliferative response to mitogens, alloantigens, and soluble antigens
   Decreased specific cytotoxicity
   Decreased helper function for pokeweed mitogen-induced B-cell immunoglobulin production
   Decreased IL-2 and IFN-γ production

Polyclonal B-Cell Activation
   Hypergammaglobulinemia and circulating immune complexes
   Inability to mount *de novo* antibody response to a new antigen
   Refractoriness to the normal signals for B-cell activation *in vitro*

Altered Monocyte or Macrophage Functions
   Decreased chemotaxis and phagocytosis
   Decreased HLA class II antigen expression
   Diminished capacity to present antigen to T cells
   Increased spontaneous secretion of IL-1, TNF-α, IL-6

From Cotran, R. S., Kumar, V., and Robbins, S. L.: Robbins Pathologic Basis of Disease. 5th ed. Philadelphia, W. B. Saunders Co., 1994, p. 226.

meningitis may develop. Clinical recovery and near normal CD4+ T-cell counts occur within 6 to 12 weeks.

2. The *middle, chronic phase,* characterized by clinical latency with smoldering low-level viral replication mainly in the lymphoid tissue, and gradual decline of CD4+ counts. Patients may develop persistent generalized lymph node enlargement, with no constitutional symptoms. This phase may last for years. Toward the end of this phase, fever, rash, fatigue, and viremia appear. The chronic phase may last from 7 to 10 years.

3. The *final, crisis phase,* characterized by rapid decline in host defenses manifested by low CD4+ counts, loss of weight, diarrhea, opportunistic infections, and secondary neoplasms. This phase is usually recognized as full-blown AIDS. CDC guidelines consider anyone with HIV infection and CD4+ T-cell count less than 200 cells/µl as having AIDS, even if all clinical features are not present.

The clinical features of full blown AIDS include:

• A variety of opportunistic infections (see also Table 6-5. *Pneumocystis carinii* pneumonia occurs in 50% of patients).
• A wide spectrum of pyogenic bacterial infections (reflecting altered humoral immunity).
• A variety of malignant neoplasms (see also Table 6-5). Aggres-

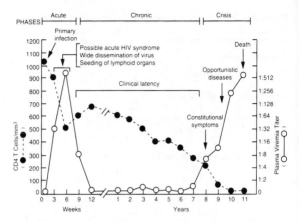

Figure 6-1. Typical course of HIV infection. During the early period after primary infection there is widespread dissemination of virus and a sharp decrease in the number of CD4+ T cells in peripheral blood. An immune response to HIV ensues, with a decrease in detectable viremia followed by a prolonged period of clinical latency. The CD4+ T-cell count continues to decrease during the following years, until it reaches a critical level below which there is a substantial risk of opportunistic diseases. (Redrawn and reproduced with permission from Pantaleo, G., Graziosi, C., and Fauci, A.S.: The immunopathogenesis of human immunodeficiency virus infection. N. Engl. J. Med. 1993, Volume 328, Page 327. Copyright 1994. Massachusetts Medical Society. All rights reserved.)

sive *Kaposi's sarcoma* occurs in 25% of patients, and for un-known reasons is more common in homosexuals than in other risk groups. Aggressive B-cell non-Hodgkin's lymphomas, espe-cially at extranodal sites, frequently involving the brain, occur at rates 60-fold higher than in the general population.
- Clinical neurologic involvement occurs in 30% to 50% of pa-tients, manifesting as (1) acute aseptic meningitis, (2) a vacuo-lar myelopathy, (3) a peripheral neuropathy, and (4) most commonly, a progressive encephalopathy designated AIDS-dementia complex.
- With AIDS, the 5-year mortality rate is 85%, and with longer intervals the rate approaches 100%.

MORPHOLOGY. *With the exception of the CNS, the tissue changes in AIDS are neither specific nor diagnostic. Basically, the pathologic features are those of the various opportunistic infections and the specific neoplasms.* These infections and those in the CNS and in AIDS-associated nephropathy are discussed elsewhere in the chapters devoted to each particular organ. Below is a description of lymph node pathology.

Lymph Nodes. Adenopathy in early HIV infection reflects the initial polyclonal B-cell proliferation and hypergammaglobuli-nemia, showing nonspecific, predominantly follicular hyperplasia with mantle zone attenuation and intense medullary plas-macytosis. HIV particles can be demonstrated in germinal cen-ters by *in situ* hybridization, localized mainly on the surface of FDCs.

- With progression to full-blown AIDS, the lymphoid follicles become involuted ("burned out"), with general lymphocyte depletion and disruption of organized FDC network.

Table 6–5. AIDS-Defining Opportunistic Infections and Neoplasms Found in Patients with HIV Infection

Infections

Protozoal and Helminthic Infections
  Cryptosporidiosis or isosporidiosis (enteritis)
  Pneumocytosis (pneumonia or disseminated infection)
  Toxoplasmosis (pneumonia or CNS infection)

Fungal Infections
  Candidiasis (esophageal, tracheal, or pulmonary)
  Cryptococcosis (CNS infection)
  Coccidioidomycosis (disseminated)
  Histoplasmosis (disseminated)

Bacterial Infections
Mycobacteriosis ("atypical," e.g., *M. avium-intracellulare,*
  disseminated or extrapulmonary; *M. tuberculosis,* pulmonary
  or extrapulmonary)
Nocardiosis (pneumonia, meningitis, disseminated)
Salmonella infections, disseminated

Viral Infections
  Cytomegalovirus (pulmonary, intestinal, retinitis, or CNS
    infections)
  Herpes simplex virus (localized or disseminated)
  Varicella-zoster virus (localized or disseminated)
  Progressive multifocal leukoencephalopathy

Neoplasms
  Kaposi's sarcoma
  Non-Hodgkin's lymphomas (Burkitt's, immunoblastic)
  Primary lymphoma of the brain
  Invasive cancer of uterine cervix

From Cotran, R. S., Kumar, V., and Robbins, S. L.: Robbins Pathologic Basis of Disease. 5th ed. Philadelphia, W. B. Saunders Co., 1994, p. 228.

- Inflammatory responses to infections may be sparse or atypical, and infectious organisms may not be apparent without special stains.
- Similar lymphoid depletion occurs in the spleen and thymus.
- Patients frequently develop diffuse high-grade malignant B-cell lymphomas (the second most common malignancy, after Kaposi's sarcoma), perhaps because of prolonged B-cell proliferation in the face of deteriorating regulatory controls.

AMYLOIDOSIS (p. 231)

Amyloid is a heterogeneous group of pathogenic fibrillar proteins that accumulate within tissues and organs, either because of excess synthesis or because of resistance to catabolism.

All these proteins share the ability to aggregate into an insoluble, "cross-beta"-pleated sheet tertiary conformation; all are deposited extracellularly in a variety of tissues, and in a large array of clinical settings. As the material accumulates, it produces pressure atrophy of adjacent parenchyma.

Depending on tissue distribution and degree of involvement, amyloid may be asymptomatic and found only as an unsuspected anatomic change, or may be life threatening.

ULTRASTRUCTURE. By EM, amyloid is composed predominantly (90%) of nonbranching fibrils of indeterminate length and a diameter of 7.5 to 10 nm. These are associated with a minor (10%) "P component," consisting of stacks of pentagonal, doughnut-shaped structures with homology to C-reactive protein.

CHEMICAL NATURE. There are two major and several minor chemically distinct classes of amyloid fibrils (Table 6–6):

- *AL (amyloid light chain protein).* Immunoglobulin light chains (or amino-terminal fragments thereof) derived from plasma cells; lambda much more often than kappa. *Frequently associated with B-cell dyscrasias (e.g., multiple myeloma).*
- *AA (amyloid-associated protein).* A nonimmunoglobulin protein derived from a 12,000-dalton serum precursor called SAA (serum amyloid-associated) protein synthesized in liver and elevated in inflammatory states.

Some less common forms of amyloid in particular clinical settings include

- *Transthyretin* (TTR). A normal serum protein that binds and transports thyroxine and retinol. A mutant form is deposited as amyloid in a group of hereditary diseases called *familial amyloid polyneuropathy.*
- A variant of transthyretin deposited in amyloidosis associated with aging.
- *Beta-2-microglobulin.* The smaller nonpolymorphic peptide component of class I MHC molecules and a normal serum protein; deposited in amyloidosis complicating long-term hemodialysis.
- *Beta-2-amyloid protein* ($A\beta_2$). A peptide found in Alzheimer's disease that forms the core of cerebral plaques and deposits within cerebral vessel walls. It derives from a transmembrane glycoprotein precursor (APP).

CLINICAL FORMS OF AMYLOIDOSIS (p. 237). Amyloidosis is subdivided into *systemic* (generalized) and *localized* (tissue-specific) forms, and is further classified on the basis of predisposing conditions (Table 6–6).

Systemic Amyloidosis. Associated with

1. *B-cell dyscrasias (also called primary amyloidosis).* The most common form in the United States. Composed of AL-type amyloid.

   - Occurs in 5 to 15% of patients with multiple myeloma.
   Tumorous plasma cells synthesize abnormal quantities of a single immunoglobulin (*M spike* on serum protein electrophoresis) or immunoglobulin light chain (*Bence Jones protein*). By virtue of their smaller size, Bence Jones proteins are frequently excreted in the urine.

     - The vast majority of cases of AL-type systemic amyloidosis are *not* associated with *overt* B-cell neoplasms. Nevertheless, they have monoclonal immunoglobulins and/or light chains.
     - Typically (but not always) involves the heart, GI tract, peripheral nerves, skin, and tongue more than other organs.

2. *Secondary or reactive amyloidosis.* Marked by AA-type amyloid. *Associated with chronic inflammatory states (infectious and noninfectious) producing protracted cell breakdown,* e.g.,

Table 6-6. Classification of Amyloidosis

Clinicopathologic Category	Associated Diseases	Major Fibril Protein	Chemically Related Precursor Protein
Systemic (Generalized) Amyloidosis			
Immunocyte dyscrasias with amyloidosis (primary amyloidosis)	Multiple myeloma and other monoclonal B-cell proliferations	AL	Immunoglobulin light chains, chiefly λ type
Reactive systemic amyloidosis (secondary amyloidosis)	Chronic inflammatory conditions	AA	SAA
Hemodialysis-associated amyloidosis	Chronic renal failure	$A\beta_2M$	β_2-Microglobulin
Hereditary amyloidosis:			
(1) Familial Mediterranean fever	—	AA	SAA
(2) Familial amyloidotic neuropathies (several types)	—	ATTR	Transthyretin
Localized Amyloidosis			
Senile cardiac	—	ATTR	Transthyretin
Senile cerebral	Alzheimer's disease	$A\beta_2$	APP
Endocrine, e.g., medullary carcinoma of thyroid	—	ACal	Calcitonin

*Transthyretin is also known as prealbumin. The transthyretins deposited as amyloid are muttant forms of normal transthyretin.
AL = amyloid light chain; AA = amyloid associated (protein); SSA = serum amyloid associated (protein).
Modified from Cotran, R. S., Kumar, V., and Robbins, S. L.: Robbins Pathologic Basis of Disease. 5th ed. Philadelphia, W. B. Saunders Co., 1994, p. 233.

rheumatoid arthritis, scleroderma, dermatomyositis, bronchiectasis, chronic osteomyelitis.

- Typically, kidneys, liver, spleen, lymph nodes, adrenals, and thyroid are involved.

3. *Hemodialysis related.* Affects up to 70% of patients on chronic hemodialysis. Due to deposition (in joints, synovium, and tendon sheaths) of beta-2-microglobulin not filtered by normal dialysis membranes.

4. *Hereditary forms.* Include many rare entities, often confined to specific geographic locations. Most common and best characterized is *familial Mediterranean fever,* a recurrent, febrile illness typically in Sephardic Jews, Armenians, and Arabs, characterized by bouts of serosal inflammation. The systemic amyloid is of AA type, suggesting that chronic inflammation plays a pivotal role. *Familial amyloidotic polyneuropathies* have autosomal dominant transmission, and show deposition of variant transthyretins principally in peripheral and autonomic nerves.

Localized Amyloidosis. Confined to amyloid in a single organ or tissue.

1. *Nodular (tumor-forming) deposits.* Often AL protein with associated plasma cell infiltrates. Occur most frequently in lung, larynx, skin, bladder, tongue, and periorbitally. May represent localized forms of B-cell dyscrasias.

2. *Endocrine amyloid.* Deposition in a variety of tumors associated with catabolism of polypeptide hormones or prohormones, e.g., thyroid medullary carcinoma (procalcitonin).

3. *Amyloid of aging.*

- *Senile cardiac amyloidosis.* Typically in the eighth and ninth decades, and most commonly due to deposition of transthyretin; sometimes due to deposition of atrial natriuretic factor.
- Besides heart, deposits may occur in lungs, pancreas, or spleen.
- *Senile cerebral amyloidosis.* $A\beta_2$ deposition in Alzheimer's disease (see above).

MORPHOLOGY. Macroscopically, affected tissues are stained blue-violet with iodine and dilute sulfuric acid. Microscopically with routine stains, amyloid is amorphous, acellular, hyaline, and eosinophilic. With special stains (e.g., Congo red), it is salmon-red, and characteristic yellow-green birefringence may be seen by means of polarized light.

Kidneys. Classically enlarged, pale gray, waxy, and firm. In advanced disease, chronic vascular occlusion (due to amyloid deposits) may result in a shrunken, contracted organ. Amyloid deposited in

- *Glomeruli,* initially mesangial and subendothelial. With continued accumulation, there is hyalinization of glomeruli.
- *Peritubular regions* begin in the tubular basement membrane and gradually extend into the interstitium.
- *Blood vessels.* Hyaline thickening of arterial and arteriolar walls with narrowing lumen, eventually causing ischemia with tubular atrophy and interstitial fibrosis.

Spleen. May be enlarged (up to 800 gm). Amyloid deposits begin between cells. With time, one of two patterns emerges:

- *"Sago" spleen.* Deposits limited to the splenic follicles, giving rise to "tapioca-like" granules on gross inspection.
- *Lardaceous spleen.* Amyloid largely spares the follicles and is deposited in the pulp. Fusion of deposits forms large geographic areas.

Liver. May induce hepatomegaly with a pale, waxy-gray, firm appearance. Microscopically, first deposits in the space of Disse, gradually encroaching on parenchyma and sinusoids to produce pressure atrophy with massive hepatic replacement.

Heart. Distinctive (although not always present) are minute, typically atrial, pink to gray subendocardial droplets representing focal amyloid accumulations. Vascular and subepicardial deposits may also occur.

Microscopically, there are interstitial and perimyocyte deposits, progressively leading to pressure atrophy.

CLINICAL FEATURES. Diagnosis is made on the basis of biopsy and characteristic Congo red stain. Favored biopsy sites are the kidney (when renal manifestations are present) and the rectum or gingiva (in systemic disease).

- Abdominal fat pad aspirates may also yield diagnostic tissue.
- In amyloidosis suspected of being associated with B-cell dyscrasias, serum and urine electrophoresis and bone marrow biopsy (for plasmacytosis) are indicated.
- In systemic amyloidosis, the prognosis is poor. Median survival after diagnosis in the setting of B-cell dyscrasias is about 14 months. Reactive amyloidosis may have a slightly better outlook, depending on the ability to control the underlying condition.

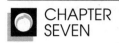

CHAPTER SEVEN

Neoplasia

A tumor is an abnormal mass of tissue, the growth of which is virtually autonomous and exceeds that of normal tissues. Unlike non-neoplastic proliferations (see Chap. 2), the growth of tumors persists after cessation of the stimuli that initiated the change. Tumors are classified into two broad categories: benign and malignant.

NOMENCLATURE (p. 242)

All tumors have two basic components: (1) the "transformed" neoplastic cells and (2) the supporting stroma composed of nontransformed elements such as connective tissues and blood vessels. Classification of neoplasms is based on the characteristics of their parenchyma.

BENIGN TUMORS. In general, their names end with the suffix "oma." For example, benign mesenchymal tumors include lipoma, fibroma, angioma, osteoma, and leiomyoma. The nomenclature of benign epithelial tumors is somewhat complex and is based on both histogenesis and architecture. Some examples follow:

- Adenomas. Benign epithelial tumors arising in glands or forming glandular patterns.
- Cystadenomas. Adenomas producing large cystic masses, seen typically in the ovary.
- Papillomas. Epithelial tumors forming microscopic or macroscopic finger-like projections.
- Polyp. A tumor projecting from the mucosa into the lumen of a hollow viscus (e.g., stomach or colon).

MALIGNANT TUMORS. These are often called cancers and are broadly divided into two categories: *carcinomas,* arising from epithelial cells, and *sarcomas,* arising from mesenchymal tissues.

The nomenclature of specific types of carcinomas or sarcomas is based on their appearance and presumed histogenetic origin. Thus, malignant epithelial tumors with glandular growth patterns are referred to as adenocarcinomas, whereas sarcomas arising from or resembling smooth muscle cells are called leiomyosarcomas.

Some tumors appear to have more than one parenchymal cell type. Two important members in this category are

- *Mixed tumors,* derived from one germ cell layer that differentiates into more than one parenchymal cell type. For example, mixed salivary gland tumor contains epithelial cells as well as myxoid stroma and cartilage-like tissue. All elements arise from altered differentiation of ductal epithelial cells.

- *Teratomas,* made up of a variety of parenchymal cell types representative of more than one germ cell layer, usually all three. They arise from totipotential cells that retain the ability to form endodermal (e.g., gut epithelium), ectodermal (e.g., skin), and mesenchymal (e.g., fat) tissues. Such tumors are found principally in the testis and ovary.

A summary of tumor nomenclature is offered in Table 7–1.

Two non-neoplastic lesions simulating tumors bear names that are deceptively similar to tumors:

- *Choristomas.* Ectopic, sometimes nodular, rests of nontransformed tissues (e.g., pancreatic cells under the small bowel mucosa).
- *Hamartomas.* Malformations that present as a mass of disorganized tissue indigenous to the particular site (i.e., a hamartomatous nodule in the lung may contain islands of cartilage, bronchi, and blood vessels).

CHARACTERISTICS OF BENIGN AND MALIGNANT NEOPLASMS (p. 245)

The distinction between benign and malignant tumors is based on appearance (morphology) and ultimately on behavior (clinical course), using four criteria: (1) differentiation and anaplasia, (2) rate of growth, (3) local invasion, and (4) metastases.

DIFFERENTIATION AND ANAPLASIA (p. 245)

Differentiation is the extent to which tumor cells resemble comparable normal cells. Cells within most benign tumors closely mimic corresponding normal cells. Thus, thyroid adenomas are composed of normal-looking thyroid acini, and the cells in lipomas look like those in normal adipose tissue. Although malignant neoplasms are in general less well differentiated than their benign counterparts, they nevertheless display patterns ranging from well differentiated to very poorly differentiated. Lack of differentiation, also called *anaplasia,* is a hallmark of malignant cells. The following cytologic features characterize anaplastic, or poorly differentiated, tumors:

- *Nuclear and cellular pleomorphism.* Wide variation in the shape and size of cells and nuclei.
- *Hyperchromatism.* Darkly stained nuclei that frequently contain prominent nucleoli.
- *Nuclear-cytoplasmic ratio.* Approaches 1:1 instead of 1:4 or 1:6, reflecting enlargement of nuclei.
- *Abundant mitoses.* Reflect proliferative activity. Mitotic figures may be abnormal (e.g., tripolar spindles).
- *Tumor giant cells* containing a single large polyploid nucleus or multiple nuclei are sometimes seen.

Poorly differentiated, anaplastic tumors also demonstrate a total disarray of tissue architecture. For example, in an anaplastic tumor of the uterine cervix the normal orientation of squamous epithelial cells with respect to each other is lost. Well-differentiated tumors, whether benign or malignant, tend to retain the functional characteristics of their normal counterparts. There may be attributes such as production of hormones in tumors of endocrine origin or keratin in squamous epithelial tumors.

Dysplasia refers to disorderly but non-neoplastic growth. It is

Table 7-1. Nomenclature of Tumors

Tissue of Origin	Benign	Malignant
I. Composed of one parenchymal cell type		
A. Tumors of mesenchymal origin		
(1) Connective tissue and derivatives	Fibroma	Fibrosarcoma
	Lipoma	Liposarcoma
	Chondroma	Chondrosarcoma
	Osteoma	Osteogenic sarcoma
(2) Endothelial and related tissues		
Blood vessels	Hemangioma	Angiosarcoma
Lymph vessels	Lymphangioma	Lymphangiosarcoma
Synovium		Synovioma (synoviosarcoma)
Mesothelium		Mesothelioma
Brain coverings	Meningioma	Invasive meningioma
(3) Blood cells and related cells		
Hematopoietic cells		Leukemias
Lymphoid tissue		Malignant lymphomas
(4) Muscle		
Smooth muscle	Leiomyoma	Leiomyosarcoma
Striated	Rhabdomyoma	Rhabdomyosarcoma
B. Epithelial tumors		
(1) Stratified squamous	Squamous cell papilloma	Squamous cell or epidermoid carcinoma
(2) Basal cells of skin or adnexa		Basal cell carcinoma

(3) Epithelial lining		
Glands or ducts	Adenoma Papilloma Cystadenoma	Adenocarcinoma Papillary carcinoma Cystadenocarcinoma
(4) Respiratory passages		Bronchogenic carcinoma Bronchial "adenoma" (carcinoid)
(5) Neuroectoderm	Nevus	Malignant melanoma
(6) Renal epithelium	Renal tubular adenoma	Renal cell carcinoma (hypernephroma)
(7) Urinary tract epithelium (transitional)	Transitional cell papilloma	Transitional cell carcinoma
(8) Placental epithelium (trophoblast)	Hydatidiform mole	Choriocarcinoma
(9) Testicular epithelium (germ cells)		Seminoma
II. More than one neoplastic cell type—mixed tumors—usually derived from one germ layer		
(1) Salivary glands	Pleomorphic adenoma (mixed tumor of salivary gland origin)	Malignant mixed tumor of salivary gland origin
(2) Breast	Fibroadenoma	Malignant cystosarcoma phyllodes
(3) Renal anlage		Wilms' tumor
III. More than one neoplastic cell type derived from more than one germ layer—teratogenous		
(1) Totipotential cells in gonads or in embryonic rests	Mature teratoma, dermoid cyst	Immature teratoma

Modified from Cotran, R. S., Kumar, V., and Robbins, S. L.: Robbins Pathologic Basis of Disease. 5th ed. Philadelphia, W. B. Saunders Co., 1994, p 244.

characterized by pleomorphism, hyperchromaticism, and loss of normal orientation. Dysplastic changes are usually encountered in epithelia, especially in the uterine cervix. When dysplastic changes are marked and *involve the entire thickness of the epithelium,* the lesion is considered a preinvasive neoplasm and is referred to as *carcinoma in situ.* This is a forerunner, in many cases, of invasive carcinoma. However, mild degrees of dysplasia, common in the uterine cervix, do not always lead to cancer and are often reversible when the inciting cause (e.g., chronic irritation) is removed.

RATE OF GROWTH (p. 248)

Most malignant tumors grow more rapidly than benign tumors. However, some cancers grow slowly for years and then enter a phase of rapid growth; others expand rapidly from the outset. Growth of cancers arising from hormone-sensitive tissues such as the uterus, for instance, may be affected by the variations in hormone levels associated with pregnancy and menopause.

Rapidly growing malignant tumors often contain central areas of ischemic necrosis because the tumor blood supply fails to keep pace with the oxygen needs of the expanding mass of cells.

LOCAL INVASION (p. 248)

- Most benign tumors grow as cohesive expansile masses that develop a rim of condensed connective tissue, or *capsule,* at the periphery.
- They do not penetrate the capsule or the surrounding normal tissues.
- The plane of cleavage between the capsule and the surrounding tissues facilitates surgical enucleation.
- Malignant neoplasms are invasive, infiltrating and destroying normal tissues surrounding them.
- A well-defined capsule and plane of cleavage are lacking, making enucleation difficult or impossible.
- Surgical treatment of such tumors requires removal of a considerable margin of healthy and apparently uninvolved tissue.

METASTASIS (p. 250)

This process involves invasion of the lymphatics, blood vessels, and body cavities by the tumor, followed by transport and growth of secondary tumor cell masses that are discontinuous with the primary tumor. This is the single most important feature distinguishing benign from malignant tumors. With the notable exception of tumors in the brain and basal cell carcinomas of the skin, almost all malignant tumors have the capacity to metastasize.

Distant spread of tumors occurs by three routes:

- *Spread into body cavities.* This occurs by seeding of surfaces in peritoneal, pleural, pericardial, and subarachnoid spaces. Carcinoma of the ovary, for example, spreads transperitoneally to the surface of the liver or other abdominal viscera.
- *Invasion of lymphatics.* This is followed by transport of tumor cells to regional nodes and, ultimately, other parts of the body, and is common in the initial spread of carcinomas. Thus, carcinomas of the breast spread to either axillary or internal mammary lymph nodes, depending on the location (and therefore lymphatic drainage) of the tumor. Lymph nodes that are

the sites of metastases are frequently enlarged. Such enlargement usually results from the growth of tumor cells in nodes, but in some cases may result primarily from a reactive hyperplasia of the lymph nodes in response to the tumor antigens.

- *Hematogenous spread.* Typical of all sarcomas but also the favored route for certain carcinomas such as those originating in the kidney. Because of their thinner walls, veins are more frequently invaded than arteries. Lung and liver are common sites of hematogenous metastases because they receive the systemic and venous outflow, respectively. Other major sites of hematogenous spread include brain and bones.

EPIDEMIOLOGY (p. 252)

A variety of factors predispose an individual or a population to the development of cancer.

GEOGRAPHIC AND ENVIRONMENTAL FACTORS (p. 253)

In the United States cancer is responsible for approximately 23% of all deaths annually. Cancers of the lung, colon, and prostate are the leading causes of cancer death in males. In females, lung, breast, and colon cancers are the most common forms.

Environmental factors significantly influence the occurrence of specific forms of cancer in different parts of the world. In Japan, for example, the death rate from cancer of the stomach is about seven times that in the United States. Conversely, carcinoma of the colon is much less common as a cause of death in Japan. In Japanese immigrants to the United States the death rates for stomach and colon cancer are intermediate between those of natives of Japan and the United States, pointing to environmental and cultural influences.

Other examples of environmental factors in carcinogenesis are

- Increased risk of certain cancers with occupational exposure to asbestos, vinyl chloride, and 2-naphthylamine.
- Association of carcinomas of the oropharynx, larynx, and lung with cigarette smoking.

AGE (p. 254)

Cancer is most common in those over 55 years of age. However, certain cancers are particularly common in children under 15 years: tumors of the hematopoietic system (leukemias and lymphomas), neuroblastomas, Wilms' tumors, retinoblastomas, and sarcomas of bone and skeletal muscle.

HEREDITY (p. 254)

Heredity plays a role in the development of cancer even in the presence of clearly defined environmental factors. Hereditary forms of cancers can be divided into three categories:

- *Inherited cancer syndromes* are characterized by inheritance of single mutant genes that greatly increase the risk of developing a tumor. The predisposition to the tumor is thus an autosomal dominant trait, as exemplified by familial retinoblastoma and familial adenomatous polyposis. These syndromes are associated with inheritance of a single mutant allele of the "cancer suppressor genes." In each of these syndromes, only specific sites or tissues are affected, and usually there is an associated "marker phenotype," e.g., the presence of multiple benign tumors in familial polyposis of colon and benign endocrine gland tumors in multiple endocrine neoplasia.

- *Familial cancers* are characterized by familial clustering of specific forms of cancer, but the transmission pattern is not clear in an individual case. Familial forms of common cancers, e.g., breast, colon, brain, and ovary, are recorded. Unlike inherited cancer syndromes, there is no marker phenotype, e.g., familial colon cancers do not arise in pre-existing polyps.
- *Autosomal recessive syndromes of defective DNA repair* are characterized by chromosome or DNA instability that greatly increases the predisposition to environmental carcinogens.

ACQUIRED PRENEOPLASTIC DISORDERS
(p. 257)

Certain clinical conditions are associated with an increased risk of developing cancers:

- Cirrhosis of the liver—hepatocellular carcinoma.
- Atrophic gastritis of pernicious anemia—stomach cancer.
- Chronic ulcerative colitis—carcinoma of the colon.
- Leukoplakia of the oral and genital mucosa—squamous cell cancers.

Certain benign tumors are also associated with the subsequent development of cancer. Although the development of cancers in benign tumors is uncommon, there are a few exceptions (e.g., villous adenomas of the colon often develop into cancer). However, most malignant tumors arise de novo.

MOLECULAR BASIS OF CANCER (p. 257)

A simplified scheme of the molecular pathogenesis of cancer is provided in Figure 7–1 and recapitulated here:

- Cancer is a genetic disease. The genetic injury may be acquired in somatic cells by environmental agents or inherited in the germ-line. Tumors develop as clonal progeny of a single genetically damaged progenitor cell. The monoclonality of tumors can be verified by study of X-linked markers, e.g., G6PD isoenzymes or X-linked RFLPs.
- Three classes of genes are the targets of genetic damage: the growth-promoting proto-oncogenes, the growth-inhibiting tumor suppressor genes, and genes that regulate apoptosis.
- Carcinogenesis is a multistep process. The attributes of malignancy, e.g., invasiveness, excessive growth, escape from the immune system, are acquired in a stepwise fashion—a process called *tumor progression*. At the genetic level, progression results from accumulation of genetic events.

ONCOGENES AND CANCER (p. 259)

- *Oncogenes* are genes whose products are associated with neoplastic transformation.
- *Proto-oncogenes* are normal cellular genes that affect growth and differentiation. They can be converted into oncogenes by (1) transduction into retroviruses (v-*onc*) or (2) changes in situ

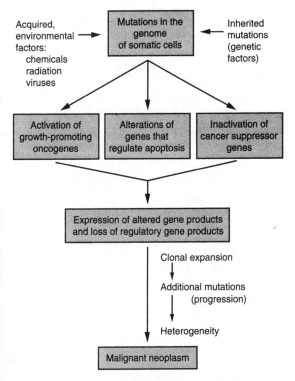

Figure 7–1. Flow chart depicts a simplified scheme of cancer pathogenesis. (From Cotran, R. S., Kumar, V., and Robbins, S. L.: Robbins Pathologic Basis of Disease. 5th ed. Philadelphia, W. B. Saunders Co., 1994, p. 258.)

that affect their expression and/or function, thereby converting them into c-*onc*.

Most human tumors are not caused by v-*onc*. The presence of c-*onc* is detected by transfection of tumor-derived DNA into the NIH/3T3 mouse fibroblast cell line. If the tumor DNA contains transforming sequences (c-*onc*), the transfected fibroblasts acquire the growth characteristics of neoplastic cells: loss of contact inhibition, growth in soft agar, and tumor formation in immunosuppressed mice. DNA transfection has revealed the presence of c-*onc* in many human tumors. Many of the transforming sequences detected by DNA transfection are homologous to known v-*onc*; others represent v-*onc* never detected in acute transforming viruses.

Protein Products of Oncogenes

To understand the transforming activity of oncogenes, it is essential to consider their functions in normal cell growth.

Stimulation of normal cell proliferation is often triggered by growth factors that bind to cell membrane receptors. The signal received on the cell membrane is transduced to the cytoplasm and ultimately to the nucleus by the generation of second messengers such as Ca^{++}. These signals activate nuclear regulatory factors that initiate DNA transcription.

The products of proto-oncogenes are grouped below and in Table 7–2 on the basis of their role in signal transduction.

- *Growth factors.* Some proto-oncogenes (e.g., c-*sis*) code for growth factors such as platelet-derived growth factor (PDGF). Many tumors that produce growth factors are also responsive to the growth-promoting effects of the secreted growth factors and hence subject to autocrine stimulation.
- *Growth factor receptors.* Several oncogenes encode growth factor receptors. Both structural alterations (mutations) and overexpression of the receptor genes have been found in association with malignant transformation. Mutations in several tyrosine-kinase type of growth factor receptors (e.g., v-*erb* B) lead to their constitutive activation without binding to their ligands. Overexpression commonly involves members of the EGF-receptor family, e.g., c-*erb* B1 is overexpressed in the majority of squamous cell carcinomas of lung; c-*erb* B2 (also called c-*neu*) is amplified in adenocarcinomas of breast, ovary, lung, stomach, and so on. In breast cancers that have amplified c-*erb* B2, the prognosis is poor, presumably because their cells are very sensitive to smaller quantities of growth factors.
- *Signal-transducing proteins.* These are biochemically heterogeneous and grouped into two major categories:

  1. *GTP-binding proteins.* To this family belongs the *ras* family of proteins and G proteins. Approximately 30% of all human tumors carry mutant *ras* proteins. Normal *ras* proteins flip back and forth between an activated (GTP-bound) signal-transmitting form and an inactive (GDP-bound) quiescent form. The conversion of active *ras* to inactive *ras* is mediated by its intrinsic GTP-ase activity, which is augmented by a family of GTP-ase–activating proteins (GAPs). Mutant *ras* proteins bind GAPs, but their GTP-ase activity fails to be augmented, and hence they are trapped in the signal-transmitting GTP-bound form.
  2. *Non–receptor-associated tyrosine kinases.* An example in this category is the c-*abl* gene, which in its normal form exerts a regulated tyrosine-kinase activity. In chronic myeloid leukemia, translocation of c-*abl* and its fusion to the *bcr* gene produce a hybrid gene with potent, unregulated tyrosine-kinase activity.

- *Nuclear regulatory proteins.* The products of *myc, jun, fos,* and *myb* oncogenes are nuclear proteins. They are expressed in a highly regulated fashion during proliferation of normal cells and they are believed to regulate transcription of growth-related genes. Their oncogenic versions are associated with persistent expression. Dysregulation of *myc* expression occurs in Burkitt's lymphoma, neuroblastomas, and small cell cancer of lung.

Activation of Oncogenes (p. 263)

Proto-oncogenes may be converted to oncogenes by one of three mechanisms: (1) point mutations, (2) translocations, or (3) gene amplification.

POINT MUTATIONS. The *ras* proto-oncogenes are activated by point mutations. Approximately 15% of all human tumors carry mutated H-*ras* or K-*ras* oncogenes. One possible mechanism of these mutations is exposure to cancer-causing chemicals.

Table 7-2. Selected Oncogenes, Their Mode of Activation, and Associated Human Tumors

Category	Proto-Oncogene	Mechanism	Associated Human Tumor
Growth Factors			
PDGF-β chain	sis	Overexpression	Astrocytoma; osteosarcoma
Fibroblast growth factors	hst-1	Overexpression	Stomach cancer
	int-2		Bladder and breast cancers; melanoma
Growth Factor Receptors			
EGF-receptor family	erb-B1	Overexpression	Squamous cell carcinomas of lung
	erb-B2	Amplification	Breast, ovarian, lung, and stomach cancers
	erb-B3	Overexpression	Breast cancers
CSF-1 receptor	fms	Point mutation	Leukemia
Proteins Involved in Signal Transduction			
GTP binding	ras	Point mutations	A variety of human cancers, including lung, colon, pancreas; many leukemias
Non-receptor tyrosine kinase	abl	Translocation	Chronic myeloid leukemia; acute lymphoblastic leukemia
Nuclear Regulatory Proteins			
Transcriptional activators	myc	Translocation	Burkitt's lymphoma
	N-myc	Amplification	Neuroblastoma; small cell carcinoma of lung
	L-myc	Amplification	Small cell carcinoma of lung

From Cotran, R. S., Kumar, V., and Robbins, S. L.: Robbins Pathologic Basis of Disease. 5th ed. Philadelphia, W. B. Saunders Co., 1994. p. 260.

TRANSLOCATIONS. Chromosomal translocations are believed to activate proto-oncogenes by one of two mechanisms:

- Placement of the genes next to strong promoter/enhancer elements. In Burkitt's lymphoma the t(8;14) translocation places the c-*myc*-containing segment of chromosome 8 in close proximity to the actively expressed immunoglobulin heavy chain (IgH) gene on chromosome 14.
- Fusion of the gene with new genetic sequences. In chronic myelogenous leukemia the t(9;22) translocation relocates the c-*abl* gene from chromosome 9 to the *bcr* locus on chromosome 22. The c-*abl*-*bcr* hybrid gene codes for a chimeric protein that exhibits tyrosine kinase activity.

GENE AMPLIFICATION. Reduplication of proto-oncogenes can lead to increased expression or activity. Examples include

- N-*myc* amplification (three to 300 copies) in neuroblastomas; there seems to be a strong correlation among N-*myc* amplification, advanced stage, and poor prognosis.
- Amplification of the c-*erb* B2 gene in 30% to 40% of breast cancers; there is a correlation between c-*erb* B2 amplification and prognosis.

CANCER SUPPRESSOR GENES (p. 265)

Cancer may arise not only by activation of growth-promoting oncogenes, but also by inactivation of genes that normally suppress cell proliferation (cancer suppressor genes, or anti-oncogenes). The *Rb* gene located on chromosome 13q14 is the prototypic cancer suppressor gene. It is relevant to the pathogenesis of the childhood tumor, retinoblastoma. Forty per cent of retinoblastomas are familial; the rest are sporadic. To account for the familial and sporadic occurrence, the "two hit" hypothesis has been proposed:

- Both normal alleles of the *Rb* locus must be inactivated (two hits) for the development of retinoblastoma.
- In familial cases, children inherit one defective copy of the *Rb* gene in the germline; the other copy is normal. Retinoblastoma develops when the normal *Rb* gene is lost in the retinoblasts as a result of somatic mutation.
- In sporadic cases, both normal *Rb* alleles are lost by somatic mutation in one of the retinoblasts.
- Cancer develops when the cells become homozygous for the mutant cancer suppressor genes. Since heterozygous cells are normal, these genes are also called "recessive cancer genes."
- The *Rb* locus may be involved in the pathogenesis of several cancers, because patients with familial retinoblastoma are at greatly increased risk of developing osteosarcomas and soft tissue sarcomas.

The mechanism of action of the *Rb* gene and other putative anti-oncogenes is not clear. Their products are nuclear proteins that may act as repressors of DNA synthesis. The *Rb* gene product is a nuclear phosphoprotein that regulates cell cycle. In its active, hypophosphorylated state, it serves to prevent cells from entering the S-phase by binding to and sequestering transcription factors. When stimulated by growth factors, *Rb* protein is phosphorylated by cyclin-dependent kinases, and the resultant hyperphosphorylated *Rb* protein releases the nuclear factors essential for cell replication. With mutations in the *Rb* gene, this orderly regulation of cell cycle is disrupted. Protein products of certain oncogenic DNA viruses, e.g., human papilloma virus, can bind to *Rb* protein and prevent the normal cell regulation.

The several other cancer suppressor genes are listed in Table 7–3. Biochemical functions of NF-1 and p53 are described briefly:

- *NF-1.* This gene is mutated in neurofibromatosis type 1. It acts in concert with the *ras* oncogene because the NF-1 gene product is a GTP-ase-activating protein (GAP). In its normal form, NF-1 favors inactivation of *ras* protein, to prevent signal transduction. With mutations, this function is lost and unchecked *ras*-activation follows.

- *p53.* Mutations of p53 are the single most common genetic alteration in human cancers. They are seen in a wide variety of tumors, including carcinomas of breast, colon, and lung. Patients who inherit a mutant p53 gene are at increased risk of developing a large variety of tumors. One function of p53, which may be important in carcinogenesis, is to prevent cells damaged by mutagenic agents from proceeding to divide. The arrest in G1 phase allows cells to repair DNA damage, and if this fails the cells undergo apoptosis. Mutant p53 fails to cause G1 arrest, and hence cells with DNA damage continue to divide and the accumulating mutations lead to neoplastic transformation.

GENES THAT REGULATE APOPTOSIS (p. 270)

The prototypic gene in this group, *bcl-2,* prevents programmed cell death, or apoptosis. Overexpression of *bcl-2* presumably extends cell survival, and if the cells are genetically damaged they continue to suffer additional mutations in oncogenes and cancer suppressor genes. The most dramatic example of *bcl-2* overexpression is seen in B cell lymphomas of the follicular type. Here a t(14;18) translocation juxtaposes *bcl-2* with transcriptionally active Ig heavy chain locus, resulting in overexpression of *bcl-2.* Other genes can also influence apoptosis. The p53 was already mentioned. In addition, if c-*myc*–driven cells do not have sufficient growth factors in their environs, they undergo apoptosis, which can be prevented by *bcl-2* overexpression.

MOLECULAR BASIS OF MULTISTEP CARCINOGENESIS (p. 271)

No single genetic alteration is sufficient to induce cancers in vivo. Multiple controls exerted by all three categories of genes—oncogenes, tumor suppressor genes, and apoptosis-regulating genes—must be lost for the emergence of cancer cells. This is best exemplified by the adenoma-carcinoma sequence in the colon. In this sequence, the evolution of benign adenomas to carcinomas is marked by increasing and additive effects of mutation, affecting *ras,* APC, p53, and DCC genes. The accumulation of mutations, resulting perhaps from genetic instability of cancer cells, may be promoted by genetic changes in master "mutator genes," such as the one mapped on chromosome 2p. This gene, in its normal form, favors repair of damaged DNA.

KARYOTYPIC CHANGES IN TUMOR CELLS (p. 272)

Many human neoplasms are associated with nonrandom chromosomal abnormalities, suggesting that certain cytogenetic abnor-

Table 7-3. Tumor Suppressor Genes Involved in Human Neoplasms

Gene	Chromosomal Location	Neoplasms Associated With Somatic Mutations	Neoplasms Associated with Inherited (Germ-Line) Mutations
Rb	13q14	Retinoblastoma; osteosarcoma; carcinomas of breast, prostate, bladder, and lung	Retinoblastoma; osteosarcoma
p53	17p13.1	Most human cancers	Li-Fraumeni syndrome; carcinomas of breast and adrenal cortex; sarcomas; leukemias; brain tumors
APC	5q21	Carcinomas of colon, stomach, and pancreas	Familial adenomatous polyposis coli; carcinomas of colon
WT-1	11p13	Wilms' tumor	Wilms' tumor
DCC	18q21	Carcinomas of colon and stomach	Unknown
NF-1	17q11	Schwannomas	Neurofibromatosis type 1: neural tumors
NF-2	22q12	Schwannomas and meningiomas	Neurofibromatosis type 2: central (acoustic) schwannomas; meningiomas
VHL	3p25	Unknown	von Hippel-Lindau disease; retinal and cerebellar hemangioblastomas; renal cell carcinomas; angiomas and cysts of many visceral organs

Data from Harris, C. C., and Hollstein, M.: Clinical implication of the *p53* tumor suppressor gene. N. Engl. J. Med. 329:1318, 1993.

malities may be important and possibly primary events in neoplastic transformation. They are also of diagnostic and prognostic significance in some cases.

Three types of nonrandom chromosomal abnormalities have been detected in cancer cells:

- *Balanced translocations.* There are two important examples in this category. First, Philadelphia (Ph¹) chromosome, comprising a reciprocal balanced translocation between chromosomes 22 and (usually) 9 [t(9;22)], is noted in over 90% of cases of chronic myeloid leukemia. In the remaining cases there is molecular evidence of c-*abl/bcr* rearrangement. Second, in over 90% of cases of Burkitt's lymphoma a t(8;14) translocation involving the c-*myc* gene is present.
- *Deletions.* These are more common in solid (nonhematopoietic) tumors. Deletion of chromosome 13, band q14, is associated with retinoblastoma; the deleted sites are often near tumor suppressor genes.
- *Gene amplification.* There are two cytogenetic manifestations of amplified genes: homogeneously staining regions (HSR) on single chromosomes, and paired fragments of chromatin unattached to any chromosome (double minutes). Gene amplification associated with these cytogenetic changes is best exemplified by neuroblastomas.

BIOLOGY OF TUMOR GROWTH (p. 272)

KINETICS OF TUMOR CELL GROWTH (p. 273)

Three variables may influence tumor cell growth:

- *Doubling time of tumor cells.* The cell cycle of transformed cells has the same five phases (G_0, G_1, S, G_2, and M) noted in normal cells. The total cell cycle time for many tumors is equal to or longer than that of corresponding normal cells. Hence, progressive and rapid tumor growth cannot be ascribed to a shortening of tumor cell cycle time.
- *Growth fraction (GF).* This refers to the proportion of cells within the tumor population that are in the replicative pool (i.e., out of G_0). Most cells within clinically detectable tumors are not in the proliferative pool. Even in some rapidly growing tumors, the GF is approximately 20%. Cells leave the replicative pool by being shed, by differentiating, and by reversion to G_0. Thus, progressive tumor growth cannot be ascribed to an inordinately high GF.
- *Cell production and loss.* Tumor cell accumulation resulting in progressive growth of tumors can best be explained by an imbalance between cell production and cell loss. In some tumors (especially those with a high GF) the imbalance is large, resulting in more rapid growth than in those in which cell production exceeds cell loss by only a small margin.

Knowledge of tumor cell kinetics has the following clinical implications:

- The rate of tumor growth depends upon the growth fraction and the degree of imbalance between tumor cell production and loss. High growth fraction, as in certain lymphomas, is associated with rapid growth.
- *Susceptibility of tumors to chemotherapy.* Because most antineoplastic agents act on dividing cells, tumors with higher growth fractions are the most susceptible to anticancer agents. They are also the most rapidly growing if left untreated.

- *Latent period of tumors.* If all descendants of an originally transformed cell remained in the replicative pool, most tumors would become clinically detectable within a few months after the initiation of tumor cell growth. However, because most tumor cells leave the replicative pool, the accumulation of tumor cells is a relatively slow process. This in turn results in a latent period of several months to years before a tumor becomes clinically detectable.

TUMOR ANGIOGENESIS (p. 275)

Because tumor cells, like normal cells, need oxygen to survive, vascularization of tumors by host-derived blood vessels has a profound influence on tumor growth. In rapidly growing tumors the rate of growth sometimes exceeds the pace of vascularization, causing areas of ischemic necrosis. Vascularization of tumors is effected by the release of tumor-associated angiogenic factors derived from tumor cells or inflammatory cells (e.g., macrophages) that enter the tumors. Such factors include TGF-α, TGF-β, EGF, PDGF, vascular-endothelial growth factor (VEGF), and heparin-binding fibroblast growth factors (FGFs). The last named are best characterized and can promote all steps of angiogenesis. By preventing the release of angiogenic factors or neutralization of the released factors, it may be possible to retard tumor growth.

TUMOR PROGRESSION AND HETEROGENEITY (p. 275)

Tumor progression refers to the phenomenon whereby tumors become progressively more aggressive and acquire greater malignant potential. Progression is related to sequential appearance within the tumor of cells that differ with respect to invasiveness, rate of growth, ability to form metastases, evade immunosurveillance, and several other attributes. Thus, a clinically detectable tumor, although monoclonal, is usually made up of phenotypically and genetically heterogeneous cells. The heterogeneity is believed to result from genetic instability of tumor cells, which are subject to a high rate of random mutations. Alternatively, the emergence of heterogeneous subclones within tumor cells may be favored by mutation in certain master "mutator genes," mentioned earlier. Tumor cell heterogeneity and progression begin well before clinical detection of tumors (latent period) and continue thereafter.

MECHANISMS OF INVASION AND METASTASIS (p. 276)

The sequential steps involved in invasion and metastasis are depicted in Figure 7–2. This sequence may be interrupted at any stage by host factors. Experimental studies in animals indicate that cells within a primary tumor are heterogeneous with respect to metastatic abilities. Only certain subclones can complete all the steps outlined in Figure 7–2 and are able to form secondary tumors at distant sites.

Invasion of Extracellular Matrix (ECM) (p. 276)

Tumor cells must attach to, degrade, and penetrate the ECM at several steps of the metastatic cascade. Invasion of ECM can be resolved into the following four steps:

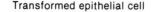

Transformed epithelial cell

↓

Clonal expansion, growth, diversification

↓

Metastatic subclone

↓

Adhesion to and invasion
of basement membrane

↓

Passage through
extracellular matrix

↓

Intravasation into blood
vessels or lymphatics

↓

Interaction with host
lymphoid cells

↓

Tumor cell embolus

↓

Adhesion to basement membrane
of blood vessels at distant site

↓

Extravasation
into tissue

↓

Metastatic deposit

Figure 7–2. The metastatic cascade. A schematic illustration of the sequential steps involved in the hematogenous spread of a tumor. (Modified from Cotran, R. S., Kumar, V., and Robbins, S. L.: Robbins Pathologic Basis of Disease. 5th ed. Philadelphia, W. B. Saunders Co., 1994, p. 277.)

- *Detachment of tumor cells from each other.* Tumor cells remain attached to each other by several adhesion molecules, including a family of glycoproteins called cadherins. In several carcinomas, there is down-regulation of epithelial (E) cadherins, presumably reducing the cohesiveness of tumor cells.
- *Attachment to matrix components.* Tumor cells bind to laminin and fibronectin via cell surface receptors. Receptor-mediated binding is an important step in invasion.
- *Degradation of ECM.* After attachment tumor cells secrete proteolytic enzymes that degrade the matrix components and create passageways for migration. In experimental systems the ability of tumor cell variants to degrade ECM can be correlated with their metastatic ability. Enzymes that are important in this respect are type IV collagenases (cleave basement membrane collagen), cathepsin D (a cysteine proteinase), and urokinase-

type plasminogen activator. These enzymes act on a large variety of substrates, including laminin, fibronectin, and protein cores of proteoglycans.

- *Migration of tumor cells.* Factors that favor tumor cell migration in the passageways created by the degradation of ECM are poorly understood. Implicated in this process are autocrine motility factors and cleavage products of the ECM.

Vascular Dissemination and Homing of Tumor Cells (p. 279)

In the circulation, tumor cells form emboli by aggregation and by adhering to circulating leukocytes, particularly platelets. Aggregated tumor cells are afforded some protection from the antitumor host effector cells.

The site where tumor cell emboli lodge and produce secondary growths is influenced by several factors:

- *Vascular and lymphatic drainage from the site of the primary tumor, as discussed earlier.*
- *Interaction of tumor cells with organ-specific receptors.* For example, certain tumor cells have high levels of an adhesion molecule, CD44, that binds to high endothelial venules in lymph nodes, thereby facilitating nodal metastases.
- *The microenvironment of the organ or site; e.g., a tissue rich in protease inhibitors might be resistant to penetration by tumor cells.*

CARCINOGENIC AGENTS (p. 280)

Radiation and many chemicals are known to be carcinogenic in animals and man, and suspicion grows ever stronger that the same is true for viruses.

CHEMICAL CARCINOGENESIS (p. 280)

Neoplastic transformation brought about by chemicals is a dynamic multistep process. It can be broadly divided into two stages: initiation and promotion.

- *Initiation.* Refers to the induction of certain irreversible changes (mutations) in the genome of cells. Initiated cells are not transformed cells; they do not have growth autonomy or unique phenotypic characteristics. However, unlike normal cells, they give rise to tumors when appropriately stimulated by promoting agents.
- *Promotion.* The process of tumor induction in previously initiated cells by chemicals referred to as promoters. The effect of promoters is relatively short-lived and reversible; they do not affect DNA and are nontumorigenic by themselves.

Mechanisms of Initiation (p. 281)

The vast majority of chemicals are referred to as procarcinogens because they require metabolic activation in vivo to produce ultimate carcinogens. Only a few alkylating and acylating agents are direct-acting carcinogens. The activation of procarcinogens in most cases is dependent on microsomal cytochrome P-450 oxygenases. Several factors such as age, sex, and hormones modulate the activity of microsomal enzymes and hence the potency of procarcinogens.

MOLECULAR TARGETS OF CHEMICAL CARCINOGENS. All direct-acting and ultimate carcinogens are highly reactive electrophilic compounds that can react with nucleophilic sites in the cell.

DNA is the primary and most important target of chemical carcinogens; thus, chemical carcinogens are mutagens that induce mutations in proto-oncogenes, cancer suppressor genes, and, possibly, genes that regulate apoptosis. As an example, the *ras* oncogene is frequently mutated in chemically induced tumors in rodents. Because specific sequences are targeted by different chemicals, an analysis of the mutations found in human tumors may allow linkage to specific carcinogens. However, carcinogen-induced changes in DNA do not necessarily lead to the initiation of carcinogenesis, since the damage to DNA can be repaired by cellular enzymes. If the ability to repair DNA is impaired, however, as in xeroderma pigmentosum, the risk of cancer development significantly increases.

Because chemical carcinogens are mutagenic, a simple in vitro test for carcinogenicity is the *Ames test,* utilizing the ability of potential carcinogens to induce mutations in selected strains of the bacterium *Salmonella typhimurium.*

Promotion of Carcinogenesis (p. 283)

As discussed earlier, the expression of the initial mutagenic event in most instances requires subsequent exposure to promoters, which can include various hormones, drugs, phenols, and phorbol esters.

Phorbol esters are the most widely used promoters in experimental systems; they are not mutagenic and seem to exert their effects by epigenetic mechanisms.

Tetradecanoyl phorbol acetate (TPA), a commonly used promoter, is a powerful activator of protein kinase C, an enzyme that is a key element in the signal transduction pathways. Activation of protein kinase C leads to a series of phosphorylation reactions that ultimately affect cell proliferation and differentiation. Thus, promoters appear to be involved in the clonal expansion and aberrant differentiation of initiated cells.

Carcinogenic Chemicals (p. 283)

- *Alkylating agents.* These include direct-acting agents, such as cyclophosphamide and busulfan, used in the treatment of cancer, as well as immunosuppressants. Patients receiving such therapy are at increased risk of developing cancer.
- *Aromatic hydrocarbons.* These are present in cigarette smoke and may therefore be relevant to the pathogenesis of lung cancer.
- *Azo dyes.* Beta-naphthylamine, an aniline dye used in the rubber industries, was in the past responsible for bladder cancers in exposed workers.
- *Naturally occurring carcinogens.* Aflatoxin B$_1$, produced by the fungus *Aspergillus flavus,* is a potent hepatocarcinogen in animals and is believed to be a factor in the high incidence of liver cancer in Africa. The fungus grows on grains and peanuts, and the toxin is ingested with contaminated foods.
- *Nitrosamines and amides.* These can be synthesized in the GI tract from ingested nitrites or derived from digested proteins, and may contribute to the induction of gastric cancer.
- *Miscellaneous agents.* Asbestos, vinyl chloride, and metals such as nickel are carcinogenic. They predispose exposed industrial

workers to the development of cancer. Saccharin and cyclamates have been implicated without definite proof as promoters of bladder cancer in humans. Hormones such as estrogens may play a role in the causation of endometrial cancer.

RADIATION CARCINOGENESIS (p. 284)

Radiant energy in the form of ultraviolet (UV) rays and ionizing radiations can cause cancer.

ULTRAVIOLET RAYS. Natural UV radiation, especially UVB, derived from the sun can cause skin cancer. At greatest risk are fair-skinned people who live in locales that receive a great deal of sunlight. Thus, carcinomas and melanomas of the exposed skin are particularly common in Australia and New Zealand. Two mechanisms may be involved in induction of cancer by UV rays:

- Damage to DNA by the formation of pyrimidine dimers.
- Immunosuppression, demonstrated only in animal models.

IONIZING RADIATION. Electromagnetic and particulate radiations are all carcinogenic. Evidence for the carcinogenicity of ionizing radiation comes from several sources:

- Miners of radioactive ores have an increased risk of lung cancer.
- The incidence of certain forms of leukemia is greatly increased in survivors of atomic bombs in Japan.
- Therapeutic radiation to the neck in children has been associated with the later development of thyroid cancer.

In man there is a hierarchy of vulnerability to radiation-induced neoplasms:

- Most common are myeloid leukemias, followed by thyroid cancer in children.
- Cancers of the breast and lung are less commonly radiation induced.
- Skin, bone, and gut are the least susceptible to radiation carcinogenesis.

The ability of ionizing radiations to cause cancer lies in their ability to induce mutations. Such mutations may result from a direct effect of the radiant energy or an indirect effect mediated by the generation of free radicals from water or oxygen. Particulate radiations (such as alpha particles and neutrons) are more carcinogenic than electromagnetic radiation (x-rays, gamma rays).

DNA REPAIR DEFECTS. Four autosomal recessive conditions: xeroderma pigmentosum, Bloom's syndrome, Fanconi's anemia, and ataxia telangiectasia are characterized by defects in DNA repair and resultant predisposition to cancer when exposed to DNA-damaging agents, including radiant energy. Best characterized is xeroderma pigmentosum, in which a defect in ability to repair DNA damage caused by UV light predisposes the patients to a high incidence of skin cancers. Xeroderma pigmentosum is genetically heterogeneous, with at least seven variants caused by mutations in different genes involved in excision repair of nucleotides.

VIRAL CARCINOGENESIS (p. 286)

A variety of DNA and RNA viruses are known to cause cancer in animals, and some are implicated in human cancer.

DNA Viruses (p. 286)

Many cause tumors in animals. Three have associations with human tumors: HPV, EBV, and HBV.

HUMAN PAPILLOMA VIRUS (HPV). Approximately 65 genetically distinct types have been identified. Some types (e.g., 1, 2, 4, and 7) definitely cause benign squamous papillomas (warts) in humans. Evidence supporting the role of HPV in human cancers is as follows:

• Squamous cell cancers of the uterine cervix contain HPV types 16 or 18 in over 90% of cases. These viruses are also contained in presumed precursors (e.g., carcinoma in situ) of the invasive cancer.
• Genital warts with low malignant potential are caused by distinct HPV types ("low risk" types), e.g., HPV-6 and HPV-11.
• Molecular analysis of HPV-associated cervical carcinomas reveals clonal integration of the viral genomes in the host cell DNA. During integration, the viral DNA is interrupted in a manner that leads to over-expression of the E6 and E7 viral proteins. These proteins have the potential to transform cells by binding to and inhibiting the functions of *Rb* and p53 tumor suppressor gene products.

EPSTEIN-BARR VIRUS (EBV). This member of the herpes family is associated with two human cancers: Burkitt's lymphoma and nasopharyngeal cancer:

• *Burkitt's lymphoma* is a tumor of B lymphocytes that is consistently associated with a t(8;14) translocation. In certain parts of Africa Burkitt's lymphoma is endemic, and virtually all these patient's tumor cells carry the EBV genome. However, it is unlikely that EBV alone can cause Burkitt's lymphoma. In normal individuals, EBV-driven B-cell proliferation is self-limited and controlled. In patients with subtle or overt immune dysregulation, EBV causes sustained B-cell proliferation. Such B cells acquire additional mutations and sometimes the translocation t(8;14), and eventually become autonomous.
• *Nasopharyngeal cancer* is endemic in southern China and some other locales, and the EBV genome is found in all such tumors. As in Burkitt's lymphoma, EBV probably acts in concert with other factors.

HEPATITIS B VIRUS (HBV). There is a close association between HBV infection and liver cancer in many parts of the world. In Taiwan, the risk of developing hepatic cancer is increased 200-fold in those infected with HBV. Cofactors other than HBV are also believed to play roles in the genesis of liver cancer.

The mechanism by which HBV causes cancer is probably multifactorial:

• By causing hepatocellular injury and resulting regenerative hyperplasia, the pool of mitotically active cells subject to mutational damage by environmental agents such as aflatoxins is increased.
• HBV encodes a regulatory element called HBx, which seems to cause transcriptional activation of several proto-oncogenes.
• HBx protein also activates protein kinase C, and thus mimics the action of tumor promoter TPA.

RNA Oncogenic Viruses (p. 289)

All oncogenic RNA viruses are retroviruses. Their genome contains three sets of genes: (1) *gag,* encoding viral coat proteins; (2) *pol,* encoding the reverse transcriptase; and (3) *env,* encoding envelope glycoproteins.

ACUTE TRANSFORMING RETROVIRUSES. These include type C viruses that cause rapid induction of tumors in animals.

- The transforming sequences of these viruses are called viral oncogenes or v-*onc.*
- The v-*onc* genes are derived from *proto-oncogenes.*
- Incorporation of proto-oncogenes into the viral genome (transduction) is associated with loss of the viral genes necessary for replication; therefore, acute transforming viruses are replication defective.

SLOW TRANSFORMING RETROVIRUSES

- These viruses do not contain v-*onc* and are replication competent. They cause transformation slowly.
- Their mechanism of transformation is referred to as *insertional mutagenesis.* The proviral DNA is always integrated near a proto-oncogene. Retroviral promoters cause increased expression of the adjacent proto-oncogene, thereby converting it into a cellular oncogene (c-*onc*).

Only one human retrovirus, HTLV-1, has been firmly implicated in carcinogenesis.

HUMAN T-CELL LEUKEMIA VIRUS TYPE 1 (HTLV-1)

- This virus has a strong tropism for CD4+ T cells and is believed to cause a leukemia/lymphoma of these lymphocytes.
- HTLV-1-associated leukemia/lymphoma is endemic in parts of Japan and the Caribbean basin. It is sporadic elsewhere, including the United States.
- HTLV-1 proviral DNA is detected in DNA of leukemic T cells. The integration shows a clonal pattern.
- The mechanism of HTLV-1-induced transformation is not clear; HTLV-1 does not contain a v-*onc,* nor is it found integrated near a proto-oncogene.
- The HTLV-1 genome contains a unique segment referred to as the *tax* region. The proteins encoded by the *tax* gene activate the transcription of the T cell growth factor IL-2 and its receptor IL-2R, thus setting up an autocrine loop. The resulting polyclonal expansion of T cells is at increased risk of developing additional mutations to give rise eventually to a monoclonal T cell tumor.

HOST DEFENSE AGAINST TUMORS (p. 290)

TUMOR ANTIGENS

These can be classified into two groups: tumor-specific antigens (TSAs), present only on tumor cells, and tumor-associated antigens (TAAs), present on tumor cells and also on some normal cells.

Tumor-specific antigens are readily demonstrated in chemically induced tumors in rodents and some human tumors. TSAs are composed of tumor-derived peptides that are presented on the cell surface by MHC class I molecules and recognized by

CD8+ T cells. There are three mechanisms by which TSAs may be formed. Some TSAs are derived from mutant forms of normal cellular proteins. Peptides generated from the mutant proteins, when presented on the cell surface by class I molecules, are recognized as nonself by CD8+ T cells; in other cases, mutations in cellular proteins alter them in such a manner that they can give rise to peptides having the structural requirements for binding to class I molecules; finally, some TSAs are generated by gene activation, i.e., during transformation a transcriptionally silent gene is activated whose protein product gives rise to an immunogenic peptide. The human melanoma-associated antigen-1 (MAGE-1) is an example of the last category. It is expressed not only in melanomas (40%) but also in 20% of breast cancers and 30% of small cell lung cancers. Mutations of proto-oncogene and tumor-suppressor genes can also give rise to peptides that can evoke a T cell response.

Tumor-associated antigens can be grouped into three categories:

- Tumor-associated carbohydrate antigens—representing abnormally glycosylated forms of several different glycoproteins.
- Oncofetal antigens—whose expression is derepressed in tumor cells, e.g., α-fetoprotein.
- Differentiation-specific antigens—that are expressed on the specific state of differentiation at which the tumor cell is arrested, e.g., CD10 (CALLA) antigen on tumors of B-progenitor cells.

These antigens are not targets of host immune response, but their detection is of value in the diagnosis of some tumors, and they can be targeted for immunotherapy.

IMMUNOSURVEILLANCE (p. 293)

A putative immunosurveillance against tumors has been hypothesized. Evidence for its existence consists of

- Increased frequency of cancers in patients with congenital or acquired (drug-induced, AIDS) immunodeficiency.
- Increased susceptibility to EBV infections and EBV-associated lymphoma in boys with X-linked immunodeficiency.

Tumors may escape immunosurveillance by

- Selective outgrowth of antigen-negative variants.
- Loss or reduced expression of histocompatibility antigens, thus becoming less susceptible to cytotoxic T-cell lysis.
- Tumor-induced immunosuppression.

Arguments against immunosurveillance are as follows:

- Tumors that develop in immunodeficient patients are mainly lymphomas, which could be the consequence of an abnormal immune system rather than failure of immunosurveillance.

CLINICAL FEATURES OF TUMORS (p. 294)
LOCAL AND HORMONAL EFFECTS (p. 294)

- Related to location. Intracranial tumors (e.g., pituitary adenoma) can expand and destroy the remaining pituitary gland, giving rise to an endocrine disorder; tumors of the GI tract

may cause obstruction of the bowel, or may ulcerate and cause bleeding.
• Hormone production. Tumors of endocrine glands may elaborate hormones; this is more common in benign than in malignant tumors.

CANCER CACHEXIA (p. 295)

Loss of body fat, wasting, and profound weakness are referred to as cancer cachexia. The basis of cachexia is multifactorial:

• Loss of appetite.
• Poorly understood metabolic changes that lead to reduced synthesis and storage of fat and increased mobilization of fatty acids from adipocytes.
• Production of cachectin (TNF-α) by activated macrophages, and possibly other humoral factors, can mimic some of the metabolic effects and hence may be involved.

PARANEOPLASTIC SYNDROMES (p. 295)

Definition Symptoms not directly related to the spread of the tumor or elaboration of hormones indigenous to the tissue from which the tumor arose. Paraneoplastic syndromes may be the earliest clinical manifestations of a neoplasm and may mimic distant spread. The most common syndromes are

• *Endocrinopathies.* Some nonendocrine cancers produce hormones or hormone-like factors (ectopic hormone production); e.g., certain cancers of the lung (small cell type) produce *Cushing's syndrome* by elaborating ACTH or related peptides.
• *Hypercalcemia,* which may occur owing to resorption of bone resulting from the elaboration of PTH-like peptides (PTH-related protein) or in some cases of TGF-α, by certain tumors (e.g., squamous cell cancer of the lung, T-cell leukemias/lymphomas).

Cancer-associated hypercalcemia also results from osteolysis induced by bony metastases; this, however, is not to be considered a paraneoplastic syndrome.

• *Acanthosis nigricans.* The acquired (nongenetic) form of this verrucous pigmented lesion of the skin is frequently associated with visceral malignancy.
• *Clubbing of fingers and hypertrophic osteoarthropathy* are associated with lung cancers.
• *Thrombotic diatheses* resulting from production of thromboplastic substance by tumor cells may manifest as disseminated intravascular coagulation or as vegetations on heart valves (nonbacterial thrombotic endocarditis).

GRADING AND STAGING OF TUMORS (p. 297)

The grade and stage of malignant neoplasms provide a semiquantitative estimate of the clinical gravity of a tumor:

• *Grading* is based on the degree of differentiation and the number of mitoses within the tumor. Cancers are classified as grades I to IV with increasing anaplasia. In general, higher-grade tumors are more aggressive than lower-grade tumors. Grading is imperfect since (1) different parts of the same tumor may display different degrees of differentiation and (2) the grade of tumor may change as the tumor grows.

- *Staging* is based on the anatomic extent of the tumor. Relevant to staging are the size of the primary tumor and the extent of local and distant spread. Two methods of staging are in current use: the TNM (*tumor, node, metastases*) and the AJC (*American Joint Committee*) systems. Both systems assign to higher stages those tumors that are larger, locally invasive, and metastatic.

Both histologic grading and clinical staging are valuable for prognostication and for planning therapy, although staging has proved to be of greater clinical value.

LABORATORY DIAGNOSIS OF CANCER (p. 297)

Histologic and Cytologic Methods

Histologic examination is the most important method of diagnosis. Proper histologic diagnosis is greatly aided by

- Availability of all relevant clinical data.
- Adequate preservation and sampling of the specimen.
- In some cases, examination of the frozen specimen to detect cell surface receptors.

In addition to the usual fixed and paraffin-embedded sections, quick-frozen sections are employed to obtain a rapid diagnosis while the patient is still under anesthesia.

FINE-NEEDLE ASPIRATION. This involves aspiration of cells and fluids from tumors/masses that occur in readily palpable sites (e.g., breast, thyroid, lymph nodes). The aspirated cells are smeared, stained, and examined.

CYTOLOGIC (PAPANICOLAOU) SMEARS. These involve examination of cancer cells that are readily shed. Exfoliative cytology is used most commonly in the diagnosis of dysplasia, carcinoma in situ, and invasive cancer of the uterine cervix and also tumors of the stomach, bronchus, and urinary bladder.

Interpretation is based chiefly on changes in the appearance of individual cells. In the hands of experts, false-positive results are uncommon, but false-negatives do occur because of sampling errors. When possible, cytologic diagnosis must be confirmed by biopsy before therapeutic intervention.

IMMUNOCYTOCHEMISTRY. This involves detection of cell products or surface markers by monoclonal antibodies. The binding of antibodies can be revealed by fluorescent labels or chemical reactions that result in the generation of a colored product. This technique is useful in the diagnosis of several carcinomas, sarcomas, and gliomas, since they possess characteristic intermediate filaments. Products of certain tumor suppressor genes (e.g., p53) and oncogenes (e.g., c-*erb* B2) can also be detected cytochemically.

DNA PROBE ANALYSIS. Currently used most extensively in the diagnosis of lymphoid neoplasms, since such tumors are associated with clonal rearrangements of T- and B-cell antigen receptor genes. Detection of oncogenes such as N-*myc* is also valuable in assessing the prognosis of certain tumors. Diagnosis of chronic myeloid leukemia can be made by detection of the *bcr-c-abl* fusion gene product, even in the absence of the Ph1 chromosome.

FLOW CYTOMETRY. Measurement of the DNA content of tumor cells by flow cytometry. With several tumors there is a relationship between abnormal DNA content and prognosis.

Flow cytometric detection of cell surface antigens is of value in the diagnosis of leukemias and lymphomas.

TUMOR MARKERS. Tumor-derived or -associated molecules that can be detected in blood or other body fluids. They are not primary methods of diagnosis but rather adjuncts to the diagnosis. They may also be of value in determining the response to therapy. Examples of tumor markers follow:

- *Carcinoembryonic antigen* (CEA), normally produced by fetal gut, liver, and pancreas, may be elaborated by cancers of the colon, pancreas, stomach, and breast. Less consistently, the levels are elevated in non-neoplastic conditions (e.g., alcoholic cirrhosis, hepatitis, and ulcerative colitis). This antigen is of value in estimating tumor burden in colorectal cancer and in detecting recurrences after surgery.
- *Alpha-fetoprotein* (AFP) is normally produced by fetal yolk sac and liver. Markedly elevated levels are noted in cancers of the liver and testicular germ cells. Non-neoplastic conditions such as cirrhosis and hepatitis are also associated with less marked elevations of AFP. Measurements of AFP levels are useful in indicating the presence of liver or testicular cancer, and in assessing recurrence and response to therapy.

CHAPTER EIGHT

Infectious Diseases

In the U.S., serious infections affect persons immunosuppressed by acquired immunodeficiency syndrome (AIDS), chronic disease, or anticancer drugs. Infectious diseases kill more than 10 million persons each year in developing countries, where mostly children die from respiratory and diarrheal infections caused by common viruses and bacteria.

Koch's postulates link a specific microorganism to a specific disease.

To understand the mechanisms of infectious disease, one must consider (1) virulence properties of the organism and (2) the host response to the infectious agent.

CATEGORIES OF INFECTIOUS AGENTS (p. 306)

VIRUSES

- Are obligate intracellular organisms.
- Contain DNA or RNA within a cylindrical or spherical protein coat or capsid, which may be surrounded by a lipid bilayer (envelope).
- Cause acute illness (e.g., colds, influenza epidemics), lifelong latency and long-term reactivation (e.g., herpesviruses), or chronic disease (e.g., HBV, HIV).

BACTERIOPHAGES AND PLASMIDS

- Are mobile genetic elements that encode bacterial virulence factors (e.g., adhesins, toxins, or antibiotic resistance).

BACTERIA

- Lack nuclei but have rigid cell walls containing two phospholipid bilayers (gram-negative species) or a single bilayer (gram-positive bacteria).
- Are major causes of severe infectious disease.
- Grow extracellularly (e.g., *Pneumococcus*) or intracellularly (e.g., *Mycobacterium tuberculosis*).

Normal persons carry 10^{12} bacteria on the skin, including *Staphylococcus epidermidis* and *Propionibacterium acnes*, and 10^{14} bacteria in the gastrointestinal tract, 99.9% of which are anaerobic.

CHLAMYDIAE, RICKETTSIAE, AND MYCOPLASMAS

- Are similar to bacteria but lack certain structures (a cell wall–mycoplasma) or metabolic capabilities (ATP synthesis-chlamydia).
- Chlamydiae cause genitourinary infections, conjunctivitis, and/or respiratory infections of newborns.
- Rickettsia are transmitted by insect vectors, including lice (epidemic typhus), ticks (Rocky Mountain spotted fever [RMSF], Q fever), and mites (scrub typhus) and cause a hemorrhagic vasculitis, pneumonia, hepatitis (Q fever), or encephalitis (RMSF).
- Mycoplasma bind to the surface of epithelial cells and cause atypical pneumonia or nongonococcal urethritis.

FUNGI

- Have thick, ergosterol-containing cell walls and grow in humans as budding yeast cells and slender tubes (hyphae).
- In otherwise healthy persons, fungi produce superficial infections (e.g., "athlete's foot" caused by tinea), and also abscesses (e.g., sporotrichosis) or granulomas (e.g., *Coccidioides, Histoplasma,* and *Blastomyces*).
- In immunocompromised hosts, opportunistic fungi (e.g., *Candida, Aspergillus,* and *Mucor*) cause systemic infections characterized by tissue necrosis, hemorrhage, and vascular occlusion.
- In AIDS patients, the opportunistic fungus-like organism *Pneumocystis carinii* causes a lethal pneumonia.

PROTOZOA

- Are single cells with a nucleus, a pliable plasma membrane, and complex cytoplasmic organelles.
- *Trichomonas vaginalis* is transmitted sexually.

  Intestinal protozoa (e.g., *Entamoeba histolytica* and *Giardia lamblia*) are infective when swallowed.
  Blood-borne protozoa (e.g., *Plasmodium* spp. and *Leishmania* spp.) are transmitted by blood-sucking insects.

HELMINTHS

- Are highly differentiated multicellular organisms with complex life cycles.
- Cause disease in proportion to the number of infecting organisms.

  Roundworms (nematodes) infect the intestines (e.g., *Ascaris,* hookworms, and *Strongyloides*) or tissues (e.g., filariae and *Trichinella*).
  Flatworms (cestodes) are segmented tapeworms in the intestines or form tissue cysts (e.g., cysticerci and hydatids).
  The most important fluke (trematode) is the blood-dwelling schistosome.

ECTOPARASITES

- Are arthropods (e.g., lice, ticks, bedbugs, fleas) that attach to and live on the skin.

- May be vectors for other pathogens (e.g., Lyme disease spirochetes transmitted by ticks).

HOST BARRIERS TO INFECTION (p. 311)

Respiratory tract: Mucociliary blanket in upper airways and macrophages and neutrophils within alveoli.

Gastrointestinal tract: Stomach acidity, the viscous mucus layer covering the gut, lytic pancreatic enzymes and bile detergents, secreted IgA antibodies, and competition with commensal bacteria in the colon.

Urogenital tract: Flushing of the urinary tract multiple times each day and vaginal acidity secondary to hyperinfection with lactobacilli.

Skin: Dryness and constant shedding of impermeable, keratinized epithelium and competition from commensal bacteria.

HOW MICROORGANISMS CAUSE DISEASE (p. 315)

Infectious agents damage tissues directly by entering cells, releasing toxins, or damaging blood vessels. Microbes also induce host cellular responses that cause additional tissue damage, including suppuration, scarring, and hypersensitivity reactions.

VIRAL INJURY TO HOST TISSUES (p. 315)

- Viruses enter host cells by (1) binding to host cell surface proteins (e.g., HIV to CD4 on helper lymphocytes), (2) translocation into the cytosol from the plasma membrane or endosomal membranes, and (3) replication via virus-specific enzymes.
- Viral infection can be abortive, latent (e.g., varicella zoster virus), or persistent (e.g., hepatitis B).
- Viruses kill host cells by inhibiting host cell DNA, RNA, or protein synthesis (e.g., poliovirus), by damaging the plasma membrane (e.g., HIV), by lysing cells (e.g., rhinoviruses and influenza viruses), and by inducing a host immune response to virus-infected cells (e.g., hepatitis B virus).

BACTERIAL INJURY TO HOST TISSUES (p. 316)

- Depends upon their ability to deliver toxins (e.g., *Vibrio cholerae*) or to adhere to host cells and enter them (e.g., *Listeria monocytogenes*).
- Bacterial adhesins include filamentous pili (e.g., *Escherichia coli* and *N. gonorrhoeae*) and hemagglutinins (e.g., *Salmonella*) that determine to which host cells the microbes will attach (bacterial tropism).
- Bacteria may reproduce within the phagolysomes (e.g., *Mycobacteria* and *Legionella*) or cytosol (e.g., *Shigella*).
- Bacterial endotoxin is a lipopolysaccharide that induces fever via host lymphokines, including tumor necrosis factor (TNF) and interleukin-1 (IL-1).
- Bacterial exotoxins are composed of a binding part and a catalytic part, which ADP-ribosylates and inactivates host proteins (e.g., diphtheria or cholera toxins) or degrades host proteins (e.g., botulinum toxin).

IMMUNE EVASION BY MICROBES (p. 319)

Microbes avoid the host immune response by

- Remaining inaccessible within the lumen of the small intestine (e.g., toxin-producing *Clostridium difficile*) or rapidly entering host cells (e.g., malaria sporozoites into the liver).
- Producing a capsule that covers antigens and prevents phagocytosis (e.g., *Streptococcus pneumoniae*).
- Changing their surface antigens (e.g., rhinoviruses, *N. gonorrhoeae*, and African trypanosomes).
- Infecting lymphocytes (e.g., HIV and EBV) and damaging the host immune system.

SPECIAL TECHNIQUES FOR DIAGNOSING INFECTIOUS AGENTS (p. 319)

Some infectious agents can be directly observed in hematoxylin and eosin-stained sections (e.g., the inclusion bodies formed by CMV and herpesvirus; bacterial clumps, which usually stain blue; *Candida* and *Mucor*, among the fungi; most protozoans; and all helminths). However, many infectious agents are best visualized after special stains that identify organisms based upon particular characteristics of their cell walls or coat (Table 8–1). In addition, cultures of lesional tissues are performed to speciate organisms and determine drug sensitivity.

SPECTRUM OF INFLAMMATORY RESPONSES TO INFECTION (p. 320)

In contrast to the vast molecular diversity of microorganisms, the tissue responses to these agents are limited to five microscopic patterns.

SUPPURATIVE INFLAMMATION (NEUTROPHILS)

- Is caused by "pyogenic" bacteria, mostly extracellular gram-positive cocci and gram-negative rods.
- Is secondary to increased vascular permeability and leukotaxis of neutrophils attracted by bacterial peptides, which contain *N*-formyl methionine residues.

Table 1. Special Techniques for Diagnosing Infectious Agents

Gram stain	Most bacteria
Acid-fast stain	Mycobacteria, Nocardia (modified)
Silver stains	Fungi, Legionella, Pneumocystis
Periodic acid-Schiff	Fungi, amebae
Mucicarmine	Cryptococci
Giemsa	Campylobacteria, Leishmania, malaria
Antibody probes	Viruses, rickettsiae
Culture	All classes
DNA probes	Viruses, bacteria, protozoa

From Cotran, R. S., Kumar, V., and Robbins, S. L.: Robbins Pathologic Basis of Disease. 5th ed. Philadelphia, W. B. Saunders Co., 1994, p. 320.

- The sizes of exudative lesions vary from tiny microabscesses formed during sepsis to diffuse involvement of the meninges (e.g., *Haemophilus influenzae*) or entire lobes of the lung (e.g., *Streptococcus pneumoniae*).

MONONUCLEAR INFLAMMATION

- Is induced by viruses, intracellular bacteria, spirochetes, intracellular parasites, or helminths.
- Includes mostly lymphocytes (e.g., chancres of primary syphilis) or macrophages (e.g., granulomas of mycobacteria), depending upon the characteristics of the organism and the host.

CYTOPATHIC-CYTOPROLIFERATIVE INFLAMMATION

- Is characterized by virus-mediated damage to individual host cells in the absence of host inflammatory response.
- May show inclusion bodies (e.g., CMV), polykaryons (e.g., measles viruses), blisters (e.g., herpesviruses), and warty changes (e.g., papilloma viruses).

NECROTIZING INFLAMMATION

- Is caused by uncontrolled viral infection (e.g., fulminant hepatitis B infection), secreted bacterial toxins (e.g., those of *Clostridium perfringens*), or contact-mediated cytolysis of host cells by protozoa (e.g., *Entamoeba histolytica*).
- Results in severe tissue necrosis in the absence of inflammatory infiltrates.

CHRONIC INFLAMMATION AND SCARRING

- Are caused by certain acute infections (e.g., gonococcal salpingitis) or chronic infections (e.g., schistosomiasis).
- May be severe despite a paucity of organisms present (e.g., *Mycobacterium tuberculosis*).

THE PATTERN OF INFLAMMATION

- May be mixed because of multiple simultaneous infections (e.g., AIDS pneumonitis with CMV, *Pneumocystis*, and mycobacteria).
- May vary based upon host response (e.g., mostly lymphocytes in tuberculoid leprosy and mostly macrophages in lepromatous leprosy).
- Should be consistent with the organisms cultured or identified by microscopy.

RESPIRATORY INFECTIONS (p. 322)

Viral respiratory disorders are the most frequent and least preventable of all infectious diseases and range in severity from the discomforting but self-limited common cold to life-threatening pneumonias.

RHINOVIRUSES (COMMON COLD)

- Are unencapsulated, icosohedral viruses that contain single-stranded RNA.

- Bind to ICAM-1 on epithelial cells of the upper respiratory tract and induce mucus secretion via bradykinin release.
- Induce serotype-specific IgG and IgA antibodies, which prevent reinfection with the same rhinovirus but not with other serotypes.

INFLUENZA VIRUSES

- Have eight single-stranded RNAs, each bound by a nucleoprotein that determines the type of influenza virus (A, B, or C).
- Have envelopes containing a hemagglutinin and neuraminidase, which project outward and determine the subtype of the virus (H1–H3; N1 or N2).
- Clearance of the primary influenza virus infection occurs when cytotoxic T cells kill virus-infected cells.
- Host antibodies to the hemagglutinin and neuraminidase prevent future infection with that flu virus.
- Remarkably, a single subtype of influenza virus A is present throughout the world at a given time.
- Epidemics of flu occur through mutations of the hemagglutinin and neuraminidase (*antigenic drift*) that allow the virus to escape most, not necessarily all, host antibodies.
- The pandemic of influenza in 1918 that killed 20 million people occurred when both the hemagglutinin and the neuraminidase were replaced, making all individuals susceptible to the new influenza virus (*antigenic shift*).
- Effects nasal channels, sinuses, eustachian tubes, tonsils, and bronchioles.
- Produces mucosal hyperemia and swelling with a predominantly lymphomonocytic and plasmacytic infiltration of the submucosa accompanied by overproduction of mucus secretions.

A major complication of viral damage to bronchial epithelium is bacterial superinfection (e.g., *Pneumococcus*, *Staphylococcus*, and *Haemophilus*).

HAEMOPHILUS INFLUENZAE (p. 323)

- Is a pleomorphic gram-negative organism, which is a major cause of life-threatening epiglottitis, laryngotracheobronchitis, and meningitis in young children.
- A polyribose capsule determines serotype and prevents opsonization by complement and phagocytosis by host cells.
- Children are vaccinated against the capsular polysaccharide b.
- Lesions feature dense, fibrin-rich exudates of polymorphonuclear cells.

TUBERCULOSIS (p. 324 and p. 700)

- Is caused by the aerobic, non–spore-forming, nonmotile bacillus *M. tuberculosis*, which has a waxy coat that stains red with acid-fast stains.
- Is the most important infectious disease, killing about 3 million persons each year.
- The vaccine BCG (bacille Calmette-Guérin) is the most widely used vaccine worldwide and the least effective (0 to 80% protective immunity).
- Urban AIDS patients in the United States frequently have florid infections with *M. tuberculosis*, which may be multidrug

resistant, and/or with *M. avium* and *M. intracellulare,* which are opportunistic pathogens.

- In primary tuberculosis, inhaled mycobacteria briefly proliferate in macrophages but are controlled in 95% of cases by T cell–mediated immune response, which is demonstrable by a positive PPD test.
- CD4+ helper T cells secrete INF-γ, which activates macrophages to kill intracellular mycobacteria via reactive nitrogen intermediates and also to form epithelioid cell granulomas.
- CD8+ suppresser T cells kill macrophages that are infected with mycobacteria, resulting in the formation of caseating (cheeselike) granulomas (delayed-type hypersensitivity reactions).
- The residual lesion is a calcified scar in the lung parenchyma and in the hilar lymph node (Ghon complex).

In secondary tuberculosis, mycobacteria associated with granulomas may remain confined to lung or may spread hematogenously throughout lungs, kidneys, meninges, marrow, and other organs.

- These granulomas, which fail to control the mycobacteria, are the major cause of tissue damage in tuberculosis.
- Cavities formed by caseating granulomas may rupture into blood vessels, causing further hematogenous spread of mycobacteria, or into airways, releasing infectious bacteria into aerosols.
- In AIDS, disseminated granulomas containing abundant *M. tuberculosis, M. avium,* and *M. intracellulare* organisms are poorly formed and are also frequent in lymph nodes and bowel.

HISTOPLASMA CAPSULATUM AND *COCCIDIOIES IMMITIS* (p. 327).

- Are dimorphic fungi, which are endemic along the Ohio and Mississippi Rivers *(Histoplasma)* and in the western United States *(Coccidioides).*
- Cause granulomatous disease, which may resemble primary and secondary tuberculosis in normal hosts and disseminated tuberculosis in AIDS patients.
- *Histoplasma,* which stain black with silver methenamine, bind to complement receptors on macrophages and reproduce within the phagolysosomes.
- 80% of persons in endemic areas have delayed-type sensitivity (response to PPD-like challenge) to *Coccidioides,* which blocks fusion of the macrophage phagosome with the lysosome.

GASTROINTESTINAL INFECTIONS (p. 328)

An overview of gastrointestinal infections is presented in Table 8–2.

VIRAL ENTERITIS

- Is caused by single-stranded RNA (Norwalk), double-stranded RNA (rotavirus), and double-stranded DNA viruses (enteric adenoviruses).
- Diarrhea results from malabsorbtion of sodium and water by blunted or destroyed villous epithelial cells.

Table 8–2. Major Infectious Causes of Diarrhea

Organism	Comment
Viruses	
Rotaviruses	Principally in children under age six. Sporadic—from contaminated water, may become epidemic; also direct fecal-oral transmission
Enteric adenoviruses	Common in infants and children, mostly sporadic
Norwalk virus	Young and old, mainly epidemic; fecal-oral
Bacteria	
Enterotoxigenic *E. coli*	Major cause of traveler's diarrhea, food- and water-borne, previously unencountered strains
Campylobacter jejuni	Major global cause, any age, mainly children, transmission by contaminated water and food
Yersinia enterocolitica	Similar to above
Shigella	Major global offender, children and adults, fecal-oral direct transmission and contaminated water and food, endemic and epidemic
Enteropathogenic *E. coli*	Children and nursery outbreaks
Salmonella spp.	Large number serotypes with range of clinical syndromes, children and adults, food- and water-borne, human and animal reservoirs
Clostridium difficile	Antibiotic-associated, hospital-acquired, mainly in predisposed adults
Vibrio cholerae	Major cause of pandemic and epidemic diarrhea in developing infections
Parasites	
Giardia lamblia	Carrier state common, major cause of traveler's diarrhea, contaminated drinking water, high infection rate in Russia, northwestern United States, other locales; may become epidemic
Entamoeba histolytica	Large reservoir of asymptomatic carriers in developed countries and endemic in developing areas, fecal-oral, sexual transmission particularly among homosexuals, and from contaminated water and food

From Cotran, R. S., Kumar, V., and Robbins, S. L.: Robbins Pathologic Basis of Disease. 5th ed. Philadelphia, W. B. Saunders Co., 1994, p. 329.

GRAM-NEGATIVE BACTERIAL ENTERITIS (p. 330)

SHIGELLA SPP. AND O-TYPE ENTEROTOXIC E. COLI

- Cause dysentery (diarrhea with blood and mucus in the stool).
- *Shigella* reproduce within the cytosol of intestinal epithelial cells and destroy them, producing numerous ulcers, featuring a fibrin- and neutrophil-rich exudate.

CAMPYLOBACTER JEJUNI (p. 330)

- Are comma-shaped bacteria that (1) secrete toxins and cause diarrhea, (2) invade the colonic epithelium and cause dysentery, or (3) reproduce in mesenteric lymph nodes and cause enteric fever.
- A related bacterium, *Helicobacter,* causes chronic gastritis and gastric ulcers.

SALMONELLA SPP. (p. 331)

- *Salmonella enteritidis*–contaminated chicken and beef are major causes of food poisoning.
- *Salmonella typhus,* which is spread from person-to-person via the fecal-oral route, causes systemic typhoid fever.
- Greater than 20 *Salmonella* virulence genes are induced by low oxygen tension in the colon and acidity within the macrophage lysosome.
- *S. typhi* multiply within macrophages of intestinal Peyer's patches (causing ulceration of the overlying mucosa), spleen, liver, and bone marrow.
- Chronic carriers of *S. typhi* (e.g., "Typhoid Mary") have asymptomatic gallbladder colonization.

VIBRIO CHOLERAE (p. 332)

- Is a noninvasive, toxin-producing bacterium that cause pandemics (long-lasting epidemics) of severe watery diarrhea, originating in India and Bangladesh.
- *V. cholerae* virulence factors include flagellar proteins important for motility and attachment and a toxin, similar in structure to the heat-labile toxin of *E. coli* that causes traveler's diarrhea.
- Cholera toxin binds to GM_1 ganglioside on epithelial cells and ADP-ribosylates host G-proteins, which activate adenyl cyclase, increase levels of intracellular cAMP, and cause massive secretion of chloride, sodium, and water.

INTESTINAL PROTOZOA (p. 333)

ENTAMOEBA HISTOLYTICA

- Causes dysentery when organisms attach via an adherence lectin to the colonic epithelium, lyse colonic epithelial cells by means of a channel-forming protein, and invade the bowel wall.
- Flask-shaped colonic ulcers contain few inflammatory cells, extensive liquefactive necrosis, and amebae, which resemble macrophages with a small single nucleus and frequently contain engulfed red blood cells.

GIARDIA LAMBLIA (p. 334)

- Is the most prevalent pathogenic gut protozoan worldwide.
- Causes acute or chronic diarrhea, when binucleate parasites adhere to the duodenal epithelium via sucker-discs.
- Causes clubbing of villi, a decreased villus-to-crypt ratio, and a mixed inflammatory infiltrate of the lamina propria.

- Produces diarrhea by blocking absorption.

GRAM-POSITIVE BACTERIAL INFECTIONS
(p. 335)

STAPHYLOCOCCUS AUREUS

- Are gram-positive cocci that form grapelike clusters and cause skin lesions (boils, carbuncles, impetigo, and scalded skin), pharyngitis, pneumonia, endocarditis, food poisoning, and toxic shock syndrome.
- Are a major cause of infection of persons with severe burns and surgical wounds and second only to *E. coli* as a cause of hospital-acquired infections.
- Virulence factors include surface proteins involved in adherence to host cells, enzymes that degrade host proteins, and toxins that lyse host cells and cause scalded skin syndrome (exotoxins), cause food poisoning (enterotoxins), and produce shock (endotoxin and toxic shock syndrome toxin).
- Whether the lesion is located in the skin, lungs, bones, or heart valves, *S. aureus* cause pyogenic inflammation, which is remarkable for its local destructiveness.

STREPTOCOCCUS SPP. (p. 337)

- Are gram-positive cocci that grow in pairs or chains, which are typed according to their surface antigens.
- *S. pneumoniae* is the major cause of community-acquired pneumonia and causes adult bacterial meningitis.
- *S. pyogenes* produces pharyngitis, scarlet fever, erysipelas (swelling skin rash), impetigo, rheumatic fever, and glomerulonephritis.
- *S. agalactiae* causes neonatal sepsis and urinary tract infections.
- *Enterococcus faecalis* and *S. viridans* cause endocarditis.
- *S. mutans* causes dental caries.

Streptococcal virulence factors include rodlike surface M-proteins and a polysaccharide capsule that prevent bacteria from being phagocytosed; exotoxins that produce the rash in scarlet fever; proteases that degrade chemotactic peptides and immunoglobulins; and lactic acid that demineralizes tooth enamel.

Streptococcal lesions are remarkable for their diffuse spreading neutrophilic infiltrates with minimal destruction of host tissues.

CLOSTRIDIUM SPP. (p. 338)

- Are gram-positive, box-shaped bacilli that grow under anaerobic conditions and produce spores frequently present in the soil.
- *C. perfringens* and *C. septicum*, which invade traumatic and surgical wounds and cause gas gangrene, also contaminate illegal abortions and cause uterine myonecrosis.
- *C. tetani*, which proliferate in puncture wounds and in the umbilical stump of newborn infants in developing countries, release a potent neurotoxin, called tetanospasmin, that causes convulsive contractions of skeletal muscles (lockjaw). Tetanus toxoid (formalin-fixed neurotoxin) is part of the DPT immunization.
- *C. botulinum* grow in inadequately sterilized canned foods and

release a potent neurotoxin that causes a severe paralysis of respiratory and skeletal muscles (botulism).
- *C. difficile* overgrow other intestinal flora in antibiotic-treated patients, release multiple toxins, and cause a pseudomembranous colitis.

Clostridial toxins block acetylcholine release at neuromuscular junctions (*C. botulinum* neurotoxin), degrade host membranes (α-toxin) and G-proteins (*C. difficile* toxins A and B), and ADP-ribosylate G-proteins (*C. botulinum* exoenzyme C3).

Clostridial cellulitis and gas gangrene are remarkable for a foul odor, marked edema or exudate with thin and discolored fluid, and wide and deep tissue destruction.

Microscopically, the extent of tissue necrosis is disproportionate to the number of neutrophils and clostridia present.

SEXUALLY TRANSMITTED INFECTIONS (p. 340)

HERPESVIRUS-1 and HSV-2

- Are large, double-stranded DNA viruses surrounded by an envelope, which are neurotropic and cause cold sores (HSV-1), genital sores (HSV-2), corneal blindness, and encephalitis (rarely).
- In primary infections, HSV-1 and HSV-2 replicate and cause vesicular lesions in the epidermis of the skin and mucous membranes.
- In secondary infections, herpesviruses, which have remained latent in the neurons, spread from the regional ganglia to the skin or to mucous membranes.
- Herpesvirus lesions show large, pink-to-purple (Cowdry type A) virion-containing intranuclear inclusions, which push darkly stained host cell chromatin to the edges of the nucleus.
- Herpesvirus also produce multinucleated syncytia, which are diagnostic in smears of fluid from intraepithelial blisters (Tzanck preparations).
- In herpes stromal keratitis, which is treated with steroids, infiltrates of mononuclear cells surround keratinocytes and endothelial cells and may lead to neovascularization, scarring, opacification of the cornea, and blindness.

CHLAMYDIA TRACHOMATIS (p. 341)

- Is an obligate intracellular pathogen of columnar epithelial cells that causes nongonococcal urethritis (NGU), lymphogranuloma venereum (LGV), and trachoma.
- In some males, *C. trachomatis* infection causes Reiter's syndrome, which is a triad of conjunctivitis, polyarthritis, and genital infection.
- Infants born to mothers with *C. trachomatis* cervicitis may develop self-limited inclusion conjunctivitis or neonatal pneumonia.
- Chlamydiae exist in two forms: elementary bodies, which never divide but are infectious, and reticulate bodies, which multiply within vacuoles of host cells but are not infectious.
- In LGV, inguinal, pelvic, and rectal lymph nodes are enlarged and contain a mixture of suppurative and granulomatous inflammation.
- In inclusion conjunctivitis, conjunctiva are hyperemic, edematous, and show a monocytic infiltrate.

NEISSERIA GONORRHOEAE (p. 343)

- Is an encapsulated, gram-negative diplococcus that causes ure-thritis ("clap"), pharyngitis, or proctitis, depending on sexual practices.
- May cause urethral strictures and chronic infections of the epididymis, prostate, and seminal vesicles.
- May infect the fallopian tubes (salpingitis), resulting in tubo-ovarian abscesses and scars, sterility, and ectopic pregnancy.
- Perinatal ophthalmic infection was a major cause of blindness before prophylactic administration of silver nitrate to neonates became routine.
- Bind to host epithelial cells via pili, which show antigenic variation based upon intragenomic recombination and upon recombination following incorporation of exogenous DNA from lysed gonococci.
- Internalization is based upon a second set of adhesins called the opacity outer membrane proteins or P.II, which also show antigenic variation.

Gonococcal lesions show exudative and purulent reactions, followed by granulation tissue, plasma cell infiltrates, and scar-ring as chronicity increases.

TREPONEMA PALLIDUM (SYPHILIS) (p. 343)

- Is a microaerophilic spirochete with an axial periplasmic fla-gella wound around a slender, helical protoplasm, all of which are covered by an outer membrane.
- Primary syphilis, which occurs approximately 3 weeks after contact with an infected individual, features a single firm, nontender, raised, red lesion (chancre) located at the site of treponemal invasion on the penis, cervix, vaginal wall, or anus.
- Secondary syphilis, which occurs 2 to 10 weeks after the pri-mary chancre, is characterized by a diffuse rash, particularly of the palms and soles, that may be accompanied by white oral lesions, fever, lymphadenopathy, headache, arthritis, and (rarely) immune complex nephritis.
- Tertiary syphilis, which occurs years after the primary lesion, is characterized by either active inflammatory lesions of the aorta, heart, and CNS or by quiescent lesions (gummas) involv-ing the liver, bones, and skin.
- Congenital syphilis causes late abortion, stillbirth, or death soon after delivery, or it may persist in latent form to become apparent only during childhood.

Whatever the stage of the disease and location of the lesions, the histologic hallmarks of syphilis are obliterative endarteritis and plasma cell infiltrates. The endarteritis is secondary to the binding of spirochetes to endothelial cells, mediated by host fibronectin molecules bound to the surface of the spirochetes.

Syphilitic gummas are white-gray and rubbery, occur singly or multiply, and vary in size from microscopic defects resembling tubercles to large, tumor-like masses.

Sequelae of congenital syphilis include an extensive cutaneous rash containing many spirochetes; osteochondritis with collapse of the bridge of the nose; periostitis with bowing of the tibia; keratitis; Hutchinson's teeth (peg-shaped incisors); and eighth nerve deafness.

TRICHOMONAS VAGINALIS (p. 346)

- Is a noninvasive anaerobic, flagellated protozoan parasite, which frequently causes vaginal itching and a profuse watery discharge containing the parasites.
- The vaginal mucosa and superficial submucosa are infiltrated by lymphocytes, plasma cells, and polymorphonuclear leukocytes.

INFECTIONS OF CHILDHOOD AND ADOLESCENCE (p. 346)

MUMPS VIRUS

- Is an RNA virus of the paramyxovirus family that includes measles virus, respiratory syncytial virus (RSV, the major cause of lower respiratory infections in infants), and parainfluenza virus (the cause of croup).
- Causes a transient inflammation and enlargement of the parotid glands and, less often, of the testes, pancreas, and central nervous system.
- Mumps lesions show interstitial edema and diffuse infiltrates of histiocytes, lymphocytes, and plasma cells.

MEASLES VIRUS (RUBEOLA) (p. 346)

- Is a paramyxovirus, which causes more than 2 million deaths per year among developing world children, who by reasons of poor nutrition are 10 to 1000 times more likely to die of measles pneumonia than Western children.
- Most children develop T cell-mediated immunity to measles virus that controls the viral infection and produces the measles rash, which is a hypersensitivity reaction to viral antigens in the skin.
- Subacute sclerosing panencephalitis and measles inclusion-body encephalitis (in immunocompromised individuals) is a rare late complication of measles, caused by hypermutated, "defective" viruses.

  Ulcerated mucosal lesions in the oral cavity near the opening of Stensen's ducts (pathognomonic Koplik spots) show necrosis, neutrophils, and neovascularization.
  The lymphoid organs typically have marked follicular hyperplasia, large germinal centers, and randomly distributed multinucleate giant cells, called Warthin-Finkeldey cells, which have eosinophilic nuclear and cytoplasmic inclusion bodies and are pathognomonic of measles.

EPSTEIN-BARR VIRUS (INFECTIOUS MONONUCLEOSIS) (p. 347)

- Is a γ-group herpesvirus that causes a benign, self-limited lymphoproliferative disease characterized by fever, generalized lymphadenopathy, splenomegaly, sore throat, and the appearance in the blood of atypical activated T lymphocytes.
- Enters the epithelial cell cytoplasm by directly fusing with the plasma membrane.
- Enters the B cell cytoplasm by fusing with endosomal membranes.
- Two EBV proteins, EBNA2 and LMP-1, are associated with

B cell immortalization, which may occur in latently infected lymphocytes.

In mononucleosis, the total white cell count increases to as many as 18,000, 95% of which are atypical T lymphocytes with an abundant, finely granular, basophilic cytoplasm, containing small fenestrations.

The lymph nodes in the posterior cervical, axillary, and groin regions are enlarged, show increased number of T cells in their paracortical zones, and contain large binucleate cells, Reed-Sternberg–like cells.

With impaired immunity, mononucleosis may become chronic and transform into B cell lymphoma.

POLIOVIRUS (p. 349)

- Is a spherical, unencapsulated RNA virus, which is a member of the enterovirus family. Other members cause childhood diarrhea, as well as rashes (coxsackievirus A), conjunctivitis (enterovirus 70), viral meningitis (coxsackievirus and echovirus), myopericarditis (coxsackievirus B), and jaundice (hepatitis A virus).
- There are three major strains of poliovirus, each of which is included in the Salk formalin-fixed (killed) vaccine and the Sabin oral, attenuated (live) vaccine.
- In 1 of 100 infected persons, poliovirus invades the CNS, replicates in motor neurons of the spinal cord (spinal poliomyelitis resulting in muscular paralysis) or brain stem (bulbar poliomyelitis possibly resulting in respiratory paralysis).

VARICELLA ZOSTER VIRUS (VZV; CHICKENPOX AND SHINGLES) (p. 349)

- Is an α-herpesvirus, which infects mucous membranes, skin, and neurons.
- Unlike HSV, VZV is transmitted in epidemic fashion by aerosols, disseminates hematogenously, and causes widespread vesicular skin lesions (chickenpox).
- VZV also infects satellite cells around neurons in the dorsal root ganglia and may recur many years after the primary infection in the form of *shingles.*
- One reason why VZV recurs less frequently than HSV is that the genes involved in reactivation in HSV are missing in VSV.

The chickenpox rash occurs approximately 2 weeks after respiratory infection and travels in multiple waves centrifugally from the torso to the head and extremities.

Each lesion progresses rapidly from a macule to a vesicle, which resembles "a dew drop on a rose petal."

Histologically, chickenpox vesicles contain intranuclear inclusions of the epithelial cells and the blisters are identical to those of HSV-1 (p. 341).

WHOOPING COUGH (p. 350)

- Is caused by the gram-negative coccobacillus *Bordetella pertussis* in persons not given the diphtheria-pertussis-tetanus (DPT) vaccine.
- Virulence factors include a filamentous hemagglutinin, pertussis toxin that ADP-ribosylate the same G-proteins as cholera toxin, and a hemolysin important in early colonization.

Laryngotracheobronchitis may include mucosal erosion, hyperemia, and copious mucopurulent exudates.

Mucosal and peribronchial lymph follicles are hypercellular and enlarged, and there is a striking peripheral lymphocytosis.

DIPHTHERIA (p. 350)

- Is caused by the gram-positive rod *Corynebacterium diphtheriae* and prevented by immunization with a formalin-fixed toxoid in the DPT vaccine.
- Phage-encoded diphtheria toxin, like *Pseudomonas* exoenzyme A, ADP-ribosylates and inactivates the ribosomal protein elongation factor-2.

Tracheal colonization may lead to mucosal erosion, formation of a suffocating pharyngeal fibrinosuppurative exudate (pseudomembrane), and toxin-mediated damage to the heart, nerves, liver, or kidneys.

OPPORTUNISTIC AND AIDS-ASSOCIATED INFECTIONS (p. 351)

Opportunistic pathogens are those that cause no or mild infections in immunocompetent individuals but may cause devastating disease in infants or in individuals with genetic or acquired immunodeficiencies.

CYTOMEGALOVIRUS (CMV)

- Is a β-group herpes virus, which causes esophagitis, colitis, hepatitis, pneumonitis, renal tubulitis, chorioretinitis, and meningoencephalitis in neonates and in persons immunosuppressed secondary to transplant chemotherapy or AIDS.
- Is spread by intrauterine or perinatal transmission at childbirth; in mother's milk, respiratory droplets, semen and vaginal fluid, blood transfusions; and by transplantation of virus-infected grafts from a donor with latent infection.

Affected infants manifest a hemolytic form of anemia, jaundice, thrombocytopenia, purpura, hepatosplenomegaly (due to extramedullary hematopoiesis), pneumonitis, deafness, chorioretinitis, and extensive brain damage.

CMV chorioretinitis is a frequent cause of blindness in AIDS patients.

Disseminated CMV in the immunoincompetent individual causes focal necrosis with minimal inflammation in virtually any organ.

Endothelial and epithelial cells infected with CMV are markedly enlarged, with large purple intranuclear inclusions surrounded by a clear halo, and smaller basophilic cytoplasmic inclusions.

PSEUDOMONAS AERUGINOSA (p. 352)

- Is an opportunistic gram-negative bacterium that is a frequent and deadly pathogen of persons with cystic fibrosis, severe burns, or neutropenia.
- Most cystic fibrosis patients die of pulmonary failure secondary to chronic infection with *P. aeruginosa.*
- *P. aeruginosa* also causes corneal keratitis in wearers of contact

lenses, endocarditis and osteomyelitis in intravenous drug abusers, external otitis (swimmer's ear) in normal individuals, and malignant external otitis in diabetics.

Distinctive virulence factors of *Pseudomonas* include:

1. Formation of mucoid colonies that are resistant to anti-LPS antibodies, complement, and phagocytes.
2. Exotoxins A and exoenzyme S that ADP-ribosylate elongation factor 2 and p21^{ras}, respectively.
3. Iron-containing compounds that are extremely toxic to endothelial cells and so may cause the vascular lesions characteristic of this bacterium.

Pseudomonas pneumonia in the neutropenic host shows necrotizing inflammation with a striking alternation of whitish necrotic and dark red hemorrhagic areas.

Microscopically, masses of organisms cloud the host tissue with a bluish haze, concentrating in the walls of blood vessels, where host cells undergo coagulation necrosis and nuclei fade away.

In cystic fibrosis, *Pseudomonas* causes mucous plugging, bronchiectasis, and chronic pulmonary fibrosis.

LEGIONELLA PNEUMOPHILA (LEGIONNAIRES' DISEASE) (p. 353)

- Is a gram-negative bacterium identified only by special stains or culture methods.
- Causes mini-epidemics of severe pneumonia in susceptible individuals exposed to aerosols from cooling systems of buildings.
- Is a facultative intracellular parasite of macrophages, in which bacteria fail to induce a respiratory burst and block phagosome fusion with the lysosome.
- Produces a multifocal pneumonia of fibrinopurulent type that is initially nodular but may become confluent or lobar.

A high ratio of mononuclear phagocytes to neutrophils is characteristic, with many destroyed phagocytes at the center of the lesions (leukocytoclasis), surrounded by intact macrophages.

CANDIDIASIS (CANDIDA ALBICANS, C. TROPICALIS) (p. 354)

- Are part of the normal flora of the skin, mouth, and gastrointestinal tract but cause disseminated visceral infections in neutropenic patients.
- Grow best on warm, moist surfaces and so frequently cause vaginitis (particularly during pregnancy), diaper rash, and oral thrush.
- Chronic mucocutaneous candidiasis occurs in persons with AIDS, in individuals with inherited or iatrogenic defects in T cell–mediated immunity, and in persons with polyendocrine deficiencies (e.g., hypoparathyroidism, hypoadrenalism, and hypothyroidism).
- Virulence factors include surface molecules that bind host cells, a proteinase that degrades host tissues, and released adenosine that blocks neutrophil oxygen radical production.

Candida infections of the oral cavity (thrush) and vagina produce superficial curdy white patches or large, almost fluffy membranes that are easily detached, revealing a reddened, irritated mucosa.

Microscopically, lesions contain yeast, hyphae, and pseudohyphae, acute and chronic inflammation, and (sometimes) granulomas.

Severe, invasive candidiasis in neutropenic persons causes microabscesses in which fungi in the centers of the lesions are surrounded by areas of necrosis.

CRYPTOCOCCUS NEOFORMANS (p. 355)

- Is a yeast acquired by inhalation that causes meningoencephalitis in AIDS patients and in persons with leukemia, lymphoma, systemic lupus, Hodgkin's disease, sarcoidosis, or organ transplants.
- High-dose corticosteroids are a major risk factor for *Cryptococcus* infection.
- *C. neoformans* virulence is associated with its capsular polysaccharide, which is stained bright red with mucicarmine in tissues or negatively stained with India ink in cerebrospinal fluid.
- In normal persons, *C. neoformans* may form a solitary pulmonary granuloma similar to the coin lesions caused by *Histoplasma*.
- In immunosuppressed patients, *Cryptococcus* forms small cysts within the gray matter (soap bubble lesions), as well as a diffuse meningitis with a chronic granulomatous reaction.

ASPERGILLUS FUMIGATUS (p. 355)

- Is a ubiquitous mold that causes allergies (brewer's lung) and colonization in otherwise healthy persons and a severe sinusitis and pneumonia in neutropenic persons.
- *Aspergillus* spp. growing on the surface of peanuts secrete the carcinogen aflatoxin, which may be a major cause of liver cancer in Africa.
- Pre-existing lesions in the lungs caused by tuberculosis, bronchiectasis, old infarcts, or abscesses may develop brownish colonies of *Aspergillus* (aspergillomas) without invasion of the tissues.
- In debilitated hosts, *Aspergillus* with septate filaments branching at acute angles causes a necrotizing pneumonia with sharply delineated, rounded gray foci with hemorrhagic borders, often referred to as target lesions.

MUCORMYCOSIS (p. 356)

- Is an opportunistic infection of neutropenic persons and ketoacidotic diabetics, caused by "bread mold fungi" including *Mucor, Absidia, Rhizopus,* and *Cunninghamella.*
- The three primary sites of *Mucor* invasion are the nasal sinuses, lungs, and gastrointestinal tract, depending on whether the spores (widespread in dust and air) are inhaled or ingested.
- In diabetics, the fungus may spread from nasal sinuses to the orbit to the brain.

In the lungs, gut, or meninges, phycomycetes, which are nonseptate with right-angle branches, cause local tissue necrosis and invade arterial walls.

PNEUMOCYSTIS CARINII
(PNEUMOCYSTIS PNEUMONIA) (p. 357)

- Is often the first opportunistic infection in HIV-1 infected persons and is the leading cause of death in AIDS.
- Is likely a fungus, based upon properties of its cell wall, the paucity of its intracellular organelles, and phylogenetic analysis of its small-subunit ribosomal RNA sequence.
- Causes a diffuse and dense pneumonia, in which the alveolar spaces are filled by a foamy, proteinaceous edema fluid, containing 4- to 6-μm-long organisms that stain with silver or Giemsa.

Frequently there is concurrent respiratory infection by opportunistic bacteria, fungi, or CMV.

CRYPTOSPORIDIOSIS
(CRYPTOSPORIDIUM PARVUM) (p. 357)

- Is a protozoan parasite, which causes a transient watery diarrhea in normal persons and a chronic and debilitating diarrhea in AIDS patients.
- *C. parvum* oocytes are not killed by chlorine but instead must be removed by filtration through sand, so that epidemics of cryptosporidiosis occur when municipal water filtration systems break down.
- Acid-fast cryptosporidia enter the cytosol of intestinal epithelial cells and cause mixed inflammation of the lamina propria.

TOXOPLASMA GONDII
(TOXOPLASMOSIS) (p. 358)

- Is an obligate intracellular protozoan, which causes a mild lymphadenopathy in normal persons yet produces severe opportunistic infections in fetuses, AIDS patients, and persons receiving bone marrow and organ transplants.
- Infects persons who ingest oocysts within cat feces or incompletely cooked lamb or pork.
- Penetrates any type of host cell, a unique property of this parasite.
- Travels through the placenta into the fetus and destroys the developing heart, brain, and lung tissues.

In AIDS patients, toxoplasma frequently causes space-occupying lesions in the CNS.

ZOONOTIC AND
VECTOR-BORNE INFECTIONS (p. 358)
RICKETTSIAE

Rickettsiae are obligate intracellular bacteria that cause epidemic typhus (*R. prowazekii*), scrub typhus (*R. tsutsugamushi*), and spotted fevers (*R. rickettsii* and others) (Table 8–3).

- Epidemic typhus, which is transmitted from person to person via body lice, is particularly associated with wars and human suffering, when persons are forced to live in close contact without changing clothes.
- Scrub typhus, transmitted by chiggers, was a major problem for U.S. soldiers in the Pacific in World War II and in Vietnam.

Table 8-3. Rickettsial Diseases and Pathogens

Disease	Agent	Transmission	Geography	Distinctive Features
	Typhus Group (No Eschar)			
Epidemic typhus	R. prowazekii	Louse feces	Worldwide (war, famine)	Endothelial infection; centrifugal type rash
Brill-Zinsser disease	R. prowazekii	Late reactivation	That of epidemic typhus	Those of epidemic typhus, but generally milder
Flying squirrel typhus	R. prowazekii	Fleas, lice of flying squirrel	Southeastern United States	Similar to epidemic typhus, but mortality is lower
Murine typhus	R. typhi (mooseri)	Rat flea feces	Worldwide (rat-related)	Similar to epidemic typhus, but mortality is lower
	Spotted Fever Group			
Rocky Mountain spotted fever	R. rickettsii	Tick bite	North and South America	Endothelia and vascular smooth muscle infected; rash is centripetal; eschar rarely seen
Boutonneuse fever	R. conorii	Tick bite	Mediterranean, India	Prominent eschar, "tache noire"
North Asian and Queensland tick typhus	R. sibirica R. australia	Tick bite	USSR, China, etc. Australia	Both diseases are typical spotted fevers commonly with eschar
Rickettsial pox	R. akari	Mite bite	United States, USSR, Korea, Africa	Prominent eschar; populovesicular rash (milder than RMSF)
Scrub Typhus	R. tsutsugamushi	Chigger bite	East Asia, Pacific	Frequent eschar and lymphadenopathy
Q Fever	Coxiella burnetti	Droplet inhalation	Worldwide	No eschar or rash; fever, pneumonia, ring granuloma
Ehrlichiosis	Ehrlichia sennetsu, E. canis	Tick bite	Not yet fully known	Fever, lymphadenopathy, no eschar or rash

From Cotran R. S., Kumar, V., and Robbins, S. L.: Robbins Pathologic Basis of Disease. 5th ed. Philadelphia, W. B. Saunders Co., 1994, p. 359.

- Rocky Mountain spotted fever (RMSF) infections, accidentally transmitted to humans by rodent and dog ticks, is actually most frequent in the Southeastern and Southwestern United States.
- Q fever, which is caused by the related organism *Coxiella burnetii* that produces pneumonia and fever, is transmitted by aerosols.

Rickettsiae predominately infect host endothelial and vascular smooth muscle cells, causing a widespread vasculitis with perivascular mixed infiltrates, which may be complicated by thrombi and hemorrhages.

In typhus fever, lesions vary from a skin rash to gangrene of the tips of fingers, nose, ear lobes, penis, and vulva.

In RMSF, an eschar at the site of the tick bite is followed by a hemorrhagic rash that extends over the entire body. Other tissues frequently involved include brain, skeletal muscle, lungs, kidneys, testes, and heart.

PLAGUE (p. 360)

- Also called the Black Death, is caused by *Yersinia pestis,* a gram-negative facultative intracellular bacterium that is transmitted by flea bites or by aerosols.
- *Y. enterocolitis* and *Y. pseudotuberculosis* are genetically similar to *Y. pestis* and cause fecal-oral transmitted ileitis and mesenteric lymphadenitis.
- A secreted protease is required for the spread of *Y. pestis* from the local site of inoculation and inflammation into the blood stream.
- *Y. pseudotuberculosis* has multiple molecules on its surface involved in attachment to and phagocytosis by host epithelial cells.
- Within host cells, *Y. pseudotuberculosis* secretes a serine/threonine kinase and a protein tyrosine phosphatase, which disrupt host signal transduction pathways.

Y. pestis causes lymph node enlargement (bubos), pneumonia, or sepsis, all with dramatic proliferation of the organisms, necrosis of tissues and blood vessels, and neutrophilic infiltrates adjacent to necrotic areas.

Y. enterocolitis and *Y. pseudotuberculosis* cause ulcerative intestinal lesions like those of typhoid fever, as well as microabscesses rimmed by activated macrophages in the submucosa.

RELAPSING FEVER (*BORRELIA* SPP.) (p. 361)

- Is caused by helical *Borrelia* spirochetes, which are transmitted from person to person by body lice (*B. recurrentis*) or from animals to man by soft ticks (*B.* spp., each named for the tick species transmitting them).
- The relapsing fever is caused by successive waves of spirochetes in the blood, each of which contains a single variant surface protein, which is eventually recognized by host antibodies (*antigenic variation*).
- Antibiotic treatment of *Borrelia* may cause a massive release of endotoxin, resulting in rigors, fall in blood pressure, and leukopenia (the Jarisch-Herxheimer reaction).

Microscopically, the spleen shows focal areas of necrosis with numerous neutrophils and borreliae.

LYME DISEASE *(BORRELIA BURGDORFERI)* (p. 361)

- Is named for the Connecticut town where in the mid-1970s there was an epidemic of arthritis associated with skin erythema, caused by the spirochete *Borrelia burgdorferi.*
- Lyme disease, which is transmitted from rodents to people by tiny, hard deer ticks, is the major arthropod-borne disease presently in the United States.
- Like syphilis, Lyme disease has three stages:

  1. An expanding area of redness with an indurated or necrotic center at the site of the tick bite (called erythema chronicum migrans).
  2. Early hematogenous spread of spirochetes, resulting in secondary annular skin lesions (erythema migrans), lymphadenopathy, migratory joint and muscle pain, cardiac arrhythmias, and meningitis, often with cranial nerve involvement.
  3. Two or three years after the initial bite, a chronic arthritis ensues, sometimes with severe damage to large joints and an encephalitis that varies from mild to debilitating. The host immune response, which is out of proportion to the scant number of organisms detectable, may be caused by antibodies to spirochete heat-shock proteins that cross-react with host tissues.

Skin lesions caused by *B. burgdorferi* contain lymphocytes and plasma cells with local edema.

In early Lyme arthritis, the synovium resembles that of early rheumatoid arthritis, with villous hypertrophy, lining cell hyperplasia, and abundant lymphocytes and plasma cells in the subsynovium.

A distinctive feature of Lyme disease is an arteritis with onion skin–like lesions.

MALARIA (*PLASMODIUM* SPP.) (p. 362)

- In its severest form is caused by the protozoan parasite *Plasmodium falciparum,* which kills 1–1.5 million persons per year and so is the major parasitic cause of death.
- *P. vivax* and *P. malariae,* which are also transmitted by *Anopheles* mosquitoes, cause mild anemia and may cause splenic rupture and nephrotic syndrome, respectively.
- *P. falciparum* parasites infect liver cells and then RBCs; cause severe anemia when RBCs lyse; and produce cerebral infarcts when infected RBCs bind to endothelial cells in the CNS.
- Genetic resistance to malaria is associated with the ability of HLA-B53 liver cells to present malaria antigens to cytotoxic T cells and the increased rate of splenic clearance of infected RBCs by individuals with the sickle trait.

P. falciparum infection initially causes congestion and enlargement of the spleen, whereas in chronic malaria infection, the spleen becomes increasingly fibrotic and brittle.

Pigmented phagocytic cells may be found dispersed throughout the bone marrow, lymph nodes, subcutaneous tissues, and lungs.

In malignant cerebral malaria caused by *P. falciparum,* brain vessels are plugged with parasitized red cells, causing ring hemorrhages.

BABESIA MICROTI (p. 363)

- Are malaria-like protozoans transmitted by the same deer ticks that carry Lyme disease.
- Parasitize RBCs and cause a mild fever and hemolytic anemia that is often subclinical except in debilitated or splenectomized individuals, who develop severe and fatal parasitemias, respectively.
- In blood smears, *Babesia* resemble *P. falciparum* ring stages, although they lack hemozoin pigment and may form tetrads, which are diagnostic.

TRICHINELLA SPIRALIS (TRICHINOSIS) (p. 364)

- Is a nematode parasite that is acquired by ingestion of improperly cooked meat from pigs that have eaten *T. spiralis*–infected rats or pork.
- In the human gut, *T. spiralis* parasites develop into adults that mate and release larvae, which penetrate into the tissues.
- Larvae disseminate hematogenously and penetrate muscle cells, causing fever, myalgias, and marked eosinophilia (frequently), and periorbital edema, dyspnea (with invasion of the diaphragm), encephalitis (with invasion of the CNS), and cardiac failure (all rarely).
- *T. spiralis* larvae, approximately 1-mm long and coiled, encyst in striated skeletal muscles (nurse cells), which are surrounded by new blood vessels and/or lymphoplasmacytic infiltrates.

CYSTICERCOSIS *(TAENIA SOLIUM)* (p. 364)

- *Taenia solium* is a cestode parasite that produces mild abdominal symptoms, caused by a solitary tapeworm in the gut lumen (hence its name) or convulsions, intracranial hypertension, and mental disturbances (cysticercosis caused by 1–100 *T. solium* cysts in brain tissues).
- Adult tapeworms result from ingestion of undercooked pork that contains *T. solium* cysticerci.
- *T. solium* tapeworms, which may be many inches long and resemble the beef tapeworm *T. saginatum* (that do not cause cerebral infections), attach to the stomach wall via hooklike scolices and release thousands of eggs in the feces each day.
- Ingested eggs cause cerebral cysticercosis when larvae hatch, penetrate the gut wall, disseminate hematogenously, and encyst in the CNS.
- Cerebral *T. solium* cysts rarely exceed 1 cm and have a cyst wall that induces little host inflammatory response.

TROPICAL INFECTIONS (p. 365)

TRACHOMA

- Is caused by *Chlamydia trachomatis;* is a chronic, suppurative eye disease and a leading global cause of blindness.
- Closely related *C. pneumoniae* and *C. psittaci* cause mild and severe pneumonias, respectively.

In progressive trachoma, there is a suppurative stage resembling inclusion conjuctivitis, followed by deeper tissue involvement with lymphoplasmacytic infiltrates.

When the conjuctiva ulcerates, penetration of the cornea leads to pannus formation, fibroblast overgrowth, scarring, and eventual blindness.

In *C. psittaci* pneumonia (also known as ornithosis) alveolar septa show edema and mononuclear infiltrates, while alveolar spaces are filled with mononuclear cells and seroproteinaceous fluid.

LEPROSY (*MYCOBACTERIUM LEPRAE*) (p. 365)

- Is a slowly progressive infection caused by *Mycobacterium leprae*, which results in unsightly or disabling deformities and peripheral neural sensory deficits.
- While *M. leprae* are for the most part contained within the skin and nerves, leprosy is believed to be transmitted from person to person via aerosols from lesions in the upper respiratory tract.
- *M. leprae* is an acid-fast obligate intracellular organism; it has not been grown in culture but can be grown in the nine-banded armadillo.

Leprosy is a bipolar disease, determined by the host cellular immune response:

1. Patients with *tuberculoid leprosy* and a normal immune response form granulomas similar to those seen in tuberculosis that contain epithelioid macrophages, giant cells, and few surviving mycobacteria. The 48-hour lepromin skin test is strongly positive, and damage to the nervous system comes from granulomas in the nerve sheaths.

2. Patients with *lepromatous leprosy* lack T cell–mediated immunity (are anergic to lepromin) and have diffuse nodular lesions containing macrophages stuffed with enormous numbers of mycobacteria, as is seen in disseminated *M. avium* or *M. intracellulare* of AIDS patients. Nodular lesions coalesce to yield a distinctive leonine facies, while peripheral nerves are symmetrically invaded with mycobacteria, with minimal inflammation, but with loss of sensation.

Because leprosy pursues an extremely slow course, spanning decades, most patients die with leprosy rather than of it.

LEISHMANIASIS (*LEISHMANIA* SPP.) (p. 367)

- Is a chronic inflammatory disease of the skin (*L. major* and *L aethiopica* in the Old World and *L. mexicana* and *L. brasiliensis* in the New World), mucous membranes (*L. brasiliensis*), or viscera (*L. donovani* in the Old World or *L. chagasi* in the New World).
- Leishmania are obligate intracellular, kinetoplastid protozoan parasites, which are transmitted through the bite of infected sandflies.
- In simple cutaneous leishmaniasis, an itchy, indurated papule changes into a shallow, slowly expanding ulcer with irregular borders, and heals by involution within 6 months without treatment. Microscopically, the lesion is granulomatous, usually with foreign body giant cells and few parasites.
- In diffuse cutaneous leishmaniasis (rare), the entire body is covered by bizarre nodular lesions, which resemble keloids and contain vast aggregates of foamy macrophages stuffed with leishmania. The patients are anergic to leishmanin and other skin antigens.

- In mucocutaneous leishmaniasis, sometimes disfiguring lesions, which contain numerous parasite-containing histiocytes, lymphocytes, and plasma cells, develop at the mucocutaneous junctions of the larynx, nasal septum, anus, or vulva.
- In visceral leishmaniasis, parasites invade macrophages throughout the reticuloendothelial system and cause severe systemic disease marked by hepatosplenomegaly, lymphadenopathy, pancytopenia, fever, and weight loss. Often there is hyperpigmentation of the skin in the extremities, which is why the disease is called kala-azar ("black fever") in Hindi.

AFRICAN TRYPANOSOMIASIS (TRYPANOSOMA RHODESIENSE, T. GAMBIENSE) (p. 369)

- Is caused by kinetoplastid parasites that proliferate as extracellular forms in the blood and cause sustained or intermittent fevers, lymphadenopathy, splenomegaly, progressive brain dysfunction (sleeping sickness), cachexia, and death.
- *Trypanosoma rhodesiense* infection is often acute and virulent, and its tsetse fly vector prefers the savannah plains of East Africa.
- *T. gambiense* infection tends to be chronic and occurs most frequently in the West African bush.
- African trypanosomes are covered by a single, very abundant, glycolipid-anchored protein called the variable surface glycoprotein (VSG), which varies in response to host antibodies.

A large, red, rubbery chancre forms at the site of the insect bite, where numerous parasites are surrounded by a dense, largely mononuclear, inflammatory infiltrate.

With chronicity, the lymph nodes and spleen enlarge due to hyperplasia and infiltration by lymphocytes, plasma cells, and macrophages, which are filled with killed parasites.

In the CNS, there is a leptomeningitis extending into the perivascular Virchow-Robin spaces and eventually a demyelinating panencephalitis.

CHAGAS' DISEASE (TRYPANOSOMA CRUZI) (p. 370)

- Caused by a kinetoplastid, intracellular protozoan parasite *T. cruzi*, is the most frequent cause of heart failure in Brazil and neighboring Latin American countries.
- *T. cruzi* parasites are transmitted from person to person via "kissing bugs" (triatomids), which hide in the cracks of rickety houses.
- *T. cruzi* resist complement by means of a surface protein homologous to the human complement regulatory protein, decay accelerating factor
- A protein called penetrin on the surface of *T. cruzi* binds the extracellular matrix proteins heparin, heparin sulfate, and collagen and mediates invasion of the parasites into host cells, where parasites escape from the phagolysosome into the cytosol.

In acute Chagas' disease, which is mild in most individuals, focal myocardial cell necrosis is accompanied by interstitial inflammatory infiltrates.

In chronic Chagas' disease, which occurs in 20% of infected

patients 5 to 15 years after initial infection and appears to be an autoimmune disease, the heart is typically dilated and contains mural thrombi. There is interstitial and perivascular mononuclear inflammatory infiltrate, which is heaviest in the right bundle branch and causes cardiac arrhythmias. Many patients with lethal carditis also have dilatation of the esophagus or colon.

SCHISTOSOMIASIS (p. 371)

- Is transmitted by fresh water snails and is the most important helminth disease, infecting ~200 million persons and killing ~250 thousand annually.
- Most of the mortality comes from hepatic granulomas and fibrosis, caused by *Schistosoma mansoni* in Latin America, Africa, and the Middle East, and *S. japonicum* and *S. mekongi* in East Asia.
- In Africa, *S. haematobium* causes hematuria and granulomatous disease of the bladder, resulting in chronic obstructive uropathy.
- Female schistosomes produce hundreds of eggs per day, around which granulomas are formed composed of macrophages, lymphocytes, neutrophils, and eosinophils.

In some 10% of heavily infected persons, schistosomes induce an exuberant periportal fibrosis, called "pipe-stem" fibrosis, or Symmer's fibrosis. In portal triads vein lumens are obliterated, causing presinusoidal portal hypertension and severe congestive splenomegaly, esophageal varices, and ascites.

In *S. haematobium* infection, granulomas may cause blood in the urine, stenoses of the ureters, and an increased rate of squamous carcinoma of the bladder.

ELEPHANTIASIS (*WUCHERERIA BANCROFTI, BRUGIA MALAYI*) (p. 373)

- Lymphatic filariasis is transmitted by mosquitoes and is caused by two closely related nematodes, *Wuchereria bancrofti* and *Brugia malayi.*
- Filariasis causes a spectrum of diseases including (1) asymptomatic microfilaremia, (2) chronic lymphadenitis with swelling of the dependent limb or scrotum (elephantiasis), and (3) tropical pulmonary eosinophilia.
- In microfilararemic individuals who appear healthy, there is a hypoimmune response to circulating parasites.
- In chronic lymphatic filariasis, there is no filaremia but instead a persistent lymphedema of the scrotum, penis, vulva, leg, or arm. Hyperkeratotic and fibrotic elephantoid skin overlies dilated lymphatics that contain adult filarial worms surrounded by eosinophils, hemorrhage, and fibrin or granulomas.
- In tropical pulmonary eosinophilia, there is an IgE-mediated hypersensitivity to microfilariae in which dead microfilariae are surrounded by stellate, hyaline eosinophilic precipitates embedded in small epithelioid granulomas (Meyers-Kouvenaar bodies).

RIVER BLINDNESS (*ONCHOCERCA VOLVULUS*) (p. 374)

- A major cause of blindness in equatorial Africa, caused by *Onchocerca volvulus,* a filarial nematode transmitted by blackflies.

- Adult parasites mate in the dermis, where they are surrounded by a mixed infiltrate of host cells that produces a characteristic subcutaneous nodule (onchocercomata).

The major pathology, which includes blindness and chronic pruritic dermatitis, is caused by large numbers of microfilariae, released by females, that accumulate in the skin and in the eye chambers.

"Leopard" skin shows foci of epidermal atrophy and elastic fiber breakdown alternating with areas of hyperkeratosis, hyperpigmentation with pigment incontinence, dermal atrophy, and fibrosis.

Degenerating microfilaria and a surrounding eosinophilic infiltrate cause blindness by means of a sclerosing keratitis, which may opacify the cornea, and cause choroid and retinal atrophy.

Environmental and Nutritional Diseases

The morbidity and mortality caused by environmental disease are staggering. Witness the toll exacted by nutritional deprivation and infectious diarrhea in Third World countries. Many environmental threats to life (e.g., water pollution, ozone depletion) are beyond our scope; here the discussions are limited to (1) adverse effects of air pollution, particularly smoking, (2) injuries induced by chemicals, including drugs, (3) hazardous physical agents, with emphasis on radiation injury, and (4) the health consequences of under- and overnutrition.

AIR POLLUTION—SMOKING (p. 380)

In industrialized countries, particularly within cities, the air is often contaminated with a variety of potentially toxic substances, including sulfur dioxide, nitrogen dioxide, carbon monoxide, ozone, and lead as well as other pollutants, some of which are mentioned in Table 9–1. But much more important is cigarette smoking (cigar and pipe smoking, although not without some risk, are much less hazardous). Cigarette smoke is a veritable "witches' brew" containing well-documented carcinogens for lower animals, (and very likely for humans, such as polycyclic hydrocarbons); cell irritants and toxins such as formaldehyde, ammonia, and oxides of nitrogen; carbon monoxide; and nicotine, to name only the most abundant. Depending on pack-years of smoking, the type of cigarette used, and personal smoking habits, the cumulative exposure to the products in cigarette smoke is very high and usually sustained for years.

ACTIVE SMOKING. Mainstream cigarette smoke increases the risk for the following disorders, correlated with intensity and duration of smoking:

- Myocardial infarction, the number one cause of death related to cigarette smoking.
- Bronchogenic carcinoma—80%–90% of these cancers attributed to cigarette smoking.
- Other cancers—lip, oral cavity, larynx, esophagus, pancreas— significantly more frequent in smokers.
- Lung diseases—chronic obstructive lung disease (acute and chronic bronchitis, emphysema), present in about 50%–70% of chronic cigarette smokers. Cigarette smoking also contributes to the development of various pneumoconioses (p. 706).
- Systemic atherosclerosis—smoking is one of the major risk factors in its development and progression.

Table 9–1. The Principal Indoor Air Pollutants and Their Sources*

Pollutant	Typical Sources	Principal Effects
SO_2, respirable particles	Tobacco smoke, wood and coal stoves, fireplaces, outside air	Irritant to respiratory epithelium
NO, NO_2	Gas ranges and pilot lights	Irritant to respiratory epithelium
CO	Gas ranges and pilot lights, outside air	Forms carboxyhemoglobin
Infectious or allergenic biologic materials	Dust mites and cockroaches, pollens, animal dander, bacteria, fungi, viruses	Allergic reactions, infections
Formaldehyde	Urea formaldehyde foam insulation, glues, fiberboard, plywood, particle board	Allergic reactions
Radon and radon daughters	Ground beneath buildings	Lung cancer
Volatile organic compounds: benzene, styrene	Outgassing from water, solvents, paints, cleaning compounds; combustion	Respiratory toxin, cancer
Semivolatile organics: chlorinated hydrocarbons and polycyclic compounds, such as benzopyrene, polychlorinated biphenyls (PCBs)	Pesticides, herbicides, combustion of wood, tobacco, and charcoal	See Table 9–5
Asbestos	Building insulation	Pneumoconiosis, cancer

*Exclusive of unique industrial pollutants that result in pneumoconioses.
From Cotran, R. S., Kumar, V., and Robbins, S. L.: Robbins Pathologic Basis of Disease. 5th ed. Philadelphia, W. B. Saunders Co., 1994, p. 382.

- Stroke—two to three times more common in cigarette smokers than in nonsmokers.
- Pregnancy—also an increased incidence of low birth weight, prematurity, spontaneous abortions, stillbirths, and infant mortality. Suggestions that it increases the likelihood of abruptio placentae, placenta previa, and premature rupture of the membranes. Whether it has adverse consequences on the intellectual development of the fetus remains controversial.

PASSIVE SMOKING. This is fairly clearly documented to be detrimental to health. Obviously, the intensity and duration of exposure to cigarette smoke determine the level of risk. It is probably highest among infants and young children of smoking mothers. The major consequences are a 1.5-fold increased risk of lung cancer, a greater prevalence of respiratory tract illnesses in the infants and children, and a somewhat increased predisposition to cardiovascular disease, particularly myocardial infarction. Whether passive smoking has a deleterious effect on the physical and intellectual development of the infant is hotly contested.

CESSATION OF SMOKING. This eventually reverses most of its deleterious effects. The increased risks of lung cancer and laryngeal cancer begin to decline within 1–2 years of smoking cessation but do not reach baseline for 20 or more years. More prompt is the reduction in the risk of MI, which begins to appear within a year or two but does not approach baseline until 5–20 years. Most promptly responsive is the predisposition to inflammations and infections of the lungs and airways (emphysema, once developed, is irreversible).

CHEMICAL AND DRUG INJURY (p. 383)

All chemicals and drugs are capable of causing injury or even death in sufficient amounts. The exposure may occur in the workplace; may be accidental, as in the child who swallows a toxic cleaning product; may be self-administered, e.g., suicide, use of "street drugs"; or may be an adverse drug reaction (ADR) to a therapeutic agent, either self- or physician-administered. Among the more than 1 million reported poisonings in the United States in 1990, 80% were accidental and occurred mostly in children under the age of 6 years. About 7% were suicidal. ADRs accounted for fewer than 1% and were responsible for only 10 of the 612 deaths attributable to chemicals and drugs.

THERAPEUTIC AGENTS (p. 383)

Adverse Drug Reactions (ADRs) (p. 384)

ADRs can be crudely defined as any unwanted response to a usual dose of a drug. A great majority of ADRs represent either (1) exaggeration of a predictable pharmacologic effect, or (2) an unpredictable response to a standard dose. An example of the first category is the potentially harmful effects on bone marrow of powerful chemotherapeutic agents used in the treatment of cancer. In the attempt to destroy all the cancer cells, the dividing marrow cells are placed at risk, and so thrombocytopenia or neutropenia sometimes appears. These complications are predictable and usually reversible but may lead to serious bleeding or infectious problems. The second category of ADR is exemplified by the totally unpredictable allergic anaphylactic reaction (potentially fatal) to a standard dose or even a skin test dose of penicillin. Some of the more common ADRs and implicated agents are presented in Table 9–2.

Although any therapeutic agent may under certain circumstances cause death, those most commonly implicated are

- Tricyclic antidepressants—widely used. Overdosage may cause central nervous system depression, convulsions, coma, and death. Concurrent alcohol consumption or barbiturates enhance their effects.
- Acetaminophen (Tylenol) is the active metabolite of phenacetin. When large amounts are taken, may induce hepatic necrosis.
- Aspirin—excessive dosages (2–4 gm in children, 10–30 gm in adults) may produce fluid and electrolyte imbalances and metabolic acidosis; chronic exposure to large doses (2–4 gm) may cause gastritis and a bleeding tendency. Prolonged exposure to proprietary preparations of analgesics containing aspirin and phenacetin as well as other analgesics has induced renal papillary necrosis.
- Halothane—anesthetic agent, has produced hepatic necrosis, sometimes massive, but the mechanism—direct toxicity or unpredictable hypersensitivity—remains uncertain.

Exogenous Estrogens and Oral Contraceptives
(p. 385)

Exogenous natural estrogens when taken with progestins, begun soon after the menopause, will retard and possibly prevent the development of postmenopausal osteoporosis and also significantly reduce the risk of myocardial infarction (relative risk: 0.5). However, there are potential adverse consequences, particularly with the prolonged use of synthetic estrogens, e.g., diethylstilbestrol. The risks of the untoward effects are reduced or neutralized with natural estrogens, particularly when coupled with progestins. Major concerns are

- *Endometrial carcinoma* with prolonged unopposed estrogens—relative risk: 1.7–2.0. Risk is reduced or neutralized when combined with progestins, albeit at the price of "pseudomenstrual" bleeding.
- *Breast carcinoma*—increased risk with high dose, unopposed synthetic estrogens; but low-dose natural steroids, particularly with cyclic progestins, no increased risk.
- *Venous thrombosis and pulmonary embolism*—increased likelihood with the use of synthetic estrogens, but low doses of natural estrogens impose no increased risk.
- *Vaginal adenosis* in adolescents whose mothers had taken stilbestrol during pregnancy (uncommonly used today). Rarely, adenosis leads to clear cell vaginal adenocarcinoma.
- *Other effects*—postmenopausal estrogens increase risk of cholesterolosis and gallbladder disease.

Oral contraceptives (OCs) have in the past been linked to an increased risk of venous thrombosis and breast cancer, but "pills" now in use have markedly reduced amounts of estrogens and are combined with progestins. The predisposition to thrombosis apparently has been completely neutralized in nonsmokers younger than 45 years of age, but there is a slight residual increase in older smokers. On the other hand, OCs protect against ovarian cancer and reduce the incidence of malignant transformation of fibrocystic changes in the breast. More contro-

Table 9–2. Some Common Adverse Drug Reactions and Their Agents

Reaction	Major Offenders
Blood Dyscrasias (feature of almost half of all drug-related deaths)	
Granulocytopenia, aplastic anemia, pancytopenia	Antineoplastic agents, immunosuppressives, and chloramphenicol
Hemolytic anemia, thrombocytopenia	Penicillin, methyldopa, quinidine
Cutaneous	
Urticaria, macules, papules, vesicles, petechiae, exfoliative dermatitis, fixed drug eruptions	Antineoplastic agents, sulfonamides, hydantoins, many others
Cardiac	
Arrhythmias	Theophylline, hydantoins
Cardiomyopathy	Doxorubicin, daunorubicin
Renal	
Glomerulonephritis	Penicillamine
Acute tubular necrosis	Aminoglycoside antibiotics, cyclosporine, amphotericin B
Tubulointerstitial disease with papillary necrosis	Phenacetin, salicylates
Pulmonary	
Asthma	Salicylates
Acute pneumonitis	Nitrofurantoin
Interstitial fibrosis	Busulfan, nitrofurantoin, bleomycin
Hepatic	
Fatty change	Tetracycline
Diffuse hepatocellular damage	Halothane, isoniazid, acetaminophen
Cholestasis	Chlorpromazine, estrogens, contraceptive agents
Systemic	
Anaphylaxis	Penicillin
Lupus erythematosus syndrome (drug-induced lupus)	Hydralazine, procainamide
Central Nervous System	
Tinnitus and dizziness	Salicylates
Acute dystonic reactions and parkinsonian syndrome	Phenothiazine antipsychotics
Respiratory depression	Sedatives

From Cotran, R. S., Kumar, V., and Robbins, S. L.: Robbins Pathologic Basis of Disease. 5th ed. Philadelphia, W. B. Saunders Co., 1994, p. 384.

versial is the effect on breast cancer and myocardial infarction. With the former, there appears to be a slightly increased risk (1.2–1.4) of cancer in women younger than 46 years who have taken combined OCs for at least 10 years, but some studies disagree. Despite the protection against myocardial infarction afforded by natural estrogens, there may be a slightly increased incidence of MI in women who are smokers and older than age 35 years. This increased risk may have been neutralized with the current use of "minipills." There is no increased risk of endometrial cancer, but there is a slightly increased risk of cervical cancer, correlated with the duration of use and level of sexual activity. The adverse reactions must be balanced against the consequences (abortions, unwanted children) of nonuse.

Other Therapeutic Agents (p. 387)

Antineoplastic agents, because they are targeted on proliferating cells, may (1) damage the bone marrow with severe anemia, leukopenia, and thrombocytopenia, as mentioned, (2) damage lymphocytes, leading to immunosuppression with its consequences, and (3) induce mutations in cells and initiate some form of cancer, particularly acute myeloid leukemia.

Immunosuppressive agents predispose to microbial infections, particularly with ever-present opportunists such as cytomegalovirus, *Pneumocystis carinii*, candida, and aspergillus. The immunosuppressed individual also is at risk for graft-versus-host disease. Uncommonly, these agents initiate some form of lymphoma, principally immunoblastic. Cyclosporine in sufficient doses is nephrotoxic, and azathioprine may cause interstitial pneumonitis.

Antimicrobial agents may (1) induce hypersensitivity reactions, (2) permit the emergence of antibiotic-resistant strains, and (3) by eradicating the normal microflora, allow opportunists to emerge, e.g., a disseminated fungal infection.

NONTHERAPEUTIC AGENTS (p. 388)

Ethyl Alcohol

Because of widespread use, is a major cause of morbidity and mortality. Has major effect on and is largely degraded in liver, and so its metabolism is discussed on p. 859. It suffices here to note that ethanol is almost completely directly absorbed in the stomach and small intestine and is metabolized mostly in the liver at the rate of 10 gm per hour in the usual adult (12 ounces of beer and 1.5 ounces of 80-proof liquor). A blood alcohol level of 20–30 mg/dl producing mild-to-moderate intoxication can result from only one or two drinks of liquor in a relatively brief time. The legal level of intoxication is set at 70–100 mg/dl in various states. Stupor can be produced by ±200 mg/dl and fatal coma at 300–400 mg/dl.

Acute alcoholism most profoundly affects the CNS but may induce acute changes in liver (fatty) and stomach (gastritis, erosions). Manifestations in CNS are mediated by its action on membrane receptors for γ-aminobutyric acid to thus block inhibitory neural pathways leading to unopposed excitatory pathways.

Chronic alcoholism has an impact on virtually all organs and tissues in the body (Table 9–3).

- *Hepatic changes* range from fatty change to alcoholic hepatitis to overt cirrhosis.
- *Central nervous system changes* conform to Wernicke's en-

Table 9–3. Major Consequences of Chronic Alcoholism

	Lesion	**Mechanism**
Liver	Fatty change	Direct toxicity
	Acute hepatitis	Direct toxicity
	Alcoholic cirrhosis (see Chapter 17)	Direct toxicity
Central nervous system	Wernicke's syndrome	Thiamine deficiency
	Korsakoff's syndrome	Combined thiamine deficiency and direct toxicity
	Cerebral atrophy (questionable)	Direct toxicity
	Cerebellar degeneration	Nutritional deficiency
Nerves	Peripheral neuropathy	Thiamine deficiency
Heart	Congestive cardiomyopathy	Direct toxicity
Skeletal muscle	Acute and chronic fiber rhabdomyolysis	Direct toxicity
Testes	Atrophy	Unclear
Pancreas	Chronic pancreatitis	Unclear
Fetal alcohol syndrome	Retardation of physical and mental development, malformations	?Direct toxicity

From Cotran, R. S., Kumar, V., and Robbins, S. L.: Robbins Pathologic Basis of Disease. 5th ed. Philadelphia, W. B. Saunders Co., 1994, p. 389.

cephalopathy, sometimes with superimposed Korsakoff's syndrome—the former with ataxia, ophthalmoplegia, and global confusion marked by symmetric foci of softening, congestion, and hemorrhages: in the paraventricular regions of the thalamus and hypothalamus; in the mammillary bodies; about the aqueduct in the midbrain and in the floor of the 4th ventricle. No new changes are seen with Korsakoff's syndrome, which apparently reflects global impairment of neuronal function, leading to a profound memory deficit.
• *Peripheral nerves* suffer a demyelinative neuropathy attributable mainly to malnourishment and thiamine deficiency.
• *Cardiovascular consequences:* may directly injure myocardium to produce dilated congestive cardiomyopathy, but moderate consumption of ethanol decreases the incidence of coronary heart disease; the reverse occurs with heavy consumption.
• *Miscellaneous changes:* increased incidence of chronic pancreatitis; cancer of the mouth, larynx, esophagus, stomach, and possibly elsewhere; and during pregnancy may adversely affect the mental and physical development of the fetus—fetal alcohol syndrome.

Lead (p. 390)

Continues to be a major environmental hazard in the United States and other industrialized countries. May be absorbed through the gastrointestinal tract, or the respiratory system when volatilized. Major source of lead, particularly for children, is flaking lead paint, but in industrialized countries lead contaminates the atmosphere (motor vehicle exhaust from leaded gasoline), water supplies from plumbing systems with lead pipes or lead-soldered joints, the soil and root vegetables. Also found in newsprint, pottery glazes, and other places.

Urban adults inhale or ingest about 100–150 μg daily and absorb only 10%. Children have a lower intake but absorb 50%. Absorbed lead is transported in the blood, and although environmental standards permit a blood level of 10 μg/dl in children and 25 μg/dl in adults, clinical surveys suggest that as little as 5–10 μg/dl may be injurious. Small daily increments are cumulative, mainly taken up by bone (80%–90%) and developing teeth in children. About 5%–10% remains in blood, and the residual is deposited in soft tissues throughout the body. Skeletal deposits that accumulate, particularly in the epiphyses, are mobilized only with the turnover of bone salts.

Lead poisons enzymes by binding to sulfhydryl groups and denatures proteins, particularly in red cell precursors involved in heme synthesis. Other possible targets may be Ca-signal transduction and inactivation of calcium pumps, as well as interference with neural adhesion molecules and possibly neural synapse formation.

Major and anatomic targets are

- *Blood*—interferes with aminolevulinic acid dehydratase and ferroketolase displacing iron from the heme molecule to form zinc protoporphyrin, thus a microcytic hypochromic anemia develops and distinctive punctate basophilic stippling of red cells.
- *Brain*—damage seen particularly in infants and children. Edema of the brain, potentially fatal in the form of global demyelination of cerebral and cerebellar white matter along with perivascular edema and sometimes hemorrhages. In the adult, CNS is uncommonly affected.
- *Peripheral nerves*—a demyelinating neuropathy typically affecting innervation of the extensor muscles of the wrist and fingers, producing *wrist and foot drop.*
- *Gastrointestinal tract*—may manifest lead "colic," but the only demonstrable anatomic changes are a "lead line" along the gingival margin, which is distinctive but not diagnostic of lead poisoning.
- *Kidney*—may develop tubulointerstitial nephritis, leading to Fanconi's syndrome. Prominent eosinophilic intranuclear inclusions in tubular epithelial cells are characteristic of lead intoxication. Made up of lead-protein complexes. With prolonged exposure to lead, normal excretion of uric acid is impaired, causing "saturnine gout." An increased incidence of renal adenomas and carcinomas.

Diagnosis rests on recognition of stippled red cells and on elevated blood lead levels.

Environmental and Occupational Carcinogens
(p. 392)

Among the myriad environmental agents proved or suspected of being carcinogenic in animals, only a relative few can be clearly implicated in humans. Some are cited in Table 9–4.

Street Drugs (p. 393)

Addiction to psychoactive drugs is on the increase in the United States and is a major social, medical, and public health problem.

Table 9–4. Some Major Environmental and Occupational Carcinogens

Agent	Type of Cancer
Arsenic (miners, insecticide manufacturers and users, chemical workers)	Skin, lung, liver carcinomas
Asbestos (see Chapter 15)	Bronchogenic carcinoma, mesothelioma, others
Benzene (rubber cement workers, distillers, dye users)	Myelogenous leukemia
Beta-naphthylamine (rubber, dye industries)	Bladder carcinoma
Cadmium (miners, processors)	Prostate, kidney carcinoma
Chromium (producers and processors)	Nasal cavity, sinus, lung, and laryngeal carcinomas
Cigarette smoke	Bronchogenic carcinoma, others
Nickel (miners and processors)	Nasal sinus, lung cancers
Nitrites (Chapter 16)	Stomach carcinoma
Uranium (miners and processors)	Lung carcinoma
Vinyl chloride (plastic industries)	Liver angiosarcoma

From Cotran, R. S., Kumar, V. , and Robbins, S. L.: Robbins Pathologic Basis of Disease. 5th ed. Philadelphia, W. B. Saunders Co., 1994, p. 393.

The three most widely used and abused are marijuana, cocaine (including crack), and heroin. Data available for 1985 indicate that there are over 25 million users of one or more of these agents in the United States. Despite the difficulties of segregating the adverse effects of one from the other because often several are taken concurrently, the following findings are reasonably well substantiated.

MARIJUANA. Once considered relatively harmless, now thought to have well-defined adverse consequences. The active product found in cannabis plants is Δ^9-tetrahydrocannabinol (THC). Hashish is the dried resin of the plant. Smoked, ingested, or extracted and injected, marijuana produces, with chronic use:

- *Behavioral and psychologic changes* in the form of cognitive and psychomotor impairments, potentially contributing to fatal auto accidents, and in a few instances, apparent psychotic breaks (either induced or unmasked).
- *Other changes* are less well established, including irritation of the respiratory tract and an increased incidence of bronchogenic carcinoma from smoking "joints"; reduced fertility (mostly in males); adverse fetal consequences (low birth weight, retarded development, increased frequency of leukemia); and possibly depressed cell-mediated and humoral immunity.

On the positive side, marijuana is effective in treatment of nausea of cancer chemotherapy, glaucoma, convulsive seizures, and asthma when other drugs have failed.

COCAINE AND CRACK. Used by 6–8 million individuals in

the United States, one-third of whom are probably confirmed addicts. It is estimated there are ± 5000 new users daily in the U.S. Extracted from the leaves of the coca plant, it is commercially available as a white powder, which is diluted with some other "look alike" e.g., talc, quinine. Extraction of the white powder yields a more potent dried resin—"crack." Cocaine is absorbed from the nasal mucosa (when snorted), the lungs (when smoked), and the gastrointestinal tract, as well as parenterally, when dissolved.

It is a potent CNS stimulant, blocking the reuptake of neurotransmitters (e.g., norepinephrine, dopamine) at synapses to increase the level of these neurotransmitters at postsynaptic receptor sites. It also increases the synthesis of norepinephrine and dopamine. Thus euphoria, hypertension, tachycardia, and vasoconstriction are induced.

Pathophysiologic consequences:

- *Intense euphoria* within minutes which soon dissipates, leaving a craving for more. The larger dosages incur risks of seizure, respiratory depression, and death.
- *Cardiovascular disease* is a serious threat, ranging from hypertension and tachycardia to arrhythmias and sudden death. Myocardial infarction has occurred, owing to the combined effects of tachycardia and coronary vasoconstriction, as well as cardiomyopathy, possibly related to hypersensitivity reaction or microvascular vasoconstriction. Another risk, rupture of the ascending aorta attributable to the hypertension.
- *Pregnancy* complications, including placental abruption, premature labor, retarded fetal development, and stillbirth.

One of the most fearsome aspects of the use of cocaine is the intense craving (virtual addiction) for repeated doses to maintain "the high," leading to psychopathic and sociopathic behavior in an effort to get the money for the habit.

HEROIN. Although less commonly used than cocaine, it is more hazardous. Derived from the poppy plant, it is marketed as a white powder diluted with some other look-alike powder. Usually taken dissolved in water, by subcutaneous or intravenous injection; in the course of preparing the "shot" the fluid is almost always contaminated, sometimes with virulent microbes. Heroin acts on the normal endogenous opioid receptors widely distributed in the body but mainly found in the CNS, endocrine, gastrointestinal, and cardiovascular systems. It produces a sense of well-being and indeed sedation, which lasts a few or more hours and then requires repeated dosages. With prolonged use habituation calls for ever larger amounts of the drug, with the following possible consequences:

- *Sudden death.* An ever-present threat, owing to possible loss of habituation (as may occur with incarceration), an unexpectedly potent drug provided by the "pusher" to "get rid of a nuisance," or confusion about the amount of drug already taken.
- *Pulmonary complications* range from sensitivity reactions with edema, septic embolism arising at the injection site, infections introduced along with the drug, and foreign body granulomas from talc used as a diluent.
- *Granulomas* may occur anywhere in the mononuclear phagocyte system as a response to injected talc silicates contained within the diluting white powder.
- *Infectious complications*, major threats, range from viral hepati-

tis transmitted by shared needles, vegetative endocarditis from introduced microbes, skin abscesses, cellulitis and ulcerations at sites of subcutaneous injections, and in the chronic addict, the development of amyloidosis secondary to the infections. Drug addicts, particularly those using heroin, constitute one of the major risk groups for AIDS.

- *Kidney disease* is a well-defined risk in the forms of focal glomerulosclerosis or renal amyloidosis.
- *Other complications* include tetanus, peripheral neuropathy, myopathy, osteomyelitis, and acute vasculitis.

OTHER NONTHERAPEUTIC AGENTS (p. 398)

Among the many that might be cited, only a few that are particularly lethal are mentioned in Table 9–5.

PHYSICAL INJURIES (p. 398)

Potential causes of physical injuries are *mechanical forces, changes in temperature, changes in atmospheric pressure,* and *radiation.*

INJURIES INDUCED BY MECHANICAL FORCE (p. 398)

Three categories: soft tissue injuries, bone injuries, and head injuries (last two covered elsewhere). Skin injuries can be classified as

- *Abrasion*—a scrape with loss of superficial epidermal cells.
- *Laceration or incision*—former is a tear from overstretching of soft tissue, may be linear or stellate, usually strands of fibrous tissue or blood vessels bridge the defect. By contrast, an incision created by a sharp cutting object (scalpel, broken glass) creates sharp margins with no fibrous or vascular bridging. Both may be superficial or deep, but both are capable of complete repair, albeit leaving a scar.
- *Contusion*—caused by a blunt force that ruptures small blood vessels to produce a hematoma without disrupting continuity of tissue. The hematoma may be superficial or deep, immediately visible, or appear only hours to days later as the partially digested red cells and hemoglobin diffuse outward.
- *Gunshot wound*—depends on many variables, including type of gun used (hand gun or rifle), caliber of bullet, type of ammunition, distance between firearm and the body, locus of injury, trajectory of the missile (at right angle to the skin or oblique), and gyroscopic stability of missile (amount of wobbling or tumbling). At close range, wound of entrance is surrounded by a grayish discoloration (fouling) resulting from heat, smoke, and burnt powder and more peripherally by a stippled halo resulting from larger particles. At a greater distance only stippling is present. Generally, the wound of entrance is smaller than the wound of exit. The wound may be circular when missile enters at right angle to the skin surface, may be oval with angled trajectory, or may be quite irregular, with a wobbling missile. Depending on mass and velocity of the bullet, it may penetrate internal viscera with fairly restricted burrowing or cause massive lacerations. Exit wound has no fouling or stippling, has everted margins, and is often irregular with radiating lacerations.

Table 9–5. Uncommon, Potentially Fatal Nontherapeutic Agents

Agent	Source	Effect	Mechanism of Injury
Methanol	Solvents, sterno, antifreezes	Inebriation, toxic necrosis of retinal ganglion cells with blindness	Metabolized to formaldehyde and formic acid
Carbon monoxide			
Acute poisoning	Fossil fuel exhaust, cigarette smoke	Cherry-red skin, mucous membranes Variable hypoxic injury to brain, liver, renal tubules	Carboxy-Hb (replaces Hb) unable to transport O_2
Chronic poisoning		Diffuse neuronal loss, particularly basal ganglia Occasionally, focal cerebral demyelination	Protracted low-level hypoxia. Once formed, carboxy-Hb is slowly replaced by mass action of O_2
Mercury			
Some organic compounds	Industrial contamination of ocean: from bacteria to fish to humans; inferior latex paint	With chronic ingestion—central nervous system disturbances, hearing loss, blindness, spasticity, paralysis (Minamata disease); acrodynia	Neuronal toxicity with focal softenings; cerebral and cerebellar atrophy
Inorganic compounds	Industrial exposure and ingestion	Membranous glomerulopathy with proteinuria, hyaline droplets to necrosis of proximal tubular epithelium	Inactivates wide variety of enzymes

Cyanide	Released by combustion of wool, silk, plastic upholstery—most likely in smoke inhalation in burning dwellings	Hypoxic injury to brain, liver, kidneys, other organs	Binds to cytochrome oxidase and inhibits cellular respiration
Mushroom poisoning	*Amanita phalloides* (potentially lethal) *A. muscaria* (rarely lethal)	Vomiting, abdominal cramps—central nervous system changes, centrilobular hepatic necrosis to massive necrosis, renal tubular necrosis	*A. phalloides* toxin inhibits RNA polymerase
Insecticides Chlorinated hydrocarbons	Agricultural and home use: DDT, chlordane, dieldrin	Hyperexcitability, delirium, convulsions, coma	Toxic neuronal injury
Organophosphates	Tri-orthocresylphosphate (TOCP)	Muscle twitching to paralysis, cardiac arrthythmias	Inhibits cholinesterase with synaptic build-up of acetylcholine

From Cotran, R. S., Kumar, V., and Robbins, S. L.: Robbins Pathologic Basis of Disease. 5th ed. Philadelphia, W. B. Saunders Co., 1994, p. 397.

INJURIES RELATED TO
CHANGES IN TEMPERATURE (p. 399)

May be produced by either hyperthermia or hypothermia.

Hyperthermic Injuries

May be superficial (*surface burns*) or have *systemic conse-quences*.

Surface cutaneous burns—the clinical significance of a cutane-ous burn depends on

- Percentage of total body surface involved.
- Depth of the burn.
- Possible presence of internal injuries from inhalation of hot gases and fumes.
- Promptness and efficacy of the postburn therapy, e.g., fluid and electrolyte replacement, prevention of shock, and control of infection.

With current effective management, there is no limit to the percentage of body surface burned and survival. More serious is depth of the burn and secondary infection. Depth is expressed by "partial thickness" or "full thickness." Former implies deeper layers of epidermis or epidermal appendages spared, from which epithelial regeneration can occur. By contrast, *full thickness* implies total destruction of epidermis and appendages, and so regeneration can occur only from margins or grafts.

Systemic consequences of a surface burn often overshadow local injury. Initially there is neurogenic shock, possibly followed by hypovolemic shock owing to loss of water, electrolytes, and protein from the burn wound. Within hours the denuded surface is colonized by organisms, most often *Pseudomonas aeruginosa,* but possibly, *Staphylococcus aureus* and fungi, in particular, candida species. Organisms proliferate wildly on necrotic tissue and inflammatory exudate. These infections may lead to throm-bophlebitis, cellulitis, endocarditis, and potentially fatal bacter-emia. Septic shock with renal failure and/or respiratory distress syndrome may now appear. These threats to life dominate the current practice of immediately providing fluids and electrolytes and an antibacterial wound cover—ideally, cultured sheets of autologous or homologous epidermal cells.

Heat Stroke (p. 400)

Heat stroke (when core body temperature exceeds 40°C) occurs in two clinical settings.

- *Exertional heat stroke* with very hot, dry skin (may be accompa-nied by sweating). May be associated with rhabdomyolysis, myoglobinemia, myoglobinuria, and acute tubular necrosis.
- *Classic heat stroke* from elevated ambient temperatures, rarely accompanied by sweating, but redistribution of blood to the skin may lead to marked hypotension, syncope, or even coma.

Abnormally Low Temperatures (p. 400)

Causes injury by the freezing of cell water, with physical disloca-tion of cells, or by slowing circulatory flow and inducing ischemic injuries. Such changes underlie "trench foot." When the whole body is exposed to low temperatures, there is slowing of meta-bolic processes and slowing of circulation. Death may occur before evident tissue injury.

INJURIES RELATED TO CHANGES IN ATMOSPHERIC PRESSURE (p. 401)

- High-altitude illness
- Blast injury
- Air or gas embolism
- Decompression disease (caisson disease)

The first two are rare and discussed in *Pathologic Basis of Disease*, so only the last two are mentioned here.

Air or gas embolism may occur with scuba diving, mechanical positive-pressure/ventilatory support, hyperbaric oxygen therapy, and rarely, decompression disease (see below). In all, there is an abnormal increase in intra-alveolar air or gas pressure, rupture of alveolar walls, and entrance of air or gas into the interstitium and small blood vessels. Pulmonary, mediastinal, and subcutaneous emphysema may follow, which are all reversible, but small air or gas emboli may gain access to the arteriolar circulation and by coalescence create obstructive emboli leading to myocardial or cerebral ischemic episodes.

Decompression (caisson) disease occurs in deep sea divers and underwater workers exposed for prolonged periods to increased atmospheric pressure. Larger and larger amounts of oxygen and accompanying gases (nitrogen or helium) dissolve in the blood and tissue fluids. Once the ambient pressure is lowered, as in ascent to the surface, bubbles form in the blood stream and tissues. Oxygen is soluble and quickly redissolved, but the other gases (nitrogen or helium) are slow to dissolve and form embolic masses in the tissues and blood. Those localizing in and about the joints cause *"the bends"*; in the respiratory passages, *"the chokes"*; in the CNS, *mental disturbances*; and in the less well-vascularized ends of bone, ischemic foci of *aseptic necrosis* may appear days later.

RADIATION INJURY (p. 402)

Radiation can injure cells or in sufficient amounts kill them (some are more vulnerable than others), and in sublethal doses induce mutations, leading to developmental abnormalities in fetuses, or to cancers in children or adults. *Radiation comprises the physical transfer of energy from its site of origin to the biologic target, inducing ionization of its atoms.* With sufficient transfer of energy, electrons can be ejected from their orbits in atoms, hence the term "ionizing radiation." But even less energetic radiation incapable of ionizing atoms or molecules, such as UV light, may be carcinogenic to the skin. Two forms of ionizing radiation: (1) electromagnetic waves, including x-rays and gamma-rays, and (2) particulate radiation, including α-particles, β-particles, protons, and others.

Mechanisms of Action

Two theories are the *"direct target effect"* and the *"indirect effect."*

The former postulates the direct impact of ionizing energy on atoms and molecules within the cell, disrupting or inactivating enzymes, structural proteins and, most importantly, DNA. The indirect theory proposes that ionizing radiation first induces radiolysis of cell water, with production of free "hot" radicals, which then interact with atoms and molecules of the cell. By either mechanism and depending on the dosage and vulnerability of particular cells, the following consequences may result:

- Reversible injury with temporary cell swelling and clumping of nuclear chromatin.
- Cell death, with nuclear pyknosis or karyorrhexis.
- Inhibition of mitotic division ("reproductive death"), sometimes is responsible for polykaryons.
- Derangement of the mitotic process, leading to abnormal nuclear morphology in cells destined to die.
- More subtle genetic injuries having delayed mutagenic, teratogenic, or carcinogenic consequences.

Factors Governing Biologic Response

Can be divided into those related to the radiation itself and those related to particular cell and tissue targets.

Those related to radiation include the type, dose, and rate of delivery—i.e., with divided doses (as is customary in radiation therapy), targeted cells may repair in the interval between radiation. Various types of radiation differ in penetrability, energy per unit of radiation, and pattern of deposition of energy. These variables can be expressed by terms LET and RBE. The LET (*linear energy transfer*) of radiation refers to the energy loss or transfer per unit of distance traveled, thus denoting the likelihood of a radiation effect within a specific target area. For example, an α-particle of large mass but low velocity will deliver most of its energy within a relatively short distance and have a high LET, yet γ-rays of high velocity penetrate deeply but generate few interactions and have a low LET. RBE (*relative biologic effectiveness*) is a measure of the effectiveness of different forms of radiation in inducing the same biologic effect. Thus, dose delivered and absorbed over a period of time and the LET and RBE values of the particular form of radiation govern its biologic potential. The size of the area exposed has systemic consequences, as discussed later.

Equally important is

- the radiosensitivity of different types of normal cells and their tumors, the cell's capacity to repair radiation damage during intervals between divided doses,
- the phase of the cell cycle during which cells are exposed, and
- the degree of vascularization and oxygenation of the cells and tissues.

In general, the *radiosensitivity* of cells and their tumors is proportional to their reproductive activity and in inverse proportion to their level of specialization. Well-differentiated neurons incapable of mitotic division and highly specialized in their differentiation are very radioresistant. However, in the case of tumors, much depends on the ability to deliver effective quantities of radiation to the neoplasm without producing unacceptable damage to intervening or surrounding normal tissues.

The *capacity to repair radiation-induced injuries* modifies the response. Individuals having genetic inability to repair DNA damage (e.g., xeroderma pigmentosum) are much more vulnerable to radiation-induced cancers, particularly skin cancers (in areas exposed to UV light).

The *phase of the cell cycle* modifies the effect, since peak sensitivity of most cells is during G_2 and mitosis. Thus, rapidly dividing populations (bone marrow, gut mucosa, and subsets of lymphocytes) are more vulnerable than highly specialized nonproliferating cells (neuron, striated muscle cells, hepatocytes).

Vascularization and oxygenation of tissues modifies vulnerability, called "the oxygen effect," which amplifies low LET radiation damage. Thus the poorly vascularized, poorly oxygenated center of large tumor masses is less vulnerable to lethal radiation injury than the better oxygenated peripheral zone.

An overview of the radiosensitivity of normal tissues and tumors is offered in Table 9–6.

Morphologic Changes in Cells and Organs—Acute Radiation Injury

First, general effects, followed by specific effects on particular tissues and structures.

In *general*, the nucleus is the prime target. It first appears swollen with clumping of chromatin. With higher levels or later, there is pyknosis and even fragmentation. All manner of abnormal nuclear morphology may appear with bizarre mitotic figures along with aneuploidy and polyploidy. There may be cell swelling, with focal plasma membrane breaks and distortion of organelles such as mitochondria.

Effects on various structures and organs. An overview of these changes is offered in Table 9–7.

Table 9–6. Radiosensitivity of Normal Tissues and Tumors

Radio-sensitivity	Normal Cells	Tumors
High	Lymphoid, hematopoietic, spermatogonia, ovarian follicles	Leukemia-lymphoma, seminoma, dysgerminoma
Fairly high	Acute reactions for gastrointestinal and mucosal epithelium, hair follicles, and lung Late reactions for lung, kidney	Squamous cell carcinoma of skin, head and neck, and cervix Adenocarcinoma of breast Neuroblastoma
Medium	Late reactions for gastrointestinal tract, endothelium, glandular epithelium of breast, glandular epithelium of pancreas, epithelium of bladder, growing cartilage, bone, and normal brain	Carcinoma of lung, esophagus, pancreas, bladder, medulloblastoma, ovarian cancer
Low	Bone, mature cartilage, muscle, peripheral nerves	Gliomas, large sarcomas, melanoma, renal cell cancer, osteosarcoma

With the gracious help of Dr. Norman Coleman, Harvard Medical School.

From Cotran, R. S., Kumar, V., and Robbins, S. L.: Robbins Pathologic Basis of Disease. 5th ed. Philadelphia, W. B. Saunders Co., 1994, p. 404.

Table 9-7. Radiation Changes in Various Organs

Organ	Early and Late Changes	Delayed Consequences
More Vulnerable Organs		
Blood vessels	Acute vascular dilatation Endothelial swelling Necrosis—endothelial and smooth muscle cells Later—intimal hyperplasia Secondary thromboses	Collagenous hyalinization of vascular walls Narrowing of lumens to complete obliteration
Skin	Mild postradiation erythema Epithelial blistering and desquamation Dermatitis with patchy increased or decreased pigmentation Dermal fibroses with atrophy—hair follicles and appendages	Atrophy of epidermis Abnormal pigmentation Ulcerations Skin cancers
Hematopoietic and lymphoid system	Shrinkage of lymph nodes and spleen Destruction of proliferating marrow precursors Lymphopenia first, then granulocytopenia and thrombocytopenia, and last, anemia	Potentially reversible with survival Residual marrow fibrosis Potential leukemogenesis
Gonads	Destruction of germinal epithelium, both sexes Sclerosis of follicles in many and loss of ova Sclerosis of seminiferous tubules in testes	Sterility
Lungs	Swelling and injury to endothelial cells of alveolar capillaries Pulmonary edema, "radiation pneumonitis"	Thickening and sclerosis of alveolar vessels Interstitial fibroses

GI tract	Mucosa of all but esophagus and rectum sensitive to radiation, with edema, hyperemia, ulcerations Atypia, dysplasia—mucosal epithelial cells	Fibrosis—bowel wall; atrophy of mucosa Cancer
Less Vulnerable Organs		
Heart	Fibrinous pericarditis, myocardial edema, "radiation cardiomyopathy"	Pericardial fibrosis, myocardial interstitial fibrosis
Kidney	Acute tubular injury, vascular sclerosis	Cortical atrophy with tubular and glomerular hyalinization, "chronic radiation nephritis"
Bladder	Acute damage to lining epithelium—"radiation cystitis"—with ulceration	Persistent mucosal atrophy, fibrosis of bladder wall
Cartilage and bone	In fetus and child, growing bone and cartilage are radiosensitive with the potential for later skeletal distortion; in the adult they are radioresistant, save for the possible development of areas of aseptic necrosis where the vascular supply is obliterated	Late-appearing osteogenic sarcoma
Central nervous system	In developing fetus, the embryonic brain is radiosensitive; mature nervous tissue is radioresistant	Areas of demyelination and neuronal degenerative changes secondary to radiation-induced ischemia
Breast		Late-appearing cancers

Less Vulnerable Organs from Cotran, R. S., Kumar, V., and Robbins, S. L.: Robbins Pathologic Basis of Disease. 5th ed. Philadelphia, W. B. Saunders Co., 1994, p. 406.

Whole Body Radiation (p. 407)

The effects of radiation on the body are materially modified by the area exposed, as well as the total dose. One hundred rads of whole body irradiation can produce significant systemic reactions, yet 4000 rads or more are often administered in divided doses to restricted fields in the radiotherapy of tumors. An overview of the consequences of whole body irradiation is presented in Table 9–8.

Late Effects of Radiation (p. 407)

As mentioned, radiation is a mutagen and may cause developmental anomalies when a fetus is exposed *in utero* or may have carcinogenic potential in the postnatal individual.

The *in utero* effects are still being debated, but there is a prevailing opinion of increased rate of stillbirths, mental retardation, and congenital malformations, as well as postnatal cancer, principally leukemias and lymphomas. Data from Hiroshima and Nagasaki, however, challenge these conclusions.

The carcinogenic potential of radiant energy is incontrovertible. Exposure of the thyroid gland in children and young adolescents to even therapeutic irradiation has led to an increased incidence of thyroid cancer years later. Survivors of the atomic bomb blasts have suffered a 20-fold increased incidence of acute leukemias and chronic myelogenous leukemia, but not chronic lymphocytic leukemia. In children younger than 10 years of age at the time of the blasts, there has been an increased incidence of breast cancer in women, thyroid cancer, lymphoma, and others.

The possible cumulative effects of small doses of radiant energy and its long latency have led to concern about the potential hazards of nuclear waste sites and nuclear reactors.

NUTRITIONAL DISEASE (p. 408)

May arise because of a grossly deficient diet or inadequate amounts of specific items, e.g., proteins and/or vitamins; but contrariwise, an excessive intake of food or specific forms of food also may be harmful. Undernutrition is a global problem. Usually caused by a lack of food (*primary malnutrition*) as is all too common in economically deprived countries, but primary malnutrition also may appear among privileged societies in pockets of poverty. Undernutrition also may occur in the midst of plenty (secondary malnutrition) for a variety of reasons, as pointed out in Table 9–9.

PROTEIN-CALORIE UNDERNUTRITION (PROTEIN-CALORIE MALNUTRITION—PCM) (p. 409)

PCM is rampant in Third World countries because of widespread starvation and because of large families with young infants deprived of breast feeding by a newborn. Much less frequently, PCM (also called protein energy malnutrition, PEM) is seen in industrialized nations among the very poor, elderly, homeless, drug addicts, and long-term hospitalized medical and surgical patients.

PCM may present as a spectrum of syndromes from *kwashiorkor* at one end, related to a lack of quality protein in the diet despite a possibly adequate caloric intake, to *marasmus* at the other end, induced by a lack of total calories (i.e., starvation). Between these extremes are many intermediate syndromes partaking of the features of both. Contributing significantly to PCM are the near-universal diarrheal infections and parasitic intestinal infestations.

Kwashiorkor is the Ga language term for "the disease of the displaced child," when a newborn requires breast feeding and displaces an older sibling. It is marked by apathy, peripheral edema, subcutaneous fat, moon face, and large, fatty liver. Often there are "flaky paint" dermatoses with areas of hyperpigmentation and depigmentation. There may also be bands of depigmentation of the hair, reflecting periods of particularly poor nutrition.

Marasmus, by contrast, implies "wasting," with stunted growth, absence of subcutaneous fat, atrophy of muscles, and pinched, wizened faces.

Central anatomic changes in PCM are (1) growth failure, more marked in marasmus than in kwashiorkor; (2) peripheral edema in kwashiorkor but not in marasmus; and (3) loss of body fat and atrophy of the muscles in marasmus. The many hybrid forms share the features of both.

The fatty *liver* in kwashiorkor is not distinctive and may be due in part to inadequate synthesis of proteins necessary for the formation of lipoproteins.

The *small bowel* in kwashiorkor reveals mucosal atrophy with loss of villi and microvilli. Many of these changes may be secondary to intestinal parasites.

The *bone marrow* in both kwashiorkor and marasmus is hypoplastic, inducing a microcytic hypochromic anemia, but a concomitant deficiency of folates may produce concurrent macrocytic changes.

The *brain* in PCM is reported by some to show cerebral atrophy, but this observation has been challenged.

With restoration of an adequate diet, physical health may be restored with "catch-up" growth; however, intellectual deficits may persist, but these may be related to social deprivation rather than diet.

VITAMINS (p. 411)

Four vitamins, A, D, E, and K, are fat soluble, and nine, C and B complex, are water soluble. Small amounts of D and K can be synthesized endogenously, but an exogenous source of all is required. Primary (dietary) deficiencies almost always involve multiple vitamins and frequently protein-calorie malnutrition as well. Secondary conditioned deficiencies, however, may be quite specific, e.g., B_{12} in pernicious anemia. However, secondary deficiencies also may involve multiple vitamins, as with fat malabsorptions. Primary deficiencies may be encountered anywhere (are much more common in Third World countries) but may . also occur in economically privileged societies among the economically deprived and those lacking knowledge of the nutritional value of foods. Secondary deficiencies occur globally and are often seen in alcoholic and elderly people, with their restricted diets. A survey of the various vitamins and their deficiency states is offered in Table 9–10.

NUTRITIONAL EXCESSES AND IMBALANCES
(p. 425)

To this point we have been considering disorders related to dietary insufficiencies, but excesses and imbalances also may be harmful.

Table 9-8. Acute Radiation Syndrome Classification

| Category | Whole-Body Dose, rem | Signs and Symptoms | | Prognosis |
		Early	Definitive	
Subclinical	≤200	Mild nausea and vomiting lasting 24 hr or less; lymphocytes < 1500/mm³	Usually asymptomatic to minimal prodromal symptoms; depression of neutrophils and platelets by week 4–5 at higher dose range	Essentially 100% survival in healthy adults; evidence of some damage at higher dose range
Hematopoietic (mild form)	200–400	Intermittent nausea and vomiting in nearly all patients for 2–4+ days; lymphocytes < 1000/mm³	Maximum hematopoietic depression at 3 weeks	Recovery in 5–6 weeks; complete recovery in 4–6 months
Hematopoietic (severe form)	400–600°	Severe hematopoietic complications; mild evidence of gastrointestinal damage on upper dose range	Severe neutrophil and platelet depression in 3–5 weeks; evidence of infection and hemorrhage may appear	Zero to 100% mortality in untreated cases; requires bone marrow transplants and other supportive measures; rarely fatal with adequate replacement therapy

Gastrointestinal	600–1000	Severe prodromal symptoms of nausea, vomiting, and diarrhea; difficult management of patient; lymphocytes < 500/mm^3	Some recovery, then return of severe diarrhea with blood and electrolyte loss; severe neutrophil and platelet depression by day 10 or earlier; hemorrhage and infection within 1–3 weeks	High mortality even among those given functional replacement therapy; progression to shock and death in 10–14 days; effectiveness of bone marrow therapy not yet evaluated
Central nervous system	≥1000	Severe, intractable nausea and vomiting; central nervous system symptoms; burning sensation at exposure and confusion; lymphocytes essentially lacking	Partial recovery, then progressive confusion and shock; central nervous system damage	100% mortality likely independent of therapy given; death in 14–36 hr; marrow therapy trial indicated

*The human whole-body LD$_{50}$ at 60 days is approximately 400–500 rem.
From Castronovo F. P.: Radiation accidents. *In* Wilkins, E. W., Jr. (ed): Emergency Medicine: Scientific Foundations and Current Practice, 3rd ed. Baltimore, Williams & Wilkins, 1989.

177

Table 9–9. Major Causes of Secondary Malnutrition

Decreased Intake
  Poor teeth
  Dysphagia
  Systemic disease inducing anorexia
  Bizarre or restricted food habits
  Anorexia nervosa

Malabsorption
  Biliary and pancreatic diseases
  Enteric malabsorption syndromes
  Vitamin B_{12} malabsorption (pernicious anemia)

Increased Requirements
  Rapid growth in infancy, in childhood, and at puberty
  Pregnancy, particularly repeated
  Trauma
  Burns
  Excessive losses, as in protein-losing enteropathies and
    nephropathies

Special categories
  Total parenteral nutrition
  Drug-induced interference with absorption
  Genetic disorders interfering with conversion or utilization of
    nutrients

From Cotran, R. S., Kumar, V., and Robbins, S. L.: Robbins Pathologic Basis of Disease. 5th ed. Philadelphia, W. B. Saunders Co., 1994, p. 408.

OBESITY (p. 425)

This is widely recognized but difficult to define and objectively diagnose, particularly its severity. Most widely used measures are

- Weight for height corrected for gender and age—body mass index (BMI).
- Skin fold measurements in specified locations—biceps, triceps, subscapular, elsewhere.
- Waist-hip circumference ratio.
- Other more elaborate systems.

Distribution of body fat tends to differ between men and women. In men, it tends to be abdominal. In women, fat tends to accumulate in the gluteal regions and upper thighs. Thus men become "apples" and women "pears."

Basis for obesity is generally held to be consumption of calories in excess of need. Lack of exercise reduces the need and often underlies the excess, but in addition there appear to be genetic factors. Children of obese parents reared by lean foster parents more often become obese than children of lean parents reared under comparable or identical circumstances. When both obese and lean individuals perform the same tasks, the obese mysteriously use up fewer calories than the lean, and so they store more calories.

Consequences of obesity are wide ranging.

- *Insulin resistance develops*—enlarged fat cells have fewer insulin receptors per unit of cell surface, and also acquire impaired glucose utilization owing to a postreceptor abnormality.

- *Diabetes mellitus*—type II adult-onset diabetes is associated with obesity in 80% of patients. Indeed, the mild diabetic state may disappear with weight loss.
- *Hypertension* is correlated with obesity.
- *Heart disease*—more prevalent among the obese than the non-obese. With obesity, blood and stroke volume and left ventricular filling pressures increase, predisposing to left ventricular hypertrophy and possible failure.
- *Coronary heart disease*—a major contributor to the higher mortality among obese people. CHD nearly 50% more common among men and women who are 30%–40% above ideal weight than among controls.
- *Other conditions*—increased incidence of cholesterol gallstones; greater difficulty breathing and greater tendency for somnolence ("pickwickian syndrome").
- *Most convincing*—caloric restriction prolongs the life of laboratory animals.

DIET AND SYSTEMIC DISEASES (p. 427)

Innumerable examples have been mentioned throughout the discussion of various disorders. A few are

- Consumption of animal fats and cholesterol and the development of atherosclerosis.
- The antiatherogenic influences of polyunsaturated fatty acids, particularly those derived from fish oils.
- Role of excess sodium in the induction of hypertension.
- Dietary deficiency of fiber or roughage as a possible predisposition to diverticulosis of the colon.
- Effect of calories and obesity on diabetes already pointed out.
- Many others.

DIET AND CANCER (p. 428)

The belief is widespread that in some way diet influences the predisposition to cancer. Most supporting evidence derives from population studies. Cancer of stomach—five times more frequent in Japan than in the U.S., but reverse is true for cancer of the colon. Families who migrate from a high incidence to a low incidence locale (or vice versa) tend to acquire over the generations the incidence rates of the new locale. These trends are attributed without hard proof to the diet. Even more convincing is laboratory evidence of reduced incidence and progression of experimentally induced neoplasms in laboratory animals on a restricted dietary intake.

Three aspects of diet are of concern: (1) potential content of exogenous carcinogens, (2) potential synthesis of endogenous carcinogens from elements of the diet, and (3) possible lack of protective factors.

Relative to exogenous carcinogens—there is a strong suspicion that aflatoxins derived from *Aspergillus flavus,* which grows on improperly stored moldy grains and ground nuts, are a major contributor to the high incidence of liver cancer in Africa. Another area of concern stemming from experiments in animals using nonphysiologic dosage is the possible roles of saccharin and cyclamates in the induction of bladder cancer in humans, but documentary evidence is lacking.

Endogenous synthesis of carcinogens points to the possible production of nitrosamines or amides from protein precursors

Table 9-10. Vitamins: Major Roles and Deficiency Syndromes

Vitamin	Roles	Deficiency Syndromes
Fat-Soluble		
Vitamin A (retinol) carotene retinoids (Synth)	Contributes critical prosthetic groups to visual pigment Required for differentiation of specialized epithelia Maintains resistance to infections ?Anticarcinogenic Antioxidant	Night blindness Squamous metaplasia, conjunctival xerophthalmia with Bitot's spots; ulceration cornea (keratomalacia); blindness Increases vulnerability to childhood infections, particularly measles ?Protects against skin cancer
Vitamin D	Facilitates intestinal absorption of Ca and PO_4 and mineralization of bone	Rickets in children—failure of mineralization in newly formed osteoid, inducing skeletal deformities in growing bone: bowing of legs, overgrowth of costochondral junction, frontal bossing, etc. Osteomalacia in adults—failure of mineralization in remodeled bone
Vitamin E Vitamin K	Major antioxidant; scavenges free radicals Cofactor in hepatic carboxylation of procoagulants—factors II (prothrombin), VII, IX, and X	Spinocerebellar degeneration Bleeding diathesis

Water-Soluble

Vitamin	Functions	Deficiency Syndromes
Vitamin B$_1$ (thiamine)	As pyrophosphate, is coenzyme in decarboxylation reactions	Dry and wet beriberi, Wernicke's syndrome
	Facilitates conduction of impulses in peripheral nerves	?Korsakoff's syndrome
Vitamin B$_2$ (riboflavin)	Converted to coenzymes flavin mononucleotide (FMN) and flavin-adenine dinucleotide (FAD), cofactors for many enzymes in intermediary metabolism	Ariboflavinosis, cheilosis, stomatitis, glossitis, dermatitis, corneal vascularization
Niacin	Incorporated into nicotinamide-adenine dinucleotide (NAD) and NAD phosphate (NADP) involved in a variety of redox reactions	Pellagra—three "Ds": dementia, dermatitis, diarrhea
Vitamin B$_6$ (pyridoxine)	Derivatives serve as coenzymes in many intermediary reactions	Cheilosis, glossitis, dermatitis, peripheral neuropathy
Vitamin B$_{12}$ (cyanocobalamin)	Requisite for normal folate metabolism and DNA synthesis	Combined system disease (megaloblastic pernicious anemia and degeneration of posterolateral spinal cord tracts)
	Maintenance of myelinization of spinal cord tracts	
Vitamin C	Serves in many oxidation-reduction (redox) reactions and hydroxylation of collagen	Scurvy
Folate	Essential for transfer and utilization of 1-carbon units in DNA synthesis	Megaloblastic anemia
Pantothenic acid	Incorporated in coenzyme A	No nonexperimental syndrome recognized
Biotin	Cofactor in carboxylation reactions	No clearly defined clinical syndrome
	Widely abundant in foods	

Water-Soluble Vitamins from Cotran, R. S., Kumar, V., and Robbins, S. L.: Robbins Pathologic Basis of Disease. 5th ed. Philadelphia, W. B. Saunders Co., 1994, p. 412.

and nitrates in the diet, but there is no clear documentation of such. Animal fats have been accused of favoring the development of colonic and breast carcinoma. Putatively, the high fat diet might increase bile acids in the gut, which favor growth of bacteroides organisms. These could then act on bile acids to produce carcinogens, but the proposition is entirely speculative. Building on the concern about synthesis of carcinogens is the absence of dietary fiber in the diet, which slows intestinal transit time and thus prolongs exposure of the intestinal mucosa to putative carcinogenic products. Intriguing as these speculations may be, they are lacking in rigorous proof.

Lack of protective factors refers particularly to inadequate fiber and inadequate amounts of vitamins A, C, and E. Another theoretic lack in the diet is selenium. How these factors protect remains unexplained, and so the line of reasoning is at best tenuous and lacking in proof.

CHAPTER TEN

Diseases of Infancy and Childhood

In general, the conditions that afflict infants and children fall into one (and frequently more) of four main categories:

- Those that are primarily a consequence of the immaturity of an organ or system(s) (e.g., hyaline membrane disease)
- Those related to the unique susceptibility of the fetus or infant to external or environmental factors (some malformations, infections)
- Those due to particular genetic or inherited "defects"
- Tumors and tumor-like conditions

INTRAUTERINE GROWTH RETARDATION (IUGR) (p. 433)

Synonymous with *small for gestational age infants* (SGA). Factors known to result in IUGR can be divided into three main categories:

- *Fetal*—Chromosomal disorders (most commonly trisomy 13, 18, and 21; liveborn monosomy X; and triploidy), congenital anomalies, congenital infections.
- *Placental*—Abruptio placentae, placenta previa, placental thrombosis and infarctions, placental infections, multiple gestations.
  Confined placental mosaicism is another cause of IUGR. Two genetic populations of cells (usually one normal and one abnormal—i.e., trisomic) are present in the placenta or fetus, depending upon when during gestation and in which cell population the genetic error occurs. The resultant phenotype may vary depending upon whether the maternal or paternal copy of the gene or chromosome is involved (*genomic imprinting*).
- *Maternal* (most common)—Underlying mechanism is decreased blood flow to the placenta. This can be caused by toxemia of pregnancy, chronic hypertension, nutritional status, maternal narcotic abuse, alcohol intake, heavy cigarette smoking, and intake of certain drugs (which may also be teratogens), such as Dilantin.

IMMATURITY OF ORGAN SYSTEMS (p. 434)

Structural and functional immaturity of organ systems is a major cause of morbidity and mortality in preterm infants, particularly those who are small for gestational age.

MORPHOLOGY

- *Lungs*—Thick-walled alveolar septa with large amounts of inter- and intralobular connective tissue resulting in a separation of the vascular supply from alveolar spaces, hindering oxygenation. Alveolar spaces frequently contain eosinophilic proteinaceous precipitate and occasional squamous epithelial cells. Development of alveoli continues after birth, with the full complement of alveoli reached at approximately 8 years of age.
- *Kidneys*—Primitive glomeruli and tubules are often present in the subcapsular zone (nephrogenic zone). Deeper glomeruli and tubules are well formed, however, and function is usually adequate, even in the premature infant.
- *Brain*—Grossly, the external surface of the brain is relatively smooth, with markedly simplified to absent convolutions (sulci and gyri). Both cell migration and myelination are incomplete, so the brain is soft and gelatinous and there is poor demarcation of white and gray matter structures. Vital brain centers are well developed enough to sustain normal function even in the very premature infant, although maintenance of homeostasis (temperature, respiration) is imperfect.
- *Liver*—The liver is large relative to the size of the preterm infant, partially due to the presence of *extramedullary hematopoiesis*. Many liver enzymes are not well developed, including those responsible for biliary excretion, partly explaining the frequent presence of physiologic jaundice in premature infants.

APGAR SCORE (p. 436)

This is a measure of the physiologic condition and responsiveness of the newborn infant, having some correlation with survival. It is calculated at 1 and 5 minutes of life based upon heart rate, respiratory effort, muscle tone, response to noxious stimulus, and skin color, each scored 0, 1, or 2.

BIRTH INJURIES (p. 436)

The risk and type of birth injury vary with the gestational age and size of the infant, with injuries most commonly involving the head, skeletal system, liver, adrenal glands, and peripheral nerves.

- *Intracranial hemorrhage* is the most common important birth injury. Predisposing factors include prolonged labor, hypoxia, hemorrhagic disorders, or intracranial vascular anomalies. Consequences of intracranial hemorrhage include increases in intracranial pressure, damage to brain substance, herniation of the medulla or base of the brain into the foramen magnum, with depression of function of the vital medullary centers.
- *Caput succedaneum,* an accumulation of interstitial fluid in the soft tissue of the scalp, resulting in a circular area of edema, congestion, and swelling at the site where the head begins to enter the lower uterine canal. If there is accompanying hemorrhage, it is referred to as a *cephalohematoma.* Both forms of injury are of little clinical significance unless associated with an underlying skull fracture.

CONGENITAL MALFORMATIONS (p. 437)

These are defined as morphologic defects present at birth, although they may not become apparent until later in life. About

3% of newborn infants have a major malformation. They represent a major cause of infant mortality and a significant cause of illness, disability, and death in the early years of life.

DEFINITIONS

Malformations

- Intrinsic abnormality occurring relatively early during the developmental process.
- They may involve single or multiple organ systems.
- Risk of recurrence varies.

Deformations

- Arise relatively late in fetal life as a result of mechanical factors.
- Usually manifest as abnormalities in shape, form, or position of the body (e.g., club feet).
- Most are associated with a much lower risk of recurrence in subsequent siblings than are malformations.
- Most common underlying factor is uterine constraint.
- Predisposing factors are both maternal (e.g., first pregnancy, uterine leiomyomas) and fetal/placental (e.g., oligohydramnios, multiple fetuses, abnormal fetal presentation).

Disruptions

- Secondary destruction or interference with an organ or body region that was previously normal in development.
- May be caused by either external or internal interferences (e.g., amniotic bands).
- Not heritable.

Sequence

- Multiple congenital anomalies resulting from a single localized aberration in organogenesis leading to secondary effects in other organs.
- Primary abnormality may be a malformation, deformation, or disruption.
- Good example is the *oligohydramnios (Potter's) sequence*: diverse factors such as renal agenesis or an amniotic leak result in decreased amniotic fluid (oligohydramnios), compression of the fetus, and a classic phenotype in the newborn infant, including flattened facies and positional abnormalities of the hands and feet.

Syndrome

- Several defects are present that are thought to be pathogenetically related but cannot be explained on the basis of a single, localized initiating anomaly.
- Most often caused by a single etiologic agent (e.g., viral infection or chromosomal abnormality) that simultaneously affects several tissues.
- When the underlying cause of a syndrome is known, such as neurofibromatosis in a child with café-au-lait spots and numerous soft tissue masses, the syndrome is referred to as a *disease*.

In contrast to the above global definitions, *organ-specific terms* include:

Agenesis Complete absence of an organ and its associated primordium

Aplasia Absence of an organ due to failure of the developmental anlage to develop

Atresia Absence of an opening, usually of a hollow visceral organ such as trachea or intestine

Hypoplasia Incomplete or underdevelopment of an organ, with decreased numbers of cells (less severe form of aplasia)

Hyperplasia Overdevelopment of an organ associated with increased numbers of cells

Hypertrophy Increase in organ size/function related to an increase in the size of individual cells

Hypotrophy Decrease in organ size/function related to a decrease in the size of individual cells

Dysplasia In the context of malformations, refers to abnormal organization of individual cells

CAUSES OF MALFORMATIONS

The exact cause is known in approximately half of cases.

Genetic

- *Karyotypic abnormalities*—present in approximately 10%–15% of liveborn infants with congenital malformations; trisomy 21 is most common, followed by Klinefelter's syndrome (47,XXY), Turner's syndrome (45,XO), and trisomy 13. Most cytogenetic aberrations arise as defects in gametogenesis and so are not familial.
- *Single gene mutations* of large effect—relatively uncommon but follow mendelian patterns of inheritance.
- *Multifactorial*—interaction of two or more genes of small effect with environmental factors.

Environmental

The presence and nature of malformations resulting from environmental factors is related to the timing of the intrauterine exposure and the differential susceptibility of various organ systems (see Figure 10–7, p. 441), of *Robbin's Pathologic Basis of Disease*).

- *Viruses*—e.g., *rubella* (infection before 16 weeks' gestation may result in cataracts, heart defects, and deafness); *cytomegalovirus* (most common fetal viral infection—highest risk for malformations occurs with infection in second trimester when organogenesis is largely complete, most commonly affects the central nervous system resulting in mental retardation, microcephaly, and deafness); and *herpes simplex.*
- *Drugs and chemicals*—probably cause less than 1% of congenital malformations; agents suspected to be teratogenic include thalidomide, folate antagonists, androgenic hormones, alcohol, anticonvulsants, and 13-*cis*-retinoic acid.
- *Radiation*—exposure to heavy doses during organogenesis can result in malformations, including microcephaly, blindness, skull defects, spina bifida.

MECHANISMS OF MALFORMATIONS

The pathogenesis of many congenital malformations is complex and poorly understood. However:

- The *timing* of the prenatal teratogenic insult has an important impact on the occurrence and type of malformation produced.
- Teratogens and genetic defects *may act at several levels,* in-

cluding cell proliferation, cell migration, differentiation, and damage to formed differentiated organs.
- Genetic defects *may cause malformations either directly or by influencing other genes;* an example of the latter is the group of morphogenesis genes, in particular the *homeobox genes* and the *paired box* or *PAX genes (see p. 442).*

PERINATAL INFECTIONS (p. 442)

Specific infections are discussed in Chapter 8.

TRANSCERVICAL OR ASCENDING INFECTIONS

- Most bacterial and a few viral infections are acquired via the cervicovaginal route.
- May be acquired either *in utero* by "inhalation" into the lungs of infected amniotic fluid or around the time of birth by passing through an infected birth canal.
- Chorioamnionitis of the placental membranes and funisitis (inflammation of the umbilical cord) are usually present.
- Pneumonia, sepsis, and frequently meningitis are the most common sequelae.

TRANSPLACENTAL OR HEMATOLOGIC INFECTIONS

- Most parasites and viral infections and a few bacterial infections gain access to the fetal blood stream via the chorionic villi.
- Infection may occur at any time during gestation or, occasionally, at the time of delivery via maternal-to-fetal transfusion.
- Sequelae are highly variable, depending upon the gestational timing and microorganism.

RESPIRATORY DISTRESS SYNDROME (RDS) (p. 444)

Also known as hyaline membrane disease, can have many etiologies including aspiration during birth of blood and amniotic fluid, feeble respiratory efforts secondary to immaturity, brain injury with failure of central respiratory centers, asphyxiating coils of umbilical cord around the neck of the infant, and excessive maternal sedation. However, idiopathic RDS is most important.

ETIOLOGY AND PATHOGENESIS

- Primarily occurs in the immature lung—60% incidence in infants born at <28 weeks' gestation and <5% incidence in infants born at >37 weeks' gestation.
- Associated with a deficiency of pulmonary surfactant, which is synthesized by type II pneumocytes most abundant after 35 weeks' gestation (Chapter 15).
- Decreased surfactant results in increased alveolar surface tension with progressive atelectasis of alveoli and a higher inspiratory pressure required to expand the alveolus (hence respiratory distress).
- Hypoxemia results in acidosis, pulmonary vasoconstriction, pulmonary hypoperfusion, capillary endothelial and alveolar epithelial damage, and leak of plasma into the alveolus, which combines with fibrin and necrotic alveolar pneumocytes to form hyaline membranes.
- Corticosteroids help prevent RDS; they induce the formation of surfactant lipids and apoprotein in fetal lung.

MORPHOLOGY

- Grossly, lungs are solid, airless, and reddish purple.
- Microscopically, alveoli are poorly developed and frequently collapsed, and pink hyaline membranes line respiratory bronchioles, alveolar ducts, and random alveoli.

CLINICAL

- Stereotypic infant is preterm but appropriate for gestational age.
- Associated with maternal diabetes and cesarean section delivery.
- Prior to delivery, assessment of amniotic fluid phospholipids (lecithin/sphingomyelin ratio) is often performed in preterm infants as an indicator of the fetal level of surfactant synthesis. When the surfactant level is low, glucocorticoids may be administered in an attempt to induce surfactant synthesis.
- At birth, infant may need to be resuscitated, but quickly establishes spontaneous rhythmic breathing and normal color for a short period of time; shortly thereafter, respiratory distress ensues, the infant becomes cyanotic, and diffuse reticulogranular densities radiographically characterize the lungs. Oxygen therapy may alleviate the symptoms, but in some cases respiratory distress persists, cyanosis increases, and the infant becomes flaccid, unresponsive, and apneic. Surfactant replacement is often administered while ventilatory assistance is provided. In uncomplicated cases, recovery begins in 3–4 days. Infants who recover are at risk for developing *bronchopulmonary dysplasia* as a direct consequence of high-concentration oxygen therapy.

ERYTHROBLASTOSIS FETALIS–HEMOLYTIC DISEASE OF THE NEWBORN (p. 446)

Hemolytic disease of the newborn infant occurs as a consequence of blood group incompatibility between mother and fetus.

ETIOLOGY AND PATHOGENESIS

The fetus inherits red blood cell antigens from the father (i.e., the D antigen of the Rh group), which the mother lacks. A small transplacental (fetal/maternal) bleed, (usually occurring at the time of delivery) allows fetal red blood cells to enter the maternal circulation and to elicit an immune response with maternal antibody production in response to this "foreign" antigen (only a minority of "foreign" blood group antigens are immunogenic). The first exposure to the specific antigenic stimulus elicits primarily production of IgM antibodies that do not cross the placenta; however, the mother is now "sensitized" to this antigen. Subsequent exposures to even small amounts of the same antigen (usually small transplacental bleeds occurring in subsequent pregnancies) elicit maternal production of IgG antibodies that *do* cross the placenta and bind to fetal red blood cells, resulting in red blood cell lysis.

Of the numerous Rh antigens, the D antigen is the major cause of Rh incompatibility (D antigen positive is referred to as Rh-positive; D antigen negative is referred to as Rh-negative). In Rh-negative mothers, immunoprophylaxis with anti-D immunoglobulin prevents sensitization and hemolytic disease of the newborn in the majority of cases. Although ABO incompatibility is more common than Rh incompatibility, hemolytic disease severe enough to require treatment is rare; this is primarily because (a) most anti-A and anti-B antibodies are of the IgM type and do not cross the placenta, (b) neonatal red cells express blood group antigens A and B poorly, and (c) many cells in addition to red cells express A and B antigens and therefore "sop up" some of the antibody that does gain access to the fetal blood stream. Depending upon the amount of IgG production and therefore fetal red blood cell lysis in erythroblastosis fetalis, the main consequences are anemia and the accumulation of bilirubin (jaundice). If hemolysis is mild, extramedullary hematopoiesis in the liver and spleen may suffice to maintain normal red cell levels. If hemolysis is marked, the presence of unconjugated bilirubin occurs; unconjugated bilirubin is water insoluble and has an affinity for lipids, binding to lipids in the brain and causing central nervous system damage referred to as *kernicterus*. If anemia is marked, hypoxic injury to the heart and liver may result in circulatory and hepatic failure and edema; when generalized edema and anasarca are present, the condition is referred to as *hydrops fetalis* (this is only one of many causes of hydrops fetalis (see Table 10–5, p. 448, in *Robbins Pathologic Basis of Disease*).

MORPHOLOGY

The morphologic findings vary with the severity of the hemolytic process.

- In general, there is evidence of abnormally increased erythropoietic activity. The red cell series in the bone marrow are hyperplastic, and there is extramedullary hematopoiesis in the liver, spleen, and frequently other tissues such as lymph nodes, kidneys, lungs, and even heart.
- In jaundiced infants, the unconjugated bilirubin appears to be particularly toxic to the central nervous system. The brain is heavy and edematous, and there is bright yellow staining (*kernicterus*) localized particularly to the basal ganglia, thalamus, cerebellum, cerebral gray matter, and spinal cord. Although neural damage rarely occurs if the serum bilirubin concentration is below 20 mg/dl, damage may occur at lower levels if the infant is premature.
- The gross presence of hydrops fetalis correlates with extensive subcutaneous and visceral edema, along with fluid in the peritoneal, pleural, and pericardial cavities.

GENETIC DISEASES, INCLUDING INBORN ERRORS OF METABOLISM

Only a few representative diseases occurring in the neonatal and childhood period are discussed in this chapter. For additional discussions, see Chapter 5 of *Robbins PBD*.

PHENYLKETONURIA (PKU) (p. 449)

- Approximately 50% of dietary phenylalanine is required for protein synthesis; the remainder is converted into tyrosine by the phenylalanine hydroxylase system.

- Homozygotes for one of several different mutations in the phenylalanine hydroxylase gene display variable degrees of phenylalanine hydroxylase deficiency and hyperphenylalanemia, accounting for several clinical variants.
- The most common mutation, "classic PKU," is relatively common in people of Scandinavian descent and uncommon in blacks and Jews.
- Affected infants are relatively normal at birth but develop rising plasma phenylalanine levels within the first few weeks of life, resulting in impairment of brain development and mental retardation.
- Screens at birth for abnormally elevated levels of various phenylalanine metabolites in the urine result in early diagnosis of PKU; dietary restriction of phenylalanine can alleviate most of the clinical sequelae.

Some mutations in the phenylalanine hydroxylase gene result in only a partial deficiency of phenylalanine hydroxylase and only moderately elevated serum levels of phenylalanine; these patients suffer no neurologic sequelae—the condition is referred to as *benign hyperphenylalanemia*. Other variants of PKU result from deficiencies in enzymes in the phenylalanine hydroxylase system other than phenylalanine hydroxylase; these patients have problems metabolizing other amino acids in addition to phenylalanine (such as tyrosine and tryptophan) and need to be diagnosed, since restriction of dietary phenylalanine is not sufficient treatment.

GALACTOSEMIA (p. 450)

Dietary lactose, present in milk, is split into glucose and galactose in the intestinal mucosa by lactase; galactose is then converted to glucose by three additional enzymes. The most common and clinically significant form of galactosemia is an autosomal recessive condition resulting from a homozygously inherited mutation(s) in galactose-1-phosphate uridyl transferase (GALT) and subsequent accumulation of galactose-1-phosphate.

The clinical picture of galactosemia is variable, probably corresponding to several different mutations in GALT, but infants fail to thrive at birth and develop vomiting and diarrhea within a few days of milk ingestion. Liver, eyes, and brain are most severely affected, and the spectrum of morphologic changes includes early fatty change in the liver and hepatomegaly, which is followed by cirrhosis; cataracts, and nonspecific alterations in the central nervous system (the latter resulting in mental retardation).

Urinary screening tests at birth reveal the presence of an abnormal reducing sugar, and antenatal diagnosis is possible. Removal of dietary galactose for at least the first 2 years of life prevents most of the clinical and morphologic sequelae.

CYSTIC FIBROSIS (CF) (p. 451)

This is the most common lethal genetic disease that affects white populations, with an incidence of 1 in 200 live births. Widespread disorder occurs in the secretory process of all exocrine glands, affecting both mucus-secreting and eccrine sweat glands throughout the body.

Etiology and Pathogenesis

- The cystic fibrosis gene on *chromosome 7* encodes a protein named CFTR (cystic fibrosis transmembrane conductance regulator) that serves as a *chloride channel.*
- Various mutations in this gene disrupt epithelial chloride transport as normal duct epithelia require chloride channels for resorption of chloride and, conversely, normal airway epithelium requires chloride channels for secretion of chloride. The inability of the sweat gland ducts to resorb chloride results in an *increased sweat chloride concentration* (forming the basis of the clinical "sweat chloride" test used in the diagnosis of CF). The inability of airway epithelia to secrete chloride into the lumen, combined with a decrease in active sodium absorption, results in increased water reabsorption from the lumen, dehydration of the mucus layer coating the mucosal cells, defective mucociliary action, and the ultimate accumulation of hyperconcentrated, viscid secretions that obstruct the airways and predispose to recurrent pulmonary infections.
- CFTR has two transmembrane domains, two nucleotide-binding domains, and a regulatory domain that contains protein kinase phosphorylation sites. Various mutations in the CF gene affect different regions of CFTR, resulting in different functional consequences ultimately manifest as differences in the severity of clinical sequelae. The most common mutations in the CF gene result in the deletion of three nucleotides coding for phenylalanine at position 508, known as *delta F508;* this results in defective processing of the CFTR protein and its degradation before it reaches the cell surface. Virtual absence of CFTR results in severe clinical disease, including early pancreatic insufficiency and various degrees of pulmonary damage. Other mutations may be involved with milder disease and some with male sterility only.

Morphology

Highly variable depending upon which glands are affected and the severity of involvement.

- *Pancreas*—abnormalities are present in approximately 90% of patients; changes range from accumulation of mucus in small ducts and mild dilatation of exocrine glands to total atrophy of the exocrine glands and ducts, leaving only the islets within a fibrofatty stroma. Absence of pancreatic exocrine secretions impairs fat absorption, and there is resulting avitaminosis A, which may be partially responsible for squamous metaplasia frequently observed in ductal structures.
- *Intestine*—thick viscid plugs of mucus may cause small intestinal obstruction in 5%–10% of infants with CF, a condition known as *meconium ileus.*
- *Liver*—plugging of bile canaliculi by mucinous material; in approximately 5% of patients this ultimately results in cirrhosis.
- *Salivary glands*—frequently involved; progressive dilatation of ducts, squamous metaplasia of ductal epithelium, and glandular atrophy.
- *Lungs*—changes are seen in most cases and are the most serious complication of this disease; there is hyperplasia of mucus-secreting cells, and thick secretions block and dilate bronchioles; superimposed infections and even pulmonary abscesses are common, frequently due to either *Staphylococcus*

aureus or *Pseudomonas aeruginosa* or both; *Pseudomonas cepacia* infections have been associated with fulminant illness.
- *Epididymis and vas deferens*—obstruction by thick secretions is responsible for azospermia and infertility in 95% of males surviving to adulthood.

Clinical Course

The molecular variability and complexity, including secondary pathogenetic mechanisms, that underlie CF results in highly variable clinical manifestations, with symptomatology ranging from mild to severe and onset occurring at birth to years later.

- Manifestations of malabsorption include large, foul stools, abdominal distention, and poor weight gain and usually appear during the first year of life.
- Faulty fat absorption results in deficiencies of the fat-soluble vitamins A, D, and/or K.
- Persistent pulmonary infections account for 80%–90% of deaths; other pulmonary problems include obstructive pulmonary disease, chronic cough, and cor pulmonale.
- Median life expectancy is approximately 26 years, but this may be modified by gene therapy (transfer of the CFTR gene to correct the chloride defect in cells) in the future.

SUDDEN INFANT DEATH SYNDROME (SIDS) (p. 454)

SIDS is officially defined as the "sudden death of an infant under 1 year of age which remains unexplained after a thorough case investigation, including performance of a complete autopsy, examination of the death scene, and review of the clinical history." Moreover, most SIDS deaths occur between 2 and 4 months of life; the infant usually dies while asleep and there is no evidence of distress or a struggle.

- Most SIDS victims have had symptoms of minor upper respiratory infection.
- Pathogenesis remains poorly understood, and SIDS is most likely a heterogeneous, multifactorial disorder; approximately 10% of cases may be due to an underlying inborn error in metabolism.
- Potential risk factors include infant sleeping in a prone position, prematurity and low birth weight, infant not firstborn or product of a multiple gestation mother, SIDS in a prior sibling, young or unmarried mother, low socioeconomic status, short intergestational interval, and maternal smoking or drug abuse.
- Current work suggests developmental *immaturity* of critical hypothalamic centers involved in cardiopulmonary function.
- Autopsy findings are usually subtle and of uncertain significance—include astrogliosis of the brain stem, thymic and epicardial petechiae, and frequently, evidence of a mild recent respiratory infection.

TUMORS AND TUMOR-LIKE LESIONS OF INFANCY AND CHILDHOOD (p. 456)

Benign tumors are much more common than malignant tumors, but cancer is the leading cause of death from disease in U.S. children between the ages of 4 and 14 years.

BENIGN TUMORS AND TUMOR-LIKE LESIONS

It is frequently difficult to distinguish between true tumors and tumor-like lesions in the infant and child, as displaced cells and masses of tissue may be present from birth that are histologically normal in appearance but nonetheless grow at approximately the same rate as the fetus and infant.

- *Heterotopia*—microscopically normal cells or tissues that are present in abnormal locations; usually of little significance but may be clinically confused with true neoplasms.
- *Hamartoma*—excessive (but focal) overgrowth of cells and tissues native to the organ/site in which it occurs; these can be thought of as the linkage between malformations and neoplasms.

Hemangiomas

Are the most common tumors of infancy; rarely become malignant. Most are located in the skin, particularly the face and scalp. They may enlarge along with the growth of the child, but not uncommonly they spontaneously regress. They may represent one facet of a hereditary disorder such as *von Hippel–Lindau disease*.

Lymphangiomas

- May occur on the skin, but also occur in the deeper regions of the neck, axilla, mediastinum, and retroperitoneal tissue. They tend to increase in size after birth and, depending upon the location, become clinically significant if they encroach upon vital structures. Histologically, they are composed of cystic and cavernous lymphatic spaces, with variable numbers of lymphocytes in the adjacent soft tissue.

Fibrous Tumors

- Histologically, range from sparsely cellular proliferations (*fibromatosis*) to richly cellular lesions indistinguishable from fibrosarcomas occurring in adults.
- In contrast to fibrous tumors occurring in adults, histology does not predict the biology of an individual tumor (e.g., "infantile fibrosarcoma" may spontaneously regress).

Teratomas

- Incidence has two peaks, one at 2 years of age, one in late adolescence.
- Most occurring in infancy/childhood arise in the sacrococcygeal region.
- 10% of sacrococcygeal teratomas are associated with congenital anomalies, primarily defects of the hindgut and cloacal region and other midline defects.
- Histologically similar to other teratomas (*see p. 243 of Robbins PBD*) in that mesodermal, endodermal, and ectodermal elements are present.
- Approximately 75% contain mature tissues only and are benign; approximately half the remainder are mixed with other germ cell malignancies (e.g., endodermal sinus tumor) and are malignant; the rest, designated immature teratomas, contain mature

and immature tissue, and the malignant potential correlates with the amount of immature tissue elements present.

MALIGNANT TUMORS

(Those not in this section are discussed in the organ system chapter from which they arise.) Childhood malignancies differ biologically and histologically from their counterparts occurring later in life.

1. There is a close relationship between abnormal development (teratogenesis) and tumor induction (oncogenesis).

2. There is a greater prevalence of an underlying familial or genetic germline aberration.

3. There is a tendency for some histologic "malignancies" occurring in the fetal or neonatal period to regress spontaneously or cytodifferentiate.

- The most frequent childhood cancers arise in the hematopoietic system (leukemia, some lymphomas), central nervous system (astrocytoma, medulloblastoma, ependymoma), adrenal medulla (neuroblastoma), retina (retinoblastoma), soft tissue (rhabdomyosarcoma), bone (Ewing's sarcoma, osteogenetic sarcoma) and kidney (Wilms' tumor).
- Leukemia accounts for more deaths in children under 15 years of age than all other tumors combined.
- Histologically, many pediatric cancers tend to have a more primitive (embryonal) rather than anaplastic/pleomorphic appearance, frequently exhibiting features of organogenesis specific to the site of tumor origin.
- Some pediatric tumors with a primitive appearance are collectively referred to as *small, round blue cell tumors*—neuroblastoma, lymphoma, rhabdomyosarcoma, Ewing's sarcoma/PNET (peripheral neuroectodermal tumor).

Neuroblastoma (p. 459)

- The vast majority occur in children younger than 5 years of age. They arise in the adrenal medulla or various ganglia and are made up of sheets of small, round blue cells within a neurofibrillary background and the presence of (Homer-Wright) pseudorosettes (p. 459). Some tumors/tumor cells display variable amounts of differentiation toward ganglion cells and, depending upon the degree of differentiation, they are called *ganglioneuroblastomas* or *ganglioneuromas*.
- Depending upon the pattern of metastases, tumors are staged I (confined to the organ of origin) through IV (disseminated metastases). Stage IVS tumors are unique; they usually occur in young infants/neonates, there is a small adrenal tumor, a markedly enlarged liver from extensive liver metastases, and tumor nodules within the skin and bone marrow (without causing bony destruction). Infants with these disseminated tumors have a >80% 5-year survival with minimal to no therapy.
- In addition to higher stage (except IVS) and older age, a worse prognosis is associated with near-diploid or near-tetraploid overall DNA content, deletions of the distal short arm of chromosome 1 (implying loss of tumor suppressor gene function), and amplification of the n-*myc* oncogene. Expression of

high levels of the *Trk receptor* also may be associated with a more favorable outcome.

Retinoblastoma (p. 461)

- Is usually diagnosed prior to 4 years of age and can be multifocal and bilateral. Patients usually present at about 2 years of age with eye pain and tenderness, poor vision, strabismus, and a whitish hue to the pupil. They can undergo spontaneous regression.
- The tumor is congenital or familial in a significant number of cases; most sporadic or nonheritable tumors (90% of cases) are unilateral and unifocal. Tumorigenesis is due to homozygous loss of the tumor suppressor Rb gene on chromosome 13q14 (see Chapter 7).
- Patients with familial retinoblastoma (and therefore a germline mutation in the Rb gene) are at increased risk for developing osteogenic sarcoma and other soft tissue tumors.
- Histologically, characterized by sheets of small, round blue cells with diagnostic true (Flexner-Wintersteiner) rosettes with a central lumen.

Wilms' Tumor (p. 462)

- Is usually diagnosed between 2 and 5 years of age, and the overall survival rate is greater than 90%.

In addition to the "sporadic" cases, there are associations with at least three groups of malformation syndromes, all involving aberrations in chromosome 11p.

1. *WAGR* (Wilms' tumor *a*niridia, genital anomalies, mental retardation)—patients with this syndrome have a 33% chance of developing Wilms' tumor; involves *deletion on chromosome 11p band 13 of the Wilms tumor 1 (WT-1) gene* and also this *aniridia gene*, which is just distal to this locus (of interest: transgenic mice lacking both copies of the WT-1 locus have renal agenesis).

2. *Denys-Drash syndrome*—patients have gonadal dysgenesis and nephropathy leading to renal failure and most develop Wilms' tumors; the genetic abnormality is a *dominant negative mutation in the WT-1 gene* that affects its DNA binding properties.

3. *Beckwith-Wiedemann syndrome*—patients have enlargement of body organs, hemihypertrophy, renal medullary cysts, adrenal cytomegaly, and a predisposition to developing Wilms' tumors and other primitive tumors; genetic abnormality (probably a deletion) is localized to *chromosome 11 band p15.5 (the Wilms tumor 2 [WT-2] gene)*; the function of the gene is unknown, but there may be a role for genomic imprinting in the pathogenesis of these cases.

Morphologically, the tumors are soft, frequently large, well-circumscribed renal masses characterized by triphasic histologic features of (1) blastema, (2) immature stroma, and (3) tubules—an attempt to recapitulate nephrogenesis. The histologic presence of *anaplasia,* observed in approximately 5% of tumors, is associated with a worse prognosis. *Nephroblastomatosis* is a "premalignant" or precursor lesion observed in the kidney.

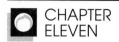

CHAPTER
ELEVEN

Blood Vessels

Pathologic changes in blood vessels have one or more basic consequences:

- Narrowing of the lumen with parenchymal ischemia and potential infarction in tissue supplied by the narrowed vessel.
- Damage to the intima with thrombosis. Alterations in flow, such as stasis, also predispose to thrombosis.
- Weakening of the wall with dilatation (aneurysm) and/or dissection, and potential rupture.

CONGENITAL ANOMALIES (p. 472)

- *Anomalous (e.g., aberrant, reduplicated) vessels,* principally of interest to surgeons.
- *Berry aneurysms* are due to congenital focal wall weakness of vessels with outpouching. They occur exclusively in cerebral vessels, occasionally with catastrophic rupture.
- *Arteriovenous fistula* is an abnormal communication between artery and vein. It may be congenital or secondary to trauma, inflammation, or healed ruptured aneurysm. Fistulas may cause left-to-right vascular shunts, increasing venous return, and predisposing to right heart failure.

ARTERIOSCLEROSIS (p. 473)

Denotes thickening and loss of elasticity of arterial walls. The three types of arteriosclerosis are atherosclerosis, Monckeberg's arteriosclerosis, and arteriolosclerosis (the latter primarily associated with hypertension and discussed in that context).

ATHEROSCLEROSIS (p. 473)

Atherosclerosis is a slowly progressive disease of arteries, marked by elevated *intimal fibrofatty plaques,* formed by lipid deposition, smooth muscle cell proliferation, and synthesis of extracellular matrix (ECM). Large to medium-sized muscular and large elastic arteries are involved, principally in the abdominal aorta, coronary arteries, popliteal arteries, descending thoracic aorta, internal carotid arteries, and circle of Willis (in descending order of frequency). Lesions initially tend to be focal, only partially involving the vessel circumference, and are patchy along its length.

Atherosclerosis typically manifests in middle age or later life either as the vessel lumen is compromised, predisposing to thrombosis, or as the underlying media are thinned, predisposing to aneurysm formation. Fifty percent of all deaths in the United States are attributed to atherosclerosis, with half of these due to myocardial infarction or sudden death in ischemic heart disease, and the remainder to cerebrovascular accidents (stroke), aneurysm rupture, mesenteric occlusion, and gangrene of the extremities.

EPIDEMIOLOGY. Risk of the development of atherosclerosis increases with age, positive family history, hypertension, diabetes, cigarette smoking, and hypercholesterolemia—the last four known as "major risk factors."

The risk is correlated with elevated serum low-density lipoprotein (LDL), formed from the catabolism of very-low-density lipoprotein (VLDL), and carrying 70% of the total serum cholesterol. Risk is *inversely* related to high-density lipoprotein (HDL) levels, perhaps because HDL helps clear cholesterol from vessel wall lesions. Hereditary defects involving the LDL receptor (e.g., in familial hypercholesterolemia) or LDL apoproteins cause elevated LDL, hypercholesterolemia and accelerated atherosclerosis. Lesser influences on the risk of atherosclerosis include obesity, sedentary or high-stress life style, and type A personality (the latter controversial).

MORPHOLOGY. The characteristic atheromatous plaque ("atheroma") is a white-yellow intimal lesion up to 1.5 cm in diameter, protruding into the vessel lumen.

Histologically, it typically is composed of a superficial *fibrous cap*, containing smooth muscle cells, leukocytes, and dense connective tissue extracellular matrix overlying a *necrotic core*, containing dead cells, lipid, cholesterol clefts, lipid-laden foam cells (macrophages and smooth muscle cells), and plasma proteins. In the periphery are proliferating small blood vessels.

- *Fatty streaks* are intimal collections of lipid-laden macrophages and smooth muscle cells, occurring in patients as young as 1 year of age. A causal relationship of fatty streaks to subsequent atheromatous plaques is suspected but has not been proved.
- *Complicated plaques* are calcified and fissured or ulcerated, predisposing to local thrombosis, hemorrhage, medial thinning, cholesterol microemboli, and aneurysmal dilatation.

PATHOGENESIS. Most theories invoke some damage to endothelium or underlying smooth muscle, with migration to the intima and subsequent proliferation of smooth muscle cells consequent to such damage.

The *response to injury hypothesis* contends that atherosclerosis is a reaction to chronic or repeated endothelial cell injury, caused by such insults as hyperlipidemia, hypertension (increased shear forces), cigarette smoking, and/or diabetic angiopathy. The endothelial injuries most important in atherosclerosis induce dysfunctional metabolic and structural changes, without actual loss of these cells. *Endothelial dysfunction* is accompanied by increased permeability to plasma constituents, including lipids, as well as adherence to the endothelium of monocytes and platelets. Monocytes emigrate into the intima, imbibe lipid (becoming "foam cells"), and also proliferate in the intima. Factors from activated platelets and monocytes (e.g., platelet-derived growth factor [PDGF]) induce smooth muscle migration from media to intima, followed by proliferation and synthesis of extracellular matrix (collagen, elastic fibers, proteoglycans). Smooth muscle cells also accumulate lipid (especially cholesterol) to become foam cells. Local oxidation of LDL renders it more easily ingested by foam cells and also accelerates atherogenesis by other mechanisms. Macrophages contribute enzymes, cytokines (e.g., IL-1, TNF) and other compounds that propagate injury. The sequence of events in the pathogenesis of atherosclerosis is summarized in Figure 11–1.

CLINICAL FEATURES. Atherosclerosis is asymptomatic for decades until it causes disease by

- Insidious narrowing of vascular lumina, e.g., gangrene of the lower leg because of stenosing atherosclerosis in the popliteal artery.
- Plaque rupture followed by superimposed thrombus causing sudden occlusion of the lumen, e.g., myocardial infarction precipitated by thrombotic occlusion of fissured coronary arterial atheroma.
- Providing a source of embolic debris, known as *atheroembolism,* e.g., renal infarction resulting from cholesterol emboli originating in an ulcerated atherosclerotic aortic plaque.
- Weakening the wall of a vessel followed by aneurysm formation and possibly rupture, e.g., an abdominal aortic aneurysm.

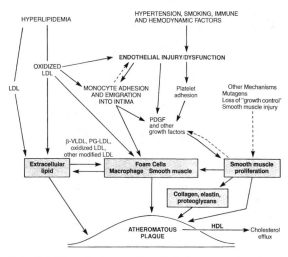

Figure 11–1. Schematic diagram of hypothetical sequence of events and cellular interactions in atherosclerosis. Hyperlipidemia, as well as other risk factors, is thought to cause endothelial injury resulting in adhesion of platelets and monocytes and release of growth factors, including platelet-derived growth factor (PDGF), which lead to smooth muscle cell migration and proliferation. Smooth muscle cells produce large amounts of collagen and proteoglycans, contributing to the atheromatous plaque. Foam cells of atheromatous plaques are derived from both macrophages and smooth muscle cells—from macrophages via the β-VLDL receptor and LDL modifications recognized by scavenger receptors (e.g., oxidized LDL), and from smooth muscle cells by less certain mechanisms. Extracellular lipid is derived from insudation from the lumen, particularly in the presence of hypercholesterolemia, and also from degenerating foam cells. Cholesterol accumulation in the plaque should be viewed as reflecting an imbalance between influx and efflux, and it is possible that HDL helps clear cholesterol from these accumulations. The diagram also depicts other postulated mechanisms for smooth muscle cell proliferation, bypassing primary endothelial injury; the action of mutagens, loss of growth control, indirect smooth muscle cell injury (such as by oxidized LDL). PG = proteoglycan. (Modified with permission from Cotran, R. S., and Munro, J. M.: Pathogenesis of atherosclerosis: Recent concepts. In Grundy, S. M., and Beam, A. G. (eds.): The Role of Cholesterol in Atherosclerosis: New Therapeutic Opportunities. Philadelphia, Hanley and Belfus, 1988, p. 5. © Merck & Co., Rahway, NJ.)

Symptomatic atherosclerotic disease most often relates to the heart, brain, kidneys, lower extremities, and small intestine.

MONCKEBERG'S ARTERIOSCLEROSIS
(MEDIAL CALCIFIC SCLEROSIS) (p. 484)

Characterized by focal calcifications in the *media* of small to medium-sized muscular arteries, without associated inflammation, largely sparing the intima and adventitia. The femoral, tibial, radial, and ulnar arteries and arteries of the genitalia are involved, typically after the age of 50 years.

The process is unrelated to atherosclerosis but may occur concurrently. The pathogenesis is unknown. The calcific deposits are nonobstructive and otherwise of little clinical significance, but they may be visualized as vascular calcifications on radiographs of the extremities of older individuals.

HYPERTENSIVE VASCULAR DISEASE
AND ARTERIOLOSCLEROSIS (p. 484)

Hypertension is the single most important risk factor in both coronary heart disease and cerebrovascular accidents; it may also lead directly to congestive heart failure (hypertensive heart disease), renal failure, and aortic dissection. When defined as diastolic pressure greater than 90 mm Hg and systolic pressure greater than 140 mm Hg, the prevalence of hypertension in the United States is about 25%.

About 90% of hypertension is primary and idiopathic (*essential*); the remaining is secondary and mostly related to renal disease or (less often) to renal artery stenosis (renovascular), endocrine abnormalities, vascular malformations, or neurogenic disorders. Causes and factors in the pathogenesis of essential and secondary hypertension are summarized in Table 11–1.

Table 11–1. Main Causes and Possible Factors in the Pathogenesis of Hypertension

Essential Hypertension
Genetic defect in renal sodium excretion
Genetic defect in sodium/calcium transport in vascular smooth muscle
Variation in genes encoding angiotensinogen and other proteins in renin-angiotensin system
Other increased vasoconstrictive influences: behavioral, neurogenic, hormonal

Secondary Hypertension
Renal disease: Increased renin secretion, sodium and fluid retention, decreased vasodilator (vasodepressor) secretion
Endocrine causes: aldosteronism, oral contraceptives, pheochromocytoma, thyrotoxicosis
Vascular causes: coarctation of the aorta, vasculitis
Neurogenic causes: psychogenic, increased intracranial pressure

From Cotran, R. S., Kumar, V., and Robbins, S. L: Robbins Pathologic Basis of Disease. 5th ed. Philadelphia, W. B. Saunders Co., 1994, p. 485.

REGULATION OF NORMAL BLOOD PRESSURE (p. 485)

Blood pressure is a complex trait that is determined by the interaction of multiple genetic and environmental factors that regulate the relationship between cardiac output and total arteriolar resistance.

- *Vasoconstriction increases vascular resistance.* Vasoconstrictors include angiotensin II, catecholamines, thromboxane, leukotrienes, and endothelin.
- Vasodilators include kinins, prostaglandins, nitric oxide, and adenosine.
- Regional *autoregulation* is also important, wherein increased blood flow leads to vasoconstriction, and vice versa.
- Cardiac output is regulated by blood volume (sodium load, mineralocorticoids, natriuretic factors), heart rate, stroke volume, and contractility.

MECHANISMS OF ESSENTIAL HYPERTENSION (p. 486)

Although unknown, the cause of essential hypertension at the most elemental level must be related either to a primary increase in cardiac output (e.g., reduced renal sodium excretion) or to an increase in peripheral resistance (e.g., due to increased release of vasoconstrictor agents, to increased sensitivity of vascular smooth muscle cells, or to behavioral or neurogenic factors), or both. In most patients, multiple defects probably contribute. Abnormalities can also occur in the renal mechanisms that regulate blood pressure, including (1) the renin-angiotensin system, (2) sodium hemostasis, and (3) production of vasodepressor substances implicated in the pathogenesis of hypertension in unilateral renal artery stenosis and renal disease. Defects in these mechanisms also may contribute to essential hypertension. For example, recent studies have suggested a propensity toward hypertension in individuals with specific molecular variants of the gene-encoding *angiotensinogen,* the physiologic substrate for renin.

VASCULAR PATHOLOGY IN HYPERTENSION (p. 488)

Hypertension accelerates atherogenesis and causes vascular structural changes that potentiate both aortic dissection and cerebrovascular hemorrhage. In addition, hypertension is associated with small vessel disease, primarily affecting arterioles and small arteries. The two basic types of arteriolosclerosis, *hyaline* and *hyperplastic,* are characterized by diffuse arteriolar wall thickening, luminal narrowing, and resultant ischemia of distal tissue.

HYALINE ARTERIOLOSCLEROSIS. Occurs typically in elderly patients, particularly those with mild hypertension and mild diabetes. The lesion is thought to reflect endothelial injury, with subsequent leakage of plasma components into arteriolar walls, and synthesis of extracellular matrix by smooth muscle cells. Microscopically, there is diffuse, pink, hyaline thickening of arteriolar walls. Hyaline arteriosclerosis is the major microscopic feature of benign nephrosclerosis *(see p. 976).*

HYPERPLASTIC ARTERIOLOSCLEROSIS. Characteristic of malignant hypertension (acute, severe elevations in blood pressure, *see p. 977*), there is concentric laminated ("onionskin") arteriolar thickening with reduplicated basement membrane and smooth muscle proliferation, frequently associated with fibrin deposition and wall necrosis—*necrotizing arteriolitis.*

INFLAMMATORY DISEASES: THE VASCULITIDES (p. 489)

Vasculitis (i.e., vascular inflammatory injury, often with necrosis) may be localized, due to direct injury (e.g., infection, trauma, toxins), or systemic, characterized by multifocal necrosis (*"necrotizing vasculitis"*) and thrombosis.

Most systemic varieties of vasculitis are thought to have an immune origin, secondary to deposition of circulating antigen-antibody complexes (e.g., acute arteritis in serum sickness and systemic lupus erythematosus [SLE]) (see p. 199), or antibody to fixed tissue antigens (e.g., Goodpasture's syndrome and Kawasaki disease) or delayed-type hypersensitivity reactions, especially in lesions with granulomas (e.g., temporal arteritis).

In many patients with vasculitis, the serum reacts with cytoplasmic antigens in neutrophils by immunofluorescence and immunochemical assays, indicating the presence of *antineutrophilic cytoplasmic autoantibodies (ANCA).* The pattern observed is either perinuclear (called P-ANCA) in which the major antigen is *myeloperoxidase,* or cytoplasmic (called C-ANCA) in which the leukocyte antigen is *proteinase 3.* C-ANCA is most characteristic of Wegener's granulomatosis; P-ANCA and C-ANCA can also be found in other vasculitides.

Classification of localized and systemic vasculitis reflects the pathogenesis, size, and site of the vessels involved, the histologic characteristics of the lesions, and the clinical manifestations (Fig. 11–2; Table 11–2).

GIANT CELL (TEMPORAL) ARTERITIS (p. 492)

The most common form of vasculitis, giant cell (temporal) arteritis is characterized by focal granulomatous inflammation of medium and small arteries, chiefly cranial vessels and most commonly the temporal arteries in elderly people. It may rarely involve the aortic arch (*giant cell aortitis*). The etiology is unknown.

Temporal arteritis typically presents with headache and facial pain; 50% of patients have systemic symptoms, including flulike syndrome with myalgias, arthralgias, and fever, called *polymyalgia rheumatica.* It may cause visual disturbances and even blindness (an acute emergency).

Morphologically, there may be one of three general appearances: (1) granulomatous vasculitis with fragmented internal elastic lamina and giant cells (two-thirds of cases); (2) nonspecific leukocytic infiltration by neutrophils, eosinophils, and lymphocytes of vessel walls; or (3) intimal fibrosis with thickening of the walls and narrowing of lumina. These three patterns may represent stages in a continuum. There often is associated thrombosis.

Biopsy may be negative in one-third of patients, presumably owing to the focality of the lesion. The disease responds well to steroids.

TAKAYASU'S ARTERITIS (p. 493)

A form of granulomatous vasculitis of medium-to-large arteries, characterized by fibrous thickening of the aortic arch with virtual

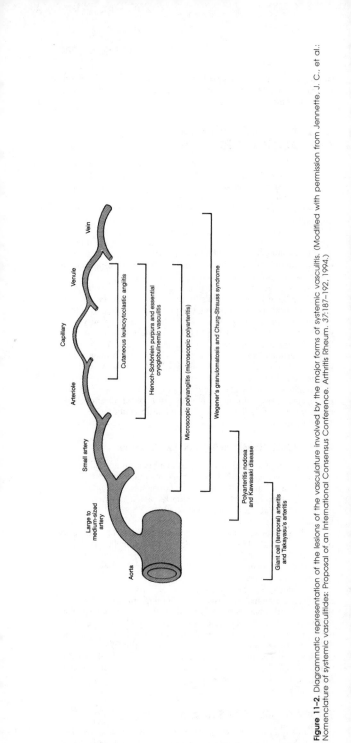

Figure 11-2. Diagrammatic representation of the lesions of the vasculature involved by the major forms of systemic vasculitis. (Modified with permission from Jennette, J. C., et al.: Nomenclature of systemic vasculitides: Proposal of an International Consensus Conference. Arthritis Rheum. 37:187–192, 1994.)

Table 11–2. Classification of Vasculitis Based on Pathogenesis

Infectious
Bacterial (e.g., *Neisseria*)
Rickettsial (e.g., Rocky Mountain spotted fever)
Spirochetal (e.g., syphilis)
Fungal (e.g., aspergillosis)
Viral (e.g., herpes)

Immunologic
Immune complex-mediated
    Henoch-Schönlein purpura
    Essential cryoglobulinemic vasculitis
    Serum sickness vasculitis
    Lupus vasculitis
    Hepatitis B microscopic polyarteritis
Direct antibody attack-mediated
    Goodpasture's syndrome (antibasement membrane
        antibodies)
    Kawasaki disease (antiendothelial antibodies)
ANCA associated (possibly ANCA mediated)
    Wegener's granulomatosis
    Microscopic polyangiitis (microscopic polyarteritis)
    Churg-Strauss syndrome
Cell-mediated
    Allograft organ rejection

Unknown
Giant cell (temporal) arteritis
Takayasu's arteritis
Polyarteritis nodosa (classic polyarteritis nodosa)

ANCA = Antineutrophil cytoplasmic antibodies.
Courtesy of J.C. Jennette, M.D., University of North Carolina.
From Cotran, R.S., Kumar, V., and Robbins, S.L.: Robbins Pathologic Basis of Disease. 5th ed. Philadelphia, W. B. Saunders Co., 1994, p. 490.

---

obliteration of the mouths of the great vessels. This results in ocular disturbances, neurologic deficits, and markedly diminished upper extremity pulses. Occasionally (one-third of cases), the disease involves the remainder of the aorta and its branches, and hypertension may occur with renal artery involvement. Another variant causes proximal aortic dilatation with aortic valvular insufficiency. The condition is most common in Asia, in women 15 to 45 years of age.

Grossly, it produces irregular thickening of the aortic wall with intimal wrinkling. *Microscopically,* early stages show adventitial perivascular (vasa vasorum) mononuclear cell infiltrate, followed in later stages by medial fibrosis, occasionally with granulomas and acellular intimal thickening. Morphologic changes may be indistinguishable from those of giant cell (temporal) arteritis.

POLYARTERITIS NODOSA GROUP (p. 494)

Polyarteritis nodosa (PAN) is a systemic disease characterized by necrotizing inflammation of small to medium-sized arteries throughout the body, primarily involving the main visceral arteries (e.g., renal, coronary, hepatic, mesenteric) and sparing the pulmonary circulation.

MORPHOLOGY. The lesions are sharply demarcated and often induce thrombosis, causing distal ischemic injury.

Microscopically, acute lesions are segmental and characterized by fibrinoid necrosis of the arterial wall with an accompanying neutrophilic infiltrate. The process is sharply circumscribed and may not involve the entire circumference of the vessel. Healing lesions show fibroblast proliferation superimposed on ongoing fibrinoid necrosis. Healed lesions show only marked fibrotic thickening of the arterial wall, with associated elastic lamina fragmentation and sometimes aneurysmal dilatation. Lesions at different histologic stages may be present concurrently.

CLINICAL FEATURES. Characteristically, PAN is a disease of young adults, with protean and nonspecific clinical signs and symptoms related to whatever tissue is involved, e.g., hematuria, albuminuria, and hypertension (kidneys); abdominal pain and melena (GI tract); diffuse myalgias; and peripheral neuritis. The most common systemic manifestations include fever, malaise, and weight loss.

PAN is frequently associated with *hepatitis B antigen,* and deposited immune complexes may play a role in pathogenesis. A specific form of anti-neutrophil cytoplasmic antibody (P-ANCA) is present in the serum of 75% of patients with PAN and correlates with disease activity.

The diagnosis is made by biopsy of affected arterial segments. Untreated, the disease is generally fatal, but a 90% cure/remission rate is achieved with immunosuppressive therapy.

A variant of PAN is *allergic granulomatosis and angiitis (Churg-Strauss syndrome),* characterized by eosinophilia and bronchial asthma, with pulmonary and splenic vessel involvement and intra- and extravascular granulomas.

KAWASAKI DISEASE (MUCOCUTANEOUS LYMPH NODE SYNDROME) (p. 495)

An acute illness of infants and children characterized by fever, lymphadenopathy, skin rash, oral/conjunctival erythema, and (in 20% of cases) coronary arteritis, often with associated aneurysms. It is endemic in Japan but considerably less common in the United States.

Patients have numerous immunoregulatory disturbances, including T cell activation, autoantibodies to endothelial cells, and circulating immune complexes, but the etiology is unknown.

Morphologically, the lesions resemble those of PAN.

The disease typically is self-limited but rarely is fatal owing to coronary arteritis with subsequent aneurysm formation, thrombosis, or rupture leading to myocardial infarction. Aspirin and intravenous gamma globulin are thought to be helpful in reducing the long-term sequelae.

MICROSCOPIC POLYANGIITIS (MICROSCOPIC POLYARTERITIS (LEUKOCYTOCLASTIC) ANGIITIS) (p. 496)

This may be distinguished from PAN by its involvement of smaller vessels (arterioles, capillaries, and venules), with lesions typically all synchronized to the same stage. This suggests an acute inciting agent (e.g., drugs, microorganisms, heterologous protein) forming immune complexes in a previously sensitized host. In general, the disease responds to removal of the offending agent.

Lesions may be confined to skin (cutaneous vasculitis) or may involve other sites, including lung, brain, heart, and kidneys. Fibrinoid necrosis often occurs, but affected vessels may reveal only fragmented neutrophilic nuclei within vessel walls and perivascularly (*leukocytoclastic angiitis*).

Specific syndromes with systemic hypersensitivity angiitis include Henoch-Schönlein purpura, essential mixed cryoglobulinemia, and vasculitis of malignancy (typically lymphoproliferative disorders).

WEGENER'S GRANULOMATOSIS (p. 496)

Consists of the following triad:

- Focal necrotizing vasculitis of the lung and upper airway.
- Necrotizing granulomas of the upper and lower respiratory tract.
- Necrotizing glomerulitis.

The vascular lesions resemble those of acute PAN but are frequently accompanied by granuloma formation.

Peak incidence is in the fifth decade. Without treatment, 80% of patients die within 1 year; in contrast, 90% respond to immunosuppression, particularly with cyclophosphamide.

Although immune complexes are occasionally seen in lesional tissue, no etiologic agent has been identified. Antineutrophilic cytoplasmic autoantibodies of the C-ANCA type, present in over 90% of patients with active disease, are a good marker of disease activity.

THROMBOANGIITIS OBLITERANS (BUERGER'S DISEASE) (p. 498)

Typically encountered in heavy smokers, often before the age of 35 years, this condition is marked by segmental, thrombosing, acute and chronic inflammation of intermediate and small *arteries and veins* in the extremities. It begins with nodular phlebitis, followed by Raynaud-like cold sensitivity and leg claudication.

Acute lesions consist of neutrophilic infiltration of the arterial wall, with mural or occlusive thrombi containing microabscesses, often with giant cell formation and secondary involvement of the adjacent vein and nerve. Late lesions show organization and recanalization. The etiology is unknown.

The vascular insufficiency can lead to excruciating pain and ultimately gangrene of the extremities.

RAYNAUD'S DISEASE (p. 499)

- *Raynaud's disease* refers to paroxysmal pallor or cyanosis of the digits of the hands or feet and infrequently the tips of the nose or ears (acral parts), caused by intense vasospasm of local small arteries or arterioles, principally of young, otherwise healthy women. Of uncertain etiology, Raynaud's disease reflects an exaggeration of normal central and local vasomotor responses to cold or emotion.
- In contrast, *Raynaud's phenomenon* refers to arterial insufficiency of the extremities *secondary to the arterial narrowing induced by various conditions, including atherosclerosis, sys-*

temic lupus erythematosus, systemic sclerosis (scleroderma), or Buerger's disease.

ANEURYSMS AND DISSECTION (p. 489)

Aneurysms are localized abnormal dilatations of vessels. A *true aneurysm* is bounded by generally complete but often attenuated arterial wall components. Most common (and significant) are abdominal aortic aneurysms, but the iliac and other large arteries are sometimes involved. In contrast, a *false aneurysm* (also called *pseudoaneurysm* or "pulsating hematoma") is an extravascular hematoma that communicates with the intravascular space; part of the vessel wall is missing. Morbidity and mortality of aneurysms are secondary to

- Rupture.
- Impingement on adjacent structures.
- Occlusion of proximate vessels by either extrinsic pressure or superimposed thrombosis.
- Embolism from mural thrombosis.

Etiologies of aneurysms include atherosclerosis and cystic medial degeneration (the two most common causes), syphilis, trauma, PAN, congenital defects, and infections (called mycotic aneurysms).

Atherosclerosis causes arterial wall thinning through medial destruction secondary to intimal plaque. *Atherosclerotic aneurysms usually occur in the abdominal aorta, most frequently between the renal arteries and the iliac bifurcation* or in the common iliac arteries. However, the arch and descending parts of the thoracic aorta can be involved as well as arteries other than the aorta.

ABDOMINAL AORTIC ANEURYSMS (p. 500)

Typically found in men over the age of 50 years. The risk of rupture increases with the diameter: minimal risk if less than 5 cm, but a risk of 5%–10% per year when more than 5 cm. Operative mortality is 5% for unruptured aneurysm but more than 50% after rupture. Since atherosclerotic peripheral vascular disease is usually accompanied by severe coronary atherosclerosis, such patients have a high incidence of ischemic heart disease.

SYPHILITIC (LUETIC) ANEURYSMS (p. 501)

An aneurysm appearing in the tertiary stage of syphilis, typically confined to the ascending aorta and arch.

These aneurysms may extend retrograde to the aortic valve ring with dilatation, causing commissural widening and narrowing and rolling of leaflets, leading to valvular insufficiency. With time, chronic left ventricular overload produces massive cardiac hypertrophy (to 1000 gm), called *cor bovinum.*

Syphilitic aortitis begins as adventitial inflammation, especially involving the vasa vasorum, with resultant obliterative endarteritis. Narrowing of the lumina causes aortic medial ischemia and results in patchy elastic fiber and smooth muscle loss, with weakening of the wall and inflammatory scarring. Affected vasa vasorum have hyperplastic thickening of the walls and a perivascular infiltrate of lymphocytes and plasma cells.

Symptoms occur via (1) the development of luetic heart disease, (2) impingement of aortic aneurysm on surrounding thoracic organs, and (3) rarely, rupture.

AORTIC DISSECTION
(DISSECTING HEMATOMA) (p. 501)

Dissection of blood along the laminar planes of the aortic media, with the formation of an intramural blood-filled channel that often ruptures, causing massive hemorrhage. Aortic dissection is not usually associated with marked dilatation of the aorta. Aortic dissection occurs principally in two groups of individuals: (1) men 40 to 60 years of age, in whom hypertension is almost invariably an antecedent (more than 90% of dissections); and (2) those with a systemic or localized abnormality of connective tissue that affects the aorta (e.g., cystic medial degeneration in Marfan's syndrome). Dissection also can be a complication of therapeutic or diagnostic arterial cannulation or other trauma.

Hypertensive patients may have degenerative histologic changes that include mild-to-moderate elastic fragmentation and excess amorphous interstitial material. More dramatic medial pathology frequently accompanies Marfan's syndrome, consisting of (1) prominent elastic tissue fragmentation and disruption, (2) focal separation of the elastic and fibromuscular elements by small, cleftlike or cystic spaces filled with material resembling amorphous extracellular matrix of connective tissue, and ultimately, (3) large-scale elastic tissue loss, without inflammation, often called *cystic medial degeneration.* The defect in Marfan's syndrome is now known to be due to decreased or loss of *microfibrillary protein* of elastic tissue.

The risk and nature of serious complications of dissection depend strongly on the level of the aorta affected. Complications include rupture of the dissection into a body cavity, extension into the great arteries of the neck or other major branches of the aorta, or retrograde dissection that disrupts the aortic valve. Thus, aortic dissections are generally classified into two types: (1) the more common (and dangerous) *proximal* lesions, involving the ascending aorta (types I and II of DeBakey's classification, often collectively called type A), and (2) *distal lesions not involving the ascending part* and usually beginning distal to the subclavian artery (DeBakey type III, often called type B). The classic clinical symptoms of aortic dissection are the sudden onset of excruciating pain, usually beginning in the anterior chest, radiating to the back, and moving downward as the dissection progresses.

There is an intimal tear (a portal of entry of blood) in the ascending aorta, within 10 cm of the aortic valve, in 90% of patients.

VEINS AND LYMPHATICS (p. 504)

Disorders of veins are common clinical problems, 90% of which comprise *varicose veins* or *phlebothrombosis.* Phlebothrombosis is an important potential source of pulmonary emboli, and both disorders contribute to secondary venous stasis, inducing passive congestion, edema, and collateral formation.

VARICOSE VEINS (p. 504)

Abnormally dilated, tortuous veins (typically the superficial veins of the lower extremities) resulting from chronic increased intraluminal pressure. The walls of varicose veins are markedly thinned at points of maximal dilatation. Although there is frequent intraluminal thrombosis, *varicosities in the superficial veins are rarely a source of clinically significant emboli.*

They occur in 10% to 20% of the general population and in women more often than men, presumably secondary to venous stasis occurring in pregnancy. Other pathogenetic influences include hereditary defects in venous wall development, obesity, prolonged dependent position of the legs, proximal intravascular thrombosis, and compressive tumor masses.

Vein dilatation or deformation renders the valves incompetent, with consequent stasis, persistent edema, and trophic skin changes, ultimately resulting in stasis dermatitis and ulceration (varicose ulcers). Affected tissues have impaired circulation and thus are vulnerable to injury, which heals poorly.

THROMBOPHLEBITIS AND PHLEBOTHROMBOSIS
(p. 505)

These terms designate the same entity. Thrombosis within a vein (*phlebothrombosis*) incites inflammation within the vein wall (*thrombophlebitis*). Predisposing factors for thrombosis include congestive heart failure, neoplasia, pregnancy, postoperative state, prolonged immobilization, or local infection.

Ninety percent occur in the deep leg veins. Other sites include the periprostatic plexus in men and ovarian and pelvic veins in women. *In contrast to thromboses in superficial leg veins, those in deep veins are common sources of emboli.*

Phlegmasia alba dolens (painful white leg; also called *milk leg*) refers to iliofemoral vein thrombosis occurring in late pregnancy and postpartum, related to compression by the gravid uterus and the hypercoagulability of pregnancy.

Migratory thrombophlebitis (Trousseau's syndrome) consists of multiple venous thrombi appearing in one place and then disappearing to crop up elsewhere; it is attributed to hypercoagulability associated with cancer, particularly visceral adenocarcinomas.

LYMPHANGITIS AND LYMPHEDEMA (p. 506)

Lymphangitis denotes infection involving the lymphatics draining a locus of inflammation, frequently (but not exclusively) due to beta-hemolytic streptococci. Lymphangitis presents as a cluster of painful subcutaneous red streaks along involved lymph channels, with regional lymphadenopathy.

Morphologically, dilated lymphatics are filled with neutrophils and histiocytes. Inflammation frequently extends into the perilymphatic tissue and may develop into cellulitis or frank abscess. It is occasionally associated with involvement of lymph nodes (*acute lymphadenitis*) and may lead to septicemia.

Lymphedema is lymphatic obstruction with lymphatic dilatation and abnormal accumulation of interstitial fluid in the affected drainage site. When prolonged, it causes interstitial fibrosis. In skin and subcutaneous tissue, it gives rise to a *"peau d'orange"* (orange peel) appearance of skin, with associated ulcers and brawny induration.

Chylous accumulations in any body cavity may occur secondary to rupture of obstructed, dilated lymphatics.

The most common causes of obstruction are malignancy, surgical resection of regional lymph nodes, postradiation fibrosis, filariasis, and postinflammatory thrombosis with lymphatic scarring.

TUMORS (p. 506)

Classically, benign vascular neoplasms are composed of *well-formed vascular channels lined by endothelial cells.* Frankly malignant tumors show few vascular channels or only abortive ones with solid, cellular, anaplastic endothelial proliferation. A few entities fall into an intermediate group. The endothelial cell origin of malignancies may be confirmed by immunohistochemistry. In addition to the true neoplasms of vessels, a few developmental anomalies—telangiectases—must be mentioned because they can simulate benign neoplasms.

BENIGN TUMORS AND TUMOR-LIKE CONDITIONS (p. 507)

Hemangioma (p. 507)

Common lesions, especially in childhood, making up 7% of all benign tumors. They encompass several histologic/clinical variants.

- *Capillary hemangiomas* usually occur in skin or mucous membranes, but also in viscera. The tumors range from 1 to 2 mm to several centimeters in diameter. All are well-defined, unencapsulated lesions composed of closely packed aggregates of capillary-sized, thin-walled vessels. They may be partially or completely thrombosed.
- *Juvenile capillary ("strawberry") hemangiomas* comprise a specific variant, are present at birth, grow rapidly for a few months, and begin regressing at age 1 to 3 years. Eighty percent disappear by age 5 years.
- *Cavernous hemangiomas* are distinguished by the formation of *large, cavernous* vascular channels, typically forming unencapsulated but discrete lesions, usually 1 to 2 cm in diameter (with rare giant forms). They have the same distribution as capillary hemangiomas but may also involve the CNS, liver, and other viscera. Cavernous hemangiomas in the cerebellum, brain stem, or eye grounds are associated with similar angiomatous or cystic neoplasms in pancreas and liver in *von Hippel–Lindau disease.*
- *Granuloma pyogenicum (granulation tissue-type hemangioma)* is an ulcerated polypoid variant of capillary hemangiomas on skin or oral mucosa, often secondary to trauma. It consists of proliferating capillaries with significant interspersed edema and inflammatory infiltrates, resembling exuberant granulation tissue. Pregnancy tumor (*granuloma gravidarum*) is essentially the same lesion, occurring in the gingiva in 1% to 5% of pregnant women.

GLOMUS TUMOR (GLOMANGIOMA) (p. 507)

A benign, extremely painful tumor of modified smooth muscle cells arising from the glomus body, a neuromyoarterial receptor sensitive to temperature that regulates arteriolar flow. Receptors and their tumors are most commonly found in the distal phalanges, especially beneath nail beds.

Grossly, the tumors are less than 1 cm in diameter and may be pinpoint. *Histologically,* they consist of branching vascular channels separated by a stroma dominated by aggregates, nests, and masses of specialized glomus cells that resemble smooth muscle cells on electron microscopy.

Vascular Ectasias (Telangiectasias) (p. 509)

An aggregation of abnormally prominent capillaries, venules, arterioles in skin or mucous membranes. They are probably not true neoplasms but rather congenital anomalies or acquired exaggerations of existing vessels.

Nevus flammeus is the term used for an ordinary birthmark. It consists of a macular cutaneous lesion that histologically shows only dermal vessel dilatation. Most eventually regress. A special variety is the *"port-wine stain,"* which persists and grows along with the child, thickening the involved skin. Facial port-wine nevi with associated leptomeningeal angiomatous masses, mental retardation, seizures, hemiplegia, and skull radiopacities characterize the *Sturge-Weber syndrome.*

Spider telangiectasias are minute focal or subcutaneous arterioles, often pulsatile, arranged in radial fashion around a central core. They typically occur above the waist and are associated with hyperestrogenic states such as pregnancy and cirrhosis.

Hereditary hemorrhagic telangiectasia (Osler-Weber-Rendu disease) is a rare, mendelian dominant disorder characterized by multiple small (<5 mm) aneurysmal lesions or telangiectasia on skin and mucous membranes. The syndrome typically presents with epistaxis, hemoptysis, or GI or GU bleeding, becoming more serious with advancing age.

Bacillary Angiomatosis (p. 509)

A potentially fatal infectious disease caused by a rickettsia-like bacteria that induces a distinct non-neoplastic proliferation of small blood vessels in the skin, lymph nodes, and visceral organs of immunocompromised patients, especially those with HIV. Grossly, skin lesions have one or more red papules and nodular subcutaneous masses histologically resembling a tumor-like capillary proliferation with atypical endothelial cells with mitoses. However, in contrast to pyogenic granuloma, Kaposi's sarcoma, or angiosarcoma, there are numerous neutrophils, nuclear dust, and purplish granular material (the bacteria).

Treatment with erythromycin cures the condition.

INTERMEDIATE-GRADE TUMORS (p. 509)

Hemangioendothelioma (p. 509)

These neoplasms lie in the interface between benign and malignant and must be distinguished from the much more aggressive angiosarcomas. Most lesions are cured by excision, although up to 40% may recur and 20% eventually metastasize.

Microscopically, vascular channels may be evident or inconspicuous, with dominant masses and sheets of somewhat pleomorphic, spindle-shaped-to-large, plump cells (especially in the *epithelioid* variant). The presence of factor VIII antigen confirms the endothelial origin.

MALIGNANT TUMORS (p. 510)

Angiosarcoma (Hemangiosarcoma) (p. 510)

Among vascular tumors, these are the most malignant. Hepatic angiosarcomas are associated with arsenicals (in some pesticides), polyvinylchloride (used in plastic manufacture), and Thorotrast (radiocontrast material used from 1928 to 1950), and in these settings are often multicentric, concomitantly arising in the spleen.

These neoplasms tend to arise in skin, soft tissue, breast, liver, and spleen. They begin as small, well-demarcated red nodules evolving into large, fleshy, gray-white, soft tissue masses. *Microscopically,* all degrees of differentiation are found, from the highly vascular variety with plump, anaplastic endothelial cells to quite undifferentiated lesions without vascular lumens and with marked cellular atypia, including giant cells.

Angiosarcomas metastasize widely and are frequently fatal.

Hemangiopericytoma (p. 511)

This is a tumor of pericytes that most commonly arises on the lower extremities or in the retroperitoneum.

Most are small, but they may be as large as 8 cm. *Microscopically,* they are composed of numerous capillary channels encased by nests and masses of spindle-shaped-to-round cells extrinsic to the endothelial basement membrane (resembling pericytes). Fifty percent metastasize.

Kaposi's Sarcoma (KS) (p. 511)

Four forms are recognized, based on epidemiology.

1. *Classic/European KS* occurs typically in elderly men of Eastern European (especially Ashkenazi Jews) or Mediterranean descent. The lesions consist of multiple red to purple cutaneous plaques and nodules on the lower extremities, with unusual visceral involvement. This form rarely causes death.

2. *African KS* is clinically similar to the classic form but occurs in younger men in equatorial Africa, where it makes up approximately 10% of all tumors.

3. *Transplant-associated KS* occurs in patients undergoing immunosuppressive therapy. There is both cutaneous and visceral systemic involvement. Lesions regress when immunosuppression is discontinued.

4. *AIDS-associated KS* occurs more commonly in homosexuals than in other risk groups. Lesions may occur anywhere in the skin and mucous membranes, lymph nodes, GI tract, or viscera. Lesions respond to cytotoxic chemotherapy or alpha-interferon.

Microscopically, the characteristic lesions consist of sheets of plump, spindle-shaped cells creating slitlike vascular spaces filled with red blood cells, intermingled with vascular channels lined by recognizable endothelium. There are also scattered microhemorrhages and hemosiderin deposits. The origin of the tumor cells remains uncertain.

TUMORS OF LYMPHATICS (p. 512)

Lymphangiomas

The lymphatic equivalent of hemangiomas, and clinically benign.

Simple (Capillary) Lymphangioma

Occurs typically in the head, neck, and axillary subcutaneous tissue but also on the trunk and within connective tissue of viscera.

Grossly, the tumors are 1- to 2-cm cutaneous nodules or

pedunculated lesions, or well-demarcated, compressible gray-pink visceral masses. *Microscopically,* they are made up of a network of endothelium-lined spaces, identifiable as lymphatics only by the absence of blood cells.

Variants include *lymphangiomyomas,* which have smooth muscle in the vessel walls.

Cavernous Lymphangioma (Cystic Hygroma)

This tumor is analogous to the cavernous hemangiomas. The masses, however, tend to be much larger (up to 15 cm), typically in the neck or axilla of children. They are difficult to resect, owing to a lack of discrete margins or encapsulation, and so tend to recur.

Microscopically, they are composed of hugely dilated cystic spaces lined by endothelium with scant stroma.

Lymphangiosarcoma (Lymphedema-Associated Angiosarcoma)

A rare malignant tumor with a poor prognosis, typically occurring in the setting of prolonged lymphatic obstruction and chronic lymphedema (e.g., after radical mastectomy or postmastectomy axillary irradiation).

Grossly, the tumors consist of multiple nodules that become confluent. *Microscopically,* vascular channels are lined by anaplastic endothelium, resembling hemangiosarcomas.

PATHOLOGY OF THERAPEUTIC INTERVENTIONS IN VASCULAR DISEASE (p. 512)

THROMBOLYSIS (p. 513)

Thrombolysis refers to therapeutic dissolution of a clot in an unwanted location. The thrombolytic agents used currently act directly or indirectly as plasminogen activators.

The major complications of thrombolytic therapy include hemorrhage caused by the systemic fibrinolytic state in 15% of patients and thrombotic re-occlusion in 15%–35%.

BALLOON ANGIOPLASTY AND RELATED TECHNIQUES (p. 513)

Balloon angioplasty is dilatation of an atheromatous stenosis of an artery by a balloon catheter. Balloon dilatation of an atherosclerotic vessel characteristically causes plaque fracture, medial dissection, and stretching of the media of the dissected segment.

The complications of balloon angioplasty and related techniques include abrupt reclosure in a small percentage of patients and proliferative restenosis in approximately one-third of patients within the first 4–6 months.

VASCULAR REPLACEMENT (p. 514)

Large-diameter (>10-cm) Dacron grafts in the aorta perform well. In contrast, small-diameter fabric vascular grafts (<6–8 mm) perform less well. Failure of small-diameter vascular prostheses of autologous saphenous vein or expanded polytetrafluroethylene (e-PTFE) is due most frequently to thrombotic occlusion or intimal fibrous hyperplasia, either generalized (in vein graft) or anastomotic only (in synthetic graft).

The long-term patency of saphenous veins used as coronary artery bypass grafts is 60% or less at 10 years, owing to pathologic changes, including thrombosis (usually early), intimal thickening (several months to several years), and atherosclerosis (>2–3 years postoperatively). Internal mammary arteries are also used with a >90% patency at 10 years.

CHAPTER TWELVE

The Heart

Heart disease is the predominant cause of morbidity and mortality in industrialized nations, accounting for 40% of all deaths in the United States. Eighty percent of cardiac deaths are attributable to *ischemic heart disease*. An additional 5% to 10% are attributable to hypertensive heart disease (including cor pulmonale), congenital heart disease, and the common valvular diseases (calcific aortic valvular stenosis, mitral valve prolapse, rheumatic heart disease, and infective endocarditis).

Abnormal circulatory function usually follows one or more general mechanisms:

- Disruption of the continuity of circulation (e.g., a gunshot wound through the thoracic aorta) that permits blood to escape.
- A disorder of cardiac conduction (e.g., heart block) or other arrhythmia (e.g., ventricular fibrillation) that leads to uncoordinated contractions of the muscular walls.
- A lesion preventing valve opening or narrowing the lumen of a vessel (e.g., aortic valvular stenosis or coarctation, respectively) that obstructs blood flow and overworks the pump behind the obstruction.
- Regurgitant flow (e.g., mitral or aortic regurgitation) that causes some of the output from each contraction to be directed backward, so that the pump repeatedly expels the same blood.
- Failure of the pump itself (congestive heart failure). This is the potential common end point of many forms of serious heart disease.

CONGESTIVE HEART FAILURE (CHF) (p. 520)

CHF is the pathophysiologic state resulting from impaired cardiac function that renders the heart unable to maintain an output sufficient for the metabolic requirements of the tissues and organs of the body. Most instances of heart failure are the consequence of progressive deterioration of myocardial contractile function (*systolic dysfunction*), as often occurs with ischemic injury, pressure or volume overload, or dilated cardiomyopathy. The damaged muscle contracts weakly or inadequately, and the chambers cannot empty properly. Sometimes, however, failure results from an inability of the heart chambers to relax sufficiently during diastole to fill the ventricle properly (*diastolic dysfunction*). This can occur with massive left ventricular hypertrophy, myocardial fibrosis, deposition of amyloid, or constrictive pericarditis. Irrespective of underlying mechanism, CHF is characterized by diminished cardiac output ("forward failure") or damming back of blood in the venous system ("backward failure"), or both.

However, with the exception of frank myocyte death, the mechanisms of myocardial decompensation in CHF are not well understood. Since adult myocytes cannot replicate, pressure or volume stress induces hypertrophy (i.e., increased heart size, due primarily to increased myocyte size). The mechanism translating physical stress into cellular changes is uncertain. Hypertrophy is initially adaptive but can make myocytes especially vulnerable to injury.

Other compensatory changes include:

- Ventricular dilatation (to improve contraction by stretching of myofibers according to the Frank-Starling law).
- Blood volume expansion by salt and water retention.
- Tachycardia.

These compensatory changes ultimately constitute further burden on cardiac function. They combine with both the primary cardiac disease and secondary hypertrophy to induce dilatation in excess of the optimal tension-generating point, leading to progressive CHF.

LEFT-SIDED HEART FAILURE (p. 522)

The major causes are ischemic heart disease, hypertension, aortic and mitral valve disease, and myocardial disease.

It is manifested most commonly by *pulmonary congestion and edema* secondary to impairment of lung vascular outflow.

- Reduced cardiac output also *causes reduced renal perfusion*, leading to

  - Further salt and water retention.
  - Ischemic acute tubular necrosis.
  - Impairment of waste excretion, causing prerenal azotemia.

- CNS perfusion is reduced, often resulting in *hypoxic encephalopathy*, with symptoms ranging from irritability to coma.

RIGHT-SIDED HEART FAILURE (p. 523)

Typically a consequence of left-sided failure. Pure right-sided failure may be caused by intrinsic disease of the lungs or pulmonary vasculature causing functional right ventricular outflow obstruction (*cor pulmonale*), or tricuspid or pulmonary valvular disease.

The major manifestations are

- Portal, systemic, and dependent peripheral (e.g., feet, ankles, sacrum) congestion and edema, and effusions (pleural and peritoneal [*ascites*])
- *Hepatomegaly* with centrilobular congestion and atrophy, producing a "nutmeg" appearance (*chronic passive congestion*). With severe hypoxia, *centrilobular necrosis* can occur, and with high right-sided pressure, sinusoidal rupture causes *central hemorrhagic necrosis.* Subsequent central fibrosis creates *cardiac sclerosis.*
- *Congestive splenomegaly* with sinusoidal dilatation, focal hemorrhages, and later hemosiderin deposits and fibrosis.
- *Renal congestion,* hypoxic injury, and acute tubular necrosis, more marked in right- than in left-sided CHF.

ISCHEMIC HEART DISEASE (IHD) (p. 524)

IHD is the generic designation for a group of closely related syndromes resulting from *ischemia*—an imbalance between the supply and demand of the heart for oxygenated blood. Ischemia comprises not only insufficiency of oxygen (*hypoxia, anoxia*), but also reduced availability of nutrient substrates and inadequate removal of metabolites.

Ischemia can be caused by

- *Reduced coronary blood flow* (the cause in over 90%); often a combination of coronary atherosclerosis with vasospasm, thrombosis, or both. Uncommon causes include arteritis, emboli, cocaine-induced vasospasm, and shock with systemic hypotension.
- *Increased myocardial demand* (e.g., tachycardia, hypertrophy) exceeding vascular supply.
- *Hypoxia due to diminished oxygen transport,* owing to severe anemia, advanced lung disease, cyanotic congenital heart disease, carbon monoxide poisoning, or cigarette smoking, is far less deleterious but may contribute to the damage if superimposed on decreased blood supply or increased demand.
- There are four general ischemic syndromes, differing largely in rate of onset and ultimate severity of ischemia.

ANGINA PECTORIS. Paroxysmal substernal/precordial pain or discomfort due to ischemia *without frank infarction.* The three somewhat distinctive patterns of angina—stable, Prinzmetal's, and unstable—are differentiated clinically on the basis of the provocation and severity of the pain. The coronary arterial pathology typically is characterized by >75% stenoses in major coronary arteries with stable angina, vasospasm in Prinzmetal's angina, and plaque disruption or fissures with variable mural thromboses in unstable angina.

MYOCARDIAL INFARCTION (MI). Death of cardiac muscle cells. See below.

CHRONIC ISCHEMIC HEART DISEASE. Typically in elderly patients with moderate-to-severe multivessel coronary atherosclerosis who insidiously develop CHF, it may result from postinfarction cardiac decompensation or slow ischemic myocyte degeneration.

- *Microscopically,* the myocardium has variable myocyte atrophy with perinuclear deposition of lipofuscin, myocytolysis of single cells or clusters, diffuse perivascular and interstitial fibrosis, and patchy-to-confluent replacement fibrosis.
- The diagnosis requires exclusion of other causes of CHF in elderly patients. Death may occur secondary to slowly progressive CHF, be due to an acute MI or an arrhythmic event, or be secondary to unrelated causes.

SUDDEN CARDIAC DEATH. When defined as unexpected cardiac death within 1 hour of symptom onset, there are 300,000 to 400,000 cases annually in the United States. It is predominantly caused by IHD; 75% to 95% of victims have marked atherosclerotic stenoses, often with acute disruption of plaque in one or more coronary arteries. In rescued patients, only about 25% develop MI. Infrequently it is a consequence of aortic valvular stenosis, hereditary or acquired conduction system abnormalities, electrolyte derangements, mitral valve prolapse, dilated or hypertrophic cardiomyopathy, or myocarditis.

The ultimate mechanism of death is a fatal arrhythmia (e.g., asystole or ventricular fibrillation), presumably triggered by conduction system scarring, acute ischemic injury, or electrical instability due to an ischemic focus or electrolytic imbalance.

MYOCARDIAL INFARCTION (MI) (p. 528)

There are two interrelated types of MI, with different morphology, pathogenesis, and clinical significance.

1. *Transmural infarct.* Infarction of full thickness of ventricular wall. Usually caused by severe coronary atherosclerosis, acute plaque disruption, and superimposed occlusive thrombosis.
2. *Subendocardial infarct.* Limited to the inner one-third to one-half of the ventricular wall (an area normally of diminished perfusion).

PATHOGENESIS. At least 90% of *transmural infarcts* are a consequence of coronary atherosclerosis with one or more severe stenosing plaques. Significant plaques typically occur in the proximal 2 cm of the left anterior descending (LAD) and left circumflex (LCX) coronary arteries, and in the proximal and distal thirds of the right coronary (RC) artery.

- Nearly all transmural MIs affect the LV; 15% simultaneously involve the RV, particularly in posterior/inferior LV infarcts. Isolated RV infarction occurs in 1% to 3% of cases.
- The initial event in most transmural MIs is ulceration, fissuring, or hemorrhagic expansion of a partially stenosing atheroma, presumably as a result of vasospasm or hemodynamic stresses.
- Thrombosis follows the acute plaque change. In a few cases, vasospasm, platelet aggregation, or both induce an MI without atherosclerotic stenosis. However, complete vessel occlusion may not necessarily cause MI, owing to collateral blood flow.
- The time interval between onset of complete myocardial ischemia and the initiation of irreversible injury is 20 to 40 minutes.
- In the absence of sudden death, thrombi may lyse spontaneously or with fibrinolytic treatment, or vasospasm may relax, thereby re-establishing flow and thus sparing some myocardium from necrosis.
- Reflow to (*reperfusion of*) precariously injured cells may restore viability but leave the cells poorly contractile ("stunned") for up to 1 to 2 days.

Subendocardial infarcts, in contrast, are usually caused by diffuse atherosclerosis and global borderline perfusion made transiently critical by increased demand, vasospasm, or hypotension, but without superimposed thrombosis. Injury is usually less than in a transmural infarct and often multifocal.

The pathogenesis of irreversible ischemic myocardial injury is summarized in Figure 12–1.

MORPHOLOGY. A myocardial infarct undergoes a characteristic sequence of gross and microscopic changes. *Grossly,*

- In 6 to 12 hours, the lesion may have a slight pallor but may be inapparent; however, changes in as early as 3 to 6 hours may be accentuated by use of histochemical techniques (e.g., triphenyl tetrazolium chloride staining for dehydrogenases colors viable myocardium red-brown but leaves nonviable areas pale).
- By 18 to 24 hours, infarcted tissue is pale to cyanotic.

POTENTIAL OUTCOMES OF ISCHEMIA

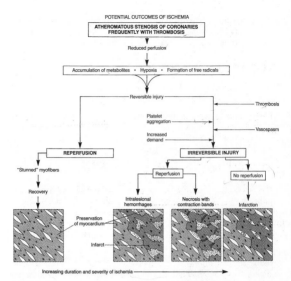

Figure 12–1. Several potential outcomes of reversible and irreversible ischemic injury to the myocardium. (From Cotran, R. S., Kumar, V., and Robbins, S. L.: Robbins Pathologic Basis of Disease. 5th ed. Philadelphia, W. B. Saunders Co., 1994, p. 538.)

- In the first week, the lesion becomes progressively more sharply defined, yellow, and softened.
- A circumferential rim of hyperemic granulation tissue appears by 7 to 10 days and progressively expands.
- Fibrous scar is usually well established by 6 weeks.

Microscopically, within 1 hour of ischemic injury there is intercellular edema, and myocytes at the edge of the infarct become wavy and buckled, attributable to stretching of these noncontractile dead fibers by adjacent viable contracting myocytes. At this stage, typical coagulative necrosis is not yet evident.

- From 12 to 72 hours postinfarction, there is a neutrophilic infiltrate into necrotic tissue, with progressive evolution of characteristic myocyte coagulative necrosis.
- Between 3 and 7 days after onset, dead myocytes begin to disintegrate and are resorbed by macrophages and enzyme proteolysis.
- Following 7 to 10 days, granulation tissue progressively replaces necrotic tissue, ultimately generating a dense fibrous scar.

CLINICAL FEATURES. Diagnosis is based mainly on symptoms (chest pain, nausea, diaphoresis, dyspnea), electrocardiographic changes, and elevation of specific myocardial enzymes (creatine kinase-MB isoenzyme, serum glutamic-oxaloacetate transaminase [SGOT], and lactate dehydrogenase [LDH-1] isoenzyme).

- Angiography, echocardiography, and perfusion scintigraphy are adjunctive.
- About 25% of patients experience sudden death after infarction, most presumably secondary to a fatal arrhythmia.

- Of patients who survive the acute event, 80% to 90% subsequently develop complications; the early mortality rate is approximately 10%.

Complications, which depend on the size and location of the necrosis, as well as the reserve of functional myocardium, consist of:

- *Arrhythmias* (75% to 95% of patients).
- *Congestive heart failure* (60%).
- *Cardiogenic shock* (10%) (usually correlates with more than 40% of LV infarcted).
- *Ventricular rupture* within the first 10 days in 1% to 5% of cases (median, 4 to 5 days). Rupture of the free wall causes pericardial hemorrhage and tamponade; rupture of the septum produces a left-to-right shunt with right heart volume overload.
- Rarely, *papillary muscle infarction* with or without rupture, often causing mitral valve dysfunction.
- *Fibrinous-to-hemorrhagic pericarditis*, common 2 to 3 days postinfarction (usually not clinically significant).
- *Mural thrombosis* in a noncontractile area, with risk of *peripheral embolization* (15% to 40%).
- Deformation of a large area of transmural infarction (*expansion*), which may heal into a *ventricular aneurysm*. Both are prone to mural thrombosis.
- Repetitive infarction (*extension*).

Overall mortality in the first year is 35%; thereafter, 5% to 10% per year.

HYPERTENSIVE HEART DISEASE (p. 541)

SYSTEMIC (LEFT-SIDED) HYPERTENSIVE HEART DISEASE (p. 541)

Minimal diagnostic criteria are

- *LV hypertrophy*, typically concentric.
- A history of hypertension.
- Absence of other lesions that might induce cardiac hypertrophy, e.g., aortic valve stenosis, coarction of aorta.

PATHOGENESIS. Myocyte hypertrophic enlargement. Thickened myocardium reduces LV compliance, impairing diastolic filling while simultaneously there is increased oxygen demand. Individual myocyte hypertrophy increases the distance for oxygen and nutrient diffusion from adjacent capillaries. Coronary atherosclerosis accompanying hypertension adds element of ischemia.

MORPHOLOGY. Thickened LV wall with increased heart weight (usually greater than 2 cm wall thickness, heart weight greater than 500 gm).

- Myocytes and nuclei are enlarged.
- In the long term, diffuse interstitial fibrosis and focal myocyte atrophy and degeneration, with LV chamber dilatation and wall thinning, may develop.

CLINICAL FEATURES. CHF is the cause of death in one-third of hypertensive patients; hypertensive hypertrophy also increases the risk of sudden cardiac death. The remainder die of renal disease, stroke, or unrelated causes.

- Therapeutic control of pressure may in time lead to regression of the myocyte hypertrophy and diminution of heart size.

PULMONARY (RIGHT-SIDED) HEART DISEASE (COR PULMONALE) (p. 542)

The right-sided counterpart to systemic hypertensive heart disease; basically RV hypertrophy or dilatation secondary to pulmonary hypertension caused by disorders affecting lung structure or function. Excluded is RV enlargement due to congenital heart disease or LV pathology.

Acute cor pulmonale refers to RV dilatation after massive pulmonary embolization.

Chronic cor pulmonale is the result of chronic RV pressure overload. Vasoconstriction in the pulmonary vascular beds incident to hypoxemia and acidosis (as would be expected with any significant primary pulmonary pathology) exacerbates baseline pulmonary hypertension.

MORPHOLOGY. *RV hypertrophy* to 1 cm or more thickness, and/or dilatation.

- RV dilatation may lead to tricuspid regurgitation.
- The left side of the heart is essentially normal.

CLINICAL FEATURES. Chronic cor pulmonale, common because chronic obstructive pulmonary disease (COPD) is widespread, is responsible for 10% to 30% of hospital admissions for cardiac decompensation. However, cardiac symptoms may be masked by those of underlying lung disease.

VALVULAR HEART DISEASE (p. 543)

DEGENERATIVE CALCIFIC AORTIC VALVE STENOSIS (p. 544)

Representing 90% of acquired aortic stenoses, these are age-related lesions that generally become clinically important in the eighth to ninth decades of life. Congenitally bicuspid valves (occurring in 1%–2% of the population) often become calcified earlier (sixth and seventh decades).

MORPHOLOGY. *Grossly,* heaped-up rigid calcific masses within sinuses of Valsalva, causing thickening and immobility of the valve cusps with narrowing of orifice. In contrast to rheumatic aortic stenosis, there is no commissural fusion. There is usually concentric LV hypertrophy from chronic pressure overload.

CLINICAL FEATURES. Need for surgical intervention is heralded by angina (hampered microcirculatory perfusion in hypertrophied myocardium), syncope (with increased risk of sudden death), or CHF.

MITRAL ANNULAR CALCIFICATION (p. 545)

Degenerative, noninflammatory, calcific deposits within the mitral annulus, usually in the elderly.

- Regurgitation may occur owing to inadequate systolic contraction of the MV ring.
- The leaflets may be unable to open over bulky deposits, causing stenosis.
- Nodular calcific deposits may cause arrhythmias by impinging on the conduction pathways; they rarely are a focus of infective endocarditis.

MITRAL VALVE PROLAPSE (MYXOMATOUS DEGENERATION OF THE MITRAL VALVE) (p. 545)

One or both MV leaflets are enlarged, myxomatous, and floppy, and they balloon back (prolapse) into the left atrium during systole, causing midsystolic click and MV insufficiency.

The disease occurs in 5%–10% of the U.S. population, typically those between 20 and 40 years of age. It is of uncertain etiology, but a developmental anomaly is suspected, perhaps affecting all connective tissues. It is common in Marfan's syndrome.

MORPHOLOGY

- *Grossly,* there is interchordal ballooning (greater than 4 mm) of the MV leaflets, and elongated, attenuated, or occasionally ruptured chordae tendineae. There is no commissural fusion.
- *Microscopically,* there is thinning and degeneration of the *fibrosa* layer (on which the strength of the leaflet depends), with myxomatous thickening of the *spongiosa*. Similar changes can be seen in the chordae.
- Secondary changes are due to injury incident to the billowing leaflets and include:

  - Fibrous thickening of valve leaflets, especially at points of contact.
  - Thickened LV endocardium at sites of friction from the prolapsing leaflets or elongated chordae.
  - Atrial thrombosis behind the ballooning cusps.
  - Calcification of the mitral annulus.

CLINICAL FEATURES.
Some patients have coincidental aortic, tricuspid, and/or pulmonary valve involvement. MV prolapse is generally asymptomatic and discovered only as a midsystolic click on auscultation. It may be associated with atypical chest pain, dyspnea, fatigue, and/or psychiatric manifestations (e.g., depression, anxiety).

Patients have an increased risk of

- infective endocarditis.
- slow, progressive mitral valvular insufficiency that may produce CHF.
- atrial and ventricular arrhythmias.
- sudden death.

RHEUMATIC FEVER (RF) AND RHEUMATIC HEART DISEASE (RHD) (p. 547)

- RF is an acute, recurrent inflammatory disease, mainly of children (ages 5 to 15 years), that typically occurs 1 to 5 weeks after a group A streptococcal infection (usually sore throat). *Most evidence suggests it is secondary to host antistreptococcal antibodies that are cross-reactive to cardiac antigens.*
- Diagnosis rests on the clinical history and the presence of two of five major (Jones) criteria.

  1. *Erythema marginatum.* In 10% to 60% of cases, as macular skin lesions with erythematous rims and central clearing, typically in a "bathing suit" distribution.
  2. *Sydenham's chorea.* A neurologic disorder with rapid, involuntary, purposeless movements.
  3. *Carditis.* Noted in 50% to 75% of children and 35% of adults; usually involves myo-, endo-, and pericardium (a *pancarditis*).

4. *Subcutaneous nodules.* In 10% to 60% of cases, giant Aschoff bodies are noted histologically (see below).
5. *Migratory large joint polyarthritis.* Seen in 90% of adults; less common in children.

Fever, arthralgia, and leukocytosis are minor criteria.

- During acute RF, death is rare, but most frequently secondary to myocarditis. Typically, myocarditis and arthritis are transient and largely resolve without complications, but the valvular involvement may lead to deformation and scarring with permanent dysfunction (*chronic RHD*) and subsequent CHF.
- Chronic RHD is more likely to occur (1) when the first attack is in early childhood, (2) when the first bout of RF is severe, or (3) with recurrent attacks.

MORPHOLOGY. *Pathognomonic* focal inflammatory nodules called *Aschoff bodies* are most characteristic in the *heart* (particularly the myocardium) but may occur elsewhere.

- Aschoff bodies constitute foci of fibrinoid necrosis, initially surrounded by lymphocytes, macrophages, and a few plasma cells, mainly about vessels, that are slowly replaced by fibrous scar.
- Aschoff bodies in the pericardium induce a fibrinous pericarditis.
- Inflammatory valvulitis (with abortive Aschoff bodies) induces formation of beady fibrinous vegetations (*verrucae*) acutely.
- The chronic (or healed) valve shows (1) fibrous thickening of leaflets with (2) bridging fibrosis across the commissures (*commissural fusion*), generating "fishmouth" or "buttonhole" stenoses, and (3) thickened, fused, and shortened mitral valve chordae.
- Calcification can occur deep in the fibrous leaflets.
- Solitary mitral involvement occurs in 65% to 70% of cases and combined aortic/mitral involvement in 20% to 25%; the tricuspid and pulmonic valves are less frequently affected.

Subendocardial collections of Aschoff nodules, usually in the left atrium, induce thickenings called *MacCallum's plaques.*

CLINICAL FEATURES. Changes secondary to tight mitral stenosis include left atrial hypertrophy and enlargement, occasionally with mural thrombi; RV hypertrophy; and CHF. Other complications include

- Increased risk of developing infective endocarditis.
- Atrial fibrillation secondary to atrial dilatation.

INFECTIVE ENDOCARDITIS (IE) (p. 550)

Colonization of heart valves with microbiologic organisms leads to the formation of friable, infected vegetations and frequently valve injury, termed infective endocarditis. Traditionally, *acute* and *subacute* forms have been distinguished.

ACUTE IE. Caused by highly virulent organisms (e.g., *Staphylococcus aureus*), often seeding a previously normal valve and producing a necrotizing, ulcerative, and invasive infection. It typically presents as a rapidly developing fever with rigors, malaise, and weakness. The larger vegetations in acute IE often cause embolic complications, and there frequently is splenomegaly. Even with treatment, death occurs in days to weeks in 50%–60% of patients.

SUBACUTE IE. Typically caused by an organism of moderate-to-low virulence (e.g., *streptococci—viridans, faecalis,* and *bovis*) seeding an abnormal or previously injured valve, causing less destruction than acute IE. This pattern of IE has an insidious onset with nonspecific malaise, low-grade fever, weight loss, and a flulike syndrome. Embolic complications are less frequent than with acute IE. The disease tends to have a protracted course even without treatment and is less often fatal than acute IE.

PATHOGENESIS. Blood-borne bacteria (bacteremia) are prerequisites for IE, acute or subacute. They may derive from an infection elsewhere in the body, intravenous drug abuse (IVDA), dental/surgical procedures, or microinjuries to gut, urinary tract, oropharynx, or skin.

- Cardiac congenital anomalies are common subsoil for IE, including tight shunts (e.g., VSD), or stenoses with jet streams. Chronic rheumatic heart disease is increasingly less common. Other risk factors include mitral valve prolapse, degenerative calcific stenosis, bicuspid aortic valve, prosthetic valves, and indwelling catheters.
- Contributory conditions include neutropenia, immunosuppressed states, and IVDA.

MORPHOLOGY. Bulky, 0.5- to 2.0-cm, friable, microbe-laden vegetations on one or more valves.

- Acute IE commonly causes erosions or perforations of leaflets, invading adjacent myocardium to produce abscess cavities, rare in subacute IE.
- With nonvalvular infections, vegetations are typically on the downstream margin of a jet lesion.
- With prosthetic valves, ring abscess is almost always present.
- With IVDA, vegetations are often acute and on right-sided valves, but left-sided valves are also frequently involved.

CLINICAL CONSEQUENCES

- Direct injury to valves (insufficiency or stenosis with CHF) or myocardium (ring abscess, perforation).
- Emboli to spleen, kidneys, brain with infarction of metastatic infection.
- Renal injury, including embolic infarction/infection, and nephrotic syndrome, renal failure, or both.
- Diagnosis is confirmed by blood cultures (with adequate sampling, positive in 80% to 95% of cases).

NONBACTERIAL THROMBOTIC ENDOCARDITIS (NBTE) (p. 554)

- Previously called marantic endocarditis.
- Small (1- to 5-mm), sterile, bland fibrin and platelet thrombi (vegetations) loosely adherent to valve leaflets (most often mitral) along the lines of closure, and without significant inflammation or valve damage.
- Characteristically (although not always) occurs in settings of cancer (particularly visceral adenocarcinomas or prolonged debilitating illness (e.g., renal failure, chronic sepsis), attributed to DIC or other hypercoagulable state.

ENDOCARDITIS ASSOCIATED WITH SYSTEMIC LUPUS ERYTHEMATOSUS (LIBMAN-SACKS ENDOCARDITIS) (p. 555)

Valvulitis of uncertain pathogenesis may appear in SLE. The mitral and tricuspid valves are most often affected with fibrinoid necrosis, mucoid degeneration, and subsequent development of small, fibrinous, sterile vegetations on *either* side of the valve leaflets.

Valve deformations may result from healing of the vegetations.

CARCINOID HEART DISEASE (p. 555)

One feature of the carcinoid syndrome *(see p. 820)* is related to elaboration by argentaffinomas of bioactive products, including serotonin, kallikrein, bradykinins, histamine, prostaglandins, and tachykinins P and K.

- The precise agent responsible for the cardiac lesions is uncertain, although it presumably is rapidly metabolized in passage through the lung, causing predominantly right heart lesions.

MORPHOLOGY. Plaquelike intimal thickenings of the endocardium of the tricuspid valve, right ventricular flow tract, and pulmonic valve are superimposed on the unaltered endocardium. The left side of the heart is usually unaffected.

COMPLICATIONS OF ARTIFICIAL VALVES (p. 556)

Prosthetic valves are of two basic types: mechanical (rigid, synthetic) and bioprosthetic (glutaraldehyde-pretreated animal valves).

Complications include

- *Paravalvular leak*—separation of the sewing ring from the valve annulus.
- *Thrombosis* and/or *thromboembolism*—a major cause of morbidity/mortality in 1% to 4% of patients per year by hindering valve function or embolizing. More common with mechanical valves. Hemorrhage can occur secondary to chronic anticoagulation therapy to prevent thrombosis.
- *Infective endocarditis*—6% of patients within 5 years of valve replacement. Difficult to cure without surgery.
- *Structural deterioration*—an uncommon problem with most mechanical valves but 20%–30% of bioprosthetic valves require re-replacement for degeneration within 10 years.
- *Others*—occlusion due to tissue overgrowth and hemolysis from mechanical trauma to erythrocytes.

MYOCARDIAL DISEASE (p. 557)

There are two broad categories of myocardial disease:

1. *Cardiomyopathy (CMP)*—defined as "heart muscle disease of unknown cause" (i.e., primary, idiopathic).
2. *Specific heart muscle disease*—defined as "heart muscle disease of known cause or associated with disorders of other systems."

- Myocardial dysfunction also occurs indirectly as a complication of ischemic, valvular, hypertensive (systemic and pulmonary), and congenital heart disease and some pericardial diseases. Thus, cardiomyopathy is not synonymous with CHF, since the latter has numerous causes.
- The clinical picture generally reflects one of three patterns (Table 12–1):
  - Dilated
  - Hypertrophic
  - Restrictive
- Endomyocardial biopsy obtained via a percutaneously inserted catheter threaded pervenously into the right ventricle allows pathologic examination of cardiac tissue.

CARDIOMYOPATHY (p. 558)

Dilated Cardiomyopathy (CMP) (p. 558)

Characterized by gradual four-chamber hypertrophy and dilatation. May occur at any age as slow, progressive CHF. Only 25% of patients survive beyond 5 years. Although the cause in a specific case is unknown, certain pathogenetic pathways are suspected to contribute to many:

- *Genetic defect.* Often with a family history. To date, however, few definite biochemical or structural abnormalities have been established.
- *Alcohol toxicity.* Attributed to direct toxicity of alcohol or a metabolite, or chronic thiamine deficiency (e.g., analogous to beriberi).
- *"Peripartum CMP."* Attributed to nutritional deficiency, hypertension, volume overload, immunologic reaction, or some metabolic derangement of pregnancy.
- *Postviral myocarditis.* Supported mostly by occasional cases in which endomyocardial biopsies have documented the progression of myocarditis to dilated CMP.

MORPHOLOGY

- Cardiomegaly (up to 900 gm), but wall thickness measurement may not reflect the degree of hypertrophy owing to dilatation.
- Poor contractile function and stasis can lead to mural thrombi.
- Valves and coronary arteries are generally usual for age.
- *Microscopic changes* are often subtle and entirely nonspecific: 25% have no significant alterations, and the remainder have diffuse myocyte hypertrophy and variable myocardial fibrosis.
- Mild-to-moderate focal endocardial thickening is sometimes seen, especially in the ventricles.

   Arrhythmogenic right ventricular cardiomyopathy (arrhythmogenic right ventricular dysplasia) is a sometimes familial disorder most commonly associated with right-sided and sometimes left-sided heart failure and various rhythm disturbances, particularly ventricular tachycardia, and sudden death. Morphologically, the right ventricular wall is severely thinned, with extensive fatty infiltration, loss of myocytes, and interstitial fibrosis.
   Death occurs (unless the patient receives a transplant) secondary to progressive CHF, embolism of mural thrombi, or fatal arrhythmias.

Table 12–1. Functional Patterns of Cardiomyopathy, Specific Heart Muscle Disease, and Indirect Myocardial Dysfunction

Functional Pattern	Cardiomyopathy (Idiopathic)	Specific (Secondary)	Indirect Myocardial Dysfunction
Dilated (systolic disorder)	Dilated cardiomyopathy	Infective myocarditis; hemochromatosis; chronic anemia; alcohol; Adriamycin; sarcoidosis	Ischemic heart disease; valvular heart disease; hypertensive heart disease; congenital heart disease
Hypertrophic (diastolic disorder)	Hypertrophic cardiomyopathy	Friedreich's ataxia; glycogen storage disease; infants of diabetic mothers	Hypertensive heart disease, especially in aged individuals; aortic stenosis
Restrictive (diastolic disorder)	Restrictive cardiomyopathy	Amyloidosis; radiation-induced fibrosis	Pericardial constriction

From Cotran, R. S., Kumar, V., and Robbins, S. L.: Robbins Pathologic Basis of Disease. 5th ed. Philadelphia, W. B. Saunders Co., 1994, p. 558.

Hypertrophic CMP (p. 560)

Also termed idiopathic hypertrophic subaortic stenosis (IHSS) and hypertrophic obstructive cardiomyopathy (HOCM).

- Characterized by a heavy, *hypercontractile*, poorly compliant heart with poor diastolic relaxation.
- Over half of cases are transmitted by autosomal dominant inheritance.
- Symptomatic disease presents usually in young adults with dyspnea, angina, near-syncope, and CHF, but the condition may be asymptomatic.
- There is an increased risk of sudden death.

MORPHOLOGY. There is marked cardiomegaly due to hypertrophy, LV more than RV, often with atrial dilatation.

- Classically, there is disproportionate thickening of the septum versus LV free wall (asymmetric septal hypertrophy [ASH]). However, some cases show concentric/symmetric hypertrophy.
- The LV cavity is compressed into a "banana-like" configuration by the asymmetrically bulging interventricular septum.
- If the basal septum is thickened at the level of the mitral valve, LV-systolic outflow may be compromised by contact of the anterior mitral leaflet with the septum (systolic anterior motion [SAM]), giving rise to *obstructive hypertrophic CMP*, reflected by a fibrous plaque on the septum.
- *Microscopically*, in addition to marked myofiber hypertrophy, 25% to 50% of the septum usually shows helter-skelter *myocyte disarray*, accompanied by myofilament disorganization within muscle cells.
- Other findings include patchy replacement fibrosis, presumably due to focal ischemic injury and abnormal thick-walled arteries of uncertain origin.

PATHOGENESIS. Families with hypertrophic CMP have been shown to have various mutations of the gene for the myosin heavy chain or other contractile proteins. However, the pathogenetic link between abnormal contractile proteins and the hypertrophic CMP phenotype remains uncertain.

CLINICAL FEATURES. The course of hypertrophic CMP is highly variable. Most patients remain unchanged for years. Only a minority progressively worsen.

- Major complications include atrial fibrillation with mural thrombus, embolization, IE, CHF, and sudden death. Outflow obstruction is seldom a major problem.

Restrictive CMP (p. 561)

A rare entity with diverse causes, resulting in a restriction of ventricular filling and thus reduced cardiac output. Interstitial myocardial fibrosis is usually present.

- *Endomyocardial fibrosis.* Found typically in children and young adults in Africa. Characterized by ventricular subendocardial fibrosis extending from the apex to the inflow tract of one or both ventricles, often with mural thrombus formation; the atrioventricular valves may be involved. Restrictive physiology occurs by reduced ventricular chamber volume. The basic cause is unknown.
- *Loeffler's endocarditis.* Characterized by endomyocardial fibrosis with large mural thrombi, similar to that described

above, but found in temperate zones. The two conditions of endomyocardiac fibrosis, however, have many overlaps. Both are frequently associated with (1) peripheral eosinophilia; (2) eosinophilic infiltration of multiple organs, including the heart; and (3) a rapidly fatal course. The cardiac changes are probably due to toxic products of eosinophils.

- *Endocardial fibroelastosis (EFE)*. An uncommon disorder of obscure etiology and possibly the end point of diverse disorders, characterized by focal-to-diffuse, cartilage-like fibroelastic thickening of the endocardium, LV more often than RV. Occurs at all ages but most commonly in patients under 2 years old. Some cases clearly have a hereditary component, but most are sporadic. Congenital cardiac anomalies are present in one-third of cases. The clinical significance depends on the extent of involvement. In most cases, there is chronic cardiac decompensation with death due to emboli or long-term CHF.

SPECIFIC HEART MUSCLE DISEASE (p. 562)

Members of the specific heart muscle disease group can cause any of the three main functional patterns described earlier.

Myocarditis (p. 562)

- Myocardial inflammation is the principal feature.
- Clinical spectrum is broad, from entirely asymptomatic to abrupt onset of arrhythmia, CHF, or even sudden death; most patients recover quickly and without sequelae.
- Etiologies include virtually all microbiologic agents, immune-mediated injury, and reaction to physical agents (heat stroke, radiation) (Table 12–2).
- Most cases are thought to be of viral origin (e.g., coxsackie-virus A and B, ECHO). Cardiac involvement occurs days to a few weeks after a primary virus infection at another site.
- Rarely of bacterial origin secondary to bacteremia, e.g., staphylococcal, tuberculous.
- *Trypanosoma cruzi*, the organism that causes Chagas' disease, affects up to 50% of the population in endemic areas of South America.
- Noninfectious myocarditis may be immune mediated, e.g., associated with rheumatic fever, SLE, or drug allergies.
- In many cases the etiology is unknown (e.g., sarcoidosis, giant cell myocarditis, and Fiedler's myocarditis, the latter two often fatal), or the microbe is unidentifiable.

MORPHOLOGY. *Gross* manifestations include a flabby ventricular myocardium with four-chamber dilatation and patchy, diffuse hemorrhagic mottling.

- Often mural thrombi arise in dilated chambers.
- Endocardium and valves are unaffected.
- After the acute stage, there may be residual dilatation/hypertrophy with small interstitial foci of fibrosis.
- *Microscopically*, there is a myocardial inflammatory infiltrate with associated myocyte necrosis or degeneration. Lesions are typically focal (and may not be seen on endomyocardial biopsy). In myocarditis associated with *viral* infections, there usually is isolated myofiber necrosis with interstitial edema and a mononuclear cell infiltrate. After the acute stage, inflammatory lesions may resolve, leaving no residua or only subtle

Table 12–2. Major Causes of Myocarditis

Infections
  Viruses (e.g., coxsackievirus, ECHO, influenza, HIV,
    cytomegalovirus)
  Chlamydia (e.g., *C. psittaci*)
  Rickettsia (e.g., *R. typhi* [typhus fever])
  Bacteria (e.g., *Corynebacterium* [diphtheria],
    Neisseria [meningococcus], *Borrelia* [Lyme
    disease])
  Fungi (e.g., *Candida*)
  Protozoa (e.g., *Trypanosoma* [Chagas' disease]),
    toxoplasmosis)
  Helminths (e.g., trichinosis)

Immune-Mediated Reactions
  Postviral
  Poststreptococcal (rheumatic fever)
  Systemic lupus erythematosus
  Drug hypersensitivity (e.g., methyldopa,
    sulfonamides)
  Transplant rejection

Unknown
  Sarcoidosis
  Giant cell myocarditis

HIV = human immunodeficiency virus.
From Cotran, R. S., Kumar, V., and Robbins, S. L.: Robbins Pathologic
Basis of Disease. 5th ed. Philadelphia, W. B. Saunders Co., 1994, p. 562.

interstitial and focal fibrosis. It may present later as dilated cardiomyopathy.

- *Bacteria and other larger parasites* produce reactions characteristic of the lesions they induce in other tissues (e.g., neutrophilic infiltrate, abscesses, granulomas).
- Myocarditis occurs in approximately two-thirds of patients with Lyme disease; myocardial spirochetes can be demonstrated in some. Lyme myocarditis is usually mild and reversible but occasionally requires a temporary pacemaker for AV block.
- In *Chagas' disease,* trypanosomes parasitize myocytes and produce acute and chronic inflammation, including eosinophils.
- In *hypersensitivity reactions,* there are predominantly perivascular mononuclear and eosinophilic infiltrates, occasionally with acute vasculitis and spotty myofiber necrosis.
- In *idiopathic giant cell myocarditis,* there is focal myocyte necrosis associated with granulomatous inflammation, including multinucleated giant cells.

OTHER SPECIFIC HEART MUSCLE DISEASE

Common morphologic changes with all cardiotoxic agents include myofiber swelling, fatty change, and individual cell lysis. Electron microscopy shows mitochondrial abnormalities, smooth endoplasmic reticulum swelling and fragmentation, and myofibril lysis. With time, delicate interstitial fibrosis and focal replacement scarring occur.

Alcohol or its metabolites (especially acetaldehyde) have a direct toxic effect on the myocardium. Nevertheless, the cause and effect relationship with alcohol alone remains tenuous, and no morphologic features distinguish alcohol-induced cardiac damage from idiopathic dilated CMP. Moreover, chronic alcoholism may be associated with thiamine deficiency, introducing an element of beri-beri heart disease (indistinguishable from dilated CMP) (*p. 558*).

The anthracycline chemotherapeutic agents doxorubicin (Adriamycin) and daunorubicin induce a dose-dependent cardiotoxicity (usually total dose >500 mg/m^2), attributed primarily to lipid peroxidation of myofiber membranes. Both the physiologic and morphologic patterns are indistinguishable from those of idiopathic dilated CMP.

Peripartum CMP is the designation given to a globally dilated heart discovered within several months before or after delivery. Although the mechanism behind this relationship is uncertain, pregnancy invokes the possibilities of hypertension, volume overload, nutritional deficiency, other metabolic derangement, or as yet poorly characterized immunologic reaction. Whatever the basis, in about half these patients proper function is restored, and dilatation of the heart disappears within months following delivery.

Iron overload can occur in hereditary hemochromatosis and hemosiderosis from multiple blood transfusions. Patients with iron storage disease present most commonly with a dilated pattern.

Amyloidosis. May occur as part of systemic amyloidosis (*see p. 231*) or may be isolated, e.g. senile cardiac amyloidosis, occurring to some extent in 50% of individuals over 70 years old. Often cardiac involvement is incidental, but it may induce arrhythmias or restrictive physiology.

Catecholamines, either administered exogenously (e.g., epinephrine) or produced endogenously (i.e., pheochromocytomas) induce tachycardia and vasomotor constriction (with superimposed platelet aggregation), resulting in diffuse but patchy ischemic necrosis. *Cocaine* may have a similar effect by blocking catecholamine reuptake at adrenergic nerve terminals.

PERICARDIAL DISEASE (p. 566)

Unusually primary; generally secondary to diseases of adjacent structures or part of a systemic disorder.

PERICARDIAL EFFUSION (p. 566)

The normal pericardial sac contains 30 to 50 ml of serous fluid. Typically, *noninflammatory* fluid accumulations rarely exceed 500 ml.

- *Serous.* The most common form. Serosa is smooth and glistening. Fluid accumulates slowly and therefore is well tolerated until very large volume compromises diastolic filling. The most common causes are CHF and hypoproteinemia.
- *Serosanguineous.* Blunt chest trauma (e.g., CPR). Rarely clinically significant.
- *Chylous.* Lymphatic obstruction (benign or malignant). Rarely clinically significant.

HEMOPERICARDIUM (p. 566)

Accumulation of pure blood in the pericardium without an inflammatory component. Usually due to traumatic perforation, myocardial rupture after a transmural MI, rupture of the intrapericardial aorta, or hemorrhage from an abscess or tumor metastasis. Escaping blood rapidly fills the sac under high pressure, and as little as 200 to 300 ml may cause tamponade.

PERICARDITIS (p. 566)

Usually secondary to disorders involving the heart or adjacent mediastinal structures (e.g., MI, surgery, trauma, radiation, tumors, infections) or (less frequently) systemic abnormalities (e.g., uremia, autoimmune diseases).

Primary acute pericarditis is rare and generally of viral origin. Chronic reactions also can occur, e.g., with tuberculosis and fungi, and healing may lead to damaging adhesions.

Acute Pericarditis (p. 567)

- *Serous pericarditis.* Usually consists of 50 to 200 ml of slowly accumulating exudate characteristically produced by nonbacterial involvements, including rheumatic fever, SLE, tumors, uremia, and primary viral infections (e.g., Coxsackie). Frequently the etiology is unknown. Microscopically, there is a scant epi- and pericardial acute and chronic inflammatory infiltration (mostly lymphocytes). The fluid resorbs if the underlying disease remits, rarely leaving any residuals.
- *Fibrinous and serofibrinous pericarditis.* The most common clinical form, seen with MI, associated with a pericardial friction rub. May also be caused by any of the aforementioned etiologies. Exudate may be completely resolved or be organized, leaving typically delicate, stringy adhesions (*adhesive pericarditis*) or plaquelike thickening, both usually inconsequential.
- *Purulent (suppurative) pericarditis.* Usually signifies bacterial, fungal, or parasitic infection, which has reached the pericardium by direct extension, by hematogenous or lymphatic spread, or during cardiotomy. Typically composed of 400 to 500 ml of a thin-to-creamy pus with erythematous, granular serosal surfaces. Presents with prominent fever, rigors, and a friction rub. Usually organizes and may produce mediastinopericarditis or *constrictive pericarditis* (see below).
- *Hemorrhagic pericarditis.* Denotes an exudate of blood admixed with fibrinous-to-suppurative effusion. Most commonly follows cardiac surgery or is associated with tuberculosis or malignancy. Usually organizes with or without calcification.
- *Caseous pericarditis.* Due to tuberculosis (typically by direct extension from neighboring lymph nodes) or, less commonly, mycotic infection. This pattern is the most frequent antecedent to fibrocalcific constrictive pericarditis.

Chronic or Healed Pericarditis (p. 568)

Healing of acute lesions can resolve or lead to pericardial fibrosis ranging from a thick, pearly, nonadherent epicardial plaque ("soldier's plaque") to thin, delicate adhesions, to massive adhesions, as described next.

- *Adhesive mediastinopericarditis.* Clinically significant—the pericardial sac is obliterated, and the parietal layer is tethered to mediastinal tissue. The heart thus contracts against all the surrounding attached structures, with subsequent hypertrophy and dilatation.
- *Constrictive pericarditis.* Clinically significant—marked by thick (up to 1-cm), dense, fibrous obliteration, often with calci-

fication of the pericardial sac that encases the heart, limiting diastolic expansion and restricting cardiac output.

RHEUMATOID HEART DISEASE (p. 568)

Rheumatoid arthritis involves the heart in 20% to 40% of severe chronic cases. The typical finding is pericarditis, marked by a mixture of fibrin and necrotic debris derived from pericardial rheumatoid granulomas. This may progress to form dense, fibrous, and potentially restrictive adhesions. Less frequently, granulomatous rheumatoid nodules occur in the myocardium, endocardium, aortic root, or valves, where they are particularly damaging. Rheumatoid valvulitis can produce changes similar to those seen in rheumatic heart disease, but classically without commissural fusion.

TUMORS (p. 569)

Primary heart tumors are rare, but cardiac metastases (hematogenous) occur in some patients who die of cancer. Metastases involve the pericardium or penetrate into the myocardium, or both. The spectrum of cardiac effects of noncardiac tumors is summarized in Table 12–3.

The following are among the many potential primary cardiac tumors:

- *Myxomas. The most common primary cardiac tumor in adults.* Usually single, 90% arise in the atria in the region of the fossa ovale; left-to-right ratio is 4:1. *Grossly* 1 to 10 cm in diameter, they are sessile-to-pedunculated and vary from globular and hard to papillary/villous and myxoid. *They may cause symptoms by physical obstruction or "wrecking-ball" trauma to the atrioventricular valves, or by peripheral embolization. Histologically,* they are composed of stellate/globular multipotential mesenchymal myxoma cells, admixed with endothelial, smooth muscle cells, and macrophages, all in an acid mucopolysaccharide matrix. The weight of evidence supports a hamartomatous origin.

Table 12–3. Cardiovascular Effects of Noncardiac Neoplasms

Direct Consequences of Tumor
Pericardial and myocardial metastases
Large vessel obstruction
Pulmonary tumor emboli
Indirect Consequences of Tumor—
Complications of Circulating Mediators
Nonbacterial thrombotic endocarditis (NBTE)
Carcinoid heart disease
Pheochromocytoma-associated heart disease
Myeloma-associated amyloidosis
Effects of Tumor Therapy
Chemotherapy
Radiation therapy

Modified from Schoen, F. J., et al.: Cardiac effects of non-cardiac neoplasms. Cardiol. Clin. 2:657, 1984.

- *Lipomas.* Circumscribed, but poorly encapsulated large polypoid accumulations of adipose tissue, more commonly in the LV, right atrium, or septum. Symptoms depend on location and on encroachment on valve function or conduction pathways. These are probably hamartomas.
- *Papillary fibroelastomas.* Usually an incidental finding at autopsy. Characteristically found on right-sided valves in children and left-sided valves in adults. Composed of clusters of 2- to 5-mm filamentous projections. *Microscopically,* filaments have a core of myxoid connective tissue with smooth muscle and fibroblasts, covered by endothelium. They probably derive from organized thrombi.
- *Rhabdomyomas.* Much less common than myxomas, but the most common primary heart tumor in children. May cause valvular or outflow tract obstruction. *Grossly,* they may be left- or right-sided gray-white ventricular wall masses up to several centimeters in diameter. *Microscopically,* they are composed of large, rounded, or polygonal cells rich in glycogen and containing myofibrils. Cytoplasmic strands radiating from the central nucleus to plasma membrane create "spider cells." Probably hamartomas; some are associated with tuberous sclerosis.
- *Angiosarcomas and rhabdomyosarcomas.* These malignant neoplasms resemble their counterparts in other locations.

CONGENITAL HEART DISEASE (p. 571)

Some abnormalities are incompatible with intrauterine survival, whereas others manifest shortly after birth as the circulation changes from fetal to postnatal configuration; still others cause cardiac malfunction only in adult life, and some are entirely inconsequential.

Twelve anomalies (Table 12–4) account for about 85% of

Table 12–4. Frequencies of Cardiac Malformations in 1000 Consecutive Children*

Malformation	% of Congenital Heart Disease
Ventricular septal defect (VSD)	33
Patent ductus arteriosus (PDA)	10
Tetralogy of Fallot	9
Aortic stenosis (AS)	8
Pulmonary stenosis (PS)	10
Coarctation of aorta	5
Atrial septal defect (ASD)	5
Transposition of great arteries	5
Atrioventricular septal defect	4
Truncus arteriosus	1
Tricuspid atresia	1
Total anomalous pulmonary venous connection (TAPVC)	1

*Combinations of lesions tabulated with dominant malformation.
  Data modified from Moller, J. H.: 1000 Consecutive children with a cardiac malformation with 26- to 37-year follow-up. Am. J. Cardiol. 70:661, 1992.

cases. Bicuspid aortic valve and mitral valve prolapse are not included.

ETIOLOGY. The causes of congenital heart disease are unknown in 90% of cases; they are very likely multifactorial with genetic and environmental inputs. There is a twofold to tenfold increase in the incidence of congenital heart disease in siblings of an affected child.

Five percent of cases are associated with well-known multisystem syndromes based on chromosomal abnormalities, e.g., trisomy 21 (Down's). *Less than 1% of congenital defects are clearly environmental,* the best documented being maternal rubella in the first trimester, which causes patent ductus arteriosus, pulmonic and aortic stenosis, tetralogy of Fallot, and other defects. Thalidomide, excessive alcohol consumption, and excessive cigarette smoking also have been strongly implicated. The most critical juncture is embryologic cardiac development in gestational weeks 3–8.

CLINICAL CONSEQUENCES. Children with significant congenital anomalies have not only direct hemodynamic sequelae, but also failure to thrive, retarded development, or cyanosis. They also are at increased risk of chronic or recurrent illness and of infective endocarditis (due to abnormal valves or to endocardial injury from jet lesions).

The various congenital anomalies are of two types: shunts or obstructions.

Shunts. Denotes abnormal communication between heart chambers, between vessels, or between chambers and vessels. Depending on pressure relationships, blood may be shunted from left to right (more common) or right to left.

Right-to-left shunts (cyanotic congenital heart disease) cause cyanosis from the outset as poorly oxygenated blood passes into the systemic circulation. They also permit emboli from venous sources to pass directly into the systemic circulation (*paradoxic embolism*).

Left-to-right shunts include chronic right heart overload with secondary pulmonary hypertension and RV hypertrophy, but eventually right-sided exceeds left-sided pressure and the shunt becomes right to left. Hence, cyanosis appears late. Once significant irreversible pulmonary hypertension develops, the structural defects of congenital heart disease are considered irreversible.

Secondary findings in long-standing cyanotic heart disease include clubbing of the fingers and toes, hypertrophic osteoarthropathy, and polycythemia.

Obstructions. Typically coarctation, valvular stenoses, or atresias. These do not cause cyanosis.

LEFT-TO-RIGHT SHUNTS: LATE CYANOSIS (p. 573)

The major anomalies in this category are atrial septal defect, ventricular septal defect, and patent ductus arteriosus.

Atrial Septal Defect (ASD) (p. 573)

An abnormal opening in the atrial septum that allows free communication of blood. ASD is the most common congenital cardiac anomaly presenting in adults and falls into three categories:

1. *Primum type.* Represents 5% of ASDs and common in Down's syndrome. It occurs low in the atrial septum, occasionally in association with mitral valve deformities.

2. *Secundum type*. Represents 90% of ASDs and occurs at the foramen ovale. The aperture may be of any size (generating a single atrial chamber if very large) and may be single, multiple, or fenestrated. It is usually isolated but sometimes associated with other anomalies.

3. *Sinus venous type*. Represents 5% of ASDs and occurs high in the septum near the superior vena cava (SVC) entrance. It is sometimes associated with anomalous right pulmonary venous drainage into the SVC or right atrium.

- Even large ASDs are usually asymptomatic until adulthood, when either right heart failure occurs or gradually increasing right-sided hypertrophy and PA pressure finally induce right-to-left shunting with cyanosis.
- Surgical correction early in life is advocated to prevent pulmonary vascular changes and paradoxic embolism.

Ventricular Septal Defect (VSD) (p. 574)

An abnormal opening in the ventricular septum that allows free communication between left and right ventricles, VSD is the most common congenital cardiac anomaly.

- Frequently associated with other structural anomalies, particularly tetralogy of Fallot, but 30% isolated. Ninety percent involve the membranous septum (membranous VSD); the remainder are muscular.
- Depending on the size of the defect, the clinical picture ranges (in decreasing order of importance) from fulminant CHF to late cyanosis, to asymptomatic holosystolic murmurs, to spontaneous closure (50% of those less than 0.5 cm in diameter).
- With a small to moderate-sized VSD, patients are at increased risk of infective endocarditis.
- Surgical correction is desirable before right heart overload and pulmonary vascular disease develop.

Patent Ductus Arteriosus (PDA) (p. 575)

- In the fetus, the ductus arteriosus permits blood flow between the aorta (distal to the left subclavian artery) and the pulmonary artery.
- At term, and under the influence of relatively high oxygen tension and reduced local PGE synthesis, muscular contraction closes the ductus within 1 to 2 days of life. Persistent patency beyond that point is generally permanent.
- About 85% to 90% of PDAs occur as isolated defects. The length and diameter (up to 1 cm) are variable. There is associated LV hypertrophy and PA dilatation.
- Although initially asymptomatic, and notable only for a prominent heart murmur (described as "machinery-like"), long-standing PDA induces pulmonary hypertension with subsequent RV hypertrophy and finally right-to-left shunting to produce late cyanosis.
- Early closure of a PDA (either surgically or with prostaglandin administration in otherwise normal infants) is therefore advocated.

RIGHT-TO-LEFT SHUNTS: EARLY CYANOSIS (p. 575)

The major anomalies in this category are tetralogy of Fallot, transposition of the great vessels, and truncus arteriosus.

Tetralogy of Fallot (p. 575)

The four cardinal features due to embryologic anteriosuperior displacement of the infundibular septum are

1. Ventricular septal defect (VSD).
2. Dextroposed aorta overriding the VSD.
3. Pulmonic stenosis with RV outflow obstruction.
4. RV hypertrophy.

Additional cardiac anomalies may be present. Cyanosis is present from birth or soon after.

- The severity of symptoms is directly related to the extent of RV outflow obstruction. With a large VSD and mild pulmonic stenosis, there is a mild left-to-right shunt without cyanosis. More severe pulmonic stenosis produces a cyanotic right-to-left shunt.
- With complete pulmonic obstruction, survival is permitted only by flow through a PDA and/or dilated bronchial arteries.
- It is reasonable to delay surgical correction, provided the child can tolerate the level of oxygenation. Pulmonic stenosis protects the lung from volume and pressure overload, and RV failure is rare owing to decompression into the LV or aorta.

Transposition of Great Arteries (p. 576)

Origin of the aorta from the right ventricle and the pulmonary artery from the right.

- Fetal development occurs as a result of mixing venous and systemic blood through the PDA and a patent foramen ovale. Therefore, postnatal life critically depends on continued patency of the ductus, as well as a VSD, ASD, or patent foramen ovale.
- Prognosis depends on the severity of tissue hypoxia and the ability of the RV to maintain aortic flow. Untreated, most children die within the first few months.
- Particularly common in children of diabetic mothers, this malformation causes cyanosis from both great arteries.

Truncus Arteriosus (p. 577)

Associated with numerous concomitant cardiac defects, this is basically a developmental failure of the aorta and PA to separate. It results in an infundibular VSD with a single vessel receiving blood from both RV and LV.

Patients present with early cyanosis due to right-to-left shunting. Eventually the flow reverses and they develop RV hypertrophy with pulmonary vascular hypertension. The anomaly carries a poor prognosis.

OBSTRUCTIVE CONGENITAL ANOMALIES (p. 577)

Coarctation of Aorta (p. 577)

- Represents a constriction of the aorta; 50% occur as isolated defects, the remainder with multiple other anomalies.
- In most cases, cardiomegaly (chronic pressure overload hypertrophy) occurs.
- Clinical manifestations depend on the location and severity of the constriction. Most occur just distal to the ductus/ligamentum arteriosus (*postductal*).

- *Preductal* coarctation manifests early in life and may be rapidly fatal. Survival depends on the ability of the ductus arteriosus to sustain blood flow to the distal aorta and lower body adequately. Even then, there tends to be lower body cyanosis. This form usually involves a 1- to 5-cm segment of the aortic root and is often associated with fetal RV hypertrophy and early right heart failure.
- *Postductal* coarctation is generally asymptomatic unless very severe. It usually leads to upper extremity hypertension but low flow in the lower extremities, causing arterial insufficiency (claudication, cold sensitivity). Collateral flow around the coarctation generally develops, with intercostal rib notching (noted on x-ray views), and internal mammary and axillary artery dilatation.
- Untreated, the mean life span is 40 years, with death secondary to CHF, aortic dissection proximal to the coarctation, intracranial hemorrhage, or infective endoaortitis at the site of narrowing.

Pulmonary Valve Stenosis or Atresia with Intact Interventricular Septum (p. 578)

- Occurs in isolation or in association with other anomalies, e.g., transposition or tetralogy.
- With *complete pulmonic atresia* there is virtually always a hypoplastic RV and an ASD with blood entering the lungs via a PDA.
- *Pulmonary stenosis,* on the other hand, generally caused by cuspal fusion, may vary from mild to severe.
- Pulmonary outflow obstructions may also be subvalvular or supravalvular and even multiple.
- Mild stenosis is generally asymptomatic. Progressively more severe stenoses cause increasing cyanosis with earlier onset.

Aortic Valve Stenosis and Atresia (p. 579)

- *Congenital complete aortic atresia* is rare and incompatible with neonatal survival. Survival with congenital *aortic valvular stenosis* (two types: valvular and subvalvular) depends on the severity of the lesion.
- Rare single-cusp aortic valves are also seen.
- Consequences include infective endocarditis, LV hypertrophy (pressure overload), poststenotic dilatation of the aortic root, and (rarely) sudden death.
- Bicuspid aortic valve is a common anomaly but is generally functionally unimportant throughout early life. However, it is prone to calcific degeneration (described earlier) and has an increased risk of infective endocarditis.

CARDIAC TRANSPLANTATION (p. 580)

Transplantation of cardiac allografts is now frequently performed, most commonly for dilated CMP and IHD. The 1-year survival is 70%–80%, and 5-year survival is over 60%.

Allograft rejection is a major postoperative problem, characterized by interstitial lymphocytic inflammation that damages adjacent myocytes. More severe stages are accompanied by extensive myocyte necrosis and frequently inflammatory vascular injury. Other postoperative problems include infection and development of malignancies, particularly lymphomas (generally related to Epstein-Barr virus). The major current limitation to the long-term success of cardiac transplantation is late, progressive, diffuse stenosing intimal proliferation of the coronary arteries (*graft arteriosclerosis*).

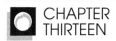

CHAPTER THIRTEEN

Red Cells and Hemostasis

ANEMIAS (p. 586)

Anemia is a reduction in the oxygen transport capacity of blood, usually due to a reduction below normal limits of the total circulating red cell mass. This is reflected by lower than normal hematocrit and hemoglobin concentrations. In most anemias erythropoietin production and erythropoiesis are increased, causing erythroid marrow hyperplasia. Increased erythropoiesis can also occur in the spleen and liver of infants (extramedullary hematopoiesis). Classification of anemias is based on the mechanism of production (Table 13–1).

ANEMIAS OF BLOOD LOSS (p. 587)

Clinical and morphologic reactions to blood loss depend on the rate of hemorrhage (acute versus chronic).

- *Acute blood loss.* Alterations reflect principally the loss of blood volume (which may lead to shock and death). After several days, if the acute episode is survived, marrow compensation is evidenced by an increase in reticulocytes.
- *Chronic blood loss.* Usually causes anemia when iron reserves are depleted, giving rise to iron deficiency anemia.

HEMOLYTIC ANEMIAS (p. 587)

Characterized by (1) premature destruction of red cells, (2) accumulation of the products of hemoglobin catabolism (e.g., bilirubin), and (3) marked increase in erythropoiesis within the marrow and associated reticulocytosis. Hemolysis may occur predominantly intravascularly or extravascularly:

- *Intravascular hemolysis* occurs when red cells are damaged by mechanical injury (e.g., microangiopathic hemolytic anemia) or by complement-mediated lysis (e.g., antibody-coated mismatched blood transfusion). It is manifested by

  - Hemoglobinemia and hemoglobinuria.
  - Hemosiderinuria.
  - Jaundice (conjugated hyperbilirubinemia).
  - Reduction in serum haptoglobin (a protein that binds free hemoglobin).

- *Extravascular hemolysis* occurs within the mononuclear phagocytic cells of the spleen and other organs. Predisposing factors

239

Table 13–1. Classification of Anemia According to Mechanism of Production

---

I. **Blood Loss**
   A. Acute: Trauma
   B. Chronic: Lesions of GI tract, gynecologic disturbances
II. **Increased Rate of Destruction (Hemolytic Anemias)**
   A. Intrinsic (intracorpuscular) abnormalities of red cells
      Hereditary
      1. Red cell membrane disorders, e.g., disorders of membrane cytoskeleton: spherocytosis, elliptocytosis
      2. Red cell enzyme deficiencies, e.g., enzymes of hexose monophosphate shunt: G6PD, glutathione synthetase
      3. Disorders of hemoglobin synthesis
         a. Deficient globin synthesis: thalassemia syndromes
         b. Structurally abnormal globin synthesis (hemoglobinopathies): sickle cell anemia, unstable hemoglobins
      Acquired
      1. Membrane defect: paroxysmal nocturnal hemoglobinuria
   B. Extrinsic (extracorpuscular) abnormalities
      1. Antibody mediated
      2. Mechanical trauma to red cells, e.g., microangiopathic hemolytic anemias, thrombotic thrombocytopenia purpura, DIC
      3. Infections: malaria
      4. Chemical injury: lead poisoning
      5. Sequestration in mononuclear phagocyte system: hypersplenism
III. **Impaired Red Cell Production**
   A. Disturbance of proliferation and differentiation of stem cells: aplastic anemia, pure red cell aplasia, anemia of renal failure
   B. Disturbance of proliferation and maturation of erythroblasts
      1. Defective DNA synthesis: deficiency or impaired utilization of vitamin B_{12} and folic acid (megaloblastic anemias)
      2. Defective hemoglobin synthesis, e.g., deficient heme synthesis: iron deficiency

---

Modified from Cotran, R. S., Kumar, V., and Robbins, S. L.: Robbins Pathologic Basis of Disease. 5th ed. Philadelphia, W. B. Saunders Co., 1994, p. 586.

are injury to the red cell membrane, reduced deformability, or opsonization of the red cells. The manifestations of extravascular hemolysis are similar to those of intravascular hemolysis except for the absence of hemoglobinemia and hemoglobinuria.

Hereditary Spherocytosis (HS) (p. 589)

Approximately 75% are autosomal dominant disorders characterized by defects in the red cell membrane that render erythrocytes spheroidal, less deformable, and vulnerable to splenic sequestration and destruction.

PATHOPHYSIOLOGY. Proteins that form the skeleton of the red cell membrane are either reduced in amount or defective in structure. A deficiency of spectrin is the most common abnormality. Spectrin-deficient red cells have unstable cell membranes, pieces of which are lost spontaneously. The resulting reduction in the cell surface causes the red cells to assume a spheroidal shape. Spherocytic red cells have reduced membrane flexibility and hence are trapped and destroyed in the splenic cords.

MORPHOLOGY

- Many red cells appear abnormally small and lack central pallor (spherocytes).
- Splenic cords of Billroth are markedly congested and exhibit prominent erythrophagocytosis.
- Marrow shows normoblastic hyperplasia.

CLINICAL FEATURES. Although there is significant clinical variability, anemia, moderate splenomegaly, and jaundice are characteristic. Intercurrent infections may trigger two types of crises: (1) hemolytic crisis associated with massive hemolysis and (2) an aplastic crisis characterized by a temporary suppression of erythropoiesis, usually triggered by intercurrent, often parvovirus, infections. Forty to 50% of adults develop gallstones due to chronic hyperbilirubinemia.

Diagnosis of HS depends on family history, hematologic findings, and laboratory evidence of spherocytosis shown by examination of peripheral smear and increased red cell osmotic fragility.

Glucose-6-Phosphate Dehydrogenase (G6PD) Deficiency (p. 591)

G6PD is an enzyme in the hexose monophosphate shunt needed to produce reduced glutathione (GSH), which is necessary to protect red cells from oxidative injuries. When G6PD-deficient cells are subjected to oxidant stresses in the form of infections or exposure to certain drugs, hemoglobin is oxidized and denatured. The altered hemoglobin precipitates within the cells in the form of Heinz bodies, which attach to the cell membrane and reduce its flexibility. Inclusion-bearing cells are susceptible to destruction by the splenic macrophages.

Inheritance of the mutant G6PD gene is X-linked. *There are several G6PD variants; only two, G6PD A$^-$ and G6PD Mediterranean, lead to clinically significant hemolysis.* A$^-$ is present in about 10% of American blacks. It is associated with progressive loss of G6PD in older red cells, which undergo hemolysis on exposure to oxidant drugs, principally the antimalarials. Because younger red cells are unaffected, hemolytic episodes are self-limited. In the Mediterranean form, the level of G6PD is much lower in all cells (young and old); thus, hemolytic anemia is more severe and persistent.

Sickle Cell Disease (p. 592)

This hereditary hemoglobinopathy, resulting from a point mutation of the globin gene, is associated with substitution of valine for glutamic acid at the sixth position of the β-globin chain. This change transforms HbA to HbS. Approximately 8% of American blacks are heterozygous for HbS.

SICKLING PHENOMENON. Upon deoxygenation, HbS molecules undergo aggregation and polymerization, leading to sickling of the red cells. In the homozygous state, irreversibly sickled cells (ISCs) can be identified in the peripheral blood.

Many factors influence sickling of the red cells:

- The amount of HbS and its interaction with other hemoglobin chains in the cell (the most important factor). In heterozygotes approximately 40% of hemoglobin is HbS; the rest is HbA, which interacts only weakly with HbS during the processes of aggregation. Therefore the heterozygote has little tendency to sickle and is said to have *sickle cell trait*. In contrast, *the homozygote has all HbS and full-blown sickle cell anemia.* Beta-globin chains other than HbA also influence the sickling process. For example, fetal hemoglobin (HbF) with its γ-globin chains also fails to interact with HbS, and hence newborns do not manifest the vaso-occlusive complications of the disease until they are 5 or 6 months of age, when the amount of HbF in the cells begins to approach adult levels.
- The mean corpuscular hemoglobin concentration (MCHC) per cell. The higher the HbS concentration within the cell, the greater are the chances of contact and interaction between HbS molecules. Thus, dehydration, which increases the MCHC, greatly facilitates sickling and may trigger occlusion of small blood vessels. Conversely, the coexistence of α-thalassemia reduces the MCHC and therefore the severity of sickling.

Consequences of Sickling

- *Chronic hemolytic state.* Sickle cells have rigid and nondeformable cell membranes and are therefore prone to sequestration and destruction. The average red cell survival is shortened to approximately 20 days and correlates with the percentage of ISCs in circulation.
- *Microvascular occlusions.* Because of their inelasticity and propensity to adhere to the capillary endothelium, sickle cells tend to occlude small blood vessels. The resultant hypoxic injury (infarction) is a clinically important and the most debilitating component of sickle cell anemia.

MORPHOLOGY

- *Spleen.* Commonly enlarged in early phases of disease owing to trapping of sickled cells in the splenic cords. Late in the course, repeated episodes of vaso-occlusion lead to progressive scarring and shrinkage in size (*autosplenectomy*).
- Bone marrow shows normoblastic hyperplasia: expansion of the marrow when severe may cause resorption of bone.
- Microvascular occlusions produce tissue damage in several organs.

CLINICAL FEATURES. Characterized by

- Chronic hemolytic anemia with its associated features (e.g., chronic hyperbilirubinemia and propensity to develop gallstones).
- Vaso-occlusive crises representing painful episodes of ischemic necroses, affecting most commonly bones, lungs, liver, brain, penis, and spleen. In children, a painful crisis affecting bones may mimic osteomyelitis.
- Aplastic crisis representing temporary marrow suppression of erythropoiesis triggered by parvovirus infections; some cases may be caused by folate deficiency.

- Increased susceptibility to infections, particularly *Salmonella* osteomyelitis, and others caused by encapsulated organisms such as *Streptococcus pneumoniae* and *Haemophilus influenzae*. Progressive splenic fibrosis and impairment of the alternate complement pathway is believed to predispose to infections.

DIAGNOSIS. Based on clinical findings, the appearance of sickle cells in the peripheral blood smear, and detection of HbS by hemoglobin electrophoresis. Prenatal detection of heterozygotes and homozygotes is possible through analysis of fetal DNA.

Thalassemia Syndromes (p. 596)

A heterogeneous group of mendelian disorders, characterized by a lack of or decreased synthesis of either the normal α- or the normal β-globin chain of hemoglobin A ($\alpha_2\beta_2$).

GENETIC DEFECTS

- *β-Thalassemia syndromes*, characterized by deficient synthesis of the β-globin chain: (1) β^0-thalassemia: total absence of β-globin chains in the homozygous state and (2) β^+-thalassemia: reduced (but detectable) β-globin synthesis in the homozygous state. Several different point mutations that affect transcription, processing, or translation of β-globin mRNA have been found to cause β^0- and β^+-thalassemia; mutations that cause aberrant splicing of mRNA are most common.
- *α-Thalassemia*, characterized by reduced synthesis of α-globin chains due to deletion of one to all four of the normally present α-globin genes.

PATHOPHYSIOLOGY. The hematologic consequences of diminished synthesis of one globin chain derive from both low intracellular hemoglobin (hypochromia) and a relative excess of the other chain.

- *β-Thalassemia*. With a decrease in the synthesis of β globin, most of the α chains produced cannot find complementary β chains to bind. The free α chains form highly unstable aggregates that produce a variety of untoward effects, the most important being cell membrane damage, leading to loss of K^+ and impaired DNA synthesis. These changes cause destruction of red cell precursors within the marrow (ineffective erythropoiesis) and hemolysis of the abnormal red cells in the spleen (hemolytic state). The resulting anemia, if severe, causes marked compensatory expansion of the erythropoietic marrow, which may encroach upon the cortical bone and cause skeletal abnormalities in growing children. Ineffective erythropoiesis is also associated with excessive absorption of dietary iron, which along with repeated blood transfusions (needed by some patients) leads to severe iron overload.
- *α-Thalassemia*. Associated with an imbalance in the synthesis of α chains and non–α chains (β, γ, or δ). The unpaired non–α chains form unstable aggregates that damage red cells and their precursors.

β-THALASSEMIA CLINICAL CLASSIFICATION. Is based on the severity of anemia, which in turn is based on the type of genetic defect (β^+ or β^0) as well as gene dosage (homozygous or heterozygous).

- *Thalassemia major*. Most common in Mediterranean countries and parts of Africa and Southeast Asia. Individuals homozygous for β-thalassemia genes have severe, transfusion-dependent anemia. Hb levels range between 3 and 6 gm per dl. Peripheral blood smear shows severe abnormalities, including marked anisocytosis with many small and virtually colorless (microcytic, hypochromic) red cells, target cells, stippled red cells, and fragmented red cells. The clinical course of β-thalassemia major is generally brief because, unless the patient is supported by transfusions, death occurs at an early age from the profound effects of anemia. Blood transfusions lessen the anemia and also suppress secondary features (bone deformities) related to excessive erythropoiesis. In multiply transfused patients, cardiac failure resulting from progressive iron overload and secondary hemochromatosis is an important cause of morbidity and mortality.

- *Thalassemia minor.* The presence of one normal gene in the heterozygote allows enough β-globin chain synthesis, so that affected individuals are usually asymptomatic. This form is more common than the thalassemia major and affects the same ethnic groups. Peripheral blood smear usually shows some minor abnormalities, including hypochromia, microcytosis, basophilic stippling, and target cells. A characteristic finding on hemoglobin electrophoresis is an increase in HbA_2, which may constitute 4 to 8% of the total hemoglobin. Recognition of β-thalassemia trait is important for genetic counseling and because it may mimic the hypochromic microcytic anemia of iron deficiency.

- *Thalassemia intermedia.* Characterized by clinical features and severity that are intermediate between the major and minor forms. These patients, as alluded to in the previous discussion, are genetically heterogeneous.

α-THALASSEMIA CLINICAL CLASSIFICATION. Made on the basis of the number of α-globin gene(s) deleted, which in turn determines the severity of anemia.

- *Silent carrier state.* Results from the deletion of a single α-globin gene; reduction in α-globin chain synthesis is barely detectable. Completely asymptomatic.

- *α-Thalassemia trait.* Deletion of two α-globin genes either from the same chromosome or from each of the two chromosomes. Both genetic patterns are identical clinically, but the position of deleted genes makes a difference in the likelihood of severe α-thalassemia (HbH disease or hydrops fetalis) in the offspring. Clinical picture is identical to that described for β-thalassemia minor.

- *Hemoglobin H (HbH) disease.* Deletion of three of the four α-globin genes. Synthesis of α chains is markedly suppressed, and unstable tetramers of excess β globin (HbH) are formed. Clinically, HbH disease resembles β-thalassemia intermedia.

- *Hydrops fetalis.* Deletion of all four α-globin genes. In the fetus, excess γ-globin chains form tetramers (Hb Barts) that have extremely high oxygen affinity but are unable to deliver the oxygen to tissues. This form is not compatible with life.

The clinical and genetic features of thalassemia are summarized in Table 13–2.

Paroxysmal Nocturnal Hemoglobinuria (PNH) (p. 601)

A rare disorder, characterized by chronic intravascular hemolysis. This is the only hemolytic anemia resulting from a membrane

Table 13-2. Clinical and Genetic Classification of Thalassemias

Clinical Nomenclature	Genotype	Disease	Molecular Genetics
A. β-Thalassemias			
I. Thalassemia major	1. Homozygous β⁰-thalassemia (β^0/β^0)	Severe, requires blood transfusions regularly	1. Rare gene deletions in β^0/β^0
	2. Homozygous β^+-thalassemia (β^+/β^+)		2. Defects in transcription, processing, or translation of β-globin mRNA
II. Thalassemia intermedia	β^0/β^+	Severe but does not require regular blood transfusions	
	β^+/β^+		
III. Thalassemia minor	β^0/β	Asymptomatic, with mild or absent anemia; red cell abnormalities seen	
	β^+/β		
B. α-Thalassemias			
I. Silent carrier	$-\alpha/\alpha\alpha$	Asymptomatic; no red cell abnormality	Gene deletions mainly
II. α-Thalassemia trait	1. $--/\alpha\alpha$ (Asian)	Asymptomatic, like β-thalassemia minor	
	2. $-\alpha/-\alpha$ (black African)		
III. HbH disease	$--/-\alpha$	Severe, resembles β-thalassemia intermedia	
IV. Hydrops fetalis	$--/--$	Lethal in utero	

From Cotran, R. S., Kumar, V., and Robbins, S. L.: Robbins Pathologic Basis of Disease. 5th ed. Philadelphia, W. B. Saunders Co., 1994, p. 599.

defect that is not inherited. Red cells have increased sensitivity to complement-mediated lysis owing to deficiency of a family of membrane proteins that regulate complement activity. These are decay accelerating factor (CD55), membrane inhibitor of reactive lysis (CD59), and C8 binding protein. These three proteins belong to a larger group of cellular proteins—the glycosyl phosphatidyl inositol (GPI)-linked proteins. Because platelets and granulocytes also have reduced activity of these proteins, their functions are affected as well; therefore, in addition to hemolysis, these patients are predisposed to infections and thrombosis, the latter involving especially the portal, cerebral, and hepatic veins.

- PNH is a clonal disorder of multipotent stem cells that sometimes transforms into other stem cell disorders such as aplastic anemia and acute leukemia. In the absence of such transformation, PNH is usually a chronic disease with a median survival of 10 years.

Immunohemolytic Anemias (p. 601)

Hemolysis in these disorders is related to emergence of anti–red cell antibodies. The major diagnostic criterion is the Coombs antiglobulin test, which detects antibodies on the surface of red cells. Classification is based on the nature of the antibodies and the presence or absence of an underlying disorder (Table 13–3). **WARM ANTIBODY HEMOLYTIC ANEMIA.** This form is idio-

Table 13–3. Classification of Immune Hemolytic Anemias

I. **Warm Antibody Type**
The antibody is of the IgG type, does not usually fix complement, and is active at 37°C.
A. *Primary* or idiopathic
B. *Secondary* to:
1. Lymphomas and leukemias
2. Other neoplastic diseases
3. Autoimmune disorder (particularly SLE)
4. Drugs

II. **Cold Agglutinin Type**
The antibodies are IgM and are most active *in vitro* at 0–4°C. Antibodies dissociate at 30°C or above. The antibody fixes complement at warmer temperatures, but agglutination of cells by IgM and complement occurs only in the peripheral cool parts of the body.
A. *Acute* (mycoplasmal infection, infectious mononucleosis)
B. *Chronic*
1. Idiopathic
2. Associated with lymphoma

III. **Cold Hemolysins (Paroxysmal Cold Hemoglobinuria)**
IgG antibodies bind to red cells at low temperature, fix complement, and cause hemolysis when the temperature is raised to 30°C.

SLE = systemic lupus erythematosus.
From Cotran, R. S., Kumar, V., and Robbins, S. L.: Robbins Pathologic Basis of Disease. 5th ed. Philadelphia, W. B. Saunders Co., 1994, p. 602.

pathic in 60% of cases. The IgG anti-red cell antibodies coat the red cells but are not complement fixing. Opsonized red cells assume a spheroidal shape owing to partial loss of red cell membrane in the process of phagocytosis by splenic macrophages. Spherocytes are eventually sequestered and destroyed in the spleen; thus, splenomegaly is characteristic.

The mechanism of antibody formation is best understood in drug-induced hemolytic anemias:

- *Hapten model.* Drugs (e.g., penicillin and cephalosporins) may act as a hapten and combine with the red cell membrane to induce antibody directed against the red cell–drug complex.
- *Immune complex model.* The drug (e.g., quinidine) serving as hapten binds to a plasma protein, and the drug-protein complex evokes antibodies. Immune complexes formed in the circulation bind to and damage the red cell membrane.
- *Autoantibody model.* The drug (e.g., the antihypertensive agent α-methyldopa) in some manner initiates production of antibodies directed against intrinsic red cell antigens.

COLD AGGLUTININ IMMUNE HEMOLYTIC ANEMIA. Caused by IgM antibodies that agglutinate red cells at low temperatures.

- *Acute.* Occurs during the recovery phase of certain infectious disorders (e.g., *Mycoplasma* pneumonia and infectious mononucleosis). This form of AHA is self-limited and rarely induces manifestations of hemolysis.
- *Chronic.* Occurs with lymphoproliferative disorders and as an idiopathic condition. Clinical symptoms result from agglutination of red cells and fixation of complement in distal body parts, where the temperature may drop below 30°C. The hemolytic anemia usually is of variable severity; vascular obstruction by agglutinated red cells results in pallor, cyanosis of the body parts exposed to cold temperatures, and Raynaud's phenomenon.

COLD HEMOLYSIN HEMOLYTIC ANEMIA. Characteristic of the disease paroxysmal cold hemoglobinuria (PCH), which manifests as acute intermittent massive intravascular hemolysis following exposure to cold. Autoantibodies are IgG in nature (Donath-Landsteiner [DL] antibody) and are directed against the P blood group antigen. They attach to the red cells and bind complement at low temperatures; when the temperature is elevated, hemolysis occurs. Most cases follow infections (e.g., *Mycoplasma* pneumonia, measles, mumps, and some ill-defined viral and "flu" syndromes).

Hemolytic Anemia Resulting from Trauma to Red Cells (p. 603)

Significant trauma to the red cells resulting in their fragmentation in the circulation can produce intravascular hemolysis. Underlying conditions are

- Prosthetic heart valves that create turbulent flow and shearing forces.
- Diffuse narrowing of the microvasculature due to deposition of fibrin, as occurs in disseminated intravascular coagulation (DIC), gives rise to microangiopathic hemolytic anemia.

The peripheral blood reveals fragmented erythrocytes in the form of burr cells, helmet cells, and triangular cells.

ANEMIAS OF DIMINISHED ERYTHROPOIESIS (p. 603)

Impaired red cell production may be caused by a variety of disorders such as deficiency of some vital substrate (iron, B_{12}, and folate) or stem cell failure.

Megaloblastic Anemias (p. 603)

These anemias, caused most commonly by a deficiency of vitamin B_{12} or folate, have the following features in common:

- Abnormally large erythroid precursors (megaloblasts) whose nuclear maturation lags behind the cytoplasmic maturation; nuclear changes such as pyknosis that are normally associated with maturation of erythroblasts are delayed or fail to occur.
- Ineffective erythropoiesis (death of megaloblasts in the marrow) associated with compensatory megaloblastic hyperplasia.
- Prominent anisocytosis (variability in cell size) is a reflection of the abnormal erythropoiesis, including abnormally large and oval red cells (macro-ovalocytes) with a mean corpuscular volume in excess of 100 m³.
- Abnormal granulopoiesis yielding giant metamyelocytes and hypersegmented neutrophils.

PATHOPHYSIOLOGY. Vitamin B_{12} and folic acid are essential coenzymes in the DNA synthetic pathway. A deficiency of these nutrients results in deranged or inadequate synthesis of DNA, but the synthesis of RNA and proteins is unaffected. Therefore, cytoplasmic enlargement and maturation occur without concomitant nuclear maturation. In addition to affecting red cell precursors, a deficiency of B_{12} and folate affects all rapidly dividing cells, including all myeloid cells and the mucosal epithelium of the GI tract. The anemia results from

- Ineffective erythropoiesis.
- Production of abnormal erythrocytes that are susceptible to accelerated hemolysis, by poorly defined mechanisms.

Ineffective granulopoiesis and thrombopoiesis as well as premature destruction may also affect granulocyte and platelet precursors, giving rise to pancytopenia.

Many pathways may lead to a vitamin B_{12} deficiency. The ultimate source of this vitamin is dietary animal products. Absorption of vitamin B_{12} occurs as follows:

- Peptic digestion releases dietary vitamin B_{12}, which is then bound to salivary and gastric B_{12}-binding proteins called R binders.
- R-B_{12} complexes transported to the duodenum are split by pancreatic proteases, and the released B_{12} attaches to intrinsic factor (IF), secreted by the parietal cells of the gastric fundic mucosa.
- IF-B_{12} complex passes to the distal ileum, where it attaches to the epithelial IF receptors, followed by absorption of vitamin B_{12}, which is then transported to the tissues by transcobalamin II.

A deficiency of vitamin B_{12} may result from

- Impaired absorption due to
  - Achlorhydria (in elderly individuals), which impairs release of B_{12} from the protein-bound form.

- Gastrectomy, which leads to loss of IF.
- Pernicious anemia, an autoimmune disorder that damages gastric parietal cells.
- Resection of the ileum (preventing absorption of IF-B$_{12}$ complex).
- Malabsorption syndromes.

- Increased requirements (e.g., pregnancy).
- Inadequate diet, uncommon since the body has large reserves of vitamin B$_{12}$.

PERNICIOUS ANEMIA (p. 605)

Caused by a lack of IF production due to chronic atrophic gastritis. The gastric mucosal atrophy is marked by a loss of parietal cells.

Pernicious anemia in all likelihood results from an autoimmune reaction against gastric parietal cells. Favoring this concept are

- The presence of autoantibodies in the serum and gastric juice of most patients with PA:

  - Antibodies that block binding of B$_{12}$ to IF (blocking antibodies).
  - Antibodies that react with both IF and B$_{12}$ (binding antibodies).
  - Antibodies that bind to the parietal cells (parietal canalicular antibodies).

- A possible autoreactive T-cell response against gastric mucosa.
- Significant association of pernicious anemia with autoimmune disorders of the adrenal and thyroid glands.

MORPHOLOGY.
Characteristic changes are found in the marrow, alimentary tract, and central nervous system:

- Bone marrow. Megaloblastic erythroid hyperplasia; giant myelocytes and metamyelocytes with hypersegmented polymorphs; large multilobed nuclei in megakaryocytes.
- Alimentary canal. Atrophic glossitis—the tongue is shiny, glazed, and red; gastric fundal atrophy with virtual absence of parietal cells; atrophic gastric mucosa replaced by mucus-secreting goblet cells (intestinalization).
- Central nervous system. Lesions found in 75% of cases; characterized by demyelination of the dorsal and lateral tracts of the spinal cord. The basis of CNS changes is obscure and possibly distinct from hematologic effects (folate deficiency produces megaloblastic anemia but neurologic changes are absent).

CLINICAL FEATURES.
Insidious onset in the fifth and sixth decades. Symptoms are those of anemia and involvement of the posterolateral spinal tracts. There is increased risk of gastric cancer. Diagnosis is based on measurement of serum B$_{12}$ levels and hematologic response (reticulocytosis) after parenteral administration of the vitamin.

ANEMIA OF FOLATE DEFICIENCY

Folic acid deficiency induces a megaloblastic anemia that is clinically and hematologically indistinguishable from that encountered in vitamin B$_{12}$ deficiency. However, the neurologic changes seen in the latter do not occur and gastric atrophy is absent.

Deficiency of folic acid may result from

- Inadequate intake; usually encountered in those who live on

marginal diets (e.g., chronic alcoholics, the elderly, and the indigent).
- Malabsorption syndromes such as tropical and nontropical sprue.
- Increased demand, as in pregnancy, infancy, and disseminated cancer.
- Administration of folate antagonists such as methotrexate, used in cancer chemotherapy.

Diagnosis of folate deficiency requires demonstration of decreased folate levels in serum or red cells.

Iron Deficiency Anemia (p. 610)

Deficiency of iron is an extremely common cause of anemia worldwide.

IRON METABOLISM. The normal Western diet contains approximately 10 to 20 mg of iron per day, most of which is in the form of heme contained in animal products. The remainder is inorganic iron found in vegetables. About 20% of heme iron (in contrast to 1 to 2% of nonheme iron) is absorbable. The duodenum is the primary site of absorption. Dietary heme iron enters the mucosal cells directly, whereas nonheme iron is transported into the cell by luminal mucins and cytosolic mobilferrin. A fraction of the absorbed iron is rapidly delivered to plasma transferrin. The remainder is bound to mucosal ferritin, some to be transferred more slowly to plasma transferrin and some to be lost with exfoliation of mucosal cells. When the body is replete with iron, most of the iron that enters the duodenal epithelium is bound to ferritin and lost with exfoliation; in iron deficiency, transfer to plasma transferrin is enhanced.

Total body iron content is in the range of 2 gm for women and 6 gm for men. Approximately 80% of functional body iron is found in hemoglobin; myoglobin and iron-containing enzymes (e.g., catalase and cytochromes). The iron storage pool, represented by hemosiderin and ferritin-bound iron, contains approximately 15 to 20% of total body iron. It is found in all tissues but particularly in liver, spleen, bone marrow, and skeletal muscle. Because serum ferritin is largely derived from the storage pool of iron, its level is a good indicator of the adequacy of body iron stores.

ETIOLOGY. Negative iron balance and consequent anemia may result from low dietary intake, malabsorption, excessive demand, and chronic blood loss.

- Low dietary intake alone is rarely the cause of iron deficiency in the United States, because the average daily dietary intake of 10 to 20 mg is more than enough for males and nearly adequate for females.
- Malabsorption may occur with sprue and celiac disease or following gastrectomy.
- Increased demands not met by normal dietary intake may occur in pregnancy and infancy.
- Chronic blood loss is the most important cause of iron deficiency anemia in the Western world; this loss may occur from the GI tract (e.g., peptic ulcers, colonic cancer, hemorrhoids, hookworm disease) or the female genital tract (e.g., menorrhagia, metrorrhagia, cancers).

CLINICAL FEATURES

- Peripheral blood. Red blood cells are pale (hypochromic) and smaller than normal (microcytic).

- Marrow. Mild hyperplasia of normoblasts, associated with loss of sideroblasts and absence of stainable iron in the reticuloendothelial cells.
- Other organs. In severe iron deficiency, depletion of essential iron-containing enzymes gives rise to changes such as alopecia, koilonychia, and atrophy of the tongue and gastric mucosa. Esophageal webs may appear, completing the *Plummer-Vinson triad* of hypochromic microcytic anemia, atrophic glossitis, and esophageal webs.

DIAGNOSIS. Rests on clinical and hematologic features along with

- Low serum iron and ferritin.
- Increased total plasma iron-binding capacity (TIBC).
- Reduced plasma transferrin saturation.

Anemia of Chronic Inflammatory States (p. 613)

Associated primarily with abnormal iron metabolism. Serum iron levels and TIBC are reduced, but there is abundant storage iron. This combination suggests that there is a defect in the reutilization of iron due to some impediment in transfer of iron from the reticuloendothelial (storage) system to the erythroid precursors. In addition, defects in erythropoietin production and shortened red cell survival have also been documented. This anemia is reversible when the primary disease is controlled.

Aplastic Anemia (p. 613)

Characterized by failure or suppression of multipotent myeloid stem cells and resultant neutropenia, anemia, and thrombocytopenia (pancytopenia).

ETIOLOGY. May be idiopathic (in 50% of cases) or caused by

- Myelotoxic drugs or chemicals, the most common cause of secondary aplastic anemia. Damage to the marrow may be dose related, predictable, and reversible or may be idiosyncratic, affecting only some of the exposed individuals and in an unpredictable manner. Best documented as predictable myelotoxins are benzene, alkylating agents, and antimetabolites (vincristine, busulfan); idiosyncratic reactions are caused by chloramphenicol, chlorpromazine, and streptomycin.
- Irradiation: when the whole body is exposed.
- Infections (e.g., non-A, non-B hepatitis).
- Inherited diseases (e.g., Fanconi's anemia, associated with multiple congenital anomalies).

PATHOGENESIS. In idiopathic cases, stem cell failure may be due to

- A primary defect in the number or function of stem cells, resulting in some cases from a somatic mutation affecting stem cells; genetically damaged stem cells may in rare cases be transformed to leukemias.
- Suppression of stem cells by immune (T cell–mediated) mechanisms.

MORPHOLOGY

- Hypocellular marrow; hematopoietic cells replaced by fat cells.
- Secondary effects of granulocytopenia (infections) and thrombocytopenia (bleeding).

CLINICAL FEATURES. Insidious onset with symptoms related to a paucity of red cells, neutrophils, and platelets. Splenomegaly is characteristically absent. In cases resulting from chemical or drug exposure, withdrawal of the inciting agent may lead to recovery. Treatment with bone marrow transplantation or immunosuppressive therapy is also of value.

Pure Red Cell Aplasia (PRCA) (p. 615)

This rare form of marrow failure results from absence or near-absence of red cell precursors. The acute form may be drug- or virus-induced or may occur as an "aplastic crisis" in chronic hemolytic states. PRCA may also appear insidiously in patients with thymomas; in this setting the anemia is cured by resection of the tumor.

Other Forms of Marrow Failure (p. 615)

- *Myelophthisic anemia.* Caused by space-occupying lesions that destroy or distort marrow architecture and depress its productive capacity. Associated with a paucity of all blood elements, and in many cases the presence of white and red cell precursors in the blood. The most common cause is metastatic cancer.
- *Diffuse liver disease* (toxic, infectious, or cirrhotic). The anemia is attributed to bone marrow failure, although other factors such as bleeding from varices and folate deficiency may also contribute.
- *Chronic renal failure.* Almost invariably associated with anemia. The basis is multifactorial, including reduced red cell production due to inadequate production of erythropoietin. Administration of recombinant erythropoietin is associated with significant improvement in the majority of cases.

POLYCYTHEMIA (p. 616)

An increased concentration of red cells that may be relative or absolute.

- *Relative.* Due to decreased plasma volume and associated with
  - Dehydration (e.g., deprivation of water or prolonged vomiting).
  - Stress polycythemia: an obscure condition of unknown etiology also called Gaisböck's syndrome.
- *Absolute*
  - Primary: increase in red cell mass due to intrinsic abnormality of myeloid stem cells. Related to myeloproliferative syndrome (*see p. 658*).
  - Secondary: increase in red cell mass in response to increased levels of erythropoietin, which may be (1) appropriate: lung disease, high-altitude living, cyanotic heart disease; or (2) inappropriate: erythropoietin-secreting tumors (e.g., renal cell carcinoma, hepatocellular carcinoma, cerebellar hemangioblastoma).

BLEEDING DISORDERS (p. 616)

Hemorrhagic diatheses may be caused by increased fragility of blood vessels, disorders of platelets, defects in coagulation, or a combination of these.

INCREASED VASCULAR FRAGILITY (p. 616)

Disorders in this category are relatively common but usually do not cause serious bleeding. Most often they induce petechial and purpuric hemorrhages. Platelet count and coagulation time are usually normal; bleeding time is variable. Conditions include

- Infections, especially meningococcemia and rickettsioses; underlying mechanisms are vasculitis or disseminated intravascular coagulation (DIC) (*see p. 257 in this volume*).
- Drug reactions. Often mediated by the deposition of immune complexes in the vessel walls with production of a hypersensitivity vasculitis.
- Poor vascular support. Results from (1) impaired formation of collagen, as occurs in scurvy and Ehlers-Danlos syndrome; or (2) loss of perivascular supporting tissue, associated with Cushing's syndrome.
- Henoch-Schönlein purpura. A systemic hypersensitivity reaction of unknown cause characterized by a purpuric rash, colicky abdominal pain, polyarthralgia, and acute glomerulonephritis. Associated with vascular and glomerular mesangial deposition of immune complexes.

THROMBOCYTOPENIA (p. 617)

Decrease in platelet number, characterized principally by petechial bleeding, most often from small vessels of the skin and mucous membranes. Thrombocytopenia must be severe, to levels of 10,000 to 20,000 platelets per mm^3 (reference range = 150,000 to 300,000 per mm^3) before the bleeding tendency becomes clinically evident.

Causes of thrombocytopenia are many, and can be classified into four major categories:

1. *Decreased production of platelets.* Occurs in generalized diseases of the bone marrow that compromise the number of megakaryocytes (e.g., aplastic anemia, disseminated cancer), as well as in ineffective megakaryopoiesis (e.g., megaloblastic states).

2. *Decreased platelet survival.* Usually results from immunologically mediated destruction of platelets; may follow drug ingestion (e.g., quinine, quinidine, methyldopa) or infections (particularly HIV infection). There is usually a compensatory megakaryocytic marrow hyperplasia. Platelet destruction can also result from mechanical injury in a manner similar to red cell fragmentation in microangiopathic hemolytic anemias.

3. *Sequestration.* May occur in the presence of splenomegaly. In these instances, splenectomy can cure the thrombocytopenia.

4. *Dilutional.* Massive transfusions may cause a relative reduction in the number of circulating platelets, because blood stored for longer than 24 hours contains virtually no viable platelets.

5. *HIV-associated.* Multifactorial because of immune complex injury, antiplatelet antibodies, and HIV-induced suppression of megakaryocytes.

The more common forms of thrombocytopenia are described below.

Idiopathic Thrombocytopenic Purpura (ITP) (p. 618)

Associated with immunologically mediated destruction of platelets. Two forms are recognized:

254 RED CELLS AND HEMOSTASIS

- *Acute ITP.* A self-limited disorder, seen most often in children after a viral infection (e.g., rubella, cytomegalovirus infection, viral hepatitis, infectious mononucleosis). Platelet destruction is probably related to formation of antigen-antibody complexes, directed against the virus, that are adsorbed onto platelets.
- *Chronic ITP.* Destruction of platelets results from the presence of platelet autoantibodies directed toward two platelet antigens—the platelet membrane glycoprotein complexes IIb/IIIa and Ib/IX. These antibodies can be demonstrated in the plasma as well as bound to platelet surface (PAIgG) in approximately 80% of patients. Destruction of antibody-coated platelets occurs in the spleen, which is also the major site of autoantibody synthesis. Splenectomy is beneficial in 75 to 80% of patients.

CLINICAL FEATURES. Chronic ITP most often occurs in adults, particularly women of childbearing age. Most commonly, there is a long history of easy bruising or nosebleed. Sometimes the onset is sudden, with a shower of petechial hemorrhages or internal bleeding (melena, hematuria). Subarachnoid or intracerebral hemorrhage is a rare but serious consequence. The idiopathic form must be distinguished from that secondary to other immunologically mediated thrombocytopenias that accompany SLE, AIDS, and drug injury.

MORPHOLOGY. The spleen is normal in size, but histologically there is congestion of the sinusoids, and splenic follicles may show prominent germinal centers. An increased number of megakaryocytes are usually seen in the bone marrow.

DIAGNOSIS. Suggested by clinical features such as petechial hemorrhages and thrombocytopenia; must be supported by demonstration of increased megakaryocytes in the marrow. As would be expected based on the low platelet count, the bleeding time is prolonged. Splenomegaly and lymphadenopathy are extremely uncommon.

Isoimmune Thrombocytopenia (p. 618)

Results from development of antibodies directed against a specific platelet isoantigen, most commonly PL^{A1}.

- Post-transfusion thrombocytopenia. When a PL^{A1}-negative individual, sensitized to PL^{A1} antigen by a previous pregnancy or blood transfusion, is transfused with PL^{A1}-positive blood, antibody-mediated destruction of platelets occurs.
- Neonatal thrombocytopenia. The pathogenesis is similar to that of the hemolytic reaction in erythroblastosis fetalis. A PL^{A1}-negative mother carrying an antigen-positive fetus develops IgG antibodies against the PL^{A1} antigens, and the resulting antibodies cross the placenta to cause thrombocytopenia in the newborn.

Thrombotic Thrombocytopenic Purpura (TTP) and Hemolytic Uremic Syndrome (HUS) (p. 619)

These rare disorders of obscure nature are characterized mainly by thrombocytopenia, microangiopathic hemolytic anemia, fever, transient neurologic deficits (TTP), and renal failure. Most of these clinical manifestations are caused by *widespread hyaline microthrombi* (composed of dense aggregates of platelets and fibrin) that are found in arterioles and capillaries.

PATHOPHYSIOLOGY. According to some investigators, perturbation of the endothelium is of primary importance. An immunologic reaction against endothelial cells or synthesis of abnormal forms of von Willebrand's factor that cause pathologic aggregation of platelets are some of the different mechanisms proposed to explain the formation of microthrombi. Unlike DIC, activation of the clotting system is not present.

CLINICAL FEATURES. Occurs more commonly in females, with peak incidence in the fourth decade. Treatment with corticosteroids (TTP) or in children (HUS) and exchange transfusions prevents an otherwise fatal outcome.

HEMORRHAGIC DISORDERS RELATED TO DEFECTIVE PLATELET FUNCTIONS (p. 620)

Characterized by prolonged bleeding time in association with normal platelet count. May be congenital or acquired.

- *Congenital*

  - *Defective platelet adhesion.* Exemplified by the autosomal recessive Bernard-Soulier syndrome, which is caused by a deficiency of a platelet membrane glycoprotein complex (GpIb/IX), the platelet receptor for von Willebrand's factor (vWF). This is necessary for platelet-collagen adhesion.
  - *Defective platelet aggregation.* Exemplified by thrombasthenia, an autosomal recessive disorder resulting from a deficiency of two platelet membrane glycoproteins (GpIIb/GpIIIa) involved in binding fibrinogen.
  - *Disorders of platelet secretion.* A group of disorders in which initial platelet aggregation with collagen or ADP is normal, but subsequent platelet responses such as secretion of prostaglandins and granule-bound ADP are impaired.

- *Acquired.* Of the many conditions associated with acquired defects, two are clinically significant:

  - *Aspirin ingestion.* Aspirin is a potent inhibitor of the enzyme cyclooxygenase and can suppress the synthesis of thromboxane A_2, which is necessary for platelet aggregation. The antiplatelet effect of aspirin forms the basis of its use in the management of myocardial infarction. In about 10% of the normal population, significant postoperative oozing may occur if aspirin is used as an analgesic.
  - *Uremia.* The pathogenesis of bleeding in uremic patients is complex and includes platelet function defects. These patients respond well to DDAVP.

HEMORRHAGIC DIATHESES RELATED TO ABNORMALITIES IN CLOTTING FACTORS (p. 620)

Bleeding seen in patients with abnormalities of the clotting factors differs somewhat from that encountered in patients with platelet deficiencies:

- The spontaneous appearance of petechiae or purpura is uncommon; more often the bleeding manifests as the development of large ecchymoses or hematomas following an injury, or as prolonged bleeding after a laceration or any form of surgical procedure.
- Bleeding into the gastrointestinal and urinary tracts, and particularly into weightbearing joints, is common.

Clotting abnormalities may occur as acquired defects or may be hereditary in origin.

ACQUIRED DEFICIENCIES. Usually characterized by multiple clotting abnormalities. Vitamin K deficiency results in depressed synthesis of factors II, VII, IX, and X and protein C. Because the liver makes virtually all the clotting factors, severe parenchymal liver disease may be associated with a hemorrhagic diathesis. DIC produces a deficiency of multiple coagulation factors.

HEREDITARY DEFICIENCIES. Typically affect a single clotting factor. The most common inherited disorders are hemophilia (A and B) and von Willebrand's disease. A review of the structure and function of factor VIII–von Willebrand's (vWF) complex will aid an understanding of these disorders.

Plasma factor VIII-vWF is a complex made up of two separate proteins (factor VIII and vWF) that can be distinguished by functional, biochemical, and immunologic criteria. One component required for activation of factor X in the intrinsic coagulation pathway is called factor VIII procoagulant protein, or factor VIII. Deficiency of factor VIII gives rise to classic hemophilia (hemophilia A). Factor VIII is linked to vWF, which forms approximately 99% of the complex and exists in the form of a series of multimers ranging in size from 4×10^3 to 12×10^6 daltons. vWF is necessary for adhesion of platelets to subendothelial collagen. GPIb serves as the major platelet membrane receptor, and it is believed that it is through this receptor that vWF bridges collagen and platelets. vWF also acts as a carrier for factor VIII.

The two components of factor VIII-vWF complex are coded by separate genes and synthesized by different cells. vWF is produced by endothelial cells and megakaryocytes. Hepatocytes are the major source of factor VIII.

von Willebrand's Disease (p. 622)

Transmitted most commonly as an autosomal dominant disorder, it is characterized by spontaneous bleeding from mucous membranes, excessive bleeding from wounds, and menorrhagia.

The classic and most common variant (type I) is characterized by a reduced quantity of circulating vWF. Synthesis of vWF is not impaired, but release of vWF multimers is inhibited by some unknown mechanism. In the less common type II variant, multimer assembly is defective, and hence the large and intermediate multimers, representing the most active form of vWF, are missing from plasma.

Levels of factor VIII may be reduced in von Willebrand's disease, because vWF stabilizes factor VIII in circulation. Therefore, patients have a compound defect involving platelet function and the coagulation pathway. This is reflected in the laboratory by a prolonged bleeding time in the presence of a normal platelet count, and prolonged partial thromboplastin time. However, except in the most severely affected patients, effects of factor VIII deficiency such as bleeding into the joints, which characterize hemophilia, are uncommon.

Factor VIII Deficiency (Hemophilia A) (p. 622)

Characterized by a reduced amount or activity of factor VIII. Inherited as an X-linked recessive trait that primarily affects males. Clinical features develop only in the presence of severe deficiency (factor VIII levels less than 1% of normal). Mild or moderate degrees of deficiency (levels between 1 and 50% of normal) are asymptomatic, although post-traumatic bleeding may be excessive. The variable degrees of deficiency in the level of factor VIII procoagulant protein result from different types of mutations in the factor VIII gene. Clinically, hemophilia is associated with

- Massive hemorrhage after trauma or operative procedures.
- "Spontaneous" hemorrhages in regions of the body normally subject to trauma, particularly the joints (hemarthroses); recurrent bleeding into joints leads to progressive, crippling deformities.
- Absence of petechiae and ecchymoses.
- Prolonged partial thromboplastin time (PTT) and normal bleeding time.

Diagnosis is possible only by assay for factor VIII. The cloning of the factor VIII gene has permitted antenatal diagnosis of hemophilia A.

Treatment consists of replacement therapy with factor VIII concentrates, which carries the risk of transmission of viral hepatitis. Before the routine screening of blood for HIV antibodies, transmission of HIV led to the development of AIDS in many hemophiliacs. With the current practice of using heat-treated factor VIII concentrates derived from the blood of HIV-seronegative donors, the risk of HIV transmission has been virtually eliminated.

Factor IX Deficiency
(Christmas Disease, Hemophilia B) (p. 623)

Clinically indistinguishable from hemophilia A; also inherited as an X-linked recessive trait, it may occur asymptomatically or with associated hemorrhage. Identification of Christmas disease is possible only by assay of factor IX levels.

DISSEMINATED INTRAVASCULAR COAGULATION
(DIC) (p. 623)

An acute, subacute, or chronic thrombohemorrhagic disorder occurring as *a secondary complication in a variety of diseases* (Table 13–4). Characterized by activation of the coagulation sequence, leading to the formation of microthrombi throughout the microcirculation. As a consequence of the thrombotic diathesis, there is consumption of platelets, fibrin, and coagulation factors, and, secondarily, activation of fibrinolytic mechanisms. Thus, DIC may present with

- Signs and symptoms relating to infarction caused by microthrombi.
- A hemorrhagic diathesis resulting from depletion of the elements required for hemostasis and activation of the fibrinolytic mechanisms.

PATHOGENESIS. There are two major mechanisms by which DIC may be triggered: (1) release of tissue factor or thromboplastic substances into the circulation and (2) widespread injury to the endothelial cells (Fig. 13–1).

- *The tissue factor/thromboplastic substances released into the circulation* may be derived from a variety of sources (e.g., placenta in obstetric complications and granules of leukemic cells in acute promyelocytic leukemia). Mucus released from

Table 13–4. Major Disorders Associated with DIC

Obstetric Complications
Abruptio placentae
Retained dead fetus
Septic abortion
Amniotic fluid embolism
Toxemia

Infections
Gram-negative sepsis
Meningococcemia
Rocky Mountain spotted fever
Histoplasmosis
Aspergillosis
Malaria

Neoplasms
Carcinomas of pancreas, prostate, lung, and stomach
Acute promyelocytic leukemia

Massive Tissue Injury
Traumatic
Burns
Extensive surgery

Miscellaneous
Acute intravascular hemolysis, snakebite, giant hemangioma,
 shock, heat stroke, vasculitis, aortic aneurysm, liver disease

---

From Cotran, R. S., Kumar, V., and Robbins, S. L.: Robbins Pathologic Basis of Disease. 5th ed. Philadelphia, W. B. Saunders Co., 1994, p. 624.

certain adenocarcinomas can also act as a thromboplastic substance. In gram-negative sepsis, bacterial endotoxins can cause release of thromboplastic substances contained within endothelial cells and the lysosomes of granulocytes and monocytes. Furthermore, activated monocytes release IL-1 and tumor necrosis factor (TNF-α), both of which increase the expression of tissue factor on endothelial cell membranes and simultaneously decrease the expression of thrombomodulin. This results in both activation of the clotting system and inhibition of coagulation control.

• *Endothelial injury* can initiate DIC by causing release of tissue factor from endothelial cells, and by promoting platelet aggregation and activation of the intrinsic coagulation pathway as a result of exposure of subendothelial connective tissue. Widespread endothelial injury may be produced by deposition of antigen-antibody complexes (e.g., SLE), temperature extremes (e.g., heat stroke, burns), or microorganisms (e.g., meningococci, rickettsiae).

MORPHOLOGY. Microthrombi, with infarctions and in some cases hemorrhages, are found in many organs and tissues. Clinically significant changes are encountered in

• Kidneys. Thrombi are found in renal glomeruli; may be associated with microinfarcts or bilateral renal cortical necrosis.
• Lungs. Microthrombi are found in alveolar capillaries; sometimes associated with a histologic picture resembling acute respiratory distress syndrome.
• Brain. Microinfarcts and fresh hemorrhages may be seen.

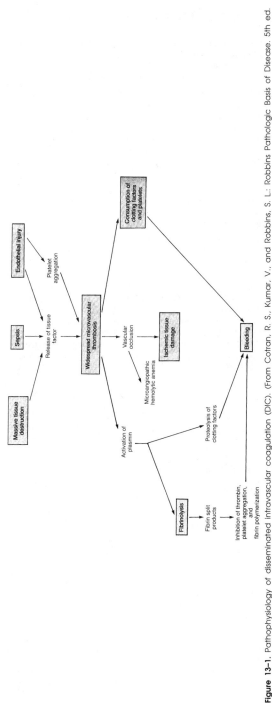

Figure 13–1. Pathophysiology of disseminated intravascular coagulation (DIC). (From Cotran, R. S., Kumar, V., and Robbins, S. L.: Robbins Pathologic Basis of Disease. 5th. ed. Philadelphia, W. B. Saunders Co., 1994, p 625.)

- Adrenals. Massive hemorrhages giving rise to the Waterhouse-Friderichsen syndrome seen in meningococcemia.
- Placenta. Widespread thrombi are noted, associated with atrophy of cytotrophoblast and syncytiotrophoblast.

CLINICAL FEATURES. About 50% of individuals with DIC are obstetric patients having complications of pregnancy; 33% have carcinomatosis. Sepsis and major trauma are responsible for most of the remaining cases. The onset may be fulminating, as in endotoxic shock or amniotic fluid embolism, or insidious, as in cases of carcinomatosis or retention of a dead fetus. There are numerous clinical manifestations. A few common patterns are as follows:

- A microangiopathic hemolytic anemia resulting from widespread microvascular occlusion.
- Respiratory symptoms (e.g., dyspnea, cyanosis, or extreme respiratory difficulty).
- Neurologic signs and symptoms, including convulsions and coma.
- Oliguria and acute renal failure.
- Circulatory failure and shock.

In general, acute DIC, associated, for example, with obstetric complications or major trauma, is dominated by bleeding diatheses, whereas chronic DIC, such as may occur in a patient with cancer, tends to present initially with thrombotic complications.

The prognosis is highly variable and depends, to a considerable extent, on the underlying disorder; each patient must be treated individually. Depending on the clinical picture, potent anticoagulants such as heparin and antithrombin III, or coagulants in the form of fresh-frozen plasma, may be administered.

CHAPTER FOURTEEN

White Cells, Lymph Nodes, and Spleen

Disorders of white cells may be associated with a deficiency of leukocytes (leukopenias) or proliferations that may be reactive or neoplastic.

LEUKOPENIA (p. 630)

May occur because of decreased numbers of any one of the specific types of leukocytes, but most often involves the neutrophils (neutropenia). Lymphopenias are much less common; they are associated with the congenital immunodeficiency diseases, and with specific clinical syndromes (e.g., Hodgkin's disease, nonlymphocytic leukemias, after corticosteroid therapy).

NEUTROPENIA (AGRANULOCYTOSIS) (p. 630)

Predisposes to serious infections. Total white cell count is reduced to 1000 cells per mm^3 of blood and, in certain instances, to levels as low as 200 to 300 cells. When the condition is of this magnitude, it is often referred to as agranulocytosis.

The neutrophil is a short-lived cell with a half-life of only 6 to 7 hours. Therefore, any impairment of granulopoiesis can induce neutropenia within hours. Causes are

- *Inadequate or ineffective granulopoiesis.*

  - Suppression of pluripotent myeloid stem cells, as occurs in aplastic anemia and a variety of leukemias and lymphomas.
  - Suppression of the committed granulocytic precursors, as occurs after exposure to drugs (discussed below).
  - Megaloblastic anemias.
  - Associated with CD8+ large granular lymphocytosis. The lymphocytes may be polyclonal or monoclonal. The mechanism of the neutropenia is not clear, but suppression of granulocytic progenitors is considered most likely.

- *Accelerated removal or destruction of neutrophils,* encountered with

  - Immunologically mediated injury to neutrophils. May be (1) idiopathic, (2) associated with a well-defined immunologic disorder (e.g., Felty's syndrome), or (3) produced by exposure to drugs.
  - Sequestration in the spleen (hypersplenism, *see p. 669*).
  - Increased peripheral utilization may occur in overwhelming infections.

The most significant neutropenias (agranulocytosis) are produced by drugs. These may be

- Dose-related. Marrow suppression occurs in a predictable, dose-related fashion, caused by alkylating agents and antimetabolites used in cancer treatment.
- Idiosyncratic and unpredictable. Caused by aminopyrine, chloramphenicol, sulfonamides, chlorpromazine, thiouracil, and phenylbutazone, among others.

MORPHOLOGY. Anatomic alterations in bone marrow depend on the underlying basis of the neutropenia:

- *Marrow hypercellularity* due to increased numbers of immature granulocytic precursors; seen when the neutropenia is caused by excessive destruction of the mature neutrophils, or in ineffective granulopoiesis such as occurs in megaloblastic anemia.
- *Marrow hypocellularity*, noted when agranulocytosis is caused by agents that affect the committed granulocytic precursors. Erythropoiesis and megakaryopoiesis usually remain at normal levels, but with certain myelotoxic drugs all marrow elements may be affected.

CLINICAL COURSE. The initial symptoms are often malaise, chills, and fever, followed in sequence by marked weakness and fatigability. Infections constitute the major problem; they commonly present as ulcerating necrotizing lesions of the gingiva, floor of the mouth, buccal mucosa, or pharynx or anywhere within the oral cavity (agranulocytic angina). All these sites often show massive growth of microorganisms with relatively poor leukocytic response.

PROGNOSIS. Very unpredictable. Before the advent of antibiotics, the mortality rate ranged between 70 and 90%. Supportive measures, such as antibiotic treatment, and efforts at increasing production, such as administration of GM-CSF, allow better survival.

REACTIVE (INFLAMMATORY) PROLIFERATIONS OF WHITE CELLS AND NODES (p. 631)
LEUKOCYTOSIS

A common reaction in a variety of inflammatory states. The particular white cell series affected varies with the underlying cause:

- *Polymorphonuclear leukocytosis* (neutrophilic granulocytosis, neutrophilia). Accompanies acute inflammation associated with infection or other stimuli such as tissue necrosis.
- *Eosinophilic leukocytosis* (eosinophilia). Characteristic of allergic disorders such as bronchial asthma, hay fever, parasitic infections, and some diseases of the skin (pemphigus, eczema, dermatitis herpetiformis). In hospitalized adult patients the most likely cause is an allergic drug reaction.
- *Monocytosis.* May be seen in (1) chronic infections, including tuberculosis, bacterial endocarditis, brucellosis, rickettsiosis, and malaria; (2) collegen vascular diseases such as systemic lupus erythematosus (SLE) and rheumatoid arthritis; and (3) inflammatory bowel disorders such as ulcerative colitis and Crohn's disease.

- *Lymphocytosis.* May accompany monocytosis in chronic inflammatory states such as brucellosis and tuberculosis. Also seen in acute viral infections such as viral hepatitis, in cytomegalovirus infections, and especially in infectious mononucleosis.

LEUKEMOID REACTIONS. In most instances, reactive leukocytosis is easy to distinguish from neoplastic proliferation of the white cells (i.e., leukemias) by the rarity of immature cells in the blood. However, in some inflammatory states many immature white cells may appear in the blood and a picture of leukemia may be simulated, giving rise to a leukemoid reaction.

ACUTE NONSPECIFIC LYMPHADENITIS

- *Localized.* Commonly caused by direct microbiologic drainage; occurs most frequently in the cervical area in association with infections of the teeth or tonsils.
- *Generalized.* Characteristic of viral infections and bacteremia, particularly in children.

MORPHOLOGY. Macroscopically, the nodes become swollen, gray-red, and engorged. Histologically, there are large germinal centers containing numerous mitotic figures. When the condition is caused by pyogenic organisms, a neutrophilic infiltrate is seen about the follicles and within the lymphoid sinuses; the centers of follicles may undergo necrosis.

CLINICAL FEATURES. Affected nodes are tender and, when abscess formation is extensive, become fluctuant. The overlying skin is frequently red and penetration of the infection to the skin may produce draining sinuses. With control of the infection the lymph nodes may revert to their normal appearance; scarring may follow the more destructive disease.

Chronic Nonspecific Lymphadenitis

May occur in the following patterns:

- *Follicular hyperplasia.* Often associated with chronic infections caused by organisms that represent B-cell antigens. Large germinal centers contain lymphocytes in which varying stages of "blast" transformation are prominent. Some causes of follicular hyperplasia are rheumatoid arthritis, toxoplasmosis, and AIDS. This form of lymphadenitis may be confused morphologically with follicular (nodular) lymphomas. Favoring a diagnosis of follicular hyperplasia are

  - Preservation of the lymph node architecture with normal lymphoid tissue between germinal centers.
  - Marked variation in the shape and size of lymphoid nodules.
  - A mixed population of lymphocytes in different stages of differentiation.
  - Prominent phagocytic activity in germinal centers.

- *Paracortical lymphoid hyperplasia.* Characterized by reactive changes within the T-cell regions of the lymph node. Parafollicular T cells undergo proliferation and transformation to immunoblasts that may efface the germinal follicles. Paracortical lymphoid hyperplasia is encountered particularly in viral infections or following smallpox vaccination, and in immunologic reactions induced by certain drugs (especially phenytoin [Dilantin]).
- *Sinus histiocytosis.* Characterized by distention and promi-

nence of the lymphatic sinusoids due to marked hypertrophy of lining endothelial cells and infiltration with histiocytes. This reaction is often encountered in lymph nodes draining cancers and may represent an immune response to the tumor or its products.

NEOPLASTIC PROLIFERATIONS OF WHITE CELLS (p. 633)

The different categories of these diseases can be briefly defined as follows:

1. *Malignant lymphomas* take the form of cohesive tumorous lesions, composed mainly of neoplastic lymphocytes, that arise in lymphoid tissue.
2. *Leukemias and myeloproliferative disorders* are neoplasms of the hematopoietic stem cells, arising in the bone marrow, that secondarily flood the circulating blood or other organs.
3. *Plasma cell dyscrasias and related disorders*, usually arising in the bones, take the form of localized or disseminated proliferations of antibody-forming cells (plasma cells).
4. *The histiocytoses* are proliferative lesions of histiocytes, including Langerhans cells.

MALIGNANT LYMPHOMAS (p. 634)

Lymphomas are malignant neoplasms derived from cells native to the lymphoid tissues (i.e., lymphocytes and their precursors and derivatives, and, rarely, histiocytes). Like other neoplasms, all lymphomas are of monoclonal origin.

Two broad groups of malignant lymphomas are recognized: Hodgkin's disease (Hodgkin's lymphoma) and the non-Hodgkin's lymphomas.

NON-HODGKIN'S LYMPHOMAS (NHLs) (p. 634)

The usual presentation of NHL is as a localized or generalized nontender lymphadenopathy. However, in about one third of cases it may be primary in other sites where lymphoid tissue is found (e.g., in the oropharyngeal region, gut, bone marrow, and skin). Although variable, all forms of lymphoma have the potential to spread from their origin in a single node to other nodes, and eventually to disseminate to the spleen, liver, and bone marrow. Some, after becoming widespread, spill over into the blood, creating a leukemia-like picture in the peripheral blood.
CLASSIFICATIONS. Multiple classifications of the NHL have been published; each of these has its own merit. However, the Working Formulation for Clinical Usage (WF) is widely accepted and will be described. Before the WF is discussed, some general principles relevant to the NHL will be presented.

- The vast majority of the NHLs (80% to 85%) are of B-cell origin; the remaining are in large part of T-cell origin. Tumors of histiocytes or macrophages are quite uncommon.
- Histologically, the lymphoma cells exhibit two different growth patterns: they are either clustered into identifiable nodules (nodular or *follicular lymphoma*) or spread diffusely throughout the node (*diffuse lymphoma*). In general, the natural his-

tory of nodular architecture is associated with a superior prognosis to that of diffuse pattern.

- Nodular lymphomas are almost exclusively B cells (apparently the follicular architecture of these lymphomas is an attempt to recapitulate the germinal centers from which these lymphomas are derived). Diffuse lymphomas may be of B cells or T cells.

The Working Formulation makes no attempt to segregate lymphomas on the basis of presumed cell of origin. Instead, NHLs are divided into three major prognostic groupings: (1) low, (2) intermediate, and (3) high grades based on survival statistics. The Working Formulation also contains a miscellaneous group that includes the rare histiocytic lymphoma, the HTLV-1–induced T-cell leukemia/lymphoma, and other T-lymphomatous disorders with prominent involvement of skin.

LOW-GRADE LYMPHOMAS (p. 636)

This category includes three tumors: (1) small lymphocytic lymphoma; (2) follicular, predominantly small cleaved cell lymphoma; and (3) follicular mixed (small cleaved and large cell) lymphoma. The two follicular lymphomas will be discussed together, since they form a distinct clinicopathologic group.

Small Lymphocytic Lymphoma (SLL)

Makes up approximately 4% of all NHLs and is the only low-grade lymphoma that does not have a follicular architecture.
MORPHOLOGY. Cells are compact, small, apparently unstimulated lymphocytes with dark-staining round nuclei, scanty cytoplasm, and little variation in size. Mitotic figures are rare and there is little or no cytologic atypia. Involvement of bone marrow is present in almost all cases, and in about 40% of patients the neoplastic cells spill over into blood, evoking a chronic lymphocytic leukemia–like picture. SLL overlaps, both clinically and morphologically, with chronic lymphocytic leukemia (CLL) and in some cases with Waldenström's macroglobulinemia. All three represent neoplasms of well-differentiated B lymphocytes.
CLINICAL FEATURES. Both CLL and SLL occur primarily in older age groups. Patients have generalized lymphadenopathy with mild-to-moderate enlargement of the liver and spleen; the associated symptoms are mild, and prolonged survival is usual.
IMMUNOPHENOTYPE. The tumor cells display surface IgM, IgD, and pan–B-cell antigen CD19, a phenotype similar to that of unstimulated B cells. However, they also express CD5, a molecule found on all T cells and a very small subset of B cells.

Follicular Lymphoma

There are two cytologic subgroups of low-grade follicular lymphomas: (1) follicular small cleaved cell and (2) follicular mixed cell type.
MORPHOLOGY

- *Follicular small cleaved cell lymphoma* is the most common form of follicular NHL. The neoplastic B cells resemble small cleaved cells seen within normal germinal centers. They are slightly larger than normal lymphocytes, with an irregular "cleaved" nuclear contour, characterized by prominent indentations and linear infoldings. Nuclear chromatin is coarse and condensed, and nucleoli are indistinct. Mitoses are infrequent.

Scattered large cleaved or noncleaved cells may be present, but do not account for more than 20% of the cells.

• *Follicular mixed small cleaved and large cell.* This term is used when the frequency of large cells exceeds 20% but is less than 50%. Follicular mixed lymphomas constitute a small proportion of all follicular tumors, and whether they form a distinct group is debatable.

CLINICAL FEATURES. Follicular lymphomas occur predominantly in older individuals and constitute approximately 40% of adult NHLs in the United States. They present with generalized painless lymphadenopathy; involvement of extranodal (e.g., visceral) sites is uncommon. The bone marrow is frequently involved (75% of cases), but peripheral blood involvement in the form of frank leukemia is uncommon.

CHROMOSOMAL CHANGES. In most patients, tumor cells reveal a translocation t(14;18); the break point on chromosome 18 involves 18q21, where a putative proto-oncogene *bcl-2* has been mapped.

PROGNOSIS. Follicular lymphomas are indolent tumors, with a median survival of 7 to 9 years that is largely unaffected by treatment. In some patients the tumors slowly progress to a diffuse high-grade histologic type representing the emergence of an aggressive subclone of neoplastic B cells. Median survival is less than 1 year after such transformation.

IMMUNOPHENOTYPE. Tumor cells express surface Ig and the B-cell antigen CD19, CD10, and CD21.

INTERMEDIATE-GRADE LYMPHOMAS (p. 638)

There are four tumors under this category of the Working Formulation, one with a follicular architecture and the other three with a diffuse pattern.

Follicular, Predominantly Large Cell Lymphoma

An uncommon tumor that represents less than 15% of all follicular NHLs. In contrast to the low-grade follicular lymphomas, most of the neoplastic cells are large, with cleaved or noncleaved nuclei. Mitotic figures are also more numerous. These tumors evolve into diffuse lymphomas early in their course and carry a poorer prognosis than the other follicular lymphomas.

Diffuse, Small Cleaved Cell Lymphoma (DSCCL)

Composed of small cleaved cells similar to those in follicular small cleaved cell lymphomas. In contrast to follicular lymphomas of similar histologic type, these tumors have a higher male-to-female ratio and more aggressive natural history (median survival of 2 to 4 years).

A phenotypically and genetically distinct subgroup of diffuse small cleaved cells, variously called "centrocytic lymphoma" and "intermediately differentiated lymphocytic lymphoma," has been identified. These tumors can be differentiated from follicular center cells (the presumed origin of most DSCCL) because, although they do express pan–B-cell antigens, these tumors do not express CD10 and do express CD5. Also, these lymphomas demonstrate a cytogenetic abnormality, t(11;14), not seen in the rest of the DSCCL.

Diffuse, Mixed Small and Large Cell Lymphoma (DM)

Contains a mixture of small cleaved cells and large cells that may be cleaved or noncleaved. The nuclei of large cleaved cells are irregular in contour, indented, and larger compared with nuclei of normal histiocytes. The nuclear chromatin is dispersed and nucleoli are inconspicuous. Cytoplasm is scant and pale. Large noncleaved cells are up to four times the size of normal lymphocytes, with a round or oval nucleus and one to two prominent nucleoli. The nuclear chromatin is vesicular and mitoses may be prominent. The amount of cytoplasm is greater than in large cleaved cells.

Diffuse, Large Cell Lymphoma (DLC)

Contains predominantly large cells of the cleaved and noncleaved types described for DM. Diffuse large cell lymphomas and the diffuse mixed variant appear to represent different morphologic expression within the spectrum of large cell lymphomas. *Although classified as intermediate-grade lymphomas, DM and DLC have clinical features akin to those of the high-grade large cell immunoblastic lymphoma described below.*

HIGH-GRADE LYMPHOMAS   (p. 640)

There are three tumors in this category: large cell immunoblastic lymphoma, lymphoblastic lymphoma, and small noncleaved cell lymphoma.

Large Cell Immunoblastic Lymphoma

Tumor cells in this neoplasm are four to five times larger than a small lymphocyte and have a round or multilobated large vesicular nucleus with one or two centrally placed prominent nucleoli. The cytoplasm is either deeply staining and pyroninophilic or clear. Some tumors have an admixture of large transformed cells and small atypical lymphocytes with contorted nuclei.

CLINICAL FEATURES. Large cell immunoblastic, diffuse large cell, and diffuse mixed lymphomas are similar in their clinical behavior, constituting 40% to 50% of adult NHLs. Collectively, these three types of lymphomas are sometimes referred to as diffuse large cell lymphoma.

They typically present with a rapidly enlarging, often asymptomatic mass at a single nodal or extranodal site. Involvement of GI tract, skin, bone, or brain may be the presenting feature. The Waldeyer's ring is involved in about 50% of these cases. Involvement of liver and spleen is not common at the time of diagnosis. Bone marrow involvement is relatively uncommon, especially at the time of diagnosis. With progressive disease, however, the marrow may be involved, and rarely a leukemic picture may emerge.

PROGNOSIS. These three diffuse lymphomas (large cell immunoblastic, diffuse large cell, and diffuse mixed) are aggressive tumors that are rapidly fatal if untreated. However, with intensive combination chemotherapy, complete remission can be achieved in 60 to 80% of patients, and up to 50% may be cured.

IMMUNOPHENOTYPE. May arise from T or B cells, but most are of B-cell origin. A reliable identification of immunophenotype (B or T) cannot be made without molecular or phenotypic studies. Most studies have failed to show any significant correlation among cytologic subtype, immunologic phenotype, and response to therapy.

Lymphoblastic Lymphoma (LL)

This clinicopathologic entity is closely related to T-cell acute lymphoblastic leukemia (T-ALL).

MORPHOLOGY. Tumor cells are fairly uniform in size, with scanty cytoplasm and nuclei somewhat larger than those of small lymphocytes. The nuclear chromatin is delicate and finely stippled, and nucleoli are either absent or inconspicuous. The nuclear membrane shows convolutions in most cases. A high mitotic rate with a "starry sky" pattern produced by the interspersed benign macrophages is typically seen.

CLINICAL FEATURES. Predominantly affects males (2:1); many patients are under 20 years of age. It constitutes less than 5% of *all* NHLs but 40% of childhood lymphomas. The presence of a prominent mediastinal mass in 50 to 70% of patients at the time of diagnosis indicates a thymic origin. Rapidly progressive early dissemination to the bone marrow and thence to blood and meninges leads to the evolution of a picture resembling T-ALL.

PROGNOSIS. Generally poor. Recent attempts to treat this tumor aggressively by utilizing protocols effective in ALL have produced encouraging results.

IMMUNOPHENOTYPE. Tumor cells resemble intrathymic T cells. Terminal deoxynucleotidyl transferase (TdT), an enzyme associated with primitive lymphoid cells, is expressed in all cases. In some patients the cells are CD2+, CD5+, and CD7+, as are early thymocytes, whereas in others CD4 and CD8 are coexpressed on tumor cells. In many cases, surface CD3 expression is lacking, but cytoplasmic CD3 is present.

Small Noncleaved Lymphoma

Within this category fall Burkitt's lymphoma, endemic in Africa, and related tumors seen outside Africa. Histologically, African and nonendemic cases are identical, although there are clinical and virologic differences. The relationship of these disorders to the Epstein-Barr virus (EBV) is discussed on *page 658*).

MORPHOLOGY. Tumor cells are monotonous, intermediate in size between small lymphocytes and large noncleaved cells, and have round or oval nuclei containing two to five nucleoli. The nuclear size approximates that of benign macrophages within the tumor. There is a moderate amount of faintly basophilic or amphophilic cytoplasm, which is intensely pyroninophilic and often contains small, lipid-filled vacuoles. These tumors have a high mitotic index associated with a "starry sky" pattern.

IMMUNOPHENOTYPE. These B-cell tumors resemble activated germinal center B cells and express surface IgM, pan–B-cell markers, and CD10.

CLINICAL FEATURES. The condition mainly affects children or young adults, accounting for approximately 30% of childhood NHLs in the United States. In African patients, involvement of the maxilla or mandible is the common mode of presentation, whereas abdominal tumors (bowel, retroperitoneum, ovaries) are more common in America.

PROGNOSIS. A 50% long-term survival rate can be expected with present methods of treatment.

MISCELLANEOUS (p. 642)

This group includes several tumors, but only two, both of T-cell origin, will be described here.

Mycosis Fungoides and Sézary's Syndrome

These T-cell tumors are characterized by involvement of the skin (cutaneous T-cell lymphomas).

MORPHOLOGY. Mycosis fungoides presents with an inflammatory premycotic phase and progresses through a plaque phase to a tumor phase. Histologically, there is infiltration of the epidermis and upper dermis by neoplastic T cells, which often have a cerebriform nucleus characterized by marked infolding of the nuclear membrane. With progressive disease, nodal and visceral dissemination appear. Sézary's syndrome is a related condition in which skin involvement is manifested clinically as a generalized exfoliative erythroderma, and in which there is an associated leukemia of "Sézary" cells that also have a cerebriform nucleus. Circulating Sézary cells can also be identified in up to 25% of cases of mycosis fungoides in the plaque or tumor phase.

IMMUNOPHENOTYPE. Both these disorders result from clonal proliferations of post-thymic CD4+ T lymphocytes.

PROGNOSIS. Median survival is 8 to 9 years.

Adult T-Cell Leukemia/Lymphoma

This T-cell neoplasm caused by infection with the HTLV-1 retrovirus is endemic in southern Japan and the Caribbean basin, but similar cases have been found sporadically elsewhere, including the southeastern United States.

Adult T-cell leukemia is characterized by skin lesions, generalized lymphadenopathy, hepatosplenomegaly, hypercalcemia, and an elevated leukocyte count with multilobed lymphocytes. The tumor cells are CD4+. This is an extremely aggressive disease with a median survival of about 8 months.

Diagnosis and Staging of NHL

The diagnosis of NHL can be suspected from the clinical features, but histologic examination of the node is required for confirmation. Definite assignment of lymphomas to T- or B-cell lineage is accomplished by immunophenotyping and by analysis of T- and B-receptor gene rearrangements.

A form of clinical staging developed for Hodgkin's disease is often used for NHL, but is much less useful in NHL since the correlation between the anatomic extent of the disease and the prognosis is less well established.

A summary of the salient clinicopathologic features of NHLs is presented in Table 14–1.

HODGKIN'S DISEASE (p. 643)

This neoplasm of the lymphoid tissues is one of the most common forms of malignancy in young adults, with an average age at diagnosis of 32 years.

Differences from NHL:

- Characterized morphologically by the presence of Reed-Sternberg (RS) cells (described below), admixed with a variable inflammatory infiltrate.

Table 14–1. Summary of Non-Hodgkin's Lymphomas

Lymphoma Type or Group	% (in Adults)	Salient Morphology	Immunophenotype	Comments
Small lymphocytic lymphoma (SLL)	3–4	Small unstimulated lymphocytes in a diffuse pattern	>95% B cells	Occurs in old age; generalized lymphadenopathy with marrow involvement and a blood picture resembling CLL; indolent course with prolonged survival
Follicular lymphomas	40	Germinal center cells arranged in a follicular pattern	B cells	Follicular small cleaved cell type most common; occur in older patients; generalized lymphadenopathy; associated with t(14;18); leukemia less common than in SLL; indolent course but difficult to cure
Diffuse large cell lymphomas°	40–50	Various cell types; predominantly large germinal center cells; some mixed with smaller cells; others with immunoblastic morphology	~80% B cells ~20% post-thymic T cells	Occur in older patients as well as pediatric age group; greater frequency of extranodal, visceral disease; marrow involvement and leukemia very uncommon at diagnosis and poor prognostic sign; aggressive tumors, but up to 60% are curable

Type		Morphology	Cell Type	Clinical Features
Lymphoblastic lymphoma	4	Cells somewhat larger than lymphocytes; in many cases, nuclei markedly lobulated; high mitotic rate; blastic chromatin pattern	>95% immature intrathymic T cells	Occurs predominantly in children (40% of all childhood lymphomas); prominent mediastinal mass; early involvement of bone marrow and progression to T-cell ALL; very aggressive
Small noncleaved (Burkitt's) lymphoma	<1	Cells intermediate in size between small lymphocytes and immunoblasts; prominent multiple nucleoli; high mitotic rate	B cells	Endemic in Africa, sporadic elsewhere; predominantly affects children; extranodal visceral involvements presenting features; rapidly progressive but responsive to therapy; t(8;14)
Mycosis fungoides and Sézary's syndrome	Uncommon	Medium to large cells with markedly convoluted (cerebriform) nucleus	CD4+ T cells	Occur in older males; proclivity for involvement of skin in both forms; tumorous masses in mycosis fungoides; Sézary's syndrome is leukemic variant
Adult T-cell leukemia/lymphoma	Rare	Very variable; cells may have cerebriform nuclei	CD4+ T cells	Associated with HTLV-1 infection; endemic in Japan and Caribbean; cutaneous lesions, leukemia, spleen and lymph node involvement; rapidly fatal

*Includes diffuse large cell, diffuse mixed, and large cell immunoblastic lymphomas of the Working Formulation. Other NHLs with diffuse pattern, e.g., lymphoblastic lymphomas, that form distinct clinicopathologic categories, are not included.

From Cotran, R. S., Kumar, V., and Robbins, S. L.: Robbins Pathologic Basis of Disease. 5th ed. Philadelphia, W. B. Saunders Co., 1994, p. 644.

- Often associated with somewhat distinctive clinical features (Table 14–2).
- The target cell of neoplastic transformation has yet to be identified with certainty.

There are four subtypes according to the *Rye classification*:

- Lymphocyte predominance (LP).
- Mixed cellularity (MC).
- Lymphocyte depletion (LD).
- Nodular sclerosis (NS).

REED-STERNBERG CELL. The common denominator among all subtypes is a large cell (15 to 45 mm in diameter), most often binucleate or bilobed or multinucleated, with abundant amphophilic cytoplasm. Prominent within the nuclei are large, inclusion-like, "owl-eyed" nucleoli generally surrounded by a clear halo.

Variants of RS cells include uninucleated cells with prominent nucleoli, and lacunar cells (associated with nodular sclerosis). The *lacunar cell* is large with single hyperlobated nucleus containing multiple small nucleoli and an abundant, pale-staining cytoplasm. In formalin-fixed tissue, the cytoplasm of these cells often retracts, giving rise to the appearance of cells lying in clear spaces or "lacunae." The RS cell and its variants are considered to be the neoplastic component in Hodgkin's disease. Their identification is necessary but not sufficient for the diagnosis of Hodgkin's disease, because cells resembling or identical to RS cells may be present in other conditions (e.g., infectious mononucleosis, NHLs, and solid tissue cancers).

MORPHOLOGY. The morphologic feature that serves to differentiate *three subgroups* (LP, MC, and LD) is the frequency of RS cells relative to the reactive elements, represented by small lymphocytes. The *fourth subgroup* (NS) appears to represent a special expression of the disease in which the collagen bands divide the lymphoid tissue into circumscribed nodules.

Lymphocyte Predominance

Characterized by a diffuse or vaguely nodular infiltrate of mature lymphocytes admixed with variable numbers of benign histiocytes. Scattered among these cells are rare RS cells. More com-

Table 14–2. Clinical Differences Between Hodgkin's and Non-Hodgkin's Lymphomas

Hodgkin's Disease	Non-Hodgkin's Lymphoma
More often localized to a single axial group of nodes (cervical, mediastinal, para-aortic)	More frequent involvement of multiple peripheral nodes
Orderly spread by contiguity	Noncontiguous spread
Mesenteric nodes and Waldeyer's ring rarely involved	Waldeyer's ring and mesenteric nodes commonly involved
Extranodal involvement uncommon	Extranodal involvement common

From Cotran, R. S., Kumar, V., and Robbins, S. L.: Robbins Pathologic Basis of Disease. 5th ed. Philadelphia, W. B. Saunders Co., 1994, p. 648.

mon are variant cells, with puffy, multilobed nuclei (popcorn cells). Many of these tumors are of B-cell origin, and hence may be considered variants of NHL.

Mixed Cellularity

A common form of Hodgkin's disease. Typical RS cells are plentiful, but there are fewer lymphocytes than in LP disease. Usually there is a heterogeneous cellular infiltrate, which includes eosinophils, plasma cells, and benign histiocytes. The prognosis is intermediate between the LP and LD variants.

Lymphocyte Depletion

This uncommon pattern is characterized by a paucity of lymphocytes and a *relative* abundance of RS cells or their pleomorphic variants. It presents in two morphologic forms: *diffuse fibrosis* and the *reticular variant*. In the former the node is hypocellular and is replaced by a disorderly, nonbirefringent connective tissue. Pleomorphic histiocytes, a few typical and atypical RS cells, and some lymphocytes are scattered within the fibrillar material. The reticular variant is cellular and contains highly anaplastic, atypical RS cells. Only a few typical RS cells can be recognized. Patients with the LD variant are usually older and have a very poor prognosis.

Nodular Sclerosis

In this variant, fine or dense collagenous bands subdivide the lymphoid tissue into circumscribed nodules. There are varying proportions of lacunar cells and lymphocytes; classic RS cells are rare. Most patients are adolescent or young females with an excellent prognosis.

CLINICAL FEATURES. Hodgkin's disease is more common in males. It usually presents with a painless enlargement of one group of lymph nodes, and spreads to anatomically contiguous nodes. Table 14-2 summarizes some of the clinical differences between HD and NHL.

The anatomic *stage* of Hodgkin's disease (Table 14-3) is of clinical importance. Generally, younger patients with the more favorable histologic types tend to present in clinical stage I or II without systemic manifestations. Patients with disseminated disease (stages III and IV) generally have the histologically less favorable variants (MC and LD) and are more likely to present with systemic complaints such as fever, weight loss, and anemia.

PROGNOSIS. With current forms of therapy, the 5-year survival rate of patients with stages I and IIA is close to 90%, and many can be cured. Even with advanced disease (stages IVA and IVB), 60% to 70% 5-year disease-free survival can be achieved. Although histologic type is a prognostic factor in Hodgkin's disease, tumor burden (i.e., *stage*) is the most important variable.

Long-term survivors of chemotherapy and radiotherapy have an increased risk of developing second cancers such as acute nonlymphocytic leukemia, lung cancer, non-Hodgkin's lymphoma, cancer of the stomach, and malignant melanoma.

ETIOLOGY AND PATHOGENESIS. The origin of the RS cells, the neoplastic component, is unclear. The general consensus seems to be that RS cells arise from activated lymphocytes (B or T) and not mononuclear phagocytes. Other inflammatory cells accumulate in response to cytokines secreted by RS cells. An infective cause of Hodgkin's disease has been suspected, and

Table 14-3. Clinical Stages of Hodgkin's and Non-Hodgkin's Lymphomas (Ann Arbor Classification)*

Stage	Distribution of Disease
I	Involvement of a single lymph node region (I) or involvement of a single extralymphatic organ or site (I_E).
II	Involvement of two or more lymph node regions on same side of diaphragm alone (II) or with involvement of limited contiguous extralymphatic organ or issue (II_E).
III	Involvement of lymph node regions on both sides of diaphragm (III), which may include spleen (III_S) and/or limited contiguous extralymphatic organ or site (III_E, III_{ES}).
IV	Multiple or disseminated foci of involvement of one or more extralymphatic organs or tissues with or without lymphatic involvement.

*All stages are further divided on the basis of the absence (A) or presence (B) of the following systemic symptoms: significant fever, night sweats, and/or unexplained weight loss of greater than 10% of normal body weight.

From Carbone, P. T., et al.: Symposium (Ann Arbor): Staging in Hodgkin's disease. Cancer Res. *31*:1707, 1971.

some studies incriminate EBV as the culprit. Clonally integrated EBV genome is found in 40% to 50% of cases, suggesting that EBV or other unknown viruses may be cofactors.

LEUKEMIAS AND MYELOPROLIFERATIVE DISEASES (p. 648)

Leukemias are malignant neoplasms of the hematopoietic stem cells, arising in the bone marrow, that flood the circulating blood or other organs. They are classified on the basis of the cell type involved (myeloid versus lymphoid) and the state of maturity of leukemia cells. *Acute leukemias* are characterized by the presence of very immature cells (called blasts) and by a rapidly fatal course in untreated patients; *chronic leukemias* are associated, at least initially, with well-differentiated (mature) leukocytes and a relatively indolent course.

ACUTE LEUKEMIAS (p. 649)

Two types are distinguished: acute myeloblastic leukemia (AML) and acute lymphoblastic leukemia (ALL).
PATHOPHYSIOLOGY. The accumulation of blasts in acute leukemia results from clonal expression of transformed stem cells and associated failure of maturation into functional end cells.

Leukemic blasts in the marrow suppress normal hematopoietic stem cells by mechanisms that are incompletely understood. This suppression has two important clinical implications.

- There is a paucity of normal red cells, white cells, and platelets; the resultant pancytopenia is responsible for the clinical manifestations.

- The aim of therapy is to reduce the population of the leukemic clone so as to allow recovery of normal stem cells.

CLINICAL FEATURES

- Abrupt, stormy onset; most patients present within 3 months of the onset of symptoms.
- Symptoms related to depression of normal marrow function: fatigue due mainly to anemia; fever, reflecting an infection due to absence of mature leukocytes; bleeding (petechiae, ecchymoses, epistaxis, and gingival bleeding) secondary to thrombocytopenia.
- Generalized lymphadenopathy, splenomegaly, and hepatomegaly, resulting from infiltration by leukemic cells; seen more commonly in ALL.
- Marrow involvement with subperiosteal bone infiltration, resulting in bone pain and tenderness.
- Leukemic infiltration of the meninges; may give rise to headache, vomiting, papilledema, cranial nerve palsies, and other CNS manifestations. Intracerebral or subarachnoid hemorrhages may also occur.

LABORATORY FINDINGS. Anemia is almost always present. The white blood cell count in about 50% of the patients is less than 10,000 cells per mm^3 of blood, whereas in about 20% it is elevated to about 100,000 cells per mm^3. The immature white cells, including "blast" forms, are found in the circulating blood and the bone marrow, where they make up 60 to 100% of all the cells. The platelet count is usually depressed to less than 100,000 per mm^3.

Acute Lymphoblastic Leukemia (ALL)

Primarily a disease of children and young adults; constitutes 80% of childhood acute leukemias with a peak incidence at approximately 4 years of age.

MORPHOLOGY. The nuclei of leukemic blasts in Wright-Giemsa stained preparations have somewhat coarse and clumped chromatin and one or two nucleoli. In contrast to the blasts of AML, the cytoplasm of ALL blasts does not contain azurophilic granules but contains large aggregates of PAS-positive material. Three morphologic subtypes, L_1, L_2, and L_3, are recognized by the FAB classification.

IMMUNOLOGIC SUBTYPES. Based on the origin of the leukemic lymphoblasts and stage of differentiation as defined by cell surface markers and antigen receptor gene rearrangements. Because immunophenotyping has prognostic implications, it is detailed in Table 14–4 and summarized below:

- About 80% of cases of ALL are of B-cell origin. The leukemic blasts of almost all these patients express CD19 (a B-cell–restricted antigen). Their nuclei contain the enzyme TdT. Most patients with B-cell–derived ALL are in either the early B or pre-B stage of B-cell maturation. Cases of ALL with the mature B-cell phenotype (expressing surface Ig but negative for the nuclear enzyme TdT) are rare (less than 2%).
- T lymphoblasts in patients with T-cell ALL are arrested at early intrathymic stages of maturation, also associated with nuclear TdT activity. T-cell ALL is related to lymphoblastic lymphoma, but distinct from other T-cell neoplasms such as adult T-cell leukemia/lymphoma and Sezary's syndrome, in

Table 14-4. Major Immunologic Subtypes of Acute Lymphoblastic Leukemia and Associated Prognosis

Subtype	Phenotype	Morphology	Approximate Frequency (%)	Prognosis[*]
Early pre-B				
CALLA (CD10) negative	DR+, sIg−, Cμ−, CD19+, CD10−	L1 or L2	5–10	Very good
CALLA positive	DR+, sIg−, Cμ−, CD19+, CD10+		55–60	
Pre-B	DR+, sIg−, Cμ+, CD19+, CD10+	L1 or L2	20	Intermediate
Mature B	DR+, sIg+, Cμ−, CD19+, CD10±	L3	1–2	Poor
Immature T	DR−, sIg−, CD19−, CD10−, T+	L1 or L2	15	Intermediate

[*]In all cases, the prognosis is worsened if there is an associated chromosomal translocation.

DR = HLA-DR (class II) antigens; sIg = surface immunoglobulin; Cμ = cytoplasmic μ chains; T = T-cell-associated antigens, e.g., CD2, CD5, CD7. CALLA = common acute lymphoblastic leukemia antigen, synonymous with CD10.

From Cotran, S. L., Kumar, V., and Robbins, S. L.: Robbins Pathologic Basis of Disease. 5th ed. Philadelphia, W. B. Saunders Co., 1994, p. 651.

which the neoplastic cells express the mature peripheral T-cell phenotype.

Prognostic differences exist among immunologic subtypes of ALL. The most favorable outcome is for patients with early, pre-B, B-cell ALL, the largest of all groups. The prognosis is intermediate for T-cell and pre–B-cell ALL, and is the poorest for surface Ig-positive B-cell ALL (leukemic phase of Burkitt's lymphoma).

CHROMOSOMAL CHANGES. Approximately 60% of patients with ALL have karyotypic abnormalities in their leukemia cells such as

- Hyperdiploidy (51 to 60 chromosomes), fairly common in early precursor B-cell ALL, and associated with good prognosis.
- A Philadelphia chromosome (Ph[1]) found in about 15% of adult cases and about 5% of childhood cases, associated with poor prognosis.
- About 20 to 25% of pre–B-cell ALLs with a t(1;19) translocation, associated with a poor prognosis.
- ALL with the mature B-cell phenotype, almost invariably associated with the t(8;14) translocation and a very poor prognosis.

PROGNOSIS. With chemotherapy, over 90% of children with ALL achieve complete remission and more than 60% are alive 5 years later. Most are likely to have been cured. Adults or children with T-cell ALL or sIg+ B-cell ALL fare less well. It may be noted that the presence of a chromosomal translocation is associated with dismal prognosis in ALL, while the prognostic correlation in AML varies.

Acute Myeloblastic Leukemia (AML)

An extremely heterogeneous group; primarily affects individuals between the ages of 15 and 39 years.

MORPHOLOGY. Wright-Giemsa stained myeloblasts reveal delicate nuclear chromatin, three to five nucleoli, and fine azurophilic granules in the cytoplasm. Distinctive red-staining intracytoplasmic rodlike structures (Auer rods) present in some cases. Blasts are generally positive for myeloperoxidase. Monocytic differentiation is associated with staining for the lysosomal nonspecific esterases. TdT is very useful in distinguishing ALL from AML, since it is present in 95% of cases of ALL and in less than 5% of AMLs.

PATHOGENESIS AND CLASSIFICATION. AMLs are of diverse origin. Some arise by transformation of multipotent (trilineage) myeloid stem cells even though myeloblasts dominate the blood and bone marrow. In others the common granulocyte-monocyte precursor is involved, giving rise to myelomonocytic disease. In the revised FAB classification (Table 14–5), AML is divided into eight categories.

CHROMOSOMAL ABNORMALITIES. High-resolution banding techniques reveal chromosomal abnormalities in approximately 90% of patients. In 50% to 70% of cases, the karyotypic changes can be detected by standard cytogenetic techniques. Many specific chromosomal abnormalities have prognostic implications. The t(15;17) translocation associated with M3 subtype is of particular interest. In these cases, the retinoic acid α-receptor (RAR-α) gene on chromosome 17 fuses with a transcription unit called PML (for promyelocytic leukemia) on chromosome 15. The fused gene encodes an abnormal retinoic acid receptor that in some manner blocks cell differentiation. However, high doses

Table 14-5. Revised FAB Classification of Acute Myeloblastic (Myelocytic) Leukemias

Class	Incidence (% of AML)	Marrow Morphology/Comments
M0 Minimally differentiated AML	2–3	Blasts lack definitive cytologic and cytochemical markers of myeloblasts (e.g., myeloperoxidase negative) but express myeloid lineage antigens and resemble myeloblasts ultrastructurally.
M1 AML without differentiation	~20	Very immature but ≥ 3% are peroxidase positive; few granules or Auer rods and little maturation beyond the myeloblast stage.
M2 AML with maturation	30–40	Full range of myeloid maturation through granulocytes; Auer rods present in most cases; presence of t(8;21) defines a prognostically favorable subgroup.
M3 Acute promyelocytic leukemia	5–10	Majority of cells are hypergranular promyelocytes often with many Auer rods per cell; patients are younger (median age 35–40 yrs) and often develop DIC; the t(15;17) translocation is characteristic.
M4 Acute myelomonocytic leukemia	15–20	Myelocytic and monocytic differentiation evident; myeloid elements resemble M2; monocytic cells positive for nonspecific esterases; the presence of chromosome 16 abnormalities defines a subset with eosinophils in the marrow and excellent prognosis.
M5 Acute monocytic leukemia	~10	Monoblasts (peroxidase-negative, nonspecific esterase-positive) and promonocytes predominate; tends to occur in older patients and characterized by very high incidence of organomegaly, lymphadenopathy, and tissue infiltration; gingival hypertrophy and skin infiltration common.
M6 Acute erythroleukemia	~5	Abnormal erythroblasts (some megaloblastoid, others with giant or multiple nuclei) predominate; some myeloblasts also present; affected persons are of advanced age.
M7 Acute megakaryocytic leukemia	~1	Blasts of megakaryocytic lineage predominate; react with platelet-specific antibodies directed against GPIIb/IIIa or vWF; myelofibrosis or increased marrow reticulin in most cases.

DIC = disseminated intravascular coagulation; vWF = von Willebrand's factor.
From Cotran, S. L., Kumar, V., and Robbins, S. L.: Robbins Pathologic Basis of Disease. 5th ed. Philadelphia, W. B. Saunders Co., 1994, p. 653.

of the vitamin A derivative all-transretinoic acid are able to overcome this block in differentiation.

PROGNOSIS. Approximately 60% of patients achieve remission with intensive chemotherapy, but only 15% to 30% remain free from disease for 5 years. Bone marrow transplantation is beneficial in some patients. Overall, prognosis is worse than that of ALL.

Myelodysplastic Syndromes (p. 654)

In this group, bone marrow is partly or wholly replaced by a clone of stem cells that retain the capacity to differentiate into mature red cells, granulocytes, and platelets, but in a manner that is both ineffective and disordered (dysplastic). The abnormal stem cell clone in the bone marrow has a tendency to lose the ability for differentiation and to transform into acute leukemia.

MORPHOLOGY. Because of the ineffective and disordered maturation, the bone marrow is hypercellular or normocellular but the peripheral blood shows pancytopenia. Abnormalities in blood and marrow include megaloblastoid erythroid precursors, hypogranular myeloid precursors, an increased proportion of blast cells in the marrow, micromegakaryocytes, agranular platelets, and unilobed and bilobed neutrophils.

CHROMOSOMAL ABNORMALITIES. Noted in up to two-thirds of patients; includes deletions or loss of chromosomes 5, 7, 20, or Y; and trisomy 8.

CLINICAL FEATURES. Most patients are males between 60 and 70 years of age who present with weakness, infections, and hemorrhages, owing to pancytopenia. Some are asymptomatic and are discovered after incidental blood tests. One third of the patients progress to frank AML. Median survival varies from 9 to 29 months.

CHRONIC MYELOID LEUKEMIA (CML) (p. 654)

This leukemia, primarily affecting adults between 25 and 60 years of age, accounts for 15 to 20% of all cases of leukemia. The peak incidence is in the fourth and fifth decades of life.

MORPHOLOGY. A markedly elevated leukocyte count, usually exceeding 100,000 cells per mm^3, is common. The circulating cells are predominantly neutrophils and metamyelocytes, but basophils and eosinophils may also be prominent. A small number of myeloblasts (<10%) can usually be detected in the peripheral blood. Approximately 50% of patients have thrombocytosis early in the course of the disease.

Differentiation of CML from a leukemoid reaction may be difficult. Helpful are

- The almost total lack of alkaline phosphatase in the granulocytes of CML.
- The presence in CML of the Ph^1 chromosome or its molecular counterpart, the *bcr*-c-*abl* rearrangement.

PATHOPHYSIOLOGY. CML is a clonal disorder of pluripotent stem cells that differentiate predominantly along the granulocytic pathway. In approximately 90% of patients the Ph^1 chromosome, representing a t(9;22) translocation, is found in all dividing progeny of multipotent myeloid stem cells (i.e., granulocytic, erythroid, and megakaryocytic precursors). In others, *bcr*-c-*abl* rearrangements can be detected. Unlike acute leukemias, differentiation of the leukemic stem cells is not blocked and the peripheral blood contains mature cells.

CLINICAL FEATURES. Initial symptoms are nonspecific and include easy fatigability, weakness, weight loss, and anorexia. A dragging sensation in the abdomen caused by extreme splenomegaly is characteristic. After about 3 years, approximately 50% of patients enter an "accelerated phase" characterized by increasing anemia, thrombocytopenia, and transformation into acute leukemia (blast crisis). In the remaining 50%, blast crises occur abruptly without an intermediate accelerated phase. In 70% of patients the blasts have features of myeloblasts. In the remaining 30% the blasts resemble early (TdT +) B cells.

PROGNOSIS. Remissions are induced with chemotherapy, but the median survival of 3 to 4 years is unaltered. Bone marrow transplantation can be curative. After the development of blast crisis, all forms of treatment become virtually ineffective.

CHRONIC LYMPHOCYTIC LEUKEMIA (CLL) (p. 655)

The most indolent of all leukemias. It accounts for 25% of all cases of leukemia in the United States and Europe, occurring typically in persons over 50 years of age (median age 60 years); males are affected as commonly as females. It is uncommon in Japan and other Asian countries.

PATHOPHYSIOLOGY. In 95% of cases CLL is a neoplasm of mature sIg-positive B cells (T-cell CLL is rare in the U.S. but fairly common in Japan and other Asian countries). Neoplastic B cells are long-lived and unable to differentiate into plasma cells; thus, patients often have hypogammaglobulinemia and increased susceptibility to bacterial infections. In 10% to 15% of patients, neoplastic B cells develop autoantibodies directed against red blood cells or platelets, resulting in hemolytic anemia or thrombocytopenia.

IMMUNOPHENOTYPE. The cells are mature B cells (sIg +, CD19 +, and CD20 +); however, these cells also express CD5, a T-cell–associated antigen expressed on a very small subset of normal B cells (*see small lymphocytic lymphoma, p. 636*).

CHROMOSOMAL ABNORMALITIES. Seen in about 50% of patients, most commonly trisomy 12; complex abnormalities involving chromosomes 14 and 11 are also found. Patients with cytogenetic changes require early treatment and have a significantly shorter survival.

MOLECULAR PATHOGENESIS. Very little is known about this in CLL; however, in about 10% to 15% of cases there is rearrangement of *bcl*-2, and, in less than 5% of cases, the *bcl*-1 gene is mutated. Because *bcl*-2 overexpression prevents apoptosis, failure of programmed cell death may account for the accumulation of B cells, at least in some cases.

CLINICAL FEATURES. Often asymptomatic, or nonspecific symptoms: easy fatigability, loss of weight, and anorexia. Generalized lymphadenopathy and hepatosplenomegaly are present in 50 to 60% of patients. The leukocyte count may be slightly or markedly (200,000 per mm^3) increased. In all cases there is absolute lymphocytosis of small, mature-looking lymphocytes.

PROGNOSIS. Extremely variable; depends primarily on the clinical stage, as determined by the number of lymphoid areas that are enlarged and the presence or absence of thrombocytopenia or anemia. Overall, median survival is 4 to 6 years. Unlike CML, transformation to acute leukemia with blast crisis is rare.

HAIRY CELL LEUKEMIA (p. 656)

- A rare form of chronic B-cell leukemia in which tumor cells have fine, hairlike projections.
- Occurs mainly in older males; symptoms result largely from infiltration of bone marrow, liver, and spleen. Splenomegaly, often massive, is the most common physical finding; lymphadenopathy is rare.
- Leukocytosis is present in only 25% of patients, but hairy cells are noted in the peripheral blood smear in most cases. Pancytopenia, resulting from marrow failure and splenic sequestration, is seen in over 50% of patients.
- Leukemic cells contain tartrate-resistant acid phosphatase (TRAP), virtually diagnostic of hairy cell leukemia. These cells also express the pan–B-cell markers CD19 and CD20 and the monocyte-associated antigen CD11c. In addition, the plasma cell–associated antigen-1 (PCA-1) is also present on the leukemic cells. Normal B cells with this cluster of antigens have not been found.
- Median survival is 4 years; splenectomy is of benefit in approximately two-thirds of patients. Interferon-α is useful.

Etiology and Pathogenesis of Leukemias and Lymphomas

Evidence implicating alterations in structure and function of proto-oncogenes in the origin of cancer was discussed in Chapter 7; only a brief recapitulation, related to neoplasms of the hematopoietic system, is offered here. In many leukemias and lymphomas, translocations shift proto-oncogenes to new locations within the genome. Such chromosomal rearrangements may alter the function or structure of several oncogenes, including c-*myc* (Burkitt's lymphoma), c-*abl* (CML), RAR-α (AML-M3), *bcl*-1 (NHL, mantle zone lymphoma), and *bcl*-2 (CLL). These genetic changes may be induced by environmental agents such as irradiation, chemicals, or therapeutic agents used to treat other forms of cancer.

CHRONIC MYELOPROLIFERATIVE DISORDERS (p. 658)

These disorders result from clonal neoplastic proliferations of the multipotent myeloid stem cells, which may differentiate along one or more pathways:

- Predominant erythroid differentiation, giving rise to polycythemia vera.
- Predominant myeloid differentiation, giving rise to CML.
- Predominant platelet differentiation, giving rise to essential thrombocythemia.
- Multilineage differentiation with marrow fibrosis, giving rise to myeloid metaplasia with myelofibrosis.

Polycythemia Vera

A clonal disorder of pluripotent stem cells associated with an absolute increase in red cell mass.
PATHOPHYSIOLOGY. Unlike secondary polycythemias, polycythemia vera is associated with virtually undetectable levels of serum erythropoietin and an absolute increase in the number of

myeloid stem cells, which are extremely sensitive to small amounts of erythropoietin.

MORPHOLOGY

- Red cells appear normal; giant platelets and megakaryocytic fragments are seen.
- Marrow is markedly hypercellular with hyperplasia of erythroid, granulocytic, and megakaryocytic elements. A moderate-to-marked increase in marrow reticulin is seen in approximately 10% of patients. With progression it may become fibrotic (myelofibrosis) or, rarely, may be replaced by blasts (leukemic transformation), as discussed below.

CLINICAL FEATURES. Red cell counts range from 6 to 10×10^6 per mm³ with hematocrit values of 60% or more; total leukocyte and platelet counts are also increased in many patients.

Polycythemia vera appears insidiously in late middle age (40 to 60 years). The major clinical features stem from increased blood volume and viscosity, vascular stasis, thrombotic tendency, and hemorrhagic diathesis. The patients are plethoric and somewhat cyanotic owing to stagnation and deoxygenation of blood in peripheral vessels. Liver and spleen may be enlarged. Headaches, dizziness, GI symptoms, hematemesis, and melena are common. Splenic or renal infarction may produce abdominal pain. There usually is intense pruritus, possibly the result of an increased release of histamine from basophils. High cell turnover gives rise to hyperuricemia, and symptomatic gout is seen in 5 to 10% of patients.

PROGNOSIS. About 30% of patients die from thrombotic complications affecting usually the brain or heart; 5% to 10% die from some hemorrhagic complication. With phlebotomies, red cell mass is reduced and median survival is 10 years. In 15 to 20% of patients there is a gradual transition to a "spent phase" during which clinical and anatomic features of myeloid metaplasia with myelofibrosis develop. A terminal acute leukemia develops in some patients, more commonly in those treated with chemotherapy and radioactive phosphorus.

Myeloid Metaplasia with Myelofibrosis

In this chronic myeloproliferative disorder, expansion of the neoplastic myeloid stem cells occurs principally in the spleen (myeloid metaplasia) in a setting of a fibrotic bone marrow (myelofibrosis). This process develops insidiously without an identifiable preceding syndrome; thus, the term "agnogenic (idiopathic) myeloid metaplasia" is sometimes used to describe this condition.

MORPHOLOGY

- Moderate-to-severe, normochromic, normocytic anemia with marked variations in red cell size and shape; characteristic (although not diagnostic) are teardrop-shaped erythrocytes (poikilocytes); numerous normoblasts and basophilic stippled red cells appear in the peripheral blood.
- The white blood cell count may be normal, reduced, or markedly elevated (80,000 to 100,000 per mm³), with a shift to the left and few immature forms. Basophils are usually prominent.
- The platelet count is normal or elevated at the onset, but thrombocytopenia supervenes with disease progression. Giant platelets are frequent, and sometimes fragments of megakaryocytes are detected.
- Bone marrow shows diffuse fibrosis and obliteration of the

normal myeloid elements; this may be preceded by hypercellularity associated with proliferation of all the myeloid elements and sometimes prominent abnormal-looking megakaryocytes.

- Spleen is markedly enlarged, sometimes up to 4000 gm owing to extramedullary hematopoiesis. Histologically, there is trilineage proliferation affecting normoblasts, granulocytic precursors, and megakaryocytes (myeloid metaplasia). The liver is often moderately enlarged, with foci of extramedullary hematopoiesis.

PATHOPHYSIOLOGY. The cause of marrow fibrosis is not clear. Proliferation of neoplastic stem cells begins within the marrow, with subsequent seeding of the spleen and other organs such as the liver. As the disease progresses, marrow fibroblasts proliferate in response to growth factors (PDGF, TGF-β) produced by the expanded pool of platelets and megakaryocytes.

CLINICAL FEATURES. Myeloid metaplasia is uncommon in individuals under 50 years of age. It usually comes to clinical attention because of progressive anemia or marked splenic enlargement, producing a dragging sensation in the left upper quadrant. Hyperuricemia and secondary gout may appear owing to rapid turnover of blood cells. Unlike the situation in the CML, there is no association with a specific chromosomal abnormality, and leukocyte alkaline phosphatase levels are normal.

PROGNOSIS. Most patients can survive for years with transfusions. Threats to life include intercurrent infections; thrombotic episodes or bleeding, related to platelet abnormalities; and, in 5 to 10% of patients, transformation to acute leukemia.

PLASMA CELL DYSCRASIAS AND RELATED DISORDERS (p. 662)

This group of disorders is characterized by the expansion of a single clone of immunoglobulin-secreting cells, and an associated increase in serum levels of a single homogeneous immunoglobulin or its fragments, hence the synonym "monoclonal gammopathies." The monoclonal immunoglobulin identified in the blood and/or urine of patients is referred to as an M component. The M component is usually a complete immunoglobulin, which in some cases is secreted along with excess light (L) or heavy (H) chains. Occasionally only L chains (Bence Jones proteins) or H chains are produced, without complete Ig. Because of its small size, Bence Jones protein is excreted in the urine.

A variety of clinicoanatomic patterns can be differentiated among monoclonal gammopathies:

- Multiple myeloma (plasma cell myeloma).
- Waldenström's macroglobulinemia.
- Heavy-chain disease.
- Primary or immunocyte-associated amyloidosis.
- Monoclonal gammopathy of undetermined significance (MGUS).

MULTIPLE MYELOMA (p. 663)

Multifocal plasma cell cancer of the osseous system; the most common of the malignant gammopathies. A total of 99% of the patients have an M protein in the serum and/or urine. In approximately 55% of patients, the M component is IgG; in 25% it is IgA, or, rarely, IgM, IgD, or IgE. In the remaining 20%

Bence Jones proteinuria alone, without serum M components, is present (light-chain disease). Sixty to 70% of patients have both plasma M components and Bence Jones proteins in the urine.

ETIOLOGY AND PATHOGENESIS. Plasma cells dominate the lesions of multiple myeloma (MM); however, phenotypic studies indicate that MM is a disease of hematopoietic stem cells. Specifically, myeloma cells express plasma cell–associated antigens such as PCA-1, B cell antigen (CD10), myelomonocytic antigen (CD33), megakaryocytes (GpIIa/IIIa), and erythroid cell antigens.

- The proliferation and differentiation of myeloma cells seem to be dependent on several cytokines, most notably IL-6.
- A variety of cytokines produced by the tumor cells, including TNF-β, IL-1, IL-6, and M-CSF have been implicated as osteoclast-activating factor causing the bone destruction typically seen in myeloma.

MORPHOLOGY

- Abnormal aggregates of plasma cells replacing 15 to 90% of the bone marrow are characteristic. The neoplastic plasma cells are mature or immature and cause multifocal destructive bone lesions, but generalized osteoporosis may also be seen. Although any bone may be involved, the vertebral column, ribs, and skull are most frequently affected.
- Renal involvement, called myeloma nephrosis, occurs in 60 to 80% of patients. The microscopic features are

  - Interstitial infiltrates of abnormal plasma cells or chronic inflammatory cells.
  - Protein casts consisting of albumin, immunoglobulins, and Tamm-Horsfall protein in distal convoluted and collecting tubules, often surrounded by multinucleated giant cells.
  - Metastatic calcifications secondary to hypercalcemia.
  - Pyelonephritis incident to the predisposition to infection.

- Systemic amyloidosis of the AL type occurs in about 10% of patients.
- Plasma cell infiltrates may be encountered in spleen, liver, lungs, nerve trunk roots, and lymph nodes, or more widely.

CLINICAL FEATURES AND COMPLICATIONS. The peak age incidence of multiple myeloma is between 50 and 60 years, and both sexes are affected equally. Clinical features stem from the effects of infiltration of organs, particularly bones and bone marrow, by the neoplastic plasma cells, and the production of excessive immunoglobulins, which often have abnormal physicochemical properties.

- Bone infiltration is manifested by pain and pathologic fractures. Hypercalcemia resulting from bone resorption may give rise to neurologic manifestations such as confusion, weakness, lethargy, constipation, and polyuria. It also contributes to renal disease.
- There are recurrent infections with encapsulated bacteria (e.g., pneumococci), resulting from severe suppression of normal immunoglobulins.
- Excessive production and aggregation of myeloma protein may lead to the hyperviscosity syndrome (see Waldenström's Macroglobulinemia) in about 7% of patients.
- Renal insufficiency occurs in up to 50% of patients. It results from multiple factors, the most important of which is excretion

of light chains believed to be toxic to the tubular epithelial cells.

PROGNOSIS. Depends on the stage of advancement at diagnosis. Patients with multiple bony lesions, increasing levels of M protein in serum, and more than 6 mg of Bence Jones proteins per dl of urine have a grave prognosis. Chemotherapy induces remission in 50 to 70% of patients, but the median survival is 2 to 3 years. Renal failure and infection are the two most common causes of death.

SOLITARY PLASMACYTOMA

About 3 to 5% of monoclonal gammopathies consist of a solitary plasmacytic lesion, in either bone or soft tissue. Elevated levels of M proteins in the blood or urine are found in a minority of patients.

- The solitary bony lesions tend to occur in the same locations as multiple myeloma, and progress to multiple myeloma in most cases.
- Extraosseous lesions are often located in the lungs, oronasopharynx, or nasal sinuses. They rarely disseminate and can usually be cured by local resection.

WALDENSTRÖM'S MACROGLOBULINEMIA (p. 665)

Constitutes about 5% of monoclonal gammopathies and shares features with myeloma and small lymphocytic lymphoma. The M protein is usually of the IgM type (macroglobulinemia).
MORPHOLOGY. There is a diffuse infiltrate of lymphocytes, plasma cells, and lymphocytoid plasma cells in the bone marrow; unlike myeloma, the cells do not occur in tumorous masses; hence, there is no bone erosion. Tumor cells are also present in the lymph nodes, spleen, or liver in disseminated disease.
CLINICAL FEATURES. Presents between the sixth and seventh decades with nonspecific complaints such as weakness, fatigability, and weight loss. Approximately 50% of patients have lymphadenopathy, hepatomegaly, and splenomegaly. Because of their size and increased concentration, the macroglobulins form large aggregates that greatly increase the viscosity of blood, giving rise to the hyperviscosity syndrome characterized by

- Visual impairment related to the striking tortuosity and distention of retinal veins, with narrowing at arteriovenous crossing, producing a "sausage-link" pattern; retinal hemorrhages and exudates may be seen.
- Neurologic problems stemming from sluggish blood flow and sludging, including headaches, dizziness, deafness, and stupor.
- Bleeding related to hyperviscosity and interference in platelet functions.
- Cryoglobulinemia. The abnormal globulins may precipitate at low temperatures, producing symptoms such as Raynaud's phenomenon and cold urticaria.

The average survival with chemotherapy is 2 to 5 years.

HEAVY-CHAIN DISEASE (HCD) (p. 666)

Extremely rare monoclonal gammopathies characterized by elevated levels in the blood or urine of a specific heavy chain. Three variants, based on the heavy chain involved, have been described. Only the most common form, alpha-chain disease, is described.

ALPHA-CHAIN DISEASE. The most common HCD is a disorder of IgA-producing cells involving mainly the sites of normal IgA synthesis. Characterized by massive infiltration of the lamina propria of the intestine and abdominal lymph nodes by lymphocytes, plasma cells, and histiocytes, giving rise to villous atrophy and severe malabsorption. Occurs most commonly in the Mediterranean area.

MONOCLONAL GAMMOPATHY OF UNDETERMINED SIGNIFICANCE (p. 666)

About 1% to 3% of asymptomatic individuals above the age of 50 years have an M protein in the serum without any of the well-defined immunoglobulin-producing disease.

- Most individuals have less than 3 gm per dl of monoclonal protein and no Bence Jones proteinuria. Other specific forms of monoclonal gammopathies must be excluded.
- The condition follows a benign clinical course most commonly; about 20% of patients develop a well-defined plasma cell dyscrasia (myeloma, macroglobulinemia, or amyloidosis).

LANGERHANS CELL HISTIOCYTOSIS (HISTIOCYTOSIS X) (p. 666)

The proliferating cell in these disorders is the Langerhans cell (LC), normally present within the epidermis and related to the mononuclear phagocyte system. These cells have Fc receptors, bear HLA-D/DR antigens, and react with anti-CD1 antibody. They have abundant, often vacuolated cytoplasm, with vesicular oval or indented nuclei. Characteristic is the presence of HX bodies, or Birbeck granules, in the cytoplasm. Under the electron microscope these are seen to have a pentalaminar, rodlike tubular structure, with characteristic periodicity and sometimes a dilated terminal end (tennis-racquet appearance).

LC histiocytoses present as three clinicopathologic entities, described below with their former designations in parentheses.

ACUTE DISSEMINATED LANGERHANS CELL HISTIOCYTOSIS (LETTERER-SIWE SYNDROME)

MORPHOLOGY. Characterized by proliferation of LC histiocytes in virtually all organs and tissues of the body, including skin, lymph nodes, spleen, liver, and particularly bone marrow, where they may cause erosive defects visible on x-ray film.

CLINICAL FEATURES. Infants and children under 2 years of age are most commonly affected. The onset is marked by fever and infections such as otitis media or mastoiditis, followed by a diffuse maculopapular eczematous or purpuric skin rash and enlargement of the spleen, liver, and lymph nodes. Pulmonary and bone lesions are frequently seen. Anemia, thrombocytopenia, and leukopenia are frequently present owing to replacement of the bone marrow. With intensive chemotherapy, 50% of patients survive 5 years.

UNIFOCAL AND MULTIFOCAL LANGERHANS CELL HISTIOCYTOSIS (EOSINOPHILIC GRANULOMA: UNIFOCAL AND MULTIFOCAL)

Both unifocal and multifocal variants are characterized by expanding, erosive accumulations of LC histiocytes, usually within the medullary cavities of bones. Histiocytes are variably admixed with eosinophils, lymphocytes, plasma cells, and neutrophils. The eosinophilic component ranges from scattered mature cells to sheetlike masses of cells.

Virtually any bone in the skeletal system may be involved, most commonly the calvarium, ribs, and femur. Similar lesions may be found in the skin, lungs, or stomach, either as unifocal lesions or as components of the multifocal disease.

UNIFOCAL (EOSINOPHILIC GRANULOMA). An indolent disorder affecting children and young adults, especially males.

The solitary bone lesions may be asymptomatic or may cause pain and tenderness, and in some instances pathologic fractures. There are no systemic manifestations such as fever or involvement of the blood or viscera.

Lesions may heal spontaneously with fibrosis or be cured by local excision or irradiation.

MULTIFOCAL (HAND-SCHÜLLER-CHRISTIAN DISEASE). Usually affects children, who present with fever; diffuse eruptions, particularly on the scalp and in the ear canals; and frequent bouts of otitis media, mastoiditis, and upper respiratory infections.

Infiltrate of LCs may lead to mild lymphadenopathy, hepatomegaly, and splenomegaly. In about 50% of patients, involvement of the posterior pituitary stalk of hypothalamus leads to diabetes insipidus. The combination of calvarial bone defects, diabetes insipidus, and exophthalmos is referred to as the Hand-Schüller-Christian triad.

Fifty per cent of patients have spontaneous regression; the other half can be treated with chemotherapy.

SPLENOMEGALY (p. 669)

The spleen may be enlarged in a variety of conditions, listed in Table 14–6.

HYPERSPLENISM (p. 669)

This complication is encountered in a minority of patients with splenic enlargement. It is characterized by (1) splenomegaly; (2) a reduction of one or more of the cellular elements of the blood, resulting from increased sequestration of the cells and the consequent enhanced lysis by splenic macrophages; and (3) correction of the cytopenia(s) after splenectomy.

NONSPECIFIC ACUTE SPLENITIS (p. 670)

Associated with enlargement of the spleen and may occur in any blood-borne infection. Grossly, the spleen is enlarged, red, and extremely soft. Microscopically, the major change is acute congestion of the red pulp, which may efface the lymphoid follicles. Reticuloendothelial hyperplasia and numerous free macrophages are prominent in the sinusoids.

Table 14–6. Disorders Associated with Splenomegaly

I. Infections
  Nonspecific splenitis of various blood-borne infections
    (particularly infective endocarditis)
  Infectious mononucleosis
  Tuberculosis
  Typhoid fever
  Brucellosis
  Cytomegalovirus
  Syphilis
  Malaria
  Histoplasmosis
  Toxoplasmosis
  Kala-azar
  Trypanosomiasis
  Schistosomiasis
  Leishmaniasis
  Echinococcosis
II. Congestive States Related to Portal Hypertension
  Cirrhosis of liver
  Portal or splenic vein thrombosis
  Cardiac failure (right-sided)
III. Lymphohematogenous Disorders
  Hodgkin's disease
  Non-Hodgkin's lymphomas
  Histiocytoses
  Multiple myeloma
  Myeloproliferative syndromes (chronic myelogenous
    leukemia, polycythemia vera, myeloid metaplasia with
    myelofibrosis)
  Chronic lymphocytic leukemia
  Acute leukemias (inconstant)
  Hemolytic anemias (autoimmune hemolytic anemia,
    hereditary spherocytosis, hemoglobinopathies)
  Thrombocytopenic purpura
IV. Immunologic-Inflammatory Conditions
  Rheumatoid arthritis
  Felty's syndrome
  Systemic lupus erythematosus
V. Storage Diseases
  Gaucher's disease
  Niemann-Pick disease
  Mucopolysaccharidoses
VI. Miscellaneous
  Amyloidosis
  Primary neoplasms and cysts
  Secondary neoplasms

From Cotran, R. S., Kumar, V., and Robbins, S. L.: Robbins Pathologic Basis of Disease. 5th ed. Philadelphia, W. B. Saunders Co., 1994, p. 669.

CONGESTIVE SPLENOMEGALY (p. 670)

Passive chronic venous congestion and enlargement may result from

• Systemic or central venous congestion encountered in cardiac decompensation involving the right side of the heart.

- Intrahepatic derangement of portal venous drainage, as occurs in various forms of cirrhosis of the liver.
- Obstruction to the extrahepatic portal vein and splenic vein, as occurs in spontaneous portal vein thrombosis, inflammatory involvement of the portal vein (pylephlebitis), and thrombosis of the splenic vein.

MORPHOLOGY. Grossly, there is moderate-to-severe enlargement of the spleen, which may weigh from 500 gm to over 1000 gm. Microscopically, the pulp is suffused with red cells during the early phases, becoming increasingly more fibrous and cellular with time. Organization of focal hemorrhages gives rise to foci of fibrosis containing deposits of iron and calcium salts (Gandy-Gamna nodules).

NEOPLASMS (p. 671)

Benign tumors include fibromas, osteomas, chondromas, lymphangiomas, and hemangiomas. Malignant tumors, most frequently of the lymphohematopoietic system, include non-Hodgkin's lymphomas or Hodgkin's disease and leukemias. There are hemangiosarcomas primary in the spleen. With secondary lesions, metastases to the spleen are not common and are usually found only in very advanced malignancies.

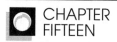

CHAPTER
FIFTEEN

The Respiratory System

CONGENITAL ANOMALIES (p. 675)

Congenital Cysts (p. 675)

Formed by abnormal detachment of a fragment of primitive foregut. Bronchogenic cysts are most common and consist of cystic spaces lined by bronchial-type epithelium. Complications include infection, with suppuration and/or abscess formation, and rupture into bronchi or the pleural cavity, causing hemorrhage/hemoptysis or pneumothorax, respectively.

Bronchopulmonary Sequestration (p. 675)

The presence of lung tissue (lobes or segments) *without* a normal connection to the airway system, and with vascular supply derived from the aorta or its branches, not the pulmonary artery.

Extralobar sequestrations are found most often in infants as abnormal mediastinal masses and in association with other congenital anomalies.

Intralobar sequestrations are found *within the lung parenchyma*. They are more common in adults and are associated with recurrent infections.

ATELECTASIS (p. 675)

Incomplete expansion or collapse of parts of or a whole lung. There are *three* basic types, all of which are reversible:

- *Obstructive atelectasis*, which follows complete obstruction of an airway (e.g., excessive bronchial secretions as in bronchial asthma or chronic bronchitis, foreign body aspiration, or bronchial neoplasms).
- *Compressive atelectasis*, when pleural space is expanded by fluid (effusions from cardiac failure or neoplasms, blood from rupture of a thoracic aneurysm) or by air (pneumothorax).
- *Patchy atelectasis* develops when there is loss of pulmonary surfactant, in neonatal respiratory distress syndrome (*see p. 444*).

PULMONARY VASCULAR DISEASE (p. 676)

PULMONARY EDEMA (p. 676)

Hemodynamic disturbances and/or changes in microvascular permeability (see ARDS below) can cause pulmonary edema (Table

Table 15–1. Classification and Causes of Pulmonary Edema

Hemodynamic Edema
Increased hydrostatic pressure
    Left-sided heart failure
    Mitral stenosis
    Volume overload
    Pulmonary vein obstruction
Decreased oncotic pressure
    Hypoalbuminemia
        Nephrotic syndrome
        Liver disease
        Protein-losing enteropathies
Lymphatic obstruction

Edema Due to Microvascular Injury
Infectious agents: viruses, *Mycoplasma,* other
Inhaled gases: oxygen, sulfur dioxide, cyanates, smoke
Liquid aspiration: gastric contents, near-drowning
Drugs and chemicals
    Chemotherapeutic agents: bleomycin, other
    Other medications: amphotericin B, colchicine, gold
    Other: heroin, kerosene, paraquat
Shock, trauma, and sepsis
Radiation
Miscellaneous
    Acute pancreatitis; extracorporeal circulation; massive fat, air,
    or amniotic fluid embolism; uremia; heat; diabetic
    ketoacidosis; thrombotic thrombocytopenic purpura (TTP);
    disseminated intravascular coagulation (DIC)

Edema of Undetermined Origin
High altitude
Neurogenic

From Cotran, R. S., Kumar, V., and Robbins, S. L.: Robbins Pathologic Basis of Disease. 5th ed. Philadelphia, W. B. Saunders Co., 1994, p. 676.

15–1). Chronic edema predisposes to infection in addition to impairing normal respiratory function.

MORPHOLOGY. Regardless of etiology, the lungs become heavy, wet, and subcrepitant. Fluid accumulates, especially in the dependent, basal regions of the lower lobes.

Histologic findings include engorged capillaries and filling of the intra-alveolar air spaces by a granular pink precipitate. In chronic congestion and edema (such as in mitral stenosis), interstitial fibrosis may occur, associated with numerous hemosiderin-laden macrophages (brown induration).

ADULT RESPIRATORY DISTRESS SYNDROME (ARDS) (p. 676)

Characterized by diffuse alveolar capillary damage, leading to severe respiratory failure and arterial hypoxemia refractory to oxygen therapy. The major causes are listed as causes of microvascular injury and edema in Table 15–1. Respiratory failure, unresponsive to oxygen therapy, develops with diffuse bilateral infiltrates on x-ray and frequent superimposed infections, resulting in over 50% mortality.

PATHOGENESIS. Basic lesion is diffuse damage to the alveolar wall, initially involving the capillary endothelium, but eventually the epithelium as well. Damage leads to the acute stage of ARDS with increased capillary permeability and edema, fibrin exudation, formation of hyaline membranes (composed of necrotic epithelial cell debris and exudative proteins), and septal inflammation.

Mechanisms of this injury include

- *Oxygen-derived free radicals*, especially in the toxicity induced by prolonged exposure to high concentrations of oxygen and/ or other toxins, e.g., paraquat.
- *Aggregation of activated neutrophils* in the pulmonary vasculature. These damage epithelium by secreting several types of injurious factors, including oxygen-derived free radicals and lysosomal enzymes (proteases), as well as arachidonic acid metabolites that augment neutrophil aggregation.
- *Activation of lung macrophages*, which release oxidants, proteases, and pro-inflammatory cytokines (e.g., IL-8).
- *Loss or damage to surfactant*, contributing to atelectasis, which (in combination with pulmonary edema) results in the stiff lungs characteristic of ARDS.

MORPHOLOGY. In the acute stage, there are diffusely firm, red, boggy, heavy lungs with acute diffuse alveolar damage (edema, hyaline membranes, acute inflammation by histology).

In the *proliferative/organizing* stage, there are patchy areas of interstitial fibrosis and type II epithelial proliferation, frequently with superimposed bacterial infection in fatal cases.

PULMONARY EMBOLISM (PE), HEMORRHAGE, AND INFARCTION (p. 679)

Occlusions of pulmonary arteries are almost always embolic; in situ thromboses are rare, occurring only with pulmonary hypertension and pulmonary atherosclerosis. However, thrombosis may complete a partial embolic occlusion.

Over 95% of PEs arise in deep veins of legs.

The frequency of PE correlates with a predisposition to thrombosis in the legs. Occurrence at autopsy ranges from 1% in the general population to 30% in hospitalized patients with severe burns, trauma, or fractures.

Potential consequences are

- Large emboli (about 5%) impacting in the major pulmonary artery(ies) or astride the bifurcation of the pulmonary artery (saddle embolus).

  - May cause instantaneous death.
  - May cause cardiovascular collapse, e.g., acute cor pulmonale (right heart failure). A shower of, or repeated, small emboli may have the same effect.
  - Hemodynamic compromise is secondary not only to vascular obstruction, but also to reflex vasoconstriction caused by such agents as TxA_2.

- Small emboli (60% to 80%).

  - May be clinically silent in patients without cardiovascular failure.
  - May cause transient chest pain and sometimes hemoptysis owing to pulmonary hemorrhage (blood in the alveoli, but no ischemic necrosis of the pulmonary parenchyma).

- In patients with compromised pulmonary circulation (cardiac failure), may give rise to infarctions generally small, manifest pathologically as peripheral, wedge-shaped hemorrhagic areas.
- Between the extremes of large and small emboli are those of middle size (about 20% to 35%) that occlude moderate-sized peripheral pulmonary branches.
  - Usually induce infarction.
- Uncommonly, overt or covert multiple small emboli produce right heart strain (chronic cor pulmonale) and eventually pulmonary hypertension and vascular sclerosis.

CLINICAL SIGNIFICANCE. Diagnosis of pulmonary emboli is often difficult; almost two-thirds of PEs, even when fatal, are not diagnosed before death. Many are silent, others are catastrophic, and even when they produce infarction they may not be clear-cut.

Even without treatment, there is usually improvement in perfusion within the first day owing to fibrinolysis and contraction of the thrombotic mass. The condition may completely resolve within weeks or months.

With diagnosis and the use of fibrinolytic agents, improvement is greatly speeded, and the mortality rate is reduced to 5% to 10%.

PULMONARY HYPERTENSION (p. 680)

Elevated pulmonary artery pressure is caused by increased pulmonary vascular resistance.

Most commonly, pulmonary hypertension is secondary to:

- Chronic obstructive or interstitial lung disease.
- Left-sided heart disease.
- Recurrent pulmonary emboli.

Primary (or idiopathic) pulmonary hypertension is uncommon, seen in children or in women aged 20 to 40, and generally progresses to severe respiratory insufficiency, cor pulmonale, and death over several years. Therapies include vasodilators and occasionally heart-lung transplantation. The etiology is unknown, but current hypotheses postulate that endothelial dysfunction and injury (which can be triggered by some chemical and dietary agents) lead to persistent vasoconstriction and subsequent intimal and medial hypertrophy, and resultant increases in vascular resistance.

MORPHOLOGY. Vascular lesions seen in all types of pulmonary hypertension include (1) atheroma in large elastic arteries and (2) intimal fibrosis/medial hypertrophy in medium-sized muscular arteries and smaller arterioles. The presence of numerous organized thrombi suggests recurrent pulmonary thromboembolism.

So-called *plexogenic arteriopathy* (tufts within capillary channels resembling a vascular plexus) is seen in severe primary pulmonary hypertension or with some congenital cardiovascular anomalies.

CHRONIC OBSTRUCTIVE PULMONARY DISEASE (COPD) (p. 683)

Diffuse pulmonary disease is classified physiologically as (1) *obstructive disease*, characterized by increased resistance to air flow, or (2) *restrictive disease* (see Interstitial Lung Disease), characterized by reduced expansion of lung parenchyma, with decreased total lung capacity.

COPD describes a spectrum of clinical diseases from pure emphysema to pure bronchitis (Table 15–2). Although there are certain differences between these two extremes, many individuals show overlapping features because of the common pathogenetic denominator, cigarette smoking.

EMPHYSEMA (p. 683)

Defined morphologically as the abnormal enlargement of air spaces distal to the terminal bronchioles, with destruction of their walls. Emphysema is further classified according to the anatomic distribution of the lesion within the acinus.

CENTRIACINAR EMPHYSEMA. Characterized by

- Destruction and enlargement of the central or proximal parts of the respiratory unit—the acinus—sparing distal alveoli.
- Predominant involvement of upper lobes and apices.

Severe lesions are seen primarily in male smokers, often in association with chronic bronchitis.

PANACINAR EMPHYSEMA. Characterized by

- Uniform destruction and enlargement of the acinus.
- Predominance in lower basal zones.
- Strong association with alpha$_1$-antitrypsin deficiency.

PARASEPTAL EMPHYSEMA. Involves mostly the distal acinus, sparing the proximal. It

- Is found near the pleura and adjacent to fibrosis or scars.
- Is often the underlying lesion of spontaneous pneumothorax.

IRREGULAR EMPHYSEMA. Irregular involvement of the acinus and associated with scarring. It is usually asymptomatic.

Other related entities are *bullous emphysema* (blebs or bullae greater than 1 cm in diameter) and *interstitial emphysema* (entrance of air into the connective tissue of the lung, mediastinum, or subcutaneous tissue).

PATHOGENESIS. The protease-antiprotease hypothesis holds that destruction of alveolar walls in emphysema stems from an imbalance between proteases and their inhibitors in the lung. The evidence is as follows:

- Individuals with a hereditary deficiency of the major protease inhibitor, alpha$_1$-antitrypsin, invariably develop emphysema, and at a younger age if they smoke.
- Pulmonary instillation of proteolytic enzymes, including neutrophil elastase, results in emphysema in experimental animals.

Tobacco smoking contributes to emphysema by

- Recruiting neutrophils into the lung by factors from smoke-activated alveolar macrophages.
- Stimulating release of elastase from neutrophils.
- Enhancing macrophage elastase activity.
- Inactivation of alpha$_1$-antitrypsin by oxidants in tobacco smoke or free radicals released by activated neutrophils.

Hence, *impaction of smoke particles in the small bronchioles leads to recruitment of inflammatory cells, increased elastase, and decreased alpha$_1$-antitrypsin, resulting in the centriacinar pattern of emphysema seen in smokers.*

Table 15–2. Disorders Associated with Airflow Obstruction: The Spectrum of COPD

Clinical Term	Anatomic Site	Major Pathologic Changes	Etiology	Signs/Symptoms
Chronic bronchitis	Bronchus	Mucous gland hyperplasia, hypersecretion	Tobacco smoke, air pollutants	Cough, sputum production
Bronchiectasis	Bronchus	Airway dilatation and scarring	Persistent or severe infections	Cough; purulent sputum; fever
Asthma	Bronchus	Smooth muscle hyperplasia, excess mucus, inflammation	Immunologic or undefined causes	Episodic wheezing, cough, dyspnea
"Small airway disease," bronchiolitis	Bronchiole	Inflammatory scarring/obliteration	Tobacco smoke, air pollutants, misc.	Cough, dyspnea
Emphysema	Acinus	Airspace enlargement; wall destruction	Tobacco smoke	Dyspnea

From Cotran, R. S., Kumar, V., and Robbins, S. L.: Robbins Pathologic Basis of Disease. 5th ed. Philadelphia, W. B. Saunders Co., 1994, p. 683.

MORPHOLOGY. With diffuse forms, lungs can become voluminous and pillowy. Microscopically, air spaces are enlarged, walls thinned, and septal capillaries compressed and bloodless. Rupture of walls may produce honeycombing.

CHRONIC BRONCHITIS (p. 688)

Defined clinically as persistent cough with sputum production for at least 3 months in at least 2 consecutive years.
MORPHOLOGY. Characterized by

* Hyperemia and edema of mucous membranes of the lung.
* Mucinous secretions or casts filling airways.
* Increase in size of the mucous glands.
* Bronchial/bronchiolar mucous plugging, inflammation, and fibrosis.
* Squamous metaplasia/dysplasia of bronchial epithelium.

Chronic irritation of the airways by inhaled substances, especially tobacco smoke, is the dominant factor in the pathogenesis of chronic bronchitis. These irritants cause bronchitis by eliciting

* Hypersecretion of mucus.
* Subsequent hypertrophy of mucous glands.
* Goblet cell metaplasia in bronchiolar epithelium.
* Bronchiolitis.

Infections are a secondary factor that maintain and promote the injury initiated by smoking.

BRONCHIAL ASTHMA (p. 689)

This is a disorder of increased responsiveness of the tracheobronchial tree to various stimuli, resulting in paroxysmal contraction of bronchial airways. Two major types are recognized: (1) extrinsic (allergen, reagin-mediated) and (2) intrinsic (idiopathic) or precipitated by various factors (see Table 15–3 and below).

Atopic (allergic) asthma, the most common type, is triggered by environmental antigens (dust, pollen, food, etc.), often with a positive family history of atopy. It is a classic type I IgE-mediated hypersensitivity reaction having

* An acute phase with binding of antigen by IgE-coated mast cells causing release of primary mediators (histamine, chemotactic factors) and secondary mediators (leukotrienes, prostaglandin D_2, cytokines, neuropeptides). *These acute-phase mediators result in bronchospasm, edema, mucus secretion, and recruitment of leukocytes.*
* An ensuing late-phase reaction mediated by recruited leukocytes (basophils, eosinophils, neutrophils, monocytes). The late phase is characterized by persistent bronchospasm and edema, leukocytic infiltration, and necrosis of epithelial cells.

Nonatopic asthma (nonreaginic), the other common type of asthma, is often triggered by respiratory tract infections, chemical irritants, and drugs, usually without a family history and with little or no evidence of IgE-mediated hypersensitivity. The primary cause of increased airway reactivity is unknown.
MORPHOLOGY. The lungs are overinflated and show patchy atelectasis, with occlusion of airways by mucous plugs.

Microscopically, the lungs exhibit edema, an inflammatory infiltrate in bronchial walls with numerous eosinophils, hypertro-

Table 15–3. Types of Asthma

Types of Asthma	Precipitating Factors°	Mechanism or Immunologic Reaction
Extrinsic		
Atopic (allergic)	Specific allergens	Type I (IgE) immune reaction
Occupational	Chemical challenge	Type I immune reactions
Allergic bronchopulmonary aspergillosis	Antigen (spores) challenge	Type I and III immune reactions
Intrinsic		
Nonreaginic	Respiratory tract infection	Unknown; hyperreactive airways
Pharmacologic (e.g., aspirin-sensitive)	Aspirin	Decreased prostaglandins, increased leukotrienes

°All types may be precipitated by cold, stress, exercise. All have hyperreactive airways.

From Cotran, R. S., Kumar, V., and Robbins, S. L.: Robbins Pathologic Basis of Disease. 5th ed. Philadelphia, W. B. Saunders Co., 1994, p. 690.

phy of bronchial wall musculature and of submucosal mucous glands, whorled mucous plugs (Curschmann's spirals), and crystalloid debris of eosinophil membranes (Charcot-Leyden crystals) within airways.

BRONCHIECTASIS (p. 692)

Represents a chronic necrotizing infection of bronchi and bronchioles leading to or associated with abnormal permanent dilatation of these airways.

Clinical features include cough, fever, and abundant purulent sputum. In severe cases, obstructive respiratory insufficiency may be seen. Complications include cor pulmonale, metastatic abscesses, and systemic amyloidosis.

Bronchiectasis is seen in association with

- Bronchial obstruction, such as by tumor or foreign bodies.
- Congenital/hereditary conditions, e.g., cystic fibrosis, intralobar sequestrations.
- Immotile cilia syndromes (e.g., Kartagener's syndrome).
- Necrotizing pneumonia.

Persistent obstruction leads to atelectasis and diminished elastic forces holding airways taut, resulting in relaxation and dilatation. These changes become irreversible if they occur during development or if added infection contributes further damage to the airway walls.

MORPHOLOGY. The most severe changes are seen in distal airways of lower lobes, with dilatations of varying shapes (*cylindrical, fusiform, or saccular*). Histology shows a spectrum of mild to necrotizing acute and chronic inflammation of the airways. Fibrosis develops in chronic cases. Extension of bronchial infection may lead to abscess formation.

PULMONARY INFECTIONS (p. 694)

Occur when normal lung or systemic defense mechanisms are impaired. Pulmonary defense mechanisms include nasal, tracheobronchial, and alveolar mechanisms to filter, neutralize, and clear inhaled organisms and particles.

Important factors interfering with normal lung defenses are

- Loss of or decreased cough reflex leading to aspiration (seen in coma, anesthesia, drug effects).
- Injury to mucociliary apparatus (as with cigarette or other smoke/gaseous inhalations).
- Decreased phagocytic/bactericidal function of the alveolar macrophage (as a result of alcohol, tobacco, oxygen toxicity).
- Edema/congestion (CHF).
- Accumulation of secretions.

BACTERIAL PNEUMONIA (p. 694)

These infections occur in two frequently overlapping morphologic patterns (bronchopneumonia and lobar pneumonia), and can be caused by a variety of gram-positive and gram-negative organisms. Depending on bacterial virulence and host resistance, the same organism may in one instance cause bronchopneumonia and in another instance lobar pneumonia, and sometimes intermediate involvements.

Bronchopneumonia (p. 694)

This pattern of bacterial pneumonia is marked by patchy exudative consolidation of lung parenchyma, caused most commonly by staphylococci, streptococci, pneumococci, *Haemophilus influenzae, Pseudomonas aeruginosa,* and coliform bacteria.

Grossly, the lungs show dispersed, elevated, focal areas of palpable consolidation and suppuration. Histologic features consist of an acute (neutrophilic) suppurative exudate filling air spaces and airways, usually about bronchi and bronchioles. Resolution of the exudate usually restores normal lung structure, but organization may occur and result in fibrous scarring in some cases, or aggressive disease may produce abscesses. A predominantly interstitial pattern of inflammation is seen in some pediatric infections, as with *Escherichia coli* or group B hemolytic streptococci.

Lobar Pneumonia (p. 695)

This pattern of acute bacterial infection involves a large portion of or an entire lobe of lung. Most lobar pneumonias are caused by pneumococci, which enter the lungs via the airways. Occasionally they are caused by other organisms (*Klebsiella pneumoniae,* staphylococci, streptococci, *H. influenzae*).

The following sequence of stages is "classic" but infrequently seen because of antibiotic therapy. However, the various stages portray the natural history of uncomplicated lobar pneumonia.

- *Congestion* predominates in the first 24 hours.
- *Red hepatization* (consolidation) describes lung tissue with

confluent acute exudation containing neutrophils and red cells, giving a red, firm, liver-like gross appearance.

* *Gray hepatization* follows, as the red cells disintegrate and the remaining fibrinosuppurative exudate persists, giving a gray-brown gross appearance.
* *Resolution* is the favorable final stage in which consolidated exudate undergoes enzymatic and cellular degradation and clearance. Normal structure is restored.

Complications of lobar pneumonia, and sometimes bronchopneumonia, are

* Abscess formation.
* Empyema (spread of infection to pleural cavity).
* Organization of exudate into fibrotic scar tissue.
* Bacteremia and sepsis, with infection of other organs.

VIRAL AND MYCOPLASMAL (PRIMARY, ATYPICAL) PNEUMONIA (p. 698)

Infections by viruses (e.g., influenza A or B, respiratory syncytial virus [RSV], adenovirus, rhinovirus, herpes simplex, cytomegalovirus) or *Mycoplasma pneumoniae* result in varied clinical and pathologic patterns, ranging from relatively mild upper respiratory tract involvements (e.g., the common cold) to severe lower respiratory tract disease.

MORPHOLOGY. Patchy or lobar areas of congestion *without* the consolidation of bacterial pneumonias (hence the term "atypical" pneumonia).

* A predominance of interstitial pneumonitis with widened, edematous alveolar walls containing a mononuclear inflammatory cell infiltrate.
* The formation of *hyaline membranes*, reflecting diffuse alveolar damage.
* Frequent superimposed bacterial infection.

Certain viruses cause necrosis of bronchial or alveolar epithelium in severe infections (herpes simplex, adenovirus, varicella), and characteristic cytopathic changes are seen with some, e.g., cytomegaly and nuclear inclusions in the cytomegalovirus infection.

LUNG ABSCESS (p. 699)

Marked by localized infectious suppurative necrosis of lung tissue. Commonly involved are staphylococci, streptococci, numerous gram-negative species, and anaerobes. Mixed infections are frequent, reflecting aspiration of oral contents.

These infections can be initiated by

* Aspiration of infective material, as in oropharyngeal surgical procedures, dental sepsis, or aspiration secondary to diminished consciousness from coma, drugs, anesthesia, and seizures.
* Antecedent primary bacterial infection.
* Septic emboli from infected thrombi or cardiac valve vegetations.
* Obstructive tumors.
* Direct traumatic punctures.
* Spread of infection from adjacent organs.

Complications include extension into the pleural cavity, hemorrhage, septic embolization, and secondary amyloidosis.

MORPHOLOGY. Abscesses vary in number (single or multiple) and size (microscopic to many centimeters in diameter). Aspiration abscesses are more common on the right, reflecting the more vertical right bronchus. They contain variable mixtures of pus and air, depending on available drainage through airways. Chronic abscesses are often surrounded by a reactive fibrous wall.

TUBERCULOSIS (pp. 324, 700)

This is the chronic, communicable disease caused by *M. tuberculosis* made distinctive by a necrotizing (caseating) granulomatous tissue response to seeded organisms.

Transmission is usually by inhalation of infected droplets produced by the coughing or sneezing of infected individuals. Predisposing factors are any debilitating or immunosuppressive condition, e.g., diabetes, alcoholism, malnutrition, chronic lung disease.

PATHOGENESIS. The cell wall lipids and carbohydrates of *M. tuberculosis* appear to enhance virulence by interfering with phagolysosomal fusion. This allows the intracellular survival of mycobacteria.

Delayed hypersensitivity (type IV) to the tubercle bacillus develops in 2 to 4 weeks after initial infection. A sensitized individual will show increased induration (greater than 5 mm) at the site of intradermal injection of purified protein derivative of *M. tuberculosis* (PPD test). However, a positive test indicates sensitivity, not active disease.

Once sensitization appears during infection, the nonspecific inflammatory response becomes granulomatous, often with central, caseous necrosis of the granulomas. A concomitant increase in resistance—the ability to inhibit intracellular replication of bacilli—occurs.

There are several forms of tuberculosis, depending on the individual's hypersensitivity and resistance.

Primary Pulmonary Tuberculosis (pp. 325, 700)

This form occurs in individuals lacking previous contact with tubercle bacilli. It begins as a single granulomatous lesion, known as a *Ghon focus*, subjacent to the pleura in the inferior upper lobe/superior lower lobe regions. Tubercle bacilli can be demonstrated histologically with acid-fast stains in early lesions. Old scarred tubercles may have no visible organisms but contain infective organisms, sometimes for decades.

The spread to draining ipsilateral bronchial or hilar lymph nodes results in a combination of lung and lymph node lesions called the *Ghon complex*.

In most cases the infection does not progress and results in local scarring and calcification. Infrequently, a progressive primary tuberculous pneumonia ensues. A further complication, miliary disseminated tuberculosis, may occur if tubercle bacilli gain access to the bloodstream.

Secondary Pulmonary Tuberculosis (p. 700)

This term denotes *active infection in a previously sensitized individual.* Most cases represent reactivation of dormant bacilli from primary lesions. Occasionally, exogenous sources of tuberculosis cause secondary disease.

Secondary tuberculosis is generally found in the apices of the lungs, reflecting the preference of *M. tuberculosis* for high pO$_2$. These lesions may progress to *cavitary fibrocaseous tuberculosis, tuberculous bronchopneumonia, or miliary tuberculosis.*

CLINICAL FEATURES. Primary tuberculosis is usually asymptomatic. The secondary form more often causes insidious fever, night sweats, weight loss, productive cough with blood-streaked sputum, or hemoptysis. Diagnosis relies on culture of the organism or demonstration of acid-fast bacilli in sputum or biopsy tissue.

Prognosis and course are variable, depending on the extent of disease, the underlying health of the individual, and other variables, but chemotherapy is effective in all but neglected cases and those caused by emerging, highly drug-resistant strains.

Disseminated Tuberculosis (p. 702)

Hematogenous spread of tubercle bacilli may produce either

- *Miliary tuberculosis* with myriad minute foci of infection in many organs, particularly liver, bone marrow, spleen, and kidneys.
- *Isolated organ tuberculosis* when disseminated organisms become established in only one or two organs, most often adrenals, kidneys, bone (tuberculous osteomyelitis), or female genital tract (salpingitis, endometritis).

INTERSTITIAL LUNG DISEASE (p. 703)

A heterogeneous group of diseases with similar clinical, radiologic, and pathologic changes.

- *Clinical.* Restrictive lung disease: dyspnea, decreased lung volumes, and compliance.
- *Radiologic.* Diffuse infiltrates, ground-glass shadows.
- *Pathologic.* Diffuse, chronic inflammation/fibrosis of alveolar interstitium. Most changes are nonspecific, but there are some characteristic features in certain diseases (e.g., asbestos bodies).

PATHOGENESIS. The pathogenetic sequence of events in this group of diseases involves initial, early, and late mechanisms.

- The *initial event* is injury to epithelium/endothelium via inhaled or blood-borne toxins/agents.
- The *early acute* changes of alveolitis follow, consisting of recruitment by chemotactic factors (e.g., IL-8) of activated inflammatory/immune cells. These cells release injurious (oxidants, cytokines) and fibrogenic (PDGF, FGF, IL-1) mediators.
- The *late effects* of the various bioactive substances result in interstitial fibrosis.

PNEUMOCONIOSES (p. 706)

Disorders caused by the inhalation of any aerosol, including mineral dusts, organic dusts, and fumes and vapors.

Factors that determine the health effects of inhaled dusts include

- The amount of dust retained, in turn determined by concentration, duration of exposure, and the effectiveness of clearance mechanisms.
- The size, shape, and buoyancy of particles: those greater than

5 μm in diameter are filtered in upper airways, and those less than 1 μm can remain suspended and be exhaled, leaving the 1- to 5-μm particles to settle in the alveoli as the most potentially dangerous particles.

- The physicochemical reactivity and solubility of particles. Quartz, for example, may injure cells directly via free radicals on the particle surface. Highly soluble particles may rapidly cause toxicity; other particles resist dissolution and may persist to invoke a chronic fibrotic reaction.

Carbon Dust–Coal Workers' Pneumoconiosis
(p. 707)

The range of pulmonary effects of carbon dust includes

- *Anthracosis*, the small harmless accumulations seen in the lungs of urban dwellers/smokers.
- *Simple coal workers' pneumoconiosis (CWP)*, with more prominent and numerous aggregates of coal dust–laden macrophages forming coal *macules*. Clinical features may include cough and blackish sputum, but no significant dysfunction is seen in uncomplicated cases.
- *Progressive massive fibrosis (PMF) or complicated CWP*, manifested by severe fibrosis and scarring in areas of dust accumulation. This pattern reflects a much heavier dust burden and results in disabling respiratory insufficiency.

Factors involved in determining the progression of simple CWP to PMF include duration and magnitude of exposure, and secretion of fibrogenic factors by coal dust–laden macrophages. **MORPHOLOGY.** In simple CWP, black coal macules composed of dust-filled macrophages 1 to 5 mm in diameter are present diffusely, especially in the upper zones of the upper and lower lobes.

In complicated CWP, large, blackened scars replace substantial portions of the lung (black lung disease), especially in the upper zones.

Silicosis (p. 708)

Prolonged *inhalation of silica particles produces a chronic, nodular, dense pulmonary fibrosis.*
Sources of silica exposure include

- Mining (gold, tin, copper, coal) and quarrying.
- Sandblasting.
- Metal grinding.
- Manufacture of ceramics.

PATHOGENESIS. Silicosis involves promotion of persistent inflammation and fibrosis by the interaction of silica particles and lung macrophages. Ingested silica leads to macrophage activation and release of oxidants, cytokines, and growth factors that ultimately cause fibroblast proliferation and collagen deposition. Injury also may be perpetuated by direct toxic effects on the macrophage, causing cell death and release of the silica—restarting the injury cycle.
MORPHOLOGY. Distinct collagenous nodules start as small lesions in the upper lung, but grow larger and more diffuse as the disease progresses. Coalescence of lesions forms large areas of dense scar. Calcification or concomitant blackening by coal dust is often present.

Microscopically, hyalinized whorls of collagen are seen with scant inflammation. Polarized light often shows birefringent silica particles within nodules.

Asbestosis (p. 709)

Asbestos is a family of fibrous silicates including curled, flexible *serpentines*, e.g., chrysotile, and brittle straight *amphiboles*, e.g., crocidolite.

Heavy occupational exposure causes diffuse interstitial fibrosis, which is morphologically nonspecific except for the presence of numerous asbestos bodies (described below) within the scarred lung.

PATHOGENESIS. Inhaled fibers that reach the alveoli are ingested by alveolar macrophages, stimulating release of C5a and other chemoattractants. Amphiboles (straight, stiff) reach the deep lung more than serpentine fibers, accounting for greater pathogenicity. Most of the inhaled asbestos is cleared by the macrophages; the rest reaches the interstitium and lymphatics. *Some ingested fibers are coated by hemosiderin and glycoproteins to form characteristic, beaded, dumbbell-shaped asbestos bodies.*

Possible mechanisms for lung injury and progressive fibrosis include

* Release of enzymes or toxic free radicals by the macrophages/ neutrophils recruited to sites of asbestos deposition.
* Release of fibrogenic cytokines and growth factors by alveolar macrophages after phagocytosis of fibers.
* Direct stimulation of fibroblast collagen synthesis by asbestos.

In addition to pulmonary fibrosis, asbestos induces *pleural reactions*, manifested by (1) benign effusions; (2) fibrous pleural adhesions; and (3) dense fibrocalcific plaques, found on the pleura or diaphragm. The plaques may sometimes be calcified; they do not contain asbestos bodies.

Asbestos exposure is also associated with increased risk of *bronchogenic carcinoma* and malignant mesothelioma.

SARCOIDOSIS (p. 712)

A relatively common disease of unknown etiology, characterized by noncaseating granulomas in virtually any tissue.

Females are affected more frequently than males, and American blacks ten times more often than American whites. There are also geographic and other ethnic variations in prevalence.

Sarcoidosis may be entirely asymptomatic and discovered only incidentally at autopsy or as bilateral hilar adenopathy on a chest radiograph obtained for other reasons. Alternatively it may present as isolated cutaneous or ocular lesions, peripheral lymphadenopathy, or hepatosplenomegaly; with the insidious onset of respiratory difficulties or constitutional symptoms (fever, night sweats, weight loss); or with an acute onset accompanied by fever, erythema nodosum, and polyarthritis.

Although elevated serum IgG and calcium, characteristic chest and phalangeal x-ray changes, and a typical clinical history may strongly suggest the diagnosis, *it can be definitively established only by biopsy (often liver or lymph node) to document noncaseating granulomas*. However, other diseases (e.g., tuberculosis, berylliosis, fungal infections) may also show the same histologic features. Diagnosis of sarcoidosis is then one of exclusion.

ETIOLOGY. The distinctive granulomatous response suggests an immune-mediated phenomenon. Immune abnormalities include

- Lymphocytic alveolitis, with numerous activated CD4 + T cells (increased IL-2 production, HLA-DR antigen proliferation, and similarly activated alveolar macrophages (increased IL-1, oxygen radical production).
- Cutaneous anergy to a wide variety of agents that normally induce a local cutaneous delayed hypersensitivity reaction (e.g., tuberculin).
- An absolute lymphopenia mainly due to reduced circulating T cells. Circulating B cells are present in normal numbers and are hyperreactive.
- Activated helper T cells and their secreted cytokines would account for the influx of monocytes and subsequent granulomas and cell-mediated injury in tissues.
- Elevated circulating γ-δ T cells (associated with mycobacterial disease) and (variably) positive PCR assays for mycobacterial DNA in sarcoidal tissue have revived interest in an infectious etiology, but the cause of sarcoidosis remains unknown.

MORPHOLOGY. Other than organomegaly (liver, spleen, lymph nodes), no macroscopic change. *Characteristic are the microscopic granulomas composed of tightly clustered epithelioid histiocytes, often including multinucleated giant cells. There is rarely central necrosis.* Also frequently present (60% of granulomas) are *Schaumann bodies* (laminated, calcified proteinaceous concretions) and *asteroid bodies* (stellate inclusions within giant cells).

Lymph nodes. Virtually always involved, most commonly in the hilar and mediastinal regions, but possibly any node. Tonsils affected 25% to 33% of the time.

Lungs. Common site of involvement. Characteristically, diffuse, scattered granulomas (showing a reticulonodular pattern on x-rays) and not grossly apparent except for foci of coalesced granulomas. Pulmonary lesions have a strong tendency to heal so that only hyalinized scars may be seen microscopically.

Spleen and Liver. Microscopically affected in up to 75% of patients. Splenomegaly occurs in only 18%. Hepatomegaly is less frequent.

Skin. Cutaneous sarcoid occurs in 33% to 50% of patients, presenting in a variety of gross forms including discrete subcutaneous nodules, erythematous scaling plaques, and lesions in the mucous membranes.

Eye. Affected in 20% to 50% of cases, as iritis, iridocyclitis, or choroid retinitis.

CLINICAL FEATURES. Sarcoid may

- Be slowly progressive.
- Pursue a remitting/resolving course.
- Spontaneously resolve (with or without steroid therapy).

In 65% to 70% of patients there are no or only minimal residual manifestations; 20% have permanent lung or ocular dysfunction; and 10% die, primarily from progressive pulmonary fibrosis and cor pulmonale.

IDIOPATHIC PULMONARY FIBROSIS (p. 714)

This is a poorly understood disorder of unknown etiology *characterized by progressive pulmonary interstitial fibrosis that results in hypoxemia.* In some cases, immune complex deposition may initiate or perpetuate lesions, but the antigen(s) are unknown. The disease is most common between 30 and 50 years of age.

MORPHOLOGY. Changes vary according to stage.

In *early stages* there is interstitial and intra-alveolar edema, interstitial infiltration by leukocytes, and type II pneumonocyte proliferation.

Interstitial and intra-alveolar fibrosis are characteristic of *intermediate stages*. In the *end stages*, the lung consists of spaces lined by epithelium and separated by inflammatory fibrous tissue (honeycomb lung).

The disease is progressive in most cases, resulting in pulmonary insufficiency, cor pulmonale, and cardiac failure.

HYPERSENSITIVITY PNEUMONITIS (p. 715)

This immunologically mediated disorder is caused by inhaled dusts or antigens, e.g.:

- Farmer's lung: spores of thermophilic actinomycetes in hay.
- Pigeon breeder's lung: proteins from bird feathers/excreta.
- Humidifier/air-conditioner lung: thermophilic bacteria.

Histologic changes include interstitial pneumonitis and fibrosis and a variable number of noncaseating, loosely formed granulomas. Early cessation of exposure to the injurious agent prevents progression to serious chronic fibrosis. The clinical manifestations are varied and include cough, dyspnea, fever, diffuse and nodular radiographic densities, and a restrictive pattern of pulmonary dysfunction.

PULMONARY EOSINOPHILIA (p. 716)

Diverse clinicopathologic conditions characterized by infiltration of eosinophils in the pulmonary interstitial and/or alveolar spaces, including

- *Simple pulmonary eosinophilia* (Loeffler's syndrome), transient, benign infiltrates with prominent eosinophilia in blood and lung.
- *Tropical eosinophilia*, caused by microfilariae.
- *Secondary chronic pulmonary eosinophilia*, induced by infections, hypersensitivity, asthma, and allergic bronchopulmonary aspergillosis.
- *Idiopathic chronic eosinophilic pneumonia*, a disorder of unknown etiology, manifested by focal consolidation of lung with prominent lymphocytes and eosinophils. It is generally steroid responsive.

BRONCHIOLITIS OBLITERANS— ORGANIZING PNEUMONIA (p. 716)

A common response to infectious or inflammatory injury of the lungs.

- Clinically associated with cough, dyspnea, and often a recent respiratory tract infection; other etiologic associations are inhaled toxins, drugs, and collagen-vascular disease.
- Major pathologic findings include loose fibrous tissue plugs within bronchioles and organizing pneumonia.
- Many patients improve gradually or with steroid therapy.

DIFFUSE PULMONARY HEMORRHAGE (p. 717)

A serious complication of some interstitial lung diseases, particularly the so-called *pulmonary hemorrhage syndromes*, which include

- *Goodpasture's syndrome*—a necrotizing, hemorrhagic interstitial pneumonitis and progressive glomerulonephritis caused by antibodies against analogous basement membrane antigens in lungs and kidneys.
- *Idiopathic pulmonary hemosiderosis*—a chronic, episodic hemorrhage of the lung, of unknown etiology, resulting in prominent hemosiderin deposition and fibrosis.
- *Vasculitis-associated hemorrhage*—seen with Wegener's granulomatosis, systemic lupus erythematosus (SLE), and hypersensitivity angitis.

PULMONARY ALVEOLAR PROTEINOSIS (p. 718)

A disease of obscure etiology and pathogenesis characterized *radiologically* by diffuse pulmonary opacification; *histologically* by accumulation of dense, amorphous, PAS-positive lipid-laden material in intracellular spaces; and *clinically* by respiratory difficulty, cough, and sputum-containing gelatinous material. *The intra-alveolar exudate consists of surfactant-like material, necrotic alveolar macrophages, and type II epithelial cells.*

The disease may occur after exposure to irritating dusts and chemicals and in immunosuppressed individuals. It is progressive in many patients, but some have a benign course with eventual resolution of the lesions.

COMPLICATIONS OF THERAPIES (p. 719)

Important complications of therapy include

- *Drug-induced lung disease*, ranging from acute bronchospasm to chronic fibrosis.
- *Radiation-induced lung disease*. Acute pneumonitis occurs 1–6 months after therapy (usually for thoracic tumors); pathology is that of diffuse alveolar damage. Chronic radiation fibrosis may follow.
- *Rejection of transplanted lungs*, including acute vascular and chronic airway forms.

TUMORS (p. 720)

BRONCHOGENIC CARCINOMA (p. 720)

Makes up 90% to 95% of lung tumors. It is the most common cause of cancer death in both men and women.

PATHOGENESIS. *Tobacco smoking is well established as the most important and common etiologic factor in the development of lung cancer.*

- *Statistically*, there is an unequivocal link between the frequency of lung cancer and the number of pack-years of smoking.
- *Clinically*, hyperplastic and atypical changes can be seen in the bronchial epithelium of smokers and in the vicinity of bronchial cancer.
- *Experimentally*, there are numerous known carcinogens in cig-

arette smoke (e.g., polycyclic aromatic hydrocarbons), but it has not been possible to induce bronchogenic cancers readily by inhalation in experimental animals.

Other etiologic factors include exposure to radiation (atomic bomb survivors, uranium miners), asbestos (especially combined with smoking), air pollution (radon, particulates), and miscellaneous occupational inhaled substances (e.g., nickel, chromates, arsenic). Genetic mechanisms implicated include dominant oncogenes (e.g., K-*ras* in adenocarcinomas) and loss of tumor suppressor genes.

HISTOLOGIC TYPES. Bronchogenic carcinomas are classified by their predominant histologic appearance (Table 15–4).

Squamous cell carcinoma has the closest correlation with smoking. Most arise in or near the hilus of the lung. The tumors are more common in males. Microscopically, they vary from well-differentiated keratinizing neoplasms to anaplastic tumors with only focal differentiation.

Adenocarcinoma is the most common lung cancer in women and is often associated with smoking. It frequently presents as a peripheral mass. The characteristic microscopic features include gland formation, usually with mucin production. There is often an adjacent desmoplastic tissue response.

Small cell carcinoma is the most malignant of lung cancers and usually presents as a central or hilar tumor. It is strongly associated with cigarette smoking. The characteristic microscopic features include small, "oat"-like cells with little cytoplasm in nests or clusters, without squamous or glandular organization. Ultrastructurally, the cancer cells may exhibit neurosecretory granules, and immunohistochemical cell stains are usually positive for neuroendocrine markers. It is these tumors that most often produce paraneoplastic syndromes (described later).

Large cell carcinoma probably represents poorly differentiated squamous cell carcinomas or adenocarcinomas. Occasionally, there are peculiar histologic elements (giant cell, clear cell, spindle cell variants).

CLINICAL FEATURES. Bronchogenic carcinomas usually present with cough, weight loss, chest pain, and dyspnea (Table 15–5). Overall 5-year survival is approximately 9%. Surgical resection of solitary (non–small cell) tumors offers some improved survival (30% to 40% 5-year) for a minority of patients with localized disease. Small cell carcinoma has almost always metastasized by

Table 15–4. Histologic Classification of Bronchogenic Carcinoma

Squamous cell (epidermoid) carcinoma
Adenocarcinoma
    Bronchial derived (acinar; papillary; solid)
    Bronchioloalveolar
Small cell carcinoma
    Oat cell (lymphocyte-like)
    Intermediate cell (polygonal)
    Combined (usually with squamous)
Large cell carcinoma (undifferentiated; giant cell; clear cell)
Combined squamous cell carcinoma and adenocarcinoma

From Cotran, R. S., Kumar, V., and Robbins, S. L.: Robbins Pathologic Basis of Disease. 5th ed. Philadelphia, W. B. Saunders Co., 1994, p. 722.

Table 15–5. Local Effects of Lung Tumor Spread

Clinical Feature	Pathologic Basis
Pneumonia/abscess/lobar collapse	Tumor obstruction of airway
Lipid pneumonia	Tumor obstruction; accumulation of cellular lipid in foamy macrophages
Pleural effusion	Tumor spread into pleura
Hoarseness	Recurrent laryngeal nerve invasion
Dysphagia	Esophageal invasion
Diaphragm paralysis	Phrenic nerve invasion
Rib destruction	Chest wall invasion
Superior vena caval (SVC) syndrome	SVC compression by tumor
Horner's syndrome°	Sympathetic ganglia invasion
Pericarditis/tamponade	Pericardial involvement

°Horner's syndrome = enophthalmos, ptosis, miosis, and anhidrosis, unilateral.

From Cotran, R. S., Kumar, V., and Robbins, S. L.: Robbins Pathologic Basis of Disease. 5th ed. Philadelphia, W. B. Saunders Co., 1994, p. 725.

the time of diagnosis, precluding surgical intervention. It is responsive to chemotherapy but ultimately recurs. Other types show disappointing responses to chemotherapy.

Paraneoplastic syndromes associated with bronchogenic carcinoma often stem from release of the following hormones:

- ADH (syndrome of inappropriate antidiuretic hormone release).
- ACTH (Cushing's syndrome).
- Parathormone or PGE (hypercalcemia).
- Calcitonin (hypocalcemia).
- Gonadotropins (gynecomastia).
- Serotonin (carcinoid syndrome).

Other paraneoplastic syndromes include myopathy, peripheral neuropathy, acanthosis nigricans, and hypertrophic pulmonary osteoarthropathy (clubbing of fingers, etc.).

BRONCHIOLOALVEOLAR CARCINOMA (p. 725)

An uncommon form of adenocarcinoma arising in the terminal bronchioloalveolar regions, almost always in the lung periphery. Macroscopic forms include single or multiple nodules or a diffuse, pneumonic consolidation with tumor. Histologically, the tumor is distinctive in that tall, columnar, often mucin-producing tumor cells line up along preserved alveolar septa, forming papillary projections within the spaces. Clinically, they occur in men and women equally and are not usually associated with smoking. Prognosis is relatively favorable after resection of a solitary nodule but dismal for those with diffuse involvement.

BRONCHIAL CARCINOID (p. 726)

Represents 1% to 5% of all lung tumors. Characterized by neuroendocrine differentiation. Surgical resection is curative in 90% to 95%. A minority (10%) are more aggressive, exhibiting local invasion or distant metastases.

Grossly, the tumors are usually intrabronchial, highly vascular, polypoid masses less than 3 to 4 cm in diameter. Microscopically, they are composed of uniform, small, round cells in nests or cords *resembling intestinal carcinoids*. Occasionally, tumors show atypia, mitoses, or pleomorphism. Neurosecretory granules are seen ultrastructurally, and neuroendocrine differentiation is confirmed by immunostaining for neuron-specific enolase, serotonin, calcitonin, or bombesin.

MISCELLANEOUS TUMORS (p. 727)

Hamartomas are relatively common, benign, nodular neoplasms composed of cartilage and admixtures of other mesenchymal tissues, e.g., fat, blood vessels, fibrous tissue.

Mediastinal tumors arise from local structures or may represent metastatic disease (Table 15–6).

Secondary involvement of the lung by metastatic tumor is common. Spread to the lung can occur via direct extension from contiguous organs or lymphatics, or hematogenous routes. Patterns of disease include discrete masses or nodules, growth within peribronchial lymphatics (lymphangitis carcinomatosa), and (rarely) multiple tumor microemboli.

DISEASES OF THE PLEURA (p. 728)

Most pleural lesions are secondary to underlying lung disease.

PLEURAL EFFUSIONS (p. 728)

Accumulations of transudate (hydrothorax) or serous exudate may appear with

- Increased hydrostatic pressure, e.g., heart failure.
- Increased vascular permeability, e.g., pneumonia.
- Decreased oncotic pressure, e.g., nephrotic syndrome.
- Increased negative intrapleural pressure, e.g., atelectasis.
- Decreased lymphatic drainage, e.g., carcinomatosis.

The various patterns of inflammatory reaction include (1) serofibrinous pleuritis, reflecting inflammatory processes in the lung, e.g., tuberculosis, pneumonia, infarcts, abscesses, or systemic diseases (such as rheumatoid arthritis, uremia); and (2) *suppurative pleuritis* or empyema, usually reflecting infection of

Table 15–6. Mediastinal Tumors

Superior Mediastinum	*Posterior Mediastinum*
Lymphoma	Neurogenic tumors
Thymoma	(schwannoma;
Thyroid lesions	neurofibroma)
Metastatic carcinoma	Lymphoma
Parathyroid tumors	Gastroenteric hernia
Anterior Mediastinum	*Middle Mediastinum*
Thymoma	Bronchogenic cysts
Teratoma	Pericardial cyst
Lymphoma	Lymphoma
Thyroid lesions	
Parathyroid tumors	

From Cotran, R. S., Kumar, V., and Robbins, S. L.: Robbins Pathologic Basis of Disease. 5th ed. Philadelphia, W. B. Saunders Co., 1994, p. 728.

the pleural space leading to accumulation of pus. Organization of these exudates with dense fibrous adhesions can affect lung expansion. *Hemorrhagic pleuritis* occurs with bleeding disorders, neoplastic involvement, and certain rickettsial diseases.

Other pleural fluid accumulations include hemothorax (a fatal complication of a ruptured aortic aneurysm) and chylothorax (a collection of milky lymph fluid, usually with neoplastic lymphatic obstruction).

PNEUMOTHORAX (p. 730)

Air or gas in the pleural cavity. Pneumothorax can be traumatic, e.g., due to air escape from the lung after rib fractures, or spontaneous, occurring in young individuals after rupture of peripheral apical blebs. *Tension pneumothorax* occurs when lung and mediastinal structures are compressed by the collected air. It represents a serious, potentially fatal complication.

PLEURAL TUMORS (p. 730)

The most common pleural tumors are metastatic from lung, breast, ovaries, or other organs. Metastases often cause a malignant effusion containing tumor cells that can be detected by cytopathologic examination.

Pleural Fibroma (p. 730)

A localized, noninvasive, fibroblastic tumor ("benign mesothelioma") composed of submesothelial fibroblasts in the pleural surfaces of the lungs. Resection is curative.

Malignant Mesothelioma (p. 730)

An uncommon tumor of mesothelial cells, this occurs most often on the pleura and rarely in the peritoneum or other organs. It is associated with occupational exposure to asbestos in 90% of cases, but only 20% of patients have actual pulmonary asbestosis. The lifetime risk in heavily exposed individuals is 7% to 10%, and the latent period between exposure and the development of mesothelioma is 25 to 45 years. Nevertheless, bronchogenic carcinoma remains the most common lung tumor found in asbestos workers.

CLINICAL FEATURES. Patients present with chest pain, dyspnea, and recurrent pleural effusions.

MORPHOLOGY. The tumor spreads diffusely over the surface of the lung and its fissures, forming a sheath of neoplastic tissue around the lung. It rarely is primary in the peritoneum.

Microscopically, the tumor consists typically of biphasic patterns of growth:

- Sarcomatoid conformation consisting of malignant, spindle-shaped cells resembling fibrosarcoma.
- Epithelioid growth composed of epithelium-like cells that form tubules and papillary projections resembling adenocarcinomas. Antigenic (keratin (positivity) and ultrastructural (microvilli) features present in mesotheliomas allow distinction from adenocarcinomas.
- Epithelioid pattern is most common (70%), followed by sarcomatoid (20%) and mixed (biphasic) (10%) tumors.

Mesotheliomas are highly malignant tumors that invade the lung and can metastasize widely. Few patients survive longer than 2 years.

CHAPTER SIXTEEN

The Gastrointestinal Tract

ESOPHAGUS

CONGENITAL ANOMALIES

Atresia and Fistulas (p. 756)

Uncommon, usually discovered soon after birth; many are incompatible with life; are often associated with congenital heart disease and other GI tract malformations.

- *Atresia*: A segment of the esophagus is only a thin, noncanalized cord, with blind pouches on either side.
- In 80% to 90% of cases, a *fistula* connects one of the pouches with the trachea or a mainstem bronchus.

Stenosis, Webs, and Rings (p. 757)

Stenosis may be congenital or acquired in adult life following severe esophageal injury (gastroesophageal reflux, radiation, scleroderma, or caustic injury). Mucosal rings are smooth ledges of mucosa with a vascularized fibrous core: when in upper esophagus, called *webs*; when at the gastroesophageal junction, called *Schatzki's rings*. Acquired lesions usually present in adult life.

- Feature of esophageal narrowing, whatever the cause: progressive dysphagia, especially to solid foods.

LESIONS ASSOCIATED WITH MOTOR DYSFUNCTION

Achalasia (p. 757)

Failure of relaxation with consequent esophageal dilatation, dysphagia, and regurgitation. Primary form presents in young adulthood or earlier, remains a problem for remainder of life. Putatively caused by abnormal innervation of esophagus. Risk of esophageal carcinoma: 2% to 7%. Other complications: candidal esophagitis, diverticula, and aspiration pneumonia.

- Manometry reveals aperistalsis; impaired relaxation of the lower esophageal sphincter (LES); increased LES resting tone.
- Secondary achalasia: caused by Chagas' disease (*Trypanosoma cruzi*), disorders of the vagal dorsal motor nuclei (polio, surgical ablation), diabetic autonomic neuropathy, infiltrative disorders (malignancy, amyloidosis, sarcoidosis).

MORPHOLOGY. Dilated esophagus above LES; thickened

(muscular hypertrophy) or thinned (distention) muscular wall; diminished myenteric ganglia; secondary mucosal damage.

Hiatal Hernia (p. 758)

Saclike dilatation of the stomach with protrusion above the diaphragm, associated with separation of the diaphragmatic crura and widening of the esophageal foramen. Two patterns:

• *Sliding* (axial) *hiatal hernia* (90%): Marked by a shortened esophagus, traction of upper stomach into thorax, bell-like dilatation of stomach within the thoracic cavity.
• *Paraesophageal hiatal hernia* (rolling hernia, <10%): Cardia of stomach dissects alongside esophagus into thorax, vulnerable to strangulation and infarction.

CLINICAL FEATURES. Reported in up to 1% to 20% of normal adults—may affect infants and children. Only 9% have symptomatology (retrosternal chest pain related to regurgitation of gastric juices). May ulcerate or strangulate, causing bleeding or perforation.

Diverticula (p. 759)

Outpouchings of one or more layers of the esophageal wall.

• *Pharyngeal (Zenker's) diverticulum*: in the upper esophagus: motor dysfunction is implicated.
• *Traction diverticulum*: more distal location, attributed to fibrosing mediastinal processes or abnormal motility.

Lacerations (Mallory-Weiss Syndrome) (p. 759)

Attributed to episodes of excessive vomiting in setting of toxic gastritis, with failure of LES relaxation. Most frequently seen in alcoholics. May lead to potentially massive hematemesis, inflammation, residual ulcer, mediastinitis, peritonitis.
MORPHOLOGY. Irregular, longitudinal tears in the esophagus at the esophagogastric junction, several mm to cm in length. May involve only the mucosa or may rarely penetrate the wall.

VARICES (p. 759)

Occur in two-thirds of cirrhotic patients, most commonly in alcoholics. Prolonged and severe portal hypertension induces formation of collateral bypass channels: through the coronary veins of the stomach into esophageal subepithelial and submucosal veins (*varices*) and thence to the azygos veins and systemic circulation. Other portosystemic shunts: rectal canal (*hemorrhoids*); falciform ligament to abdominal wall (*caput medusa*).
MORPHOLOGY. Tortuous, dilated veins lying primarily within the submucosa of distal esophagus and proximal stomach, with irregular protrusion of overlying mucosa into lumen. May develop superficial ulceration, resulting in inflammation, adherent blood clot, and potential rupture.
CLINICAL FEATURES. Clinically silent until rupture, with catastrophic hematemesis (40% fatality for each episode of bleeding, 90% chance of recurrence within a year in survivors).

• Massive hematemesis in patients with varices also may be caused by gastritis, esophageal laceration, peptic ulcer.

ESOPHAGITIS (p. 761)

PREDISPOSING CONDITIONS

- *Reflux of gastric contents (reflux esophagitis).*
- Prolonged gastric intubation.
- Ingestion of irritants: alcohol, corrosive acids or alkalis, excessively hot fluids, smoking.
- Uremia.
- Bacteremia or viremia; herpes; cytomegalovirus infection.
- Fungal infection: candida, mucormycosis, aspergillosis.
- Radiation.
- Cytotoxic anticancer therapy.
- Systemic desquamative disorders: pemphigoid, epidermolysis bullosa.
- Graft-versus-host disease.

PATHOGENESIS. Gastric regurgitation (most often related to hiatal hernia or disordered motility but other possible causes as well) leads to exposure of esophageal mucosa to acid, bile acids, and/or lysolecithin in regurgitated fluid; immunologic debilitation; direct toxic damage by ingested material. These influences individually or collectively contribute to mucosal damage.

MORPHOLOGY (from mild to severe). Hyperemia and edema; thickening of basal zone and thinning of superficial layers of stratified squamous epithelium; mucosal polymorphonuclear leukocyte infiltrate; eventually superficial necrosis and ulceration with adherent inflammatory exudate.

CLINICAL FEATURES. Reflux esophagitis is usually encountered in adults but may be seen in children and infants. Symptoms include dysphagia, heartburn, regurgitation of sour brash, hematemesis, and melena. Complications are stricture and Barrett's esophagus.

Barrett's Esophagus (p. 762)

Marked by *metaplasia of the distal esophageal squamous epithelium to a columnar epithelium, in response to prolonged injury.* Most common in adults but may be seen in children and infants.

PATHOGENESIS (proposed). Long-standing gastroesophageal reflux leads to inflammation and ulceration of squamous mucosa; healing is by re-epithelialization by pluripotent stem cells, which in the setting of low pH differentiate into more resistant gastric-type or intestinal epithelium.

MORPHOLOGY. *Gross:* Red, velvety mucosa existing as an irregular circumferential band at the gastroesophageal junction; may also take the form of linear streaks or isolated patches of metaplastic mucosa in the distal esophagus. *Microscopic:* A mixture of gastric and intestinal-type columnar epithelial cells (mucin-secreting and absorptive). Substantial risk of ulceration, stricture, and adenocarcinoma (30 times the normal risk of cancer).

TUMORS

Benign Tumors (p. 764)

- *Intramural or submucosal tumors:* leiomyoma, fibroma, lipoma, hemangioma, neurofibroma, lymphangioma.
- *Mucosal tumors* include: squamous papilloma, fibrovascular polyp (bland fibrovascular core with overlying epithelium), inflammatory polyp (severely inflamed mesenchyme with overlying epithelium).

They rarely exceed 3 cm in diameter.

Malignant Tumors (p. 764)

- Esophageal carcinomas make up 6% of all cancers of GI tract, but cause a disproportionately high death rate.
- Malignant stromal tumors (of smooth muscle or fibroblast origin) are rare.

Squamous Cell Carcinoma (p. 764)

EPIDEMIOLOGY. Adults over age 50 years; more often in men; incidence varies considerably among geographic areas, highest in Northern China, Iran, Russia, South Africa; blacks are at greater risk than whites.

PATHOGENESIS. Multifactorial, with synergistic interaction of environmental and dietary factors, perhaps modified by genetic factors (Table 16–1).

MORPHOLOGY. Begin as *in situ* lesions: gray-white, plaque-like thickenings or elevations of mucosa. With progression, the lesions extend longitudinally along the esophageal axis, circumferentially, and deep (with invasion).

- Distribution (in thirds): upper esophagus 20%, middle esophagus 50%, lower esophagus 30%.
- Gross patterns: *polypoid* (60%), *necrotic and excavating* (25%), *diffusely infiltrative* (15%). Early, *superficial* carcinoma denotes invasion no deeper than submucosa.
- Usually moderately to well-differentiated, with or without keratinization.
- Tend to spread via the rich submucosal lymphatic network to nearby lymph nodes and locally by deep extension into adjacent mediastinal structures.

CLINICAL FEATURES. Insidious in onset. Symptoms that develop late in the course are dysphagia, esophageal obstruction, weight

---

Table 16–1. Factors Associated with the Development of Esophageal Squamous Cell Carcinoma

---

Dietary
Vitamin deficiency (A, C, riboflavin, thiamine, pyridoxine)
Deficiency of trace metals (zinc, molybdenum)
Fungal contamination of foodstuffs
High content of nitrites/nitrosamines

Lifestyle
Alcohol consumption
Tobacco usage

Esophageal Disorders
Long-standing esophagitis
Achalasia
Plummer-Vinson syndrome

Predisposing Influences
Long-standing celiac disease
Ectodermal dysplasia, epidermolysis bullosa
Genetic (racial) predisposition

Modified from Cotran, R. S., Kumar, V., and Robbins, S. L.: Robbins Pathologic Basis of Disease. 5th ed. Philadelphia, W. B. Saunders Co., 1994, p. 764.

loss, hemorrhage, sepsis secondary to ulceration, and fistula formation into respiratory tree with aspiration.

- Curative resection is possible in many cases when discovered as part of screening programs.
- Five-year survival: superficial 75%; advanced "resectable" 25%; but only 5% for all patients with esophageal cancer.

Adenocarcinoma (p. 765)

Represents one-quarter of esophageal cancers. The primary risk factor is Barrett's mucosa, since cancer appears to evolve through a dysplastic change in Barrett's mucosa.

MORPHOLOGY. *The vast majority arise from areas of dysplasia in Barrett's mucosa*—most are in distal third of esophagus. *Gross*: may be exophytic nodule or excavated and deeply infiltrative. *Microscopic*: mucin-producing glandular tumors with intestinal features or diffusely infiltrative signet ring cells; rarely adenosquamous or small cell type.

CLINICAL FEATURES. Arise in Barrett's patients over age 40 years, more common in men than women, symptoms as in squamous cell carcinoma. Previous symptoms of gastroesophageal reflux are present in fewer than half of patients. Overall 5-year survival is 15%; screening programs detect disease earlier.

STOMACH

CONGENITAL ANOMALIES

Diaphragmatic Hernias (p. 769)

- Weakness or defect in diaphragm (usually on the left) but does not involve the hiatal orifice, thus not a "hiatal" hernia.
- Usually a portion (or all) of the stomach herniates *in utero*, occasionally small bowel, liver. If hernia is large, respiratory impairment with pulmonary hypoplasia threatens life.

Pyloric Stenosis (p. 769)

Congenital hypertrophic pyloric stenosis consists of hypertrophy and possibly hyperplasia of circular muscle of the muscularis propria of the pyloris. Occurs in 1:300 to 1:900 live births, males:females 4:1. Peristalsis is visible and a firm, ovoid mass is palpable by physical examination.

- Multifactorial inheritance, high concordance in twins.
- Mucosal edema and inflammation aggravate narrowing.
- Regurgitation and vomiting by third week of life.
- Full-thickness muscle-splitting incision (pyloromyotomy) is curative.

Acquired pyloric stenosis may result from long-term chronic antral gastritis, peptic ulcers close to the pylorus, or malignancy (carcinoma, lymphoma, pancreatic carcinoma).

GASTRITIS (p. 770)

Defined as *inflammation of the gastric mucosa*.

Acute Gastritis (p. 770)

An acute mucosal inflammatory process, usually transient.
PATHOGENESIS. Associations: chronic and heavy use of

NSAIDs, particularly aspirin; excessive alcohol consumption; heavy smoking; cancer chemotherapy; uremia; systemic infection; severe stress (burns, trauma, surgery); ischemia and shock; ingestion of acid, alkali; gastric irradiation; mechanical trauma; following distal gastrectomy.

Proposed causal mechanisms, acting singly or in combination: increased acid production with back-diffusion; decreased production of surface bicarbonate buffer; reduced mucosal blood flow; disruption of mucous layer; direct damage to mucosal epithelium.

MORPHOLOGY. Moderate mucosal edema and hyperemia with entry of neutrophils into the epithelial layer (*"activity"*). Sloughing of the superficial epithelium (*erosion*) and hemorrhage constitute *acute hemorrhagic erosive gastritis*.

CLINICAL FEATURES. Asymptomatic or minor abdominal pain; or acute abdominal pain with hematemesis.

Chronic Gastritis (p. 771)

Defined as *the presence of chronic mucosal inflammatory changes leading eventually to mucosal atrophy and epithelial metaplasia*. Constitutes a background for carcinoma.

PATHOGENESIS. Etiologic associations are

- Immunologic (*autoimmune gastritis*): antibodies to parietal cells (including the H^+,K^+-ATPase) cause parietal cell atrophy and destruction; decreased production of intrinsic factor may lead to pernicious anemia.
- Chronic infection, especially *Helicobacter pylori*.
- Toxic: alcohol and tobacco usage.
- Postsurgical: postantrectomy reflux of bile.
- Motor/mechanical: e.g., obstruction, atony.
- Radiation.
- Granulomatous conditions: e.g., Crohn's disease.
- Graft-versus-host disease, uremia, amyloidosis.

Helicobacter pylori. This S-shaped gram-negative rod colonizes over 50% of Americans over age 50 years. The theory is that *colonization of gastric mucosa damaged by other events leads to a state of retarded healing and chronic mucosal inflammation*; *H. pylori* per se does not necessarily cause chronic gastritis by itself.

MORPHOLOGY. Reddened and coarse-textured mucosa, may be boggy or exhibit flattening; has variable distribution depending on the origins of inflammation:

- *Autoimmune*: diffuse damage of body-fundic mucosa.
- *Environmental causes* (including *H. pylori*): more patchy distribution in antrum, or antrum and corpus.

Microscopic: An inflammatory infiltrate of lymphocytes and plasma cells in the lamina propria, either involving the superficial portion or entire mucosal thickness. Modifying features are activity (intraepithelial neutrophils); regenerative change; variable atrophy; metaplasia to an intestinal-type of epithelium; and dysplasia in some cases of long-standing chronic gastritis. *H. pylori*, when present, are found nestled in the superficial mucous layer but do not invade.

CLINICAL FEATURES. Usually few symptoms—maybe nausea, vomiting, and upper abdominal discomfort. Rarely, overt pernicious anemia develops in autoimmune gastritis. Laboratory abnormalities: gastric hypochlorhydria, serum hypergastrinemia. Long-term risk of cancer is 2% to 4%.

GASTRIC ULCERATION (p. 773)

An ulcer is defined as *a defect in the mucosa of the alimentary tract that extends through the muscularis mucosa into the submucosa or deeper.*

Peptic Ulcers (p. 773)

Chronic, most often solitary, ulcers in any portion of the alimentary tract arising from exposure to acid-peptic juices. Ninety-eight percent of the ulcers are found in the duodenum and stomach, in a ratio of 4:1, respectively.

EPIDEMIOLOGY. The lifetime likelihood of peptic ulcer is 10% for American men, 4% for women, most often in middle-aged to older adults. Even with healing, the propensity to ulcers remains. There are no genetic tendencies. Duodenal ulcer is more frequent in patients with alcoholic cirrhosis, chronic obstructive pulmonary disease, chronic renal failure, or hyperparathyroidism.

MORPHOLOGY. *Gross:* Sharply punched out defect with overhanging mucosal borders, smooth and clean ulcer base. *Microscopic:* Four layers can be identified in the ulcer base: a thin superficial layer of necrotic debris sits on a zone of inflammation, which is underlaid by a layer of granulation tissue, beneath which is a fibrous scar in long-standing lesions. The surrounding mucosa usually exhibits chronic gastritis.

PATHOGENESIS. *Peptic ulcers are produced by an imbalance between the gastroduodenal mucosal defense mechanisms and damaging forces.*

- *Mucosal defense mechanisms:* surface mucus secretion; bicarbonate secretion into mucus, mucosal blood flow, apical epithelial cell transport systems, and epithelial regeneration. Prostaglandins play an uncertain role. Mucosal defense is impaired by ischemia and shock; delayed gastric emptying; or duodenal-gastric reflux.
- *Damaging forces:* gastric acid and pepsin, *H. pylori* infection, NSAIDs and aspirin, cigarettes, alcohol, impaired regulation of acid secretion (for unclear causes). The roles of *personality* and *psychologic stress* are uncertain.
- *H. pylori* plays major role: the organism is present in the gastric mucosa of 90% to 100% of patients with duodenal ulcer and 70% of those with gastric ulcer. Bacterial *urease* and *protease* presumably damage the mucosa, predisposing to inflammation, which perpetuates the mucosal injury.

CLINICAL FEATURES. Typical symptoms are epigastric gnawing, burning, or aching pain that is worse at night or 1 to 3 hours after meals; nausea; vomiting; bloating; belching; and/or weight loss. Complications include anemia (from occult bleeding), frank hemorrhage, perforation, or obstruction (from surrounding edema and scar in a pyloric channel ulcer). Malignant transformation is rare and related to the underlying gastritis.

Acute Gastric Ulceration (p. 777)

Defined as focal, acutely developing gastric mucosal defects appearing during severe stress ("stress ulcer"). Encountered in *shock, extensive burns, or severe trauma (Curling's ulcers), or elevated intracranial pressure, as from trauma or surgery (Cushing's ulcers).* NSAID use also may cause acute ulceration.

Acute gastric ulceration falls in a continuum with acute erosive gastritis, depending on the depth of mucosal damage.

PATHOGENESIS. Unclear, possibly related to impaired mucosal oxygenation, systemic acidosis, or excessive stimulation of vagal nuclei and gastric hypersecretion (in the setting of elevated intracranial pressure).

MORPHOLOGY. Ulcers are usually <1 cm in diameter, multiple, and shallow. The ulcer base is brown (blood); the adjacent mucosa is normal (both gross and microscopic).

CLINICAL FEATURES. The primary sign of acute gastric ulceration is upper gastrointestinal hemorrhage. This lesion occurs in 5% to 10% of intensive care unit patients. The single most important determinant of outcome is *the ability to correct the underlying disease condition(s)* (e.g., trauma, sepsis).

MISCELLANEOUS CONDITIONS

Hypertrophic Gastropathy (p. 778)

Several forms, but all marked by giant cerebriform enlargement of gastric rugal folds. Caused by hyperplasia of mucosal epithelial cells.

- *Menetrier's disease*: hyperplasia of surface mucosal cells.
- *Hypertrophic-hypersecretory gastropathy*: hyperplasia of parietal and chief cells.
- *Gastric gland hyperplasia* can occur secondary to excessive gastrin secretion by a gastrinoma; the condition of excessive stimulation of peptic secretions with ensuant peptic ulceration is called *Zollinger-Ellison syndrome*.

CLINICAL FEATURES. Hypertrophic gastropathies mimic diffuse gastric cancer or lymphoma on radiographic studies; patients are at risk for peptic ulceration. Excess secreted protein may cause hypoalbuminemia and a *protein-losing gastroenteropathy*. The hyperplastic mucosa may become dysplastic, with a modestly increased risk of adenocarcinoma.

Gastric Varices (p. 778)

Develop near the gastroesophageal junction in setting of portal hypertension; they are less common than esophageal varices and almost always coexist with esophageal varices.

TUMORS

Gastric Polyps (p. 779)

The term "polyp" refers to any nodule or mass that projects above the level of the surrounding mucosa; the term is generally restricted to *mass lesions arising from the mucosa*.

- The majority of gastric polyps (90%) are *hyperplastic/inflammatory polyps*: smooth-surfaced, sessile, or pedunculated polyps composed of epithelial tubules and cysts, interspersed with an inflamed stroma. They are often multiple and are seen in the setting of chronic gastritis. They are regarded as having no malignant potential *per se*.
- *Gastric adenoma*: a true neoplasm with *proliferative dysplastic epithelium*; and thereby an adenoma has malignant potential. They are usually single, and may be *sessile* (without a stalk) or *pedunculated* (with a stalk). Adenomas are much more common in the colon.

The incidence of gastric adenomas increases with age. Up to 40% of adenomas harbor carcinoma at the time of diagnosis. They arise sporadically in the background of chronic gastritis or in the setting of genetic polyposis syndromes.

Gastric Carcinoma (p. 779)

EPIDEMIOLOGY. Ninety per cent to 95% of gastric malignancies are carcinomas (versus lymphomas, carcinoids, spindle cell tumors). The worldwide distribution is widely variable. The incidence has decreased 4-fold over the last 60 years for unclear reasons, but the prognosis is dismal; gastric cancer still represents 3% of all cancer deaths in the United States.

MORPHOLOGY. Variably classified according to:

- *Depth of invasion:* early gastric carcinoma is confined to the mucosa and submucosa, regardless of the presence or absence of lymph node metastases. *Advanced gastric carcinoma* has extended beyond the submucosa.
- *Macroscopic growth pattern:* (1) exophytic; (2) flat or depressed; or (3) excavated. Uncommonly, (4) diffuse invasion throughout the stomach wall creates a rigid, thickened stomach, called *linitis plastica.*
- *Histologic subtype* according to the *Lauren classification: Intestinal:* gland-forming columnar epithelium, usually mucin-producing. This form usually exhibits a polypoid expansile growth pattern, almost always associated with intestinal metaplasia; mean age of diagnosis is 55 years, male:female 2:1; this form is decreasing in incidence. *Diffuse:* poorly differentiated, single signet-ring cells, mucin-producing (as in type 4 above); mean age of diagnosis is 48 years, male:female 1:1; this form has exhibited no change in incidence.
- Dissemination of gastric cancer to ovaries generates so-called ovarian *Krukenberg tumors.*

CLINICAL FEATURES. Gastric cancer is an insidious disease and is initially asymptomatic. Abdominal pain, anorexia, nausea, and vomiting initially mimic the symptoms of chronic gastritis; altered bowel habits, dysphagia, anemia, hemorrhage, and weight loss then develop. Spread is via lymphatics, via local invasion into adjacent structures, and vascular spread, especially to the liver. Prognosis depends only on the *depth of invasion:* 90% to 95% 5-year survival for resected early gastric cancer (even with positive lymph nodes), 10% survival for advanced disease.

SMALL AND LARGE INTESTINES
CONGENITAL ANOMALIES

Meckel's Diverticulum (p. 786)

A *diverticulum* is a mucosa-lined blind pouch leading off the alimentary tract, whose lumen communicates with the lumen of the gut. Meckel's diverticulum is the prototype congenital diverticulum, arising from persistence of a segment of the vitelline duct (which connects the yolk sac with the gut lumen). A solitary diverticulum is found 30 cm from the ileocecal valve (in the adult), consisting of a *pouch of mucosa, submucosa, and muscularis propria. Included heterotopic gastric (or pancreatic) mucosa may generate symptoms of peptic ulceration or "appendicitis."* The diverticulum may also intussuscept, incarcerate, or perforate. It is present in 2% of the normal population but is usually asymptomatic.

Congenital Aganglionic Megacolon— Hirschsprung's Disease (p. 786)

Arrested migration of neural crest cells into the gut (proximal to distal) generates an aganglionic distal colonic segment with functional obstruction, and colonic dilatation proximal to the affected segment.

MORPHOLOGY. Marked by the absence of ganglion cells and ganglia in the muscle wall (Auerbach's plexus) and submucosa (Meissner's plexus) of the affected segment. The rectum is always affected; proximal involvement is more variable. Progressive dilatation and hypertrophy of the unaffected proximal colon (megacolon) develop over time.

CLINICAL FEATURES. The incidence is 1 in 5000 to 8000 live births; male:female 4:1. Associated with Down's syndrome and neurologic abnormalities. Hirschsprung's disease manifests as a failure to pass meconium in the neonate, or abdominal distention with difficulty to pass stools in the young child. There is a risk of perforation, sepsis, or enterocolitis with ensuing fluid derangements.

Megacolon may also be acquired: Chagas' disease (infection and destruction of visceral ganglion cells), distal bowel obstruction, inflammatory bowel disease, psychosomatic disorders.

Atresia and Stenosis (p. 787)

May arise from developmental failure (e.g., intrauterine vascular accidents) or intussusception early in life; the duodenum is most commonly affected. A rare cause of obstruction is failure of the cloacal diaphragm to rupture, which leads to *imperforate anus*.

VASCULAR DISORDERS
Ischemic Bowel Disease (p. 787)

Predisposing conditions are

- *Arterial thrombosis*, secondary to atherosclerosis, vasculitis, dissecting aneurysm, angiography, surgery, or hypercoagulable states.
- *Arterial embolism* arising from cardiac thrombi (postmyocardial infarction), cardiac valve vegetations, aortic atheroembolism, or following aortic angiography.
- *Venous thrombosis* occurring in hypercoagulable states, cirrhosis, sepsis, surgery (and abdominal trauma), and neoplasms invasive into the portal vein (e.g., hepatocellular carcinoma).
- *Nonocclusive ischemia* resulting from cardiac failure, shock, dehydration, and vasoconstrictive drugs.
- *Miscellaneous causes*: radiation, volvulus, stricture, herniation.

MORPHOLOGY. Takes one of several patterns:

- *Transmural infarction*: Sudden and total occlusion of a major vessel leads to infarction of all bowel layers. The bowel segment becomes hemorrhagic, owing to blood reflow into damaged area from adjacent vascularized segments. The bowel appears rubbery and dusky and may be swollen (by edema) or flaccid. Superimposed bacterial proliferation produces gangrene, and perforation may develop within days.

- *Mural and mucosal infarction*: Incomplete necrosis or necrosis of the mucosa only may be due to any cause of vascular compromise (occlusive or nonocclusive). The bowel mucosa appears hemorrhagic, but the serosa may be normal. This form is frequently patchy in distribution, and the degree of inflammation depends on the duration of injury.
- *Chronic ischemia*: Chronic vascular insufficiency causes mucosal inflammation and possibly ulceration, in a segmental patchy distribution. Mural fibrosis and stricture may develop.

Transmural infarction is more common in the small bowel, which is completely dependent on the mesenteric blood supply; the large bowel has posterior abdominal wall collaterals in several places.

CLINICAL FEATURES. Total infarction imparts a 50% to 75% death rate and usually occurs in severely ill patients. It presents with severe abdominal pain and tenderness, bloody diarrhea or gross melena, nausea, vomiting, bloating, and abdominal wall rigidity. Incomplete infarction produces nonspecific abdominal complaints, which are easily confused with acute and chronic inflammatory conditions.

Angiodysplasia (p. 789)

Consists of tortuous, abnormal dilatations of the submucosal veins in the cecum and ascending colon, which extend into the lamina propria. Lesions range from small, focal ectasias to large, dilated, tortuous venous formations. They have a propensity for bleeding, which may be massive.

PATHOGENESIS. These are acquired ectasias occurring mostly in elderly people and are attributed to long-term partial intermittent occlusion of submucosal veins in the cecum and ascending colon, the site of maximal wall tension due to its greater diameter (Laplace's Law).

Hemorrhoids (p. 789)

Consist of variceal dilatation of anal and perianal submucosal venous plexuses, affecting 5% of the adult population. Associated with constipation (straining at stool), venous stasis of pregnancy, and cirrhosis (portal hypertension).

MORPHOLOGY. Ectasia of the inferior hemorrhoidal plexus below the anorectal line produces external hemorrhoids; in the superior hemorrhoidal plexus, internal hemorrhoids result— these may coexist. Complications include secondary thrombosis (with recanalization), strangulation, and/or ulceration with fissure formation.

ENTEROCOLITIS

Diarrhea and Dysentery (p. 790)

Diarrhea is roughly defined as *daily stool production in excess of 250 gm, containing 70% to 95% water*, resulting in an *increase in stool volume, fluidity, and/or frequency*. Low-volume, painful, bloody diarrhea is known as *dysentery*. The basic forms of diarrhea are

- *Secretory diarrhea*: net intestinal fluid secretion >500 ml/day, which is isotonic with plasma and persists during fasting; due to intrinsic intestinal secretions.
- *Osmotic diarrhea*: osmotic forces exerted by luminal solutes

lead to >500 ml stool/day; abates during fasting and exhibits an osmotic gap (stool osmolality exceeds electrolyte concentration by >50 mOsm).
- *Exudative diseases*: purulent, bloody stools that persist during fasting; frequent stools but variable in volume.
- *Malabsorption*: voluminous, bulky stools with excess fat and osmolarity; diarrhea abates on fasting.
- *Deranged motility*: variable in stool content and in frequency; other causes must be excluded before invoking deranged motility as a potential cause.

Major causes for each form of diarrhea are given in Tables 16–2 and 16–3; contributing mechanisms may overlap.

Infectious Enterocolitis (p. 791)

A major cause of morbidity and mortality worldwide:

- More than 12,000 deaths *per day* of children of developing countries, causing one-half of all childhood deaths before age 5 years worldwide.
- Attack rates in industrialized nations are one to two illnesses *per person per year*, afflicting 40% of United States population annually.
- Parasitic and protozoal diseases affect more than *one-half of the world's population* on a chronic or recurrent basis—see Chapter 8.

Viral Gastroenterocolitis (p. 791)

Major gastrointestinal viral infections include

- *Rotavirus (Group A)*: A 70-nm double-stranded (ds) DNA virus, exhibiting person-to-person transmission via food and water, affecting infants of 6 to 24 months; 140 million cases and 1 million deaths worldwide per year. Minimal infective inoculum: 10 particles. Outbreaks are characteristic.
- *Norwalk-like viruses*: 27-nm single-stranded (ss) RNA viruses, person-to-person transmission via cold food, water, raw shellfish; affects school-age children to adults. Outbreaks may occur after exposure to a common food source.
- *Enteric adenoviruses*: 80-nm dsDNA virus, person-to-person transmission, affects children less than 2 years old.
- *Caliciviruses* and *astroviruses*: ssRNA viruses affecting children, exhibiting person-to-person transmission via water, cold foods, and raw shellfish.

MORPHOLOGY. The small intestine exhibits modestly shortened villi, lamina propria inflammation, and damage to surface cells; viral particles sometimes are seen by electron microscopy.
CLINICAL FEATURES. Incubation periods range from hours to several days, and the acute illness lasts from 1 to 7+ days, depending on the virus. In addition to diarrhea, anorexia, headache, and fever may develop.

Bacterial Enterocolitis (p. 792)

Pathogenesis of gastrointestinal bacterial illnesses includes

- *Ingestion of preformed toxin* in contaminated food, including the toxins of *Staphylococcus aureus*, vibrios, and *Clostridium perfringens*. Note that botulinus toxin is neurotoxic, not diarrhea-producing.

Table 16–2. Major Causes of Diarrheal Diseases

Secretory Diarrhea
Infectious: viral damage to surface epithelium
    Rotavirus
    Norwalk virus
    Enteric adenoviruses
Infectious: enterotoxin-mediated
    Vibrio cholerae
    Escherichia coli
    Bacillus cereus
    Clostridium perfringens
Neoplastic: tumor elaboration of secretagogues
    Thyroid medullary carcinoma (calcitonin, prostaglandin)
    Carcinoid (serotonin, ?prostaglandins)
    Pancreatic cholera syndrome (VIP, others)
    Ganglioneuroma, ganglioneuroblastoma, neurofibroma (VIP, prostaglandins)
    Villous adenoma in distal colon (nonhormone-mediated)
Excess laxative use
Defects in intraluminal digestion and absorption
    Bile salt malabsorption
    Excess delivery of free fatty acids to colon

Osmotic Diarrhea
Disaccharidase deficiencies
Lactulose therapy (for hepatic encephalopathy, constipation)
Prescribed gut lavage (Na_2SO_4, polyethylene glycol)
Antacids ($MgSO_4$ and other magnesium salts)
Galactose-glucose malabsorption, fructose malabsorption
Mannitol, sorbitol ingestion (as from chewing gum)
Generalized malabsorption

Exudative Diseases
Idiopathic inflammatory bowel disease
Infectious diarrhea
    Shigella
    Salmonella
    Campylobacter
    Entamoeba histolytica

Deranged Motility
Decreased intestinal transit time
    Pyloroplasty, hemigastrectomy
    Short gut syndrome (following bypass or resection)
    Irritable bowel syndrome
    Colonic resection, ileocecal valve resection
    Hyperthyroidism
    Diabetic neuropathy
    Carcinoid syndrome
    Bowel irritation during active inflammation
Decreased motility
    Small intestinal diverticula
    Blind loop syndrome
    Bacterial overgrowth

Malabsorption
Further classified in Table 16–3

From Cotran, R. S., Kumar, V., and Robbins, S. L.: Robbins Pathologic Basis of Disease. 5th ed. Philadelphia, W. B. Saunders Co., 1994, p. 791.

Table 16–3. Classification of Malabsorption Syndromes

Defective Intraluminal Hydrolysis or Solubilization
Primary pancreatic insufficiency
Secondary pancreatic insufficiency
Deficiency of intraluminal bile salts
Bacterial overgrowth
  Blind intestinal loops
  Multiple strictures and jejunal diverticula
  Fistulas
Postgastrectomy
Scleroderma and neuromuscular dysfunction

Primary Mucosal Cell Abnormalities
Disaccharidase deficiency and monosaccharide malabsorption
Abetalipoproteinemia
Vitamin B_{12} malabsorption
  Parietal cell loss (pernicious anemia)
  Ileal dysfunction or resection
Cystinuria and Hartnup's disease

Reduced Small Intestinal Surface
Gluten-sensitive enteropathy (celiac sprue)
Refractory sprue
Whipple's disease
Short gut syndrome
Crohn's disease
Allergic and eosinophilic gastroenteritis
Lymphoma-associated diffuse enteritis

Infection
Acute infectious enteritis
Parasitic infestation
Tropical sprue

Lymphatic Obstruction
Lymphoma
Tuberculosis and tuberculous lymphadenitis
Lymphangiectasia

Iatrogenic
Subtotal or total gastrectomy
Distal ileal resection or bypass
Radiation enteritis

Drug-Induced
Cholestyramine
Colchicine
Irritant laxatives
Neomycin
p-Aminosalicylic acid
Phenindione

Unexplained
Hypogammaglobulinemia
Carcinoid syndrome
Diabetes mellitus
Mastocytosis
Hyperthyroidism, hypothyroidism, hypoadrenocorticism, and
  hypoparathyroidism

From Cotran, R. S., Kumar, V., and Robbins, S. L.: Robbins Pathologic Basis of Disease. 5th ed. Philadelphia, W. B. Saunders Co., 1994, p. 796.

- *Infection by toxigenic organisms*, which then proliferate in the gut lumen and elaborate an enterotoxin.
- *Infection by enteroinvasive organisms*, which proliferate, invade, and destroy mucosal epithelial cells.

Key bacterial properties involved in disease production:

- *Bacterial adhesion and replication*: In order to produce disease, ingested organisms must adhere to the mucosal epithelial cells; otherwise they will be swept away. Adherence is dependent on plasmid-encoded adhesins, which are proteins expressed on the bacterial surface.
- *Bacterial enterotoxins*, which are polypeptides that cause diarrhea by one of two mechanisms: *secretagogues* (e.g., *cholera toxin* from *Vibrio cholerae*) stimulate fluid secretion by activation of endogenous secretion systems; and *cytotoxins* (e.g., *Shiga toxin*) cause direct tissue damage through epithelial cell necrosis. *E. coli* produces both forms of toxins.
- *Bacterial invasion*: Microbe-stimulated endocytosis permits intracellular proliferation, cell lysis, cell-to-cell spread, and spread to the circulation. This mechanism is typical of enteroinvasive *E. coli, Shigella, Salmonella,* and *Yersinia enterocolitica*.

MORPHOLOGY. Bacterial enterocolitis exhibits extremely variable morphology. Nonspecific features common to many infections are surface epithelial damage, increased epithelial mitotic rate, lamina propria hyperemia and edema, and neutrophilic infiltration of lamina propria and epithelium. Features characteristic of some forms of infection are

- *Salmonella* involves the ileum and colon with Peyer's patch involvement. The "typhoid fever" of *S. typhimurium* consists of bacteremia and dissemination to the biliary tree, joints, bones, and meninges.
- *Shigella* causes colonic inflammation, erosion, and a fibrinopurulent exudate.
- *Campylobacter jejuni* and other species affect the small intestine, appendix, and colon, causing ulcers, inflammation, and a fibrinopurulent exudate.
- *Yersinia enterocolitica* and *Y. pseudotuberculosis* affect the ileum, appendix, colon, Peyer's patches, and mesenteric lymph nodes with granulomas; infection results in the systemic spread of organisms.
- *Vibrio cholerae* causes no significant morphologic changes.
- *Clostridium perfringens* causes a usually mild disease, although some strains cause a severe necrotizing enterocolitis ("pigbel").
- *Escherichia coli:* Enterotoxigenic *E. coli* produces a choleralike toxin; *enterohemorrhagic E. coli* produces a shiga-like toxin; *enteropathogenic E. coli* attaches and effaces epithelium but does not invade; *enteroinvasive E. coli* causes a disease like shigellosis. All *E. coli* pathogens potentially cause traveler's diarrhea.

CLINICAL FEATURES. Symptoms depend on the disease mechanism:

- *Ingestion of preformed toxins* leads to explosive diarrhea and abdominal pain within hours.
- *Infection with enteric pathogens* requires an incubation period of hours to days, followed by *diarrhea and dehydration* or *dysentery*, depending on the subsequent pathogenic process.
- *Insidious infection* with *Yersinia* and mycobacteria leads to a chronic illness. All enteroinvasive organisms can mimic (or coexist with) acute onset of inflammatory bowel disease.

Necrotizing Enterocolitis (NEC) (p. 794)

Acute, necrotizing inflammation of the small intestine and colon can occur in premature neonates or those of low birth weight. The presumed contributing mechanisms are ischemia, colonization with pathogenic organisms, excessive protein intake (placing stress on the immature gut), and functional immaturity.

MORPHOLOGY. Mucosal edema, hemorrhage, and necrosis involve the terminal ileum and proximal colon or entire gut.

CLINICAL FEATURES. NEC presents as a mild gastrointestinal illness or fulminant illness with gangrene, perforation, sepsis, and shock. When severe, massive resection of bowel may be required.

Antibiotic-Associated Colitis (p. 795)

Consists of an acute colitis characterized by *the formation of an adherent, inflammatory "membrane" (pseudomembrane) overlying sites of mucosal injury*, usually caused by toxins of *Clostridium difficile* elaborated in the setting of antibiotic therapy.

MORPHOLOGY. Fibrinopurulent-necrotic debris and mucus adhere to damaged colonic mucosa in a plaque-like fashion. These "pseudomembranes" of inflammatory debris also may form following any severe mucosal injury, as from ischemia, volvulus, and enteroinvasive infection.

CLINICAL FEATURES. An acute or chronic diarrheal illness develops while on antibiotic therapy, with *C. difficile* toxin detectable in the stool. Response to appropriate antibiotic therapy is prompt.

MALABSORPTION SYNDROMES (p. 796)

Malabsorption is characterized by suboptimal absorption of fats, fat-soluble and other vitamins, proteins, carbohydrates, electrolytes, minerals, and water and is the result of disturbed

- *Intraluminal digestion* by secreted enzymes, or lipid emulsification by biliary bile salts.
- *Terminal digestion* by enzymes of enterocyte membranes.
- *Transepithelial transport* through the enterocyte.

Table 16–3 presents a classification of malabsorption syndromes. Deficiencies in nutrients and vitamins lead to the following clinical consequences:

- *Alimentary tract*: diarrhea; flatus; pain; weight loss; passage of bulky, frothy, greasy stools. Excessive diarrhea may be life-threatening.
- *Hematopoietic system*: anemia, bleeding.
- *Musculoskeletal system*: osteopenia, tetany.
- *Endocrine system*: amenorrhea, impotence, infertility, hyperparathyroidism.
- *Skin*: purpura and petechiae, edema, dermatitis.
- *Nervous system*: peripheral neuropathy.

The most common causes in the United States are celiac sprue, chronic pancreatitis, and Crohn's disease.

Celiac Sprue (p. 797)

Consists of a chronic disease with a characteristic small intestinal mucosal lesion and impaired nutrient absorption, which improves on withdrawal of wheat gliadins and related grain proteins from the diet. Also called *gluten-sensitive enteropathy, nontropical sprue, celiac disease*. Generally is a disease of whites, with a prevalence of 1:2000 to 3000.

PATHOGENESIS. Due to immunologic sensitivity to gluten, which contains the gliadin protein component, shared by wheat, oat, barley, and rye. Contributing causes are

- *Genetic susceptibility*, based on evidence of familial clustering, and increased DQw2 (and HLA B8) histocompatibility antigen frequency.
- *Immune-mediated injury*, as evidenced by serum antibodies to gliadin, and an infiltrate of gliadin-sensitized B cells in intestinal wall mucosa.

MORPHOLOGY. Sprue is a *diffuse enteritis* with flattened (atrophic) villi, elongated regenerative crypts, surface epithelial damage with intraepithelial lymphocytes, and robust lamina propria inflammation (lymphocytes, plasma cells, macrophages). It exhibits decreased severity from proximal to distal in the small intestine and reverts to near normal upon withdrawal of dietary gluten.

CLINICAL FEATURES

- *Symptoms* consist of diarrhea, flatulence, weight loss, and fatigue. Presents from infants up to mid-adult life. Responds to withdrawal of dietary gluten.
- *Complications* develop from nutritive, iron, and vitamin deficiencies; there is a 10% to 15% lifetime risk of gastrointestinal B-cell or T-cell lymphoma.

Tropical Sprue (Postinfectious Sprue) (p. 798)

Occurs almost exclusively in people living in or visiting the tropics. Unknown etiology, perhaps enterotoxigenic *E. coli*. Responds to long-term, broad-spectrum antibiotic therapy.

MORPHOLOGY. Extremely variable intestinal changes, ranging from normal to resembling celiac disease.

- Unlike celiac disease, brunt of injury is distal.
- Lamina propria has abundant lymphocytes and more eosinophils than celiac disease.

Whipple's Disease (p. 799)

A rare, systemic condition principally involving the intestine, central nervous system, and joints. Attributed to infection by *Tropheryma whippelii*, a gram-positive actinomycete.

MORPHOLOGY. The small intestinal mucosa is laden with distended macrophages in the lamina propria, containing rod-shaped bacilli seen by electron microscopy. Similar macrophages are present in lymphatics, lymph nodes, joints, brain, elsewhere. Inflammation is essentially absent.

CLINICAL FEATURES. Salient features include

- Malabsorption with diarrhea, steatorrhea, abdominal cramps, distention, fever, and weight loss; migratory arthritis and heart disease may be presenting problems.
- Usually whites in fourth to fifth decade; male:female 10:1.
- Usually responds to antibiotic therapy.

Bacterial Overgrowth Syndrome (p. 799)

Pathologic colonization of proximal small intestine by an abnormally large population of both anaerobic and aerobic organisms similar to those in the colon leads to malabsorption.

- Predisposing conditions include *luminal stasis* caused by strictures, fistulas, diverticula, blind loops, reduplications, or motility disorders; gastric *hypochlorhydria* or *achlorhydria*; and *immune deficiencies* or *impaired mucosal immunity*.
- Excess bacterial load competes for essential nutrients; bacteria deconjugate and dehydroxylate luminal bile salts; bacteria damage surface enterocytes and also inactivate luminal lipase.

Disaccharidase Deficiency (p. 800)

- Disaccharidase is an apical membrane enzyme of surface absorptive cells, which cleaves lactose.
- With enzyme deficiency, lactose remains in the lumen and exerts an osmotic pull, leading to diarrhea and malabsorption.
- A rare congenital deficiency produces explosive, frothy stools; and abdominal distention in infants exposed to milk, or milk products.
- The acquired form is common among North American blacks, occurring especially in the setting of enteric infections. Symptoms are much milder.
- No morphologic abnormalities are seen in the mucosa or mucosal epithelial cells.

Abetalipoproteinemia (p. 800)

A congenital lack of betalipoprotein, which is required for enterocyte export of chylomicrons.

- Exhibits familial, autosomal recessive inheritance.
- The inability to synthesize apoproteins required for lipoprotein export from mucosal cells leads to triglyceride retention in enterocytes, with lipid vacuolation.
- Severe hypolipoproteinemia results from depressed levels of chylomicrons, prebetalipoproteins (VLDL), and betalipoproteins (LDL). The defective lipid membranes of circulating erythrocytes create a "burr cell" appearance.
- Presents in infancy with failure to thrive, diarrhea, and steatorrhea.

IDIOPATHIC INFLAMMATORY BOWEL DISEASE (IBD) (p. 800)

Two conditions are *chronic, relapsing intestinal inflammatory disorders of obscure origin*:

- *Crohn's disease* (CD): granulomatous disease affecting any portion of the gut, most often the small intestine and colon.
- *Ulcerative colitis* (UC): a colonic disease exhibiting no granulomas.

Salient differences are given in Table 16–4)

ETIOLOGY AND PATHOGENESIS. Both diseases remain unexplained, i.e., are *idiopathic*. Potential mechanisms for their pathogenesis are

- *Genetic*: familial aggregations are well documented, but there are no dominant HLA types among IBD patients.
- *Infectious*: there are no proved pathogens; many agents are capable of mimicking IBD in symptomatology and mucosal damage.
- *Mucosal structure*: possible susceptibility factors among patients and their relatives include increased intestinal permeability and synthesis of altered muciproteins.

Table 16-4. Distinctive Features of Crohn's Disease and Ulcerative Colitis

Feature	Crohn's Disease—SI	Crohn's Disease—C	Ulcerative Colitis
Macroscopic			
Bowel region	Ileum ± colon	Colon ± ileum	Colon only
Distribution	Skip lesions	Skip lesions	Diffuse
Stricture	Early	Variable	Late/rare
Wall appearance	Thickened	Thin	Thin
Dilatation	No	Yes	Yes
Microscopic			
Pseudopolyps	No to slight	Marked	Marked
Ulcers	Deep, linear	Deep, linear	Superficial
Lymphoid reaction	Marked	Marked	Mild
Fibrosis	Marked	Moderate	Mild
Serositis	Marked	Variable	Mild to none
Granulomas	Yes (50%)	Yes (50%)	No
Fistulas/sinuses	Yes	Yes	No
Clinical			
Fat/vitamin malabsorption	Yes	Yes, if ileum	No
Malignant potential	Yes	Yes	Yes
Response to surgery	Poor	Fair	Good

SI, Crohn's disease of the small intestine; C, Crohn's disease of the colon. Features not all present in a single case.
From Cotran, R. S., Kumar, V., and Robbins, S. L.: Robbins Pathologic Basis of Disease. 5th ed. Philadelphia, W. B. Saunders Co., 1994, p. 807.

329

- *Abnormal host immunoreactivity*: it is postulated that patients mount an abnormal immune response to otherwise innocuous luminal (dietary or infectious) antigens.
- *Inflammation as final common pathway*: IBD ultimately results from *activation of inflammatory cells, whose products cause tissue injury*. While the mechanism(s) for such activation remains unclear, treatment modalities attempt to downregulate the host inflammatory process.

Crohn's Disease (CD) (p. 801)

CD is characterized by sharply delimited and typical transmural involvement of the bowel by an inflammatory process with mucosal damage. Salient features include the presence of noncaseating granulomas; fissuring and fistula formation; and systemic manifestations.

EPIDEMIOLOGY

- Annual incidence in United States: 1 to 3 per 100,000.
- Presents at any age: young childhood to advanced age.
- Peak incidence: second and third decades of life.
- Females more than males, whites more than nonwhites.

MORPHOLOGY. The visceral distribution is small intestine alone (40%), small intestine and colon (30%), colon (30%). CD is uncommon in the duodenum, stomach, esophagus, and mouth. Perianal involvement is more common.

   Gross features of intestinal segments involved with CD include a granular intestinal serosa with adherent "creeping" mesenteric fat; a rubbery, thick intestinal wall with edema, inflammation, fibrosis, muscular hypertrophy, and often stricture; punched-out mucosal "aphthous" ulcers and linear ulcers; a tendency to fistula and sinus tract formation; and *sharply demarcated involved bowel segments with intervening normal areas* ("skip lesions"). Multiple segments may be involved.

   Microscopic features of CD are

- *Mucosal inflammation* with intraepithelial neutrophils and crypt abscesses (neutrophils within crypt lumens), lamina propria mononuclear inflammation.
- *Ulceration.*
- *Chronic mucosal damage*—villus blunting, atrophy, metaplasia, architectural disarray.
- *Transmural inflammation* with *lymphoid aggregates; noncaseating granulomas* in about half of cases—they may be present throughout the gut, even in uninvolved segments.
- *Fibrosis.*
- Muscle and neural hypertrophy.
- Occasional mural vasculitis.

CLINICAL FEATURES. The symptomatology is dominated by intermittent attacks of diarrhea, fever, abdominal pain, anorexia, and weight loss, with intervening asymptomatic periods. Complications develop from fibrotic strictures; fistulas to adjacent viscera, abdominal and perineal skin, bladder, vagina, and so on; malabsorption and malnutrition; and loss of albumin (in the form of a protein-losing enteropathy).

- With extensive terminal ileal involvement, vitamin B_{12} deficiency may develop, leading to pernicious anemia; bile salt malabsorption may lead to steatorrhea.
- Extraintestinal manifestations include migratory polyarthritis, sacroiliitis, ankylosing spondylitis, erythema nodosum, uveitis,

cholangitis, amyloidosis, and a mildly increased risk of bowel cancer.

Ulcerative Colitis (UC) (p. 804)

An ulceroinflammatory disease limited to the colon, affecting only the mucosa and submucosa except in the most severe cases. Unlike CD, *UC extends in a continuous fashion proximally from the rectum, and granulomas are absent.*

EPIDEMIOLOGY

- Annual incidence in United States: 4 to 6 per 100,000.
- Generally presents in adolescence to older adulthood.
- Peak incidence: 20 to 25 years of age.
- Females more than males, whites more than nonwhites.

MORPHOLOGY. UC involves the rectum and extends proximally in a retrograde fashion to involve the entire colon (pancolitis); the distal ileum may show some inflammation.

- *Gross*: UC is a disease of continuity with no "skip" lesions. The mucosa may be reddened, granular, and friable with inflammatory "pseudopolyps" and may exhibit extensive ulceration; alternatively, the mucosa may be atrophic and flattened. Mural thickening and stricture do not occur.
- *Microscopic*: UC exhibits *mucosal inflammation* similar to that of CD, including *ulceration* and *chronic mucosal damage*. With treated or inactive disease, regions may appear almost normal by microscopy.
- The *epithelial dysplasia* that can occur in UC may progress to *carcinoma*; the risk of dysplasia (and carcinoma) increases with increasing extent of colonic involvement and increased duration of disease.

CLINICAL FEATURES. Patients typically experience intermittent attacks of bloody, mucoid diarrhea and abdominal pain; UC rarely presents as explosive illness with severe electrolyte disturbances and toxic megacolon.

- Extraintestinal manifestations include migratory polyarthritis, sacroiliitis, ankylosing spondylitis, uveitis, pericholangitis, primary sclerosing cholangitis, and skin lesions such as erythema nodosum.
- *Risk of carcinoma arising from dysplasia*: the highest risk is in patients with pancolitis of >10 years' duration (10- to 20-fold higher than controls), but the rate of progression of UC to dysplasia and carcinoma is still slow, and many patients do not develop dysplasia.

COLONIC DIVERTICULOSIS (p. 806)

Unlike the congenital Meckel's diverticulum (discussed earlier), *acquired diverticula* may occur in the esophagus, stomach, small intestine, and colon. Acquired *colonic diverticula* ("diverticulosis") are uncommon under age 30 years but are present in 50% of Western populations over age 60 years.

MORPHOLOGY. Colonic diverticula are multiple, flask-like outpouchings 0.5 to 1 cm in diameter, usually in the distal colon. They protrude alongside taeniae coli and dissect into appendices epiploicae. They possess a thin wall lined by mucosa and submucosa and an attenuated-to-absent muscularis propria. The muscularis of intervening bowel wall is hypertrophic. The primary complications are *bleeding* and *diverticulitis*—typically the diverticulitis follows obstruction or perforation of one or more outpouchings.

PATHOGENESIS. The presumed mechanism for formation of diverticula is

- *Focal anatomic weakness in the bowel wall* at sites of penetrating vasa recta.
- *Increased intraluminal pressure* resulting from exaggerated peristaltic contractions (possibly the result of decreased bulk in the diet). Focal mucosal and submucosal protrusion through the pre-existing sites of mural weakness.

CLINICAL FEATURES. Diverticula are usually asymptomatic but may be associated with cramping, abdominal discomfort, and constipation. Diverticulitis may lead to pericolic abscesses, sinus tracts, peritonitis, and chronic blood loss.

BOWEL OBSTRUCTION (p. 808, Table 16–5)

Hernias (p. 808)

Weakness or a defect in the wall of the peritoneal cavity permits protrusion of a peritoneal sac; denoted a *"hernial sac."* Segments of viscera may become trapped in one (*external herniation*); stasis and edema may then lead to *incarceration*; further vascular compromise leads to *strangulation*. Typical sites are the inguinal (internal and external) and femoral canals, umbilicus, surgical scars, and into the retroperitoneal space.

Adhesions (p. 808)

Localized peritoneal inflammation (*peritonitis*) may develop after surgery, infection, endometriosis, or radiation; healing leads to fibrous bridges between viscera. Complications of adhesions include *internal herniation* (trapping of intestine by adhesions, within the abdominal cavity), intestinal obstruction, and strangulation of viscera. Rarely, adhesions are congenital in origin.

Table 16–5. Major Causes of Intestinal Obstruction

Mechanical Obstruction
Adhesions
Hernias, internal or external
Volvulus
Intussusception
Tumors
Inflammatory strictures
Obstructive gallstones, fecaliths, foreign bodies
Congenital strictures; atresias
Congenital bands
Meconium in mucoviscoidosis
Imperforate anus

Pseudo-Obstruction
Paralytic ileus (e.g., postoperative)
Vascular—bowel infarction
Myopathies and neuropathies (e.g., Hirschsprung's)

From Cotran, R. S., Kumar, V., and Robbins, S. L.: Robbins Pathologic Basis of Disease. 5th ed. Philadelphia, W. B. Saunders Co., 1994, p. 808.

Intussusception (p. 809)

Occurs when one segment of intestine telescopes into the immediately distal segment, usually small bowel. In infants and children, intussusception is usually spontaneous and reversible. In adults, the point of traction is usually a tumor. Vascular compromise of the trapped segment may lead to infarction, if corrective steps are not taken.

Volvulus (p. 809)

Consists of complete twisting of a bowel loop about its mesenteric base, and leads to obstruction and infarction. Volvulus occurs most often in the small bowel or in redundant loops of sigmoid colon.

TUMORS OF THE SMALL AND LARGE INTESTINES
(p. 809, Table 16–6)

The colon (including the rectum) is the segment of the GI tract most affected by tumors. Benign tumors, primarily epithelial, are present in 25% to 50% of older adults. Some relevant terminology is as follows:

- *Polyp*: a tumorous mass that protrudes into the lumen of the gut. *Pedunculated*: with stalk. *Sessile*: without stalk.
- *Non-neoplastic*: polyps resulting from abnormal mucosal maturation, inflammation, or architecture; no malignant potential.
- *Neoplastic*: polyps arising from proliferative *dysplasia*, termed *adenomas*. *Adenomas are precursors to carcinoma.*

Non-Neoplastic Polyps (p. 810)

These generally innocuous lesions represent 90% of epithelial polyps in colon.

Table 16–6. Tumors of the Small and Large Intestines

Non-Neoplastic (Benign) Polyps	**Mesenchymal Lesions**
Hyperplastic polyps	Benign lesions
Hamartomatous polyps	Leiomyoma
Juvenile polyps	Lipoma
Peutz-Jegher polyps	Neuroma
Inflammatory polyps	Angioma
Lymphoid polyps	Malignant lesions
	Leiomyosarcoma
Neoplastic Epithelial Lesions	Liposarcoma
Benign polyps	Malignant spindle cell tumor
Tubular adenoma°	Kaposi's sarcoma
Tubulovillous adenoma°	
Villous adenoma°	**Lymphoma** (malignant)
Malignant lesions	
Adenocarcinoma°	
Carcinoid tumor	
Anal zone carcinoma	

°Denotes the benign and malignant counterparts of the same neoplastic process.
From Cotran, R. S., Kumar, V., and Robbins, S. L.: Robbins Pathologic Basis of Disease. 5th ed. Philadelphia, W. B. Saunders Co., 1994, p. 809.

- *Hyperplastic polyp*: Found in more than one half of persons over 60 years old. Nipple-like hemispheric protrusions usually <5 mm in diameter, composed of well-formed mature glands, and scant lamina propria. Origin: delayed shedding of surface epithelial cells.
- *Juvenile polyp*: A focal hamartomatous malformation of the small intestine and colon, usually sporadic. The vast majority occur in children less than 5 years old, and most are in the rectum. The rare *juvenile polyposis syndrome* exhibits autosomal dominance, numerous polyps, and risk of adenomas and adenocarcinoma. Juvenile polyps are large (1 to 3 cm), rounded, pedunculated polyps with cystically dilated glands and abundant lamina propria.
- *Peutz-Jeghers polyp*: Hamartomatous polyps of the small intestine and colon, often sporadic. The rare *Peutz-Jeghers syndrome* exhibits autosomal dominance, melanotic pigmentation of mucosal and skin surfaces, and increased risk of carcinomas of pancreas, breast, lung, ovary, uterus. These are large, pedunculated, lobulated polyps with arborizing smooth muscle surrounding normal abundant glands. Rarely, patients with this syndrome develop coexisting adenomas, with attendant risk of adenocarcinoma.
- *Other polyps*: *Lymphoid aggregates* (normal); *inflammatory polyps* in inflammatory bowel disease; smaller isolated hamartomatous polyps (*retention polyps*) found in the colon of adults.

Neoplastic Epithelial Lesions

Adenomas (p. 811)

Adenomas are the most common neoplasm of humans; the prevalence of adenomas approaches 50% after age 60 years, and they are frequently multiple. *All adenomas arise as the result of epithelial proliferative dysplasia; adenocarcinoma generally arises from adenomas*. Three histologic appearances are characteristic:

- *Tubular adenoma*: tubular glands, smooth surface.
- *Villous adenoma*: villous frond-like projections.
- *Tubulovillous adenoma*: a mixture of the above two.

Most tubular adenomas are small and become pedunculated as they enlarge, whereas most villous adenomas are large and remain sessile during growth. *The risk of coexistent malignancy is correlated with three interdependent features: polyp size, histologic architecture, and severity of dysplasia*. Larger and/or villous adenomas are more likely to harbor severe dysplasia and/or carcinoma. *Adenomas are slow-growing; their doubling time is approximately 10 years*. Thus, detection and removal of adenomas is central to reducing the incidence of colorectal carcinoma. **MORPHOLOGY.** Most (90%) adenomas are in the colon; essentially identical lesions may occur in the stomach and small intestine. They may be single or multiple. By definition, all adenomas are made of a *dysplastic epithelium*: tall, hyperchromatic disorderly cells with increased nuclear/cytoplasmic ratio and cigar-shaped nuclei. The dysplastic cells line the entire colonic crypt and mucosal surface. The degree of dysplasia may be mild (nuclei still basally oriented, mucin production maintained) to severe (stratified nuclei over full thickness of epithelium, no mucin production). Although the risk may vary, *all adenomas may harbor intramucosal carcinoma* (confined to lamina propria) *or invasive carcinoma* (invasive into submucosa or deeper), *regardless of size or histologic type.*

- *Tubular adenomas* begin as smooth, contoured bumps in the mucosa involving only a few adjacent crypts; with growth they become bulky neoplasms (up to 4 cm in diameter) and protrude into the lumen. Traction creates a submucosal stalk lined by normal mucosa. Branching dysplastic glands are embedded in lamina propria.
- *Villous adenomas* tend to be larger when discovered, and may carpet up to 10 cm of colonic mucosa. Finger-like projections are lined by dysplastic epithelium with a lamina propria core.
- *Tubulovillous adenomas* are typically intermediate in size, are likely to have a stalk, and are a mixture of tubular and villous architecture.

CLINICAL FEATURES. Adenomas are usually asymptomatic, or cause anemia and occult bleeding. In the small intestine they may cause obstruction or intussusception. Rarely, large villous adenomas in the distal colon may hypersecrete copious amounts of mucus rich in protein and potassium, leading to excessive protein loss. The following considerations pertain:

- *Severe dysplasia* ("high-grade dysplasia," "carcinoma in situ") cannot yet metastasize and is not yet malignant.
- *Intramucosal carcinoma* is still confined to the mucosa, where lymphatic channels are absent (in the colon); it has little to no metastatic potential.
- *Invasive adenocarcinoma* is a malignant lesion with metastatic potential, since it has crossed into the submucosa, which contains lymphatics. Nevertheless, *endoscopic removal of a pedunculated polyp is adequate therapy, provided that* (a) the invasive adenocarcinoma is superficial and does not approach the margin; (b) no vascular or lymphatic invasion is present; and (c) the carcinoma is not poorly differentiated.
- *Invasive adenocarcinoma arising in a sessile polyp cannot be adequately resected by polypectomy*: further surgery is required.
- *The only adequate treatment for any adenoma is resection*, regardless of whether carcinoma is present. Any residual adenomatous tissue is still a premalignant lesion or may yet harbor invasive adenocarcinoma.

Familial Adenomatous Polyposis (FAP) (p. 813)

FAP is the archetype of *autosomal dominant* polyposis syndromes, exhibiting innumerable adenomatous polyps in the colon (and elsewhere); the risk of progression to adenocarcinoma is virtually 100%.

- Minimum of 100 colon adenomas is required for diagnosis.
- Prophylactic colectomy is curative for the colonic risk of cancer; adenomas elsewhere create continued problems.
- *Gardner's syndrome*: An FAP variant also exhibiting multiple osteomas (mandible, skull, long bones), epidermal cysts, fibromatosis (desmoid tumors), abnormal dentition, and a higher frequency of duodenal and thyroid cancer.
- FAP and Gardner's syndrome are felt to represent variants of the same genetic condition. *Turcot's syndrome* is much rarer, exhibiting alimentary adenomas and central nervous system tumors (gliomas). A *flat adenomatosis syndrome* also exists.
- For all these polyps, the average age of onset is the second to

third decade, with progression to cancer in 10 to 15 years without surgery.

Adenoma-Carcinoma Sequence (p. 814)

Evidence for an adenoma-carcinoma progression comes from

- *Epidemiology*: the populations at risk are similar.
- *Topology*: the colorectal distributions of adenomas and adenocarcinomas are similar.
- *Chronology*: the peak incidence years of adenomas slightly precede those of adenocarcinoma.
- *Histology*: adenomas commonly harbor adenocarcinoma.
- *Numerology*: the risk of adenocarcinoma is related to the number of polyps in the patient.
- *Intervention*: screening programs with removal of adenomas reduce the incidence of colorectal carcinoma.

Genetic alterations in adenomas and colon carcinomas constitute a paradigm for human carcinogenesis:

- FAP and Gardner's syndrome patients exhibit a somatic mutation in chromosome 5q21 (*APC gene*: Adenomatous Polyposis Coli). APC gene mutations also are found in the malignant tissue of sporadic cancers.
- *DNA hypomethylation* occurs early in colonic adenomas.
- *Ras gene* and other oncogenes are mutated with increasing frequency as adenoma size increases, and mutations are detectable in carcinomas.
- Allelic loss on 18q is common in colon cancer: the loss is localized to the *DCC locus* (Deleted in Colon Cancer), which codes for a cell adhesion protein.
- Losses at 17p (site of *p53 gene*) are common in cancers.
- *Instability of microsatellite DNA* on chromosome 2 and other chromosomes may underlie a genetic predisposition to mutations in neoplastic tissues.

The accumulation of these *alterations in the genome appear to lead to progressive increases in size, level of dysplasia, and invasive potential of neoplastic lesions*. No single sequence of events is critical (e.g., genetic steps 1 through 6 above), but a *multihit* genetic mechanism appears to be operative.

Colorectal Carcinoma (p. 815)

EPIDEMIOLOGY. Colonic carcinoma (58,000 deaths per year) is second only to bronchogenic carcinoma in the United States; 98% of colon cancers are adenocarcinomas. The peak age of incidence is 60 to 70 years, except in young adults with polyposis syndromes. Male:female ratio is the same except for the rectum; here males are more common. Colon cancer has a worldwide distribution, which is higher in industrialized countries.

PATHOGENESIS

- *Diet*: The risk of cancer is associated with low vegetable fiber intake, high content of refined carbohydrates, high fat content, and decreased intake of "protective micronutrients" (vitamins A, C, E). Altered diet may promote increased exposure to bile acids and bacterial degradative byproducts. *Causal relationships are unproved.*
- *Genetics*: A somatic genetic cause is established only for the polyposis syndromes.
- Most, perhaps all, arise in pre-existing adenomas.

MORPHOLOGY. The colonic distribution used to be predominantly distal but is now shifting to a more even colonic distribution. Colon cancers may be *polypoid, fungating masses* (especially in the capacious cecum and right colon), or *annular, encircling masses* with "napkin ring" obstruction (characteristic of the distal colorectum). Both forms penetrate the bowel wall over years.

Microscopic features are the same regardless of site: tall, columnar cells resembling the neoplastic epithelium of adenomas but now invasive into the submucosa and muscularis propria. Alternatively, cancers contain poorly differentiated cells with limited resemblance to a columnar epithelium. Invasive tumors incite a *desmoplastic stromal response*, consisting of inflammation and fibrosis of the mesenchyme. A minority of tumors produce copious mucin. Less commonly, there are foci of neuroendocrine differentiation, signet ring features, or squamous differentiation.

CLINICAL FEATURES. Colon cancers are asymptomatic for years, but eventually cause fatigue, weakness, iron deficiency anemia, abdominal discomfort, progressive bowel obstruction, or liver enlargement (due to metastases). The *prognosis is based on extent of invasion at diagnosis*: the Astler-Coller staging system for colon and rectal carcinoma is

A Limited to mucosa.
B1 Extending into muscularis propria but not penetrating through it; uninvolved lymph nodes.
B2 Penetrating through muscularis propria; uninvolved lymph nodes.
C1 Extending into muscularis propria but not penetrating through it; involved lymph nodes.
C2 Penetrating through muscularis propria; involved lymph nodes.
D Distant metastatic spread.

The 5-year survival: Stage A (100%), B1 (67%), B2 (54%), C1 (43%), C2 (23%). Surgery is the only hope for cure.

Small Intestinal Neoplasms (p. 817)

The small intestine represents 75% of the length of the GI tract yet contributes only 3% to 6% of tumors: the malignant-to-benign ratio is 1.5:1. Benign lesions include leiomyomas, adenomas, lipomas, neuromas, vascular malformations, and hamartomatous lesions.

Adenocarcinomas typically exhibit a napkin ring encircling pattern or are polypoid fungating masses. They present with obstruction (cramping pain, nausea, vomiting), weight loss, or bleeding. Spread is to mesentery, regional lymph nodes, and the liver as with colonic adenocarcinoma; the histology is the same as that of colon tumors. Five-year survival is 70% with wide *en bloc* excision.

Carcinoid Tumors (p. 818)

Tumors of neuroendocrine cells are termed "carcinoid," based on their slow growth rate. Most arise in the gut but also occur in the pancreas, lungs, biliary tree, liver. Peak age of incidence is the sixth decade. Carcinoids represent one-half of small intestine malignancies.

- *Appendiceal, rectal carcinoids infrequently metastasize.*
- *Ileal, gastric, colonic carcinoids are frequently aggressive,* spreading to regional lymph nodes and the liver.

AMBROSIA

As they arise from neuroendocrine cells, many elaborate bioactive products (e.g., hormonally active amines or peptides).

MORPHOLOGY. Carcinoids arise as submucosal or intramural masses, and are small, firm, and yellow-tan. Appendiceal and rectal carcinoids tend to be solitary; elsewhere carcinoids tend to be multiple. Carcinoids may cause kinking and obstruction of intestine. Metastases tend to be in the form of small and dispersed nodules.

Microscopy: Carcinoids are made of discrete islands, trabeculae, glands, or sheets of monotonous uniform epithelial cells with scant, pink, granular cytoplasm and an oval stippled nucleus; a fibrous stroma is the basis for their firmness.

CLINICAL FEATURES. Carcinoids are usually asymptomatic but may cause local symptoms from obstruction or bleeding. Inconstant secretory products include gastrin (causing the *Zollinger-Ellison syndrome* with peptic ulceration); adrenocorticotropic hormone (causing Cushing's syndrome); insulin (causing hyperinsulinism); and others. *Carcinoid syndrome* arises from tumor secretion of serotonin and other bioactive amines, and features

- *Vasomotor disturbances*: flushing, cyanosis.
- *Intestinal hypermotility*: diarrhea, cramps, nausea, vomiting.
- *Asthmatic bronchoconstriction*: cough, wheezing, dyspnea.
- *Systemic fibrosis*: pulmonic and tricuspid valve thickening and stenosis, endocardial fibrosis, retroperitoneal and pelvic fibrosis, and collagenous pleural and intimal aortic plaques.
- *Hepatomegaly*: in the case of intestinal carcinoids, hepatic metastases are required if bioactive products are to reach the systemic circulation, since the normal liver clears the portal circulation of such chemicals.
- Carcinoid syndrome is diagnosed by documenting excess 5-hydroxyindoleacetic acid (5-HIAA) in urine; this is the breakdown product of 5-hydroxytryptamine (5-HT; serotonin).

The 5-year survival rate for carcinoids (excluding appendiceal and rectal) is 90%. When hepatic metastases are present, the 5-year survival is 50%.

Gastrointestinal Lymphoma (p. 820)

The gut is the most common location of the 40% of lymphomas arising in sites other than lymph nodes. Although they usually arise as sporadic neoplasms (1% to 3% of gut malignancies), *primary gastrointestinal lymphomas occur more frequently in patients with chronic sprue-like malabsorption syndromes; in natives of the Mediterranean region; in patients with congenital immunodeficiency states or HIV infection; or following organ transplantation with immunosuppression.*

- *Sporadic lymphoma* is the most common form of gut lymphoma in the Western Hemisphere. They are B-cell lymphomas, presumably arising from Mucosa-Associated Lymphoid Tissue (MALT). The distribution is stomach (55% to 60%), small intestine (25% to 30%), colon (20% to 25%), and they affect primarily adults. Their origin may be related to chronic mucosal lymphoid activation, as in *Helicobacter*-associated chronic inflammation of the stomach.
- *Sprue-associated lymphoma* affects younger individuals (30 to 40 years of age), following the long duration of a malabsorptive disorder. They are often T cell, and the prognosis is poor.
- *Mediterranean lymphoma* is a B-cell lymphoma of children and young adults of Mediterranean ancestry, arising from a

background of chronic, diffuse mucosal plasmacytosis. Also called *immunoproliferative small intestinal disease* and has a poor prognosis.

MORPHOLOGY. Early lymphomas are plaque-like lesions of the mucosa and submucosa. Advanced lymphomas become full-thickness mural lesions or are polypoid, fungating masses that protrude into the lumen. *Microscopic*: lymphomas exhibit atypical lymphocytes infiltrating the mucosa and wall and replacing normal structures. Extreme numbers of lymphocytes may populate the epithelium (*lymphoepithelial lesion*). B-cell lesions (95%) may be low or high grade; T-cell lesions are all high grade.

CLINICAL FEATURES. Most sporadic lymphomas are amenable to surgical resection. The clinical outcome depends on size, grade, and invasiveness of tumor at time of resection.

Mesenchymal Tumors (p. 821)

- *Lipomas*: generally submucosal, in small intestine and colon; they are the most common gastrointestinal mesenchymal tumor.
- *Gastrointestinal stromal tumors (GIST)*: spindle cell lesions generally of smooth muscle phenotype; may also exhibit neural or histiocytic features. There are benign and malignant forms (e.g., leiomyoma, leiomyosarcoma).
- *Kaposi's sarcoma*: visceral involvement is common (especially in AIDS).

CLINICAL FEATURES. Most mesenchymal tumors are asymptomatic. Larger lesions may cause mucosal ulceration with bleeding (especially in stomach), obstruction, or intussusception.

APPENDIX
ACUTE APPENDICITIS (p. 823)

This is the most common acute abdominal condition requiring surgery. The differential diagnosis includes virtually every acute process that can occur in the abdomen, and some in the thorax.

PATHOGENESIS. Obstruction of the lumen (fecalith, calculus, tumor, worms—*Oxyuriasis vermicularis*) predisposes to build-up of intraluminal pressure, ischemic injury (exacerbated by edema and exudate), and bacterial invasion.

MORPHOLOGY. Early acute appendicitis exhibits scant neutrophil exudations throughout the mucosa, submucosa, and muscularis; congestion of subserosal vessels; and perivascular neutrophil emigration. The serosa is dull, granular, and red. Advanced acute appendicitis (*acute suppurative appendicitis*) exhibits more severe neutrophilic infiltration; fibrinopurulent serosal exudate; and luminal abscess formation with ulceration and suppurative necrosis. Further worsening leads to gangrenous necrosis (*acute gangrenous appendicitis*), followed by *rupture*.

CLINICAL FEATURES. Appendicitis is mainly a disease of adolescents and young adults but can occur in any age group. Classic symptoms are periumbilical pain then localizing to the right lower quadrant; nausea or vomiting; abdominal tenderness; mild fever; and leukocytosis >15,000 cells per mm³. However, symptoms are only variably present and deceptively absent in the very young and elderly. Surgically removed appendices may be histologically normal; a false-positive clinical diagnosis rate of

20% to 25% is felt to outweigh the 2% mortality of appendiceal perforation.

- *Complications*: perforation, pylephlebitis, and thrombosis of portal venous drainage; liver abscess; and bacteremia.
- *Mimics of appendicitis*: enterocolitis, mesenteric lymphadenitis secondary to enterocolitis, systemic viral infection, acute salpingitis, ectopic pregnancy, mittelschmerz, cystic fibrosis, Meckel's diverticulitis.

TUMORS OF THE APPENDIX (p. 824)

Mucocele and Pseudomyxoma Peritonei

Mucocele is a dilatation of appendiceal lumen by mucinous secretions, caused by

- *Mucosal hyperplasia*, with non-neoplastic elongated columnar mucous cells producing copious amounts of mucin.
- *Mucinous cystadenoma*, which is a neoplastic mucin-producing columnar epithelium. Mechanical distention may lead to appendiceal rupture and spillage of mucin and neoplastic cells into the abdomen; this does not constitute malignant spread to the peritoneum.
- *Mucinous cystadenocarcinoma* is indistinguishable from cystadenomas except for the presence of *invasion of the appendiceal wall by neoplastic cells and spread beyond the appendix as peritoneal implants*. The peritoneal cavity becomes distended with tenacious, semisolid mucin, called *pseudomyxoma peritonei*. The presence of anaplastic adenocarcinomatous cells distinguishes this cancer from mucinous spillage, but malignant cells may be very hard to find in the abundant mucin, making clinical distinction sometimes difficult.

The potentially lethal outcome of appendiceal mucinous cystadenocarcinoma is identical to that of similar ovarian cancers that spread to the peritoneum.

Carcinoma and Other Tumors (p. 824)

Carcinoid is the most common tumor and is almost always a bland, incidental lesion found at the time of appendectomy. Adenocarcinomas and mesenchymal tumors resemble their intestinal counterparts.

PERITONEUM

Sterile Peritonitis (p. 825)

Sterile inflammation of the peritoneal surfaces (peritonitis) is caused by chemical irritation, as from bile (via rupture or perforation of the biliary system), pancreatic juices (from pancreatitis, especially the acute hemorrhagic form), surgically introduced material, and gynecologic processes (e.g., blood from endometriosis, ruptured dermoid cysts).

Peritoneal Infection (p. 825)

Peritoneal bacterial infection may develop from appendicitis, ruptured peptic ulcer, cholecystitis, diverticulitis, bowel strangulation, acute salpingitis, abdominal trauma, peritoneal dialysis, or perforated inflammatory conditions of intestines. Spontaneous bacterial peritonitis can develop in setting of ascites, seen in children with nephrotic syndrome and adult cirrhotic patients.

MORPHOLOGY. Peritoneal infection transforms the normally glistening peritoneal membranes into dull gray surfaces. This is followed by development of an exudate and outright suppuration. Localized subhepatic or subdiaphragmatic abscesses may develop. Inflammation tends to remain superficial. *Tuberculous peritonitis* produces a plastic exudate with myriad minute granulomas.

CLINICAL FEATURES. Peritoneal infections may heal spontaneously or with therapy. Residual, walled-off abscesses may persist, serving as foci for new infection. The exudate may organize, leaving fibrous adhesions.

Sclerosing Retroperitonitis (p. 826)

Consists of dense fibromatous overgrowth of retroperitoneal tissues. The fibrous overgrowth is infiltrative, but the accompanying infiltrate of lymphocytes, plasma cells, and neutrophils suggests an inflammatory rather than neoplastic disease. The fibrous process may encroach on the ureters (leading to hydronephrosis) or bowel segments. Although usually sporadic, sclerosing retroperitonitis also is seen in settings of methysergide use (for migraine headaches), and fibrosing disorders (mediastinal fibrosis, sclerosing cholangitis, Riedel's fibrosing thyroiditis).

Mesenteric Cysts (p. 826)

Cystic masses arising from (1) sequestered lymphatic channels, (2) pinched-off enteric diverticula of developing foregut or hindgut, (3) cysts of developing urogenital origin, (4) cysts from walled-off infections or pancreatic pseudocysts, and (5) cysts of malignant origin from other sites.

Tumors (p. 826)

- *Primary*: the rare mesothelioma is similar to that of the pleura and pericardium.
- *Secondary* malignancies are common, resulting from any form of advanced cancer that extends into the peritoneum. When such invasion occurs, there is a tendency for diffuse seeding of peritoneal surfaces.

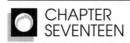

CHAPTER
SEVENTEEN

Liver, Biliary System, and Pancreas

LIVER

MORPHOLOGIC PATTERNS OF HEPATIC INJURY (p. 833)

The liver is vulnerable to metabolic, toxic, microbial, circulatory, and neoplastic insults. The enormous functional reserve masks clinical impact of early liver damage. The limited responses are

- *Necrosis:* Coagulative necrosis (ischemia) or *apoptosis* (Councilman bodies) from toxic or immunologic causes. Lesions may be focal (scattered through the parenchyma), zonal, submassive or massive, or geographic.
- *Degeneration:* Swelling and edema of hepatocytes. Accumulation of specific material: e.g, retained bile pigments, iron, copper, viral particles.
- *Inflammation (hepatitis):* Influx of acute or chronic inflammatory cells. Granulomas may be incited by foreign bodies, organisms, or drugs.
- *Regeneration:* Occurs in all but the most fulminant diseases. May produce thickened hepatocyte cords.
- *Fibrosis:* Develops in response to inflammation or direct toxic insult. Continuing fibrosis leads to cirrhosis.

CIRRHOSIS (p. 834)

Defined by three characteristics:

- *Fibrosis:* Delicate bands or broad septa.
- *Nodules* created by regeneration of hepatocytes.
- *Disruption of parenchymal architecture of the entire liver.*

The fibrosis is generally irreversible and is accompanied by reorganization of the vascular architecture, with formation of abnormal interconnections between inflow and outflow.

Classification is best on the basis of etiology. Once cirrhosis has developed, it is often impossible to establish an etiologic diagnosis. The major causes in Western nations are

Alcoholic liver disease	60%–70%
Viral hepatitis	10%
Biliary diseases	5%–10%
Primary hemochromatosis	5%
Wilson's disease	rare

Alpha$_1$-antitrypsin (α_1-AT) deficiency rare
Cryptogenic cirrhosis 10%–15%

PATHOGENESIS. Interstitial collagen (types I and III) is normally in portal tracts and around central veins; occasional bundles are in the space of Disse. A delicate reticulin (collagen type IV) is in the space of Disse. In cirrhosis, types I and III collagen are deposited in all portions of the lobule, and sinusoidal endothelial cells lose fenestrations ("capillarization" of sinusoids). Major source of excess collagen is the Ito cell. Normally vitamin A fat-storage cells, Ito cells may become activated and transform into myofibroblast-like cells. Collagen synthesis is stimulated by

- Chronic inflammatory conditions, with cytokine generation.
- Release of cytokines by Kupffer cells.
- Disruption of the normal extracellular matrix.
- Direct toxic stimulation of collagen synthesis.

PORTAL HYPERTENSION (p. 835)

Increased resistance to portal blood flow develops from

- *Prehepatic:* Obstructive thrombosis and narrowing of the portal vein, or massive splenomegaly with shunting of blood into the splanchnic circulation.
- *Intrahepatic:* Cirrhosis, schistosomiasis, veno-occlusive disease, massive fatty change, diffuse fibrosing granulomatous disease, nodular regenerative hyperplasia.
- *Posthepatic:* Severe right-sided heart failure, constrictive pericarditis, hepatic vein outflow obstruction (Budd-Chiari syndrome).

   Major clinical consequences of portal hypertension are

- Ascites, especially in cirrhosis.
- Formation of portosystemic venous shunts.
- Congestive splenomegaly.
- Hepatic encephalopathy.

Ascites (p. 836)

Defined as the collection of excess serous fluid in the peritoneal cavity. Pathogenesis involves

- Hepatic sinusoidal hypertension.
- Percolation of hepatic lymph into the peritoneal cavity.
- Renal retention of sodium and water.

Portosystemic Shunts (p. 837)

Principal sites for portal-systemic venous bypasses are

- Cardioesophageal junction (*esophagogastric varices*). Rupture and bleeding cause massive hematemesis and death in one-half of cirrhotics.
- Rectum (hemorrhoids).
- Retroperitoneum.
- Falciform ligament and umbilicus (*caput medusae*).

Splenomegaly (p. 837)

Caused by long-standing congestion and may induce hematologic abnormalities attributable to hypersplenism.

BILIRUBIN AND HEPATIC BILE FORMATION

JAUNDICE AND CHOLESTASIS (p. 838)

Yellow discoloration of the skin and sclerae (*jaundice, icterus*) is due to systemic retention of bilirubin. *Cholestasis* is retention of bilirubin as well as other biliary solutes, e.g., bile salts, and cholesterol.

Jaundice occurs when bilirubin production exceeds hepatic clearance capacity, via the following mechanisms:

Unconjugated Hyperbilirubinemia

* Excessive production of bilirubin.
* Reduced hepatic uptake.
* Impaired hepatic conjugation.

Conjugated Hyperbilirubinemia

* Decreased hepatic excretion of bilirubin conjugates.
* Impaired intra- or extrahepatic bile flow.

More than one mechanism may operate to produce jaundice, but generally one mechanism predominates in a given disease state. *Cholestasis* may result from hepatocellular dysfunction or biliary obstruction. Symptoms include jaundice, *pruritus* from retention of bile acids, or *xanthomas* (skin accumulations of cholesterol).

MORPHOLOGY OF CHOLESTASIS

* Accumulation of bile pigment within the parenchyma of the liver: Dilated bile canaliculi, foamy degeneration of hepatocytes, Kupffer cell phagocytosis of bile.
* With biliary obstruction, portal tracts exhibit distended and proliferating bile ducts, edema, periductular neutrophils.
* Prolonged obstruction leads to *portal tract fibrosis* and eventually cirrhosis. Necrotic parenchymal foci may coalesce to form *bile lakes.*

CLINICAL FEATURES

* *Cholestasis of intrahepatic origin* (hepatocellular dysfunction or intrahepatic bile duct disease) cannot be benefited by surgery, short of transplantation.
* *Cholestasis due to extrahepatic obstruction* may be amenable to surgical correction.

HEREDITARY HYPERBILIRUBINEMIAS (p. 840)

Unconjugated hyperbilirubinemia occurs when >80% of serum bilirubin is unconjugated.

* *Bilirubin overproduction:* Hemolytic disease, resorption of major hemorrhages, intramedullary hemolysis (ineffective erythropoiesis).
* *Reduced hepatic uptake of bilirubin:* Gilbert's syndrome, some drugs (rifampin).

Gilbert's syndrome (?autosomal dominant): common, benign inherited condition with decreased levels of bilirubin glucuronosyltransferase (UGT). Occurs in 7% of the population. Characterized by mild, fluctuating subclinical hyperbilirubinemia, typically occurring in association with stress. No clinical consequences.

* *Impaired hepatic conjugation of bilirubin:* Transient deficiency of bilirubin UGT in newborns (*neonatal jaundice*); or may be genetic:

- *Crigler-Najjar syndrome Type I* (autosomal recessive): total absence of UGT, fatal.
- *Crigler-Najjar syndrome Type II* (autosomal dominant): less severe deficiency, nonfatal.

Conjugated hyperbilirubinemia occurs when >50% of serum bilirubin is conjugated. Is typically associated with cholestasis. Two inherited conditions:

- *Dubin-Johnson syndrome* (autosomal recessive): Defective canalicular secretion of bilirubin conjugates. Liver is brown, with accumulation of pigment granules in hepatocytes (polymers of epinephrine metabolites). Most patients are asymptomatic but jaundiced; normal life expectancy.
- *Rotor's syndrome* (autosomal recessive): Ill-characterized, asymptomatic conjugated hyperbilirubinemia.

HEPATIC FAILURE (p. 841)

Failure develops only with loss of more than 80% to 90% of hepatic function. Clinical features are shown in Table 17–1. Often, intercurrent disease places a greater demand on hepatic function and tips the balance toward decompensation: GI hemorrhage, systemic infection, electrolyte disturbances, severe physiologic stress. Few survive with supportive measures; hepatic transplantation may enable survival. Overall mortality is 70% to 95%. Conditions leading to hepatic failure are

- *Chronic liver disease:* Relentless chronic hepatitis, cirrhosis, inherited metabolic disorders.
- *Massive hepatic necrosis:* Fulminant viral hepatitis, massive toxic damage (acetaminophen, halothane, mushroom poisoning).
- Rare *ultrastructural lesions* without overt necrosis: Reye's syndrome, acute fatty liver of pregnancy, tetracycline.

HEPATIC ENCEPHALOPATHY (p. 842)

A metabolic disorder of the CNS and neuromuscular system, with minor morphologic changes in brain (edema, astrocytic

Table 17–1. Major Clinical Features of Hepatic Failure

Jaundice
Hypoalbuminemia
Coagulopathy
Disseminated intravascular coagulation
Hyperammonemia
Fetor hepaticus
Increased serum levels of hepatic enzymes LDH, alanine and serine aminotransferases
Gynecomastia, testicular atrophy, palmar erythema, spider angiomas of skin
Hepatic encephalopathy
Hepatorenal syndrome
Coma

Adapted from Cotran, R. S., Kumar, V., and Robbins, S. L.: Robbins Pathologic Basis of Disease. 5th ed. Philadelphia, W. B. Saunders Co., 1994, p. 841.

reaction). Pathogenesis unclear, possibly shunting of blood around liver, severe loss of hepatocellular function. Clinical features: disturbances in consciousness (behavioral abnormalities, confusion, stupor, coma, death), EEG changes, limb rigidity and hyperreflexia, seizures, asterixis (flapping tremor of extended hands).

HEPATORENAL SYNDROME (p. 842)

The appearance of renal failure in patients with severe liver disease, in whom there are no intrinsic renal disturbances. Kidney function promptly improves if hepatic failure is reversed. Pathophysiology unclear, possibly related to decreased renal blood flow with decreased glomerular filtration rate. Clinical features: drop in renal output, rising blood urea nitrogen (BUN) and creatinine. Urine is hyperosmolar, devoid of proteins or sediment, and *low in sodium.*

INFLAMMATORY DISORDERS

VIRAL HEPATITIS (p. 843)

Any blood-borne infection may involve the liver, whether systemic or abdominal in origin, including bacterial, fungal, and parasitic infections (discussed in Chapter 8). Systemic viral infections that may involve the liver include infectious mononucleosis (Epstein-Barr virus), cytomegalovirus, herpes virus, and, rarely, rubella, adenovirus, enterovirus infections, and yellow fever. However, *unless otherwise specified, "viral hepatitis" refers to infection of the liver caused by a small group of hepatotropic viruses.* All produce similar patterns of clinical and morphologic acute hepatitis but vary in their potential to induce chronic or fulminant disease or the carrier state.

Hepatitis A Virus (HAV) (p. 843)

Originally called "infectious hepatitis." Causes a benign, self-limited disease, incubation period 14–45 days. Accounts for 20% to 25% of acute hepatitis in the developing world. Fecal-oral spread. Does not cause chronic disease or the carrier state. Fulminant hepatitis is rare (fatality rate less than 0.1%). Small, nonenveloped, icosahedral capsid 27 nm in diameter, member of a single-stranded RNA picornavirus family. Acute infection marked by anti-HAV IgM in serum; IgG appears as IgM declines (within a few months) and can persist for years, conferring immunity.

Hepatitis B Virus (HBV) (p. 844)

Originally called "serum hepatitis"; the initial antigen discovery termed *Australia antigen (HAA).* Plays an important role in the development of hepatocellular carcinoma. Can produce

- An asymptomatic carrier state.
- Acute hepatitis with possible complete recovery.
- Chronic hepatitis, either indolent or progressive.
- Progression to cirrhosis in less than 1% of cases.
- Fulminant hepatitis with massive liver necrosis.

Spread mainly by parenteral routes (transfusion, blood products, needle-stick accidents, shared needles among drug addicts, and to newborn infants during parturition), or via body fluids (saliva, semen, and vaginal fluid), hence the risk of sexual transmission.

MOLECULAR BIOLOGY. Member of *hepadnavirus* family. DNA virus, spherical, 42-nm diameter (*Dane particle*), 3200-nucleotide double-stranded DNA circle. Viral coat contains surface antigen (HBsAg). Nucleocapsid has HBV-DNA, DNA polymerase, hepatitis B core antigen (HBcAg). HBeAg is elaborated in serum during viral replication and consists of HBcAg plus a "pre-core" region. HBV mutants may lack the ability to form HBeAg.

INCUBATION PERIOD. Four to 26 weeks (typically 6 to 8 weeks).

PATHOGENESIS. Immunologically mediated hepatocyte necrosis by sensitized cytotoxic T cells, attributed to cellular expression of viral antigens during the episomal phase of viral replication (*proliferative phase*). With integration of HBV-DNA into the host genome (*integrative phase*), viral replication ceases, infectivity ends, and active liver damage subsides.

SERUM MARKERS. HBsAg appears before symptoms, peaks during overt disease, declines over months, is a marker of active infection. HBeAg, HBV-DNA, and DNA-polymerase appear soon after HBsAg, before onset of acute disease. HBeAg usually declines within weeks; persistence indicates probable progression to chronic disease. IgM anti-HBc is usually the first antibody to appear, followed shortly by anti-HBe; IgG anti-HBc slowly replaces the IgM. Anti-HBs signifies the end of acute disease and persists for years, conferring immunity. In HBV mutants not expressing serum HBeAg, the inability to form anti-HBeAb carries the risk of more fulminant disease.

Hepatitis C Virus (HCV) (p. 846)

- Causes 90% to 95% of transfusion-associated hepatitis.
- Carries a 50% risk of chronic progressive hepatitis and an overall 25% risk of cirrhosis. *Persistent infection and chronic hepatitis are the hallmarks of HCV infection.*
- Primary risk groups are hemophiliacs, intravenous drug abusers, hemodialysis patients, and homosexuals. Sexual transmission is absent to rare. Fifty percent of cases are sporadic with no known exposure risk.

MOLECULAR BIOLOGY. Small, enveloped, single-stranded RNA virus of flavi/pesti virus family, 30- to 60-nm diameter. Single, ~3010-amino acid polypeptide is processed into nucleocapsid protein, envelope protein, five nonstructural proteins. Genomic variability constitutes a major obstacle to vaccine development.

INCUBATION PERIOD. Two to 26 weeks, mean 6 to 12 weeks.

PATHOGENESIS. Probably immunologically mediated liver damage.

SERUM MARKERS. HCV-RNA is detectable in blood for 1 to 3 weeks during active infection and persists in many patients despite the presence of neutralizing antibodies. Episodic elevations in serum transaminases are seen in chronic disease states. *Elevated titers of anti-HCV IgG following active infection do not confer effective immunity, either against reactivation of endogenous HCV or against infection with a new HCV strain.*

Hepatitis D Virus (HDV) (p. 848)

A small, defective RNA virus that can replicate and cause infection only when encapsulated by HBsAg. Hence, *HDV infection can develop only when there is concomitant HBV infection.*

- *Acute coinfection* by HDV and HBV: mild to fulminant hepatitis; chronicity rarely develops.
- *Superinfection* of chronic HBV by HDV: eruption of acute hepatitis, conversion of mild chronic disease into fulminant disease or into chronic disease terminating in cirrhosis.

Endemic in Africa, the Middle East, Italy, and elsewhere; in the United States, primarily drug addicts and male homosexuals.
MOLECULAR BIOLOGY. Virus has the appearance of a "Dane particle" with an HBV envelope, but an internal, 24-kD HDV virus-specific polypeptide (*delta antigen*, HDV Ag), and a 1689-base circular molecule of genomic single-stranded RNA.
SERUM MARKERS. HDV-RNA in blood and liver just before and in early acute symptomatic infection. IgM anti-HDV indicates recent HDV exposure. Differentiating acute coinfection from superinfection requires correlation with HBV markers.

Hepatitis E Virus (HEV) (p. 849)

Enterically transmitted, water-borne infection, endemic in Asia, Indian subcontinent, and elsewhere. *High mortality rate in pregnant women (20%).* Self-limiting disease, average incubation period of 6 weeks, no chronic disease tendency.
MOLECULAR BIOLOGY. Unenveloped, single-stranded RNA calicivirus, 32 to 34 nm in diameter, with 7.6-kb genome. Antigen (HEV Ag) in hepatocytes during active infection.

Clinicopathologic Syndromes (p. 849)

The Carrier State (p. 849)

A "carrier" is an individual without manifest symptoms who harbors and therefore can transmit an organism. Two types: those with little or no adverse effects ("healthy carriers") and those with chronic disease but few or no symptoms.

- HAV and HEV: Do not produce a carrier state.
- HBV: 90% to 95% of infants infected at birth become carriers, 1% to 10% of individuals infected as adults, especially individuals with impaired immunity.
- HCV: Can clearly induce a carrier state, estimated at 0.2% to 0.6% of the general United States population.
- HDV: Low risk of post-transfusion HDV infection.

MORPHOLOGY OF "HEALTHY" HBV CARRIERS. Normal liver architecture and hepatocytes. Isolated cells or clusters show a finely granular, eosinophilic cytoplasm ("ground glass") that stains positive for HBsAg. Tubules and spheres of HBsAg in the cytoplasm seen by electron microscopy. The "carrier" state of HCV does not exhibit ground glass cells.

Acute Viral Hepatitis (p. 850)

Similar for all hepatitis viruses: incubation period is of variable length depending on the causative agent (see previous discussion). Disease course consists of an asymptomatic preicteric phase, symptomatic icteric phase, and convalescence. A fulminant course with high mortality occurs in <1% of cases.

MORPHOLOGY. Can be mimicked by drug reactions. Liver slightly enlarged and more or less green. Necrosis of scattered hepatocytes, clumps, or an entire lobule; necrotic hepatocytes are eosinophilic and rounded-up (*apoptosis, Councilman bodies*) or swollen. Lymphocytes are variably present adjacent to necrotic cells. Macrophages engulf necrotic hepatocytes. Lobular architecture is disrupted by necrosis (*lobular disarray*). Connection of portal-to-central tracts (*bridging necrosis*) is a harbinger of more severe disease.

Ancillary features: Hypertrophy and hyperplasia of Kupffer cells and sinusoidal lining cells, portal tract inflammation (mainly lymphocytes and macrophages), hepatocellular regeneration, occasional cholestasis.

Chronic Viral Hepatitis (p. 851)

Symptomatic, biochemical, or serologic evidence of continuing inflammatory hepatic disease for more than 6 months without steady improvement. Major etiologies: viral hepatitis, Wilson's disease, α_1-antitrypsin deficiency, alcohol, drugs, autoimmunity. Morphologic patterns of chronic viral damage have been classified since 1968 as *chronic persistent hepatitis* (portal tract inflammation), *chronic lobular hepatitis* (lobular inflammation), and *chronic active hepatitis* (inflammation spilling from portal tracts into lobule). This classification is no longer used, since the primary determinant of disease progression is etiology. The likelihood of chronic hepatitis is

- HAV: Extremely rare.
- HBV: Greater than 90% in infected neonates, 5% of adults.
- HCV: *Develops in more than 50% of infected patients, of whom half progress to cirrhosis.*
- HDV: Rare in acute HBV/HDV coinfection but is the most frequent outcome of HDV superinfection.
- HEV: Does not produce chronic hepatitis.

MORPHOLOGY. Ranges from exceedingly mild to severe to eventual cirrhosis. Mild: chronic inflammatory infiltrate limited to portal tracts. The hallmark of progressive disease (formerly "chronic active hepatitis") is *piecemeal necrosis:* extension of chronic inflammation from portal tracts into parenchyma, with necrosis of hepatocytes; linking of portal-to-portal and portal-to-central tracts constitutes *bridging necrosis. Continued loss of hepatocytes results in fibrous septum formation which, accompanied by regeneration, eventuates in cirrhosis.*

CLINICAL FEATURES. Symptoms: fatigue, malaise, anorexia, bouts of jaundice. Occasional findings: spider angiomas, palmar erythema, mild hepatosplenomegaly, hepatic tenderness. Laboratory: persistently elevated serum liver enzymes, prolonged prothrombin time, hyperglobulinemia, hyperbilirubinemia.

Unpredictable clinical course: spontaneous remission, indolent disease without progression, rapidly progressive disease to cirrhosis within a few years. Death from complications of cirrhosis or hepatocellular carcinoma (develops in <0.1% of HBV-infected individuals in the United States, and an unknown percentage of HCV-infected individuals).

AUTOIMMUNE HEPATITIS (p. 853)

A chronic hepatitis of unknown etiology, which responds dramatically to immunosuppressive therapy.

- Marked by female predominance; absence of viral serologic markers; elevated serum IgG levels; high serum titers of autoantibodies in 80% of cases—antinuclear (ANA), anti–smooth muscle (SMA), antimitochondrial (AMA), anti–liver and kidney microsome (LKM) antibodies.
- Increased frequency of HLA B8 or DRw3.
- Associated with other autoimmune diseases: rheumatoid arthritis, thyroiditis, Sjögren's syndrome, ulcerative colitis.
- May progress to cirrhosis in some individuals.

MORPHOLOGY. Similar to chronic viral hepatitis, with robust portal infiltrate of lymphocytes and plasma cells.

FULMINANT HEPATITIS (p. 853)

Fulminant hepatic failure is hepatic insufficiency progressing from onset to death (or hepatic transplantation) within 2 to 3 weeks. Subfulminant hepatic failure denotes a course of up to 3 months. Causes listed in Table 17–2. May present with jaundice, encephalopathy, fetor hepaticus, coagulopathy and bleeding, cardiovascular instability, renal failure, adult respiratory distress syndrome, electrolyte and acid-base disturbances, and sepsis. Mortality is 25% to 90% without transplantation.

Table 17–2. Causes of Fulminant or Subfulminant Hepatic Failure

---

Acute viral hepatitis (50% to 65%)
    Acute hepatitis A
    Acute hepatitis B
    Acute hepatitis C
    Acute hepatitis D (delta)
        Coinfection with HBV
        Superinfection of HBV
    Acute hepatitis E
    Acute hepatitis due to infection with herpes or other viruses
Acute drug-induced hepatitis
Acute hepatitis due to poisoning
    Amanita phalloides (mushroom)
Other causes
    Ischemic liver cell necrosis
    Obstruction of the hepatic veins
        Budd-Chiari syndrome
        Veno-occlusive disease
    Massive malignant infiltration
    Wilson's disease
    Microvesicular steatosis
        Acute fatty liver of pregnancy
        Reye's syndrome
        Drug-induced microvesicular steatosis
    Autoimmune chronic hepatitis
    Reactivation of chronic hepatitis B
    Hyperthermia (heat stroke)
    Liver transplantation
    Partial hepatectomy

Adapted with permission from Bernau, J., et al.: Fulminant and subfulminant liver failure: Definitions and causes. Seminars in Liver Disease, 6(2):98, 1986. Thieme Medical Publishers, Inc.

MORPHOLOGY. The entire liver, or just portions, may be involved. Affected areas are soft, muddy-red or bile stained; liver is shrunken. Entire lobules are destroyed, leaving cellular debris and a collapsed reticulin network; inflammation may be minimal. With massive destruction, regeneration is disorderly and scar may form, producing coarsely lobulated *postnecrotic cirrhosis*.

POSTNECROTIC CIRRHOSIS (p. 855)

Progressive chronic hepatitis of any etiology inexorably transforms a normal liver into a patchwork of variably sized nodules alternating with broad septal scars. Most common cause is viral infection, but etiology cannot be deduced from morphology. Death is from usual complications of cirrhosis, or from hepatocellular carcinoma.

LIVER ABSCESSES (p. 856)

Common in developing countries, from parasitic infections, e.g., amebic, echinococcal, other protozoal or helminthic organisms. Uncommon in developed countries; usually bacterial or candidal spread from an infection elsewhere.

- Sources of infection: Intra-abdominal via the portal vein; systemic via arterial supply; biliary tree (*ascending cholangitis*); direct extension; penetrating injuries.
- Histologic features are nonspecific abscess formation, although parasitic fragments may be identifiable in tissue sections.

DRUG-INDUCED AND TOXIN-INDUCED LIVER DISEASE (p. 856)

Exposure to a toxin or therapeutic agent should be included in the differential diagnosis of any form of liver disease. Injury is caused by direct drug toxicity, hepatic conversion of a xenobiotic to an active toxin, and/or injury via immune mechanisms. Injury may be immediate or develop over weeks to months. Injury may take the form of *hepatocyte necrosis, cholestasis,* or *insidious onset of liver dysfunction. Drug-induced chronic hepatitis is clinically and histologically indistinguishable from chronic viral hepatitis.* Examples are given in Table 17–3.

ALCOHOLIC LIVER DISEASE (p. 857)

Alcohol abuse constitutes the major form of liver disease in most Western countries. The metabolism of ethanol is described in Figure 9–5 (p. 388) of *Pathologic Basis of Disease*, 5th edition. There are three distinctive, albeit overlapping, forms of liver disease, characterized by morphology.

HEPATIC STEATOSIS (FATTY LIVER) (p. 857)

Small (*microvesicular*) lipid droplets accumulate in hepatocytes with even moderate intake of alcohol. With chronic alcohol intake, lipid accumulates in *macrovesicular* droplets, displacing the nucleus. At first centrilobular, fatty change may involve entire lobule over time. The liver becomes enlarged and is soft and yellow. Little to no fibrosis at the outset, but this may develop.

Table 17–3. Drug-Induced and Toxin-Induced
Hepatic Injury

Hepatocellular Damage
Microvesicular fatty change
  Tetracycline, salicylates, yellow phosphorus
Macrovesicular fatty change
  Ethanol, methotrexate, amiodarone
Centrilobular necrosis
  CCl_4, acetaminophen, halothane, rifampin, bromobenzene
Diffuse or massive necrosis
  Halothane, isoniazid, acetaminophen, α-methyldopa,
    trinitrotoluene, *Amanita phalloides* (mushroom) toxin
Hepatitis, acute and chronic
  α-Methyldopa, isoniazid, nitrofurantoin, phenytoin,
    oxyphenisatin
Fibrosis-cirrhosis
  Ethanol, methotrexate, amiodarone, most drugs that cause
    chronic hepatitis
Granuloma formation
  Sulfonamides, α-methyldopa, quinidine, phenylbutazone,
    hydralazine, allopurinol
Cholestasis (with or without hepatocellular injury)
  Chlorpromazine, anabolic steroids, erythromycin estolate,
    oral contraceptives, organic arsenicals

Vascular Disorders
Veno-occlusive disease
  Cytotoxic drugs, pyrrolizidine alkaloids (bush tea)
Hepatic or portal vein thrombosis
  Estrogens (and oral contraceptives), cytotoxic drugs
Peliosis hepatis
  Anabolic steroids, oral contraceptives, danazol

Hyperplasia and Neoplasia
Adenoma
  Oral contraceptives
Hepatocellular carcinoma
  Vinyl chloride, aflatoxin, Thorotrast
Cholangiocarcinoma
  Thorotrast
Angiosarcoma
  Vinyl chloride, inorganic arsenicals, Thorotrast

From Cotran, R. S., Kumar, V., and Robbins, S. L.: Robbins Pathologic
Basis of Disease. 5th ed. Philadelphia, W. B. Saunders Co., 1994, p. 857.

ALCOHOLIC HEPATITIS (p. 858)

Characterized by *liver cell necrosis*, particularly in centrilobular
region; *Mallory body* formation (eosinophilic clumped intermediate filaments); *neutrophilic reaction* to degenerating hepatocytes;
inflammation in portal tracts spilling into lobule; and
fibrosis—sinusoidal, pericentral, and periportal.

ALCOHOLIC CIRRHOSIS (p. 858)

The final and irreversible outcome of alcoholic liver disease. The
liver is transformed from a fatty and enlarged organ to a brown,
shrunken, nonfatty organ. Regenerative nodules may be promi-

nent or buried in dense fibrous scar. End stage resembles postne-crotic cirrhosis.

PATHOGENESIS OF ALCOHOLIC
LIVER DISEASE (p. 859)

- *Steatosis* results from shunting of substrates toward lipid bio-synthesis, impaired lipoprotein assembly and secretion, and increased peripheral catabolism of fat. Ethanol also displaces other nutrients as a *caloric source.*
- *Induction of cytochrome P-450* augments biotransformation of other drugs to toxic metabolites, which cause liver injury.
- *Free radicals* are generated by the microsomal ethanol oxidiz-ing system (MEOS) involved in the metabolism of ethanol.
- Ethanol directly affects *microtubule* and *mitochondrial* func-tion and *membrane fluidity.* Ethanol also induces *immunologic attack* on hepatic neoantigens by unclear mechanisms.
- *Acetaldehyde,* an intermediate metabolite of ethanol catabo-lism, induces lipid peroxidation and adduct formation.

CLINICAL COURSE (p. 861)

Hepatic steatosis: Asymptomatic or mild elevation of serum bili-rubin and alkaline phosphatase. *Alcoholic hepatitis:* acute onset of mild to fulminant hepatic failure. *Alcoholic cirrhosis:* manifests like any other form of cirrhosis. Proximate causes of death are hepatic coma (most common), massive gastrointestinal hemor-rhage, intercurrent infection, hepatorenal syndrome, and hepato-cellular carcinoma (in 3% to 6% of patients).

INBORN ERRORS OF METABOLISM AND
PEDIATRIC LIVER DISEASE
HEMOCHROMATOSIS (p. 861)

Defined as *the excessive accumulation of body iron, most of which is deposited in the parenchymal cells of various organs,* particularly liver and pancreas. *Hereditary hemochromatosis* (HHC; also *primary* or *idiopathic hemochromatosis*) is a homo-zygous recessive heritable disorder. *Secondary hemochromatosis:* denotes disorders with identifiable sources of excess iron (Table 17–4).

Features of fully developed HHC: micronodular cirrhosis, diabetes mellitus, skin pigmentation, arthritis. Most common cause of death: hepatocellular carcinoma. Frequency of HHC allele is 6% in white populations of Northern European descent; homozygosity in 0.45% and heterozygosity in 11%.

PATHOGENESIS. Hemochromatosis gene on short arm of chro-mosome 6, close to HLA locus. Associated with HLA A3, B7, B14, or Bw35. Fundamental defect appears to be unregulated intestinal absorption of iron. Fundamental disease mechanism is direct iron toxicity to innocent bystander host tissues. Mecha-nisms of toxicity: free radical formation with lipid peroxidation, stimulation of collagen formation, interactions of iron with DNA. Effects are potentially reversible with treatment, unless cirrhosis has already developed.

MORPHOLOGY. Iron accumulates as ferritin and hemosiderin in parenchymal tissues (liver, pancreas, myocardium, endocrine glands), and in synovial joint linings. The liver initially is histolog-

Table 17–4. Classification of Iron Overload

Increased iron absorption
    Idiopathic primary hemochromatosis
    Dyserythropoietic anemias
        β-Thalassemia
        Sideroblastic anemia
        Pyruvate kinase deficiency
    Liver disease
        Postportocaval anastomosis
        Porphyria cutanea tarda
    Increased oral intake of iron
        Dietary iron overload in the Bantu
        Prolonged excessive medicinal iron ingestion
    Congenital atransferrinemia
Parenteral iron administration
    Blood transfusions
    Iron dextran injections
    Chronic hemodialysis
Iron redistribution
    Alcoholic liver disease

From Nichols, G. M., and Bacon, B. R.: Iron metabolism and disorders of iron overload. *In* Kaplowitz, N. (ed.): Liver and Biliary Diseases. Baltimore, Williams & Wilkins, 1992, p. 311, with permission.

ically normal, but with years becomes progressively fibrotic, eventuating in cirrhosis. The pancreas develops diffuse interstitial fibrosis with atrophy. Diffuse myocardial interstitial fibrosis leads to a cardiomyopathy, with progressive heart enlargement. A slate-blue color is imparted to the skin due to deposition of hemosiderin in dermal macrophages and fibroblasts. The testes become atrophic, and joint synovitis develops with synovial hemosiderin deposition and calcium pyrophosphate precipitation.

The Prussian blue reaction (potassium ferrocyanide and hydrochloric acid) highlights tissue hemosiderin in all involved tissues. *Biochemical determination of hepatic iron content in unfixed tissue is the standard for quantifying liver iron.* Normal is less than 1000 µg/gm dry weight of liver. Adult patients with HHC exceed 10,000 µg/gm dry weight.

WILSON'S DISEASE (p. 863)

Autosomal recessive disorder of copper metabolism, marked by the accumulation of toxic levels of copper in liver, brain, and eye (*hepatolenticular degeneration*).

PATHOGENESIS. Genetic defect on chromosome 13, in linkage with esterase D locus. Allele frequency is 1:200 to 1:400; disease incidence of 1:200,000. Unclear disease mechanism: there is normal copper absorption and delivery to liver but diminished export from liver into the circulation. Underlying defect may be related to *defective mobilization of copper from hepatocellular lysosomes for biliary excretion.* Proposed mechanisms of tissue injury: poisoning of hepatic enzymes, abnormal binding of copper to serum proteins, and formation of free radicals.

Biochemical diagnosis is based on *a decrease in serum ceruloplasmin* (a copper-binding serum protein), *increase in hepatic copper content,* and *increased urinary excretion of copper.*

MORPHOLOGY. May range from minor to severe liver damage, e.g., *fatty change; acute and chronic hepatitis* resembling viral hepatitis but with Mallory bodies, fatty change, and copper accumulation; *cirrhosis* with features of chronic hepatitis; and *massive liver necrosis*, fortunately rare.

ALPHA₁-ANTITRYPSIN (α_1-AT) DEFICIENCY (p. 864)

Autosomal recessive disorder with abnormally low serum levels of this major protease inhibitor ("Pi"); deficiency leads to pulmonary disease (emphysema, *see p. 685*, PBD 5th ed.), and hepatic disease (cholestasis or cirrhosis).
PATHOGENESIS. α_1-AT is 394-amino acid serum protease inhibitor synthesized primarily in the liver. Gene is on chromosome 14, with over 75 gene products. Most common allele is PiM, and genotype PiMM. Homozygotes for the PiZ allele (genotype PiZZ) have circulating α_1-AT levels 10% of normal. Gene frequency of PiZ in the North American white population is 0.0122, with homozygote frequency of 1:7000.

PiZ exhibits a Glu_{342} to Lys_{342} substitution: the nascent polypeptide misfolds and cannot be secreted normally. Impaired hepatic α_1-AT secretion leads to its accumulation in hepatocytes (within the endoplasmic reticulum); mechanism of liver damage is unclear.
MORPHOLOGY. Lesions include *neonatal hepatitis* (active inflammation with cholestasis), *childhood* and *adult cirrhosis;* hepatocellular carcinoma is a rare complication. Diagnosed by PAS-diastase–resistant cytoplasmic globules of retained α_1-AT in hepatocytes.

REYE'S SYNDROME (p. 865)

An acute disorder usually of childhood, occurring 3 to 5 days after a viral illness, heralded by pernicious vomiting, irritability, and lethargy. Microvesicular steatosis and disruption of mitochondrial ultrastructure in hepatocytes, skeletal muscle, kidneys, and heart. In severe cases, cerebral edema occurs with swelling of astrocytes and formation of myelin blebs. Pathogenesis believed to involve mitochrondrial biochemical derangements; some patients may possess an underlying disorder in fatty acid metabolism. Associated with administration of salicylates (aspirin) during viral syndrome. Fatality is 10%–40%; recovery is usually complete. Disease frequency has markedly decreased in recent years, with discontinuance of aspirin use for febrile illness in children.

NEONATAL HEPATITIS (p. 866)

Nonspecific term for a variety of hepatic disorders (Table 17–5) in the neonate involving prolonged conjugated hyperbilirubinemia (*neonatal cholestasis*), hepatomegaly, and variable degrees of hepatic dysfunction such as hypoprothrombinemia.
MORPHOLOGY. Hepatocytes: necrosis and lobular disarray, panlobular giant cell transformation, prominent cholestasis. Inflammation of portal tract, Kupffer cell reaction, extramedullary hematopoiesis. To be distinguished from the bile duct proliferation seen in obstructive bile duct disease (biliary atresia).

Table 17–5. Causes of Neonatal Cholestasis

Neonatal hepatitis
  Idiopathic
  Viral
    Cytomegalovirus
    Rubella
    Reovirus 3
    Herpesviruses
    Enteroviruses
    Coxsackievirus
    ECHO virus
    Parvovirus
    Adenovirus
    Hepatitis B,C
  Bacterial and parasitic
    Bacterial sepsis
    Listeriosis
    Tuberculosis
    Syphilis
    Toxoplasmosis

Bile duct obstruction
  Extrahepatic biliary atresia
  Anomalies of the extrahepatic biliary tree
  Inspissated bile/mucus plug
  Cholelithiasis
  Tumors

Idiopathic syndromes of intrahepatic cholestasis

Toxic
  Drugs
  Parenteral nutrition

Metabolic diseases

Amino acid	Tyrosinemia
Lipid	Niemann-Pick disease
	Gaucher's disease
	Wolman's disease
Carbohydrate	Galactosemia
	Fructosemia
	Type IV glycogenosis
Bile acid metabolism	
Miscellaneous	α_1-Antitrypsin deficiency
	Cystic fibrosis
	Neonatal hemochromatosis
	Hypothyroidism
	Hypopituitarism

Miscellaneous
  Shock/hypoperfusion
  Intestinal obstruction
  Histiocytosis X
  Indian childhood cirrhosis
  Erythrophagocytic lymphohistiocytosis
  Autosomal trisomies
  Neonatal lupus erythematosus

Adapted from Suchy, F. J., Schneider, B. L.: Neonatal jaundice and cholestasis. *In* Kaplowitz, N. (ed.): Liver and Biliary Diseases. Baltimore, Williams & Wilkins, 1992, p. 445.

INTRAHEPATIC BILIARY TRACT DISEASE

SECONDARY BILIARY CIRRHOSIS (p. 867)

Most common causes: obstruction from extrahepatic cholelithiasis (stones), biliary atresia, malignancies of biliary tree and head of pancreas, strictures from previous surgical procedures.

MORPHOLOGY. *Cholestasis* may be severe but is reversible. *Periportal fibrosis* eventually leads to *cirrhosis,* which is irreversible. End stage liver is yellow-green and finely divided by fibrous tissue. Small and large bile ducts are distended and contain inspissated bile; ascending bacterial infection (cholangitis) incites neutrophilic infiltration of bile ducts and abscess formation.

PRIMARY BILIARY CIRRHOSIS (PBC) (p. 868)

A chronic, progressive cholestatic liver disease characterized by destruction of intrahepatic bile ducts, portal inflammation and scarring, and eventual cirrhosis and liver failure. Presymptomatic phase may span two or more decades. Primarily a disease of middle-aged women. Onset is insidious, with pruritus and hepatomegaly; jaundice and xanthomas (from retained cholesterol) develop later, eventuating in general hepatic failure.

Laboratory: Elevated serum alkaline phosphatase and cholesterol; serum antimitochondrial antibodies (AMA; especially M2 subtype) positive in 90% of patients. Associated conditions: Sjögren's syndrome (dry eyes and mouth), scleroderma, thyroiditis, rheumatoid arthritis, Raynaud's phenomenon, membranous glomerulonephritis, and celiac disease. Autoimmune pathogenesis.

MORPHOLOGY. Best described as

- *Portal tract lesion:* Destruction of interlobular and septal bile ducts by granulomatous inflammation; inflammatory infiltrate of portal tracts;
- *Progressive lesion:* Global involvement of hepatic portal tracts, secondary obstructive changes with eventual cirrhosis; and
- *End stage:* Indistinguishable from other forms of cirrhosis.

PRIMARY SCLEROSING CHOLANGITIS (PSC) (p. 869)

A chronic, progressive cholestatic liver disease characterized by inflammation, obliterative fibrosis, and segmental dilatation of the intrahepatic and extrahepatic bile ducts. Commonly seen in association with inflammatory bowel disease (70% of cases), particularly chronic ulcerative colitis. More common in middle-aged men. Pathogenesis is unknown; autoantibodies are usually absent.

MORPHOLOGY. Segmental inflammation and concentric fibrosis around bile ducts, progressive atrophy, and obliteration of the bile duct lumen; culminates in biliary cirrhosis (and hepatic failure).

ANOMALIES OF THE BILIARY TREE (p. 870)

Altered architecture of the intrahepatic biliary tree:

- *Von Meyenburg complexes:* Small clusters of dilated bile ducts in a fibrous stroma; an incidental portal tract lesion.
- *Polycystic liver disease:* Few to hundreds of biliary epithelium-lined cystic lesions 0.5 to 4 cm in diameter, seen in association with polycystic kidney disease.

- *Congenital hepatic fibrosis:* Incomplete involution of embryonic ductal structures; liver is subdivided by dense fibrous septa with embedded, irregular biliary structures. Portal hypertension with esophageal varices may develop.
- *Caroli's disease:* Segmental dilatation of larger ducts of intrahepatic biliary tree; complicated by cholelithiasis, hepatic abscesses, and cholangiocarcinoma.

CIRCULATORY DISORDERS (p. 871)

- *Obstruction to inflow of blood.* Extrahepatic: portal vein thrombosis, postsurgical compromise of hepatic artery. Intrahepatic: thrombosis with infarction, idiopathic fibrosing obliterative portal vein lesions.
- *Compromise to sinusoidal blood flow.* Sinusoidal occlusion: disseminated intravascular coagulation (e.g., eclampsia), sickle cell disease, sarcoidosis. Systemic compromise: systemic hypoperfusion (e.g., shock).
- *Hepatic vein outflow obstruction:* Passive congestion (e.g., constrictive pericarditis), hepatic vein thrombosis (Budd-Chiari syndrome), veno-occlusive disease.

LIVER INFARCTION (p. 871)

Rare, may arise from embolism, neoplasia, polyarteritis nodosa, sepsis with localized thrombosis, or surgical procedures.

PORTAL VEIN OBSTRUCTION AND THROMBOSIS (p. 872)

Portal vein thrombosis: Hypercoagulable conditions, cirrhosis, following neonatal umbilical transfusions or transplantation. *Pylephlebitis:* Peritoneal infections. *Splenic vein thrombosis:* Secondary to pancreatitis. *Retrograde propagation of intrahepatic tumor,* especially hepatocellular carcinoma.

PASSIVE CONGESTION AND CENTRILOBULAR NECROSIS (p. 872)

The two represent a morphologic and clinical continuum, manifesting as elevated serum transaminases.

- Cardiac decompensation with right-sided failure leads to *congestion:* enlarged, tense, and cyanotic liver, which oozes blood on cut section. Soft and dusky centrilobular areas are surrounded by paler portal areas (the *"nutmeg liver"*); centrilobular congestion and hepatocyte atrophy.
- Left-sided heart failure or shock may lead to hepatic hypoperfusion and hypoxia; centrilobular hepatocytes undergo ischemic *necrosis.*
- The synergistic combination of passive congestion and hypoperfusion generates *centrilobular hemorrhagic necrosis.*

Cardiac Sclerosis (p. 873)

Chronic severe congestive heart failure may lead to centrilobular fibrosis of the liver. Cirrhosis *per se* is rare.

PELIOSIS HEPATIS (p. 873)

Primary dilatation of hepatic sinusoids associated with exposure to anabolic steroids, rarely oral contraceptives and danazol. Liver is mottled and blotchy with irregular blood-filled lakes. Microscopic lesions consist of irregular blood-filled cystic spaces, with or without a lining endothelium.

HEPATIC VEIN THROMBOSIS (BUDD-CHIARI SYNDROME) (p. 874)

Develops in thrombotic conditions: polycythemia vera, pregnancy and the postpartum state, oral contraceptive use, paroxysmal nocturnal hemoglobinuria, intra-abdominal cancers (e.g., hepatocellular carcinoma). Membranous webs of inferior vena cava may give rise to obstruction.

Characterized by hepatomegaly, weight gain, ascites, abdominal pain. May be acute or more chronic. In acute cases, liver is swollen and red-purple; parenchyma has profound centrilobular congestion and necrosis. Subacute or chronic cases may develop superimposed fibrosis.

VENO-OCCLUSIVE DISEASE (p. 874)

Originally described in Jamaican drinkers of pyrrolizidine alkaloid–containing bush tea; now occurs primarily in bone marrow transplant population as a toxic complication of drug treatment. Clinical features are the same as those of Budd-Chiari syndrome. Characterized by patchy obliteration of hepatic vein radicles by varying amounts of endothelial swelling and collagen.

HEPATIC DISEASE ASSOCIATED WITH PREGNANCY

PRE-ECLAMPSIA AND ECLAMPSIA (p. 875)

Pre-eclampsia is defined as hypertension, proteinuria, peripheral edema, coagulation abnormalities, and varying degrees of disseminated intravascular coagulation. *Eclampsia* is defined as hyperreflexia and convulsions occurring in the setting of pre-eclampsia. The *HELLP* syndrome (*h*emolysis, *e*levated *l*iver enzymes, and *l*ow *p*latelets) is common in pre-eclampsia. Definitive treatment is termination of pregnancy.

MORPHOLOGY. *Gross:* small, red hemorrhagic patches, with occasional yellow or white patches of infarction. *Microscopic:* Fibrin deposits in periportal sinusoids; periportal necrosis and hemorrhage. Coalescence of hemorrhagic areas leads to hepatic hematomas and potentially fatal intra-abdominal rupture.

ACUTE FATTY LIVER OF PREGNANCY (p. 875)

Incipient hepatic failure in the third trimester, leading to bleeding, nausea and vomiting, jaundice, coma, and death. Diagnosis is based on *demonstration of microvesicular fatty transformation of hepatocytes*. Pathogenesis unknown. Definitive treatment is termination of pregnancy.

INTRAHEPATIC CHOLESTASIS OF PREGNANCY
(p. 876)

Onset of pruritus and jaundice in third trimester of pregnancy; pathophysiology related to estrogenic hormones. Liver shows cholestasis; generally benign, but pruritus may be severe.

TRANSPLANTATION (p. 876; Tables 17–6 and 17–7)
DRUG TOXICITY FOLLOWING BONE MARROW TRANSPLANTATION (p. 876)

Administration of cytotoxic drugs prior to transplantation leads to hepatic dysfunction in up to one-half of patients; heralded by weight gain, tender hepatomegaly, edema, ascites, hyperbilirubinemia, and a fall in urinary sodium excretion. *Clinical features are indistinguishable from those of veno-occlusive disease.* Morphologic features are nonspecific (hepatocyte necrosis and cholestasis). Outcome is dependent on severity of hepatic injury.

GRAFT-VERSUS-HOST DISEASE (GVHD) AND LIVER REJECTION (p. 876)

GVHD is characterized by *direct attack of lymphocytes on epithelial cells of the liver. Acute GVHD* generates a picture of hepatitis (parenchymal inflammation and hepatocyte necrosis), vascular lymphocytic inflammation and intimal proliferation (*endothelialitis*), and *destruction of bile ducts. Chronic GVHD* en-

Table 17–6. Major Indications for Liver Transplantation

Fulminant hepatic failure
  Viral hepatitis
  Acute poisoning
  Metabolic liver disease
  Acute fatty liver of pregnancy
Cirrhosis arising from
  Alcoholic liver disease
  Viral hepatitis
  Autoimmune chronic active hepatitis
  Chronic drug-induced injury
  Cryptogenic cirrhosis
End stage cholestatic disorders
  Biliary atresia
  Primary biliary cirrhosis
Metabolic disorders
  Alpha$_1$-antitrypsin deficiency
  Crigler-Najjar syndrome
  Glycogen storage disease
  Wilson's disease
Hepatic malignancies
  Primary liver cancer
Vascular disorders
  Budd-Chiari syndrome
  Veno-occlusive disease
Miscellaneous
  Biliary tree malformations
  Severe trauma

Table 17–7. Hepatic Complications of Bone Marrow and Liver Transplantation

---

Bone Marrow Transplantation
Pretransplant
    Viral hepatitis
    Malignant involvement
    Drug toxicity
    Veno-occlusive disease
    Opportunistic infection
    Biliary tract disease
Post-transplant (listed in approximate order of early to late
    complications)
    Drug toxicity
    Veno-occlusive disease
    Graft-versus-host disease (acute or chronic)
    Opportunistic infection
    Viral hepatitis (hepatotropic)
    Nodular regenerative hyperplasia
    Toxicity from total parenteral nutrition
    Epstein-Barr virus–induced lymphoproliferative disorders

Liver Transplantation (listed in approximate order of early to
    late complications)
    Primary graft nonfunction
    Technical problems (e.g., vascular anastomoses)
    Hyperacute rejection
    Acute rejection
    Drug toxicity
    Opportunistic infections
    Technical problems (e.g., biliary anastomosis)
    Nonspecific cholestasis
    Chronic vascular rejection
    Vanishing bile duct syndrome
    Hepatic artery thrombosis
    Portal vein thrombosis
    Recurrent disease
    Viral hepatitis (hepatotropic)
    Epstein-Barr virus–induced lymphoproliferative disorders

Based on Cotran, R. S., Kumar, V., and Robbins, S. L.: Robbins Pathologic Basis of Disease. 5th ed. Philadelphia, W. B. Saunders Co., 1994, p. 877.

genders portal tract inflammation, bile duct destruction, and fibrosis.

Acute rejection of liver allografts exhibits portal tract inflammation and vascular changes typical of all solid organ transplants. *Chronic rejection* may lead to obliteration of arteries and bile ducts and eventual loss of the graft.

TUMORS AND TUMOROUS CONDITIONS (p. 878)

Hemangiomas and biliary cysts are common benign lesions.

NODULAR HYPERPLASIAS (p. 878)

Solitary or multiple benign hepatocellular nodules in the absence of cirrhosis; putative etiology is focal obliteration of hepatic vasculature, with compensatory hypertrophy of well-vascularized lobules. *Focal nodular hyperplasia* occurs in young to middle-aged adults and is an irregular, unencapsulated tumor containing a central stellate fibrous scar. *Nodular regenerative hyperplasia* is a diffuse nodular transformation of the liver *without fibrosis,* occurring in association with virtually any systemic inflammatory condition; may pose problems from portal hypertension.

ADENOMAS (p. 878)

Liver cell adenomas are benign neoplasms of hepatocytes up to 30 cm in diameter occurring in younger women, typically on oral contraceptives. Adenomas may be confused with malignancy, may rupture with massive hemorrhage, and rarely may harbor hepatocellular carcinoma. Composed of sheets and cords of hepatocytes, with arteries and veins; *portal tracts with bile ducts are absent.*

MALIGNANT TUMORS (p. 879)

Most tumors involving the liver are metastatic. Most primary liver cancers are hepatocellular carcinomas. Rare variants are *hepatoblastoma:* tumor of young childhood, exhibiting *epithelial* features of the fetal liver, or *mixed* features of epithelial and mesenchymal differentiation; *angiosarcoma:* similar to those occurring elsewhere, associated with exposure to vinyl chloride, arsenic, and Thorotrast (a thyroid contrast agent of the 1950s).

Primary Carcinoma of the Liver (p. 879)

Hepatocellular carcinoma (HCC): 90% of primary liver cancer, arises in the middle to late decades of life, male:female ratio of 3–4:1. A strong causal relationship has been established between hepatotropic viral infection (especially HBV) and HCC.
EPIDEMIOLOGY OF HCC. Global distribution is closely linked to distribution of HBV infection. Represents 40% of all cancers in high-incidence locales (Africa, Southeast Asia), and 2%–3% in United States and Western Europe. Strongly associated with protracted HBV infection, particularly when acquired early in life, presumably following integration of HBV into the hepatocellular genome. Chronic HCV infection also strongly implicated. Other associated environmental influences: cirrhosis (alcoholism, primary hemochromatosis, tyrosinemia), environmental and iatrogenic carcinogens (aflatoxin B_1 from *Aspergillus,* Thorotrast).
MORPHOLOGY. *Gross:* unifocal mass, multifocal nodules, or as a diffusely infiltrative cancer, with massive liver enlargement. More often occurs in cirrhotic livers in the United States. Pale pink-yellow or bile-stained; intrahepatic metastasis and vascular invasion (especially of hepatic veins and portal vein radicles) are common.

May range from well-differentiated to highly anaplastic undifferentiated lesions. *Well-differentiated:* hepatocytes arranged in trabecular (sinusoidal) or acinar (tubular) pseudoglandular patterns. *Poorly differentiated:* markedly pleomorphic giant cells; small, completely undifferentiated cells; spindle cells; or completely anaplastic cells. Hepatocellular features include formation of bile (by light microscopy) or bile canaliculi (by electron microscopy); cytoplasmic inclusions resembling Mallory bodies; staining for alpha-fetoprotein and alpha$_1$-antitrypsin.
CLINICAL FEATURES. Hepatomegaly, right upper quadrant pain,

weight loss, or elevated serum levels of alpha-fetoprotein. Prognosis depends on the resectability of the tumor. In Western countries, survival is dismal; death within 6 months of diagnosis. **Fibrolamellar Variant of HCC.** Arises in the absence of identifiable risk factors or underlying liver disease in children, adolescents, and young adults. More often resectable; 60% survival at 5 years. Usually a single, sometimes encapsulated multinodular mass. Contains prominent fibrous bands separating trabeculae of large, eosinophilic polygonal hepatocytes. Cytoplasmic hyalin globules and PAS-positive inclusions may be present.

Cholangiocarcinoma. Arises from elements of the intrahepatic biliary tree. Causal associations: prior treatment with Thorotrast, protracted parasitic infection of the biliary tree with *Clonorchis* (*Opisthorchis sinensis*) and its close relatives, and Caroli's disease. Cirrhosis not usually present, unlike HCC. As with HCC, may appear as a unifocal large mass, multifocal, or diffusely infiltrative. Extensive intrahepatic nodular metastases and spread to regional lymph nodes, distant metastasis to lungs, other viscera. Unlike HCC, tumor is typically pale (since biliary epithelium does not secrete bilirubin pigment) and firm, and is composed of bile ductular elements that may be well- or more poorly differentiated, resembling adenocarcinomas elsewhere in the alimentary tract. Mixed variants of *hepatocellular cholangiocarcinoma* may rarely occur. Clinical outlook is dismal, as they are rarely resectable.

METASTATIC TUMORS (p. 882)

The liver and lung are the visceral organs most often involved in the metastatic spread of cancers. Thus, the overwhelming majority of hepatic malignancy is metastatic in origin, most commonly from carcinomas of the breast, lung, and colon—any cancer in any site of the body may spread to the liver, including those of the blood-forming elements. Typically, multiple implants are present, with massive enlargement of the liver. Metastases that outgrow their blood supply become centrally necrotic. Massive involvement of the liver may be present before hepatic failure develops.

BILIARY SYSTEM

CONGENITAL ANOMALIES (p. 884)

Normal anatomy of biliary tree: pancreatic duct and common bile duct join to form a common intrapancreatic channel; or the ducts enter the duodenum separately. Abnormal variants of gallbladder: folded fundus (*phrygian cap*), congenitally *absent* or *duplicated, bilobed* or *aberrant location*.

DISORDERS OF THE GALLBLADDER
CHOLELITHIASIS (GALLSTONES) (p. 884)

Bile is a carrier fluid for the hepatic elimination of cholesterol (as free cholesterol and as bile salts), bilirubin, and xenobiotics from the body. Bile salts emulsify dietary lipid, facilitating intestinal lipid digestion and absorption. Cholesterol is solubilized by bile salts and cosecreted lecithin; supersaturation of bile with cholesterol or bilirubin salts predisposes to stone formation. Two kinds of stones: *cholesterol* (more than 50% crystalline cholesterol monohydrate) and *pigmented* (predominantly bilirubin calcium salts).

PREVALENCE AND RISK FACTORS. Gallstones afflict 10% to 20% of adult populations in developed countries. Patients with cholesterol gallstones exhibit these risk factors:

- Native Americans, adults in industrialized countries.
- Increasing age, male:female ratio 1:2.
- Estrogenic influences, clofibrate, obesity, rapid weight loss.
- Gallbladder stasis: spinal cord injury, pregnancy.
- Hypercholesterolemic syndromes.

Patients with pigmented gallstones exhibit these risk factors:

- Asian more than Western, rural more than urban.
- Chronic hemolytic syndromes, biliary tract infection (as with bacteria or parasites).
- Ileal disease (resection or bypass), cystic fibrosis with pancreatic insufficiency.

PATHOGENESIS. *Three conditions necessary for formation of cholesterol stones:* (1) *Bile must be supersaturated with cholesterol;* (2) *nucleation must occur,* typically around a calcium salt crystal nidus; and (3) *cholesterol crystals must remain in the gallbladder long enough to agglomerate into stones.* Nucleation is promoted by microprecipitates of calcium salts (inorganic or bilirubin salts) and inhibited by luminal muciproteins. Gallbladder stasis promotes agglomeration.

The pathogenesis of pigmented stones is based on the presence in the biliary tree of unconjugated bilirubin (which is poorly soluble in water), *and precipitation of calcium bilirubin salts.* Infection of biliary tract with *Escherichia coli, Ascaris lumbricoides,* or the liver fluke *Opisthorchis sinensis* promotes deconjugation of bilirubin glucuronides secreted by the liver, and generation of unconjugated bilirubin. Chronic hemolytic conditions also promote formation of unconjugated bilirubin in the biliary tree.

MORPHOLOGY. *Cholesterol stones* arise exclusively in the gallbladder and are pale yellow and hard. Single stones are ovoid, multiple stones tend to be faceted. Bilirubin salts may impart black color. *Pigmented stones* are classified as *black* and *brown.* Black pigment stones are found in sterile gallbladders, brown stones in infected intrahepatic or extrahepatic bile ducts. Both are soft and usually multiple; brown stones are greasy. Based on calcium content, cholesterol stones are more often radiolucent and pigment stones more often radiopaque.

CLINICAL FEATURES. Seventy per cent to 80% of gallstone patients remain asymptomatic throughout life. *Asymptomatic patients convert to symptomatic ones at the rate of 1% to 3% per year, and the risk diminishes with time.* Symptom: spasmodic, "colicky" pain, owing to obstruction of bile ducts by passing stones. Gallbladder obstruction *per se* generates right upper abdominal pain.

More severe complications:

- Gallbladder inflammation (*cholecystitis*), empyema, perforation, fistulas, biliary tree inflammation (*cholangitis*).
- Obstructive cholestasis or pancreatitis.
- Erosion of a gallstone into adjacent bowel (*gallstone ileus*).
- Clear mucinous secretions in an obstructed gallbladder are called *mucocele.*

CHOLECYSTITIS

Acute Calculous Cholecystitis (p. 888)

Gallbladder inflammation almost always develops in the setting of gallstones, typically with obstruction of the neck or cystic duct. *Symptoms:* An attack of right upper quadrant or epigastric pain, mild fever, anorexia, tachycardia, diaphoresis, nausea, and vomiting. Jaundice suggests common bile duct obstruction.

PATHOGENESIS. Acute inflammation is not initiated by infection; may be secondary to release of inflammatory mediators (lysolecithin, prostaglandins), chemical irritation by bile acids, ischemia. Bacterial contamination is a later complication.

MORPHOLOGY. Enlarged, tense gallbladder, bright red to blotchy green-black with a serosal covering of fibrin. Luminal contents may be turbid or outright purulent.

Complications include

- Bacterial superinfection with cholangitis and sepsis.
- Gallbladder perforation or rupture.
- Enteric fistula formation.
- Aggravation of pre-existing illness.

Acute Acalculous Cholecystitis (p. 888)

About 10% of inflamed gallbladders are free of stones. *Predisposing conditions:* After major surgery, severe trauma, severe burns, multisystem organ failure, sepsis, prolonged intravenous hyperalimentation, the postpartum state. Clinical symptoms and morphology are similar to those of acute calculous cholecystitis but are usually masked. An indolent form may develop in patients with systemic vasculitis, severe atherosclerotic disease, and acquired immunodeficiency syndrome (AIDS) with microbial complications.

Chronic Cholecystitis (p. 889)

May arise from repeated bouts of symptomatic acute cholecystitis, or in the absence of antecedent attacks. Although gallstones are usually present, they may not play a direct role in the initiation of inflammation. Patient populations and symptoms are the same as for the acute form.

MORPHOLOGY. Gallbladder may be contracted (from fibrosis), normal in size, or enlarged (from obstruction). The wall is variably thickened and gray-white. Mucosa is generally preserved, but may be atrophied. Stones are frequent. Inflammation in the mucosa and wall is variable; mucosal outpouchings through the wall (*Rokitansky-Aschoff sinuses*) may be present. Rare findings are mural dystrophic calcification (*porcelain gallbladder*) and a fibrosed, nodular gallbladder with marked histiocytic inflammation (*xanthogranulomatous cholecystitis*).

DISORDERS OF THE EXTRAHEPATIC BILE DUCTS

BILIARY ATRESIA (p. 890)

Extrahepatic biliary atresia (EHBA) is complete obstruction of bile flow owing to destruction or absence of all or part of the extrahepatic bile ducts; occurs in 1 in 10,000 live births.

PATHOGENESIS. Intact biliary tree at birth, progressive inflammatory destruction following birth. Cause is unknown.

MORPHOLOGY. Inflammation and fibrosing stricture of both extrahepatic and, with progression of disease, intrahepatic biliary tree. Liver shows florid features of bile duct obstruction: marked bile ductular proliferation, portal tract edema, and fibrosis progressing to cirrhosis within 3 to 6 months.

CLINICAL FEATURES. Neonatal cholestasis in an infant of normal birth weight and postnatal weight gain. If untreated, death occurs within 2 years of birth; liver transplantation is curative.

CHOLEDOCHOLITHIASIS AND ASCENDING CHOLANGITIS (p. 891)

Choledocholithiasis is the presence of stones within the biliary tree. Western nations: Almost all stones are derived from the gallbladder and are cholesterol stones. Asia: Stones are usually primary in the ducts and are pigmented. Symptoms include those from obstruction, pancreatitis, cholangitis, hepatic abscess, secondary biliary cirrhosis, and acute calculous cholecystitis.

Cholangitis refers to bacterial infection of the bile ducts; usually arises in the setting of choledocholithiasis. Uncommon causes include indwelling stents or catheters, tumors, acute pancreatitis, benign strictures. Infections are usually from ascending bacteria (e.g., *E. coli, Klebsiella,* other coliforms) entering the biliary tract through the sphincter of Oddi.

CHOLEDOCHAL CYSTS (p. 891)

Congenital dilatations of the common bile duct, presenting most often in children before age 10 years with nonspecific symptoms of jaundice and/or recurrent abdominal pain. Predispose to stone formation, stenosis and stricture, pancreatitis, obstructive biliary complications, and bile duct carcinoma in the adult.

TUMORS

The primary neoplasms of the gallbladder are epithelial. Adenomas are described in Chapter 16.

CARCINOMA OF THE GALLBLADDER (p. 891)

Fifth most common cancer of the digestive tract, slightly more common in women, most often in seventh decade. Gallstones coexist in 60% to 90% of patients in Western nations; less common in Asian populations, where pyogenic and parasitic disease dominate.

MORPHOLOGY. Two patterns of growth: (1) *infiltrating* (diffuse thickening and induration of gallbladder), and (2) *fungating* (growth into the lumen as an irregular, cauliflower-like mass). Most are adenocarcinomas, with histologic patterns of papillary and/or infiltrating architecture, moderately to poorly differentiated to undifferentiated, and rarely squamous or adenosquamous, carcinoid, mesenchymal. *Patterns of spread:* Local invasion of liver, extension to cystic duct and portohepatic lymph nodes, seeding of peritoneum, viscera, lungs. Usually unresectable when discovered.

CLINICAL FEATURES. *Symptoms:* Insidious and indistinguishable from those caused by cholelithiasis. Prognosis is poor.

CARCINOMA OF THE EXTRAHEPATIC
BILE DUCTS (p. 892)

Distinctly uncommon malignancies of the extrahepatic biliary tree down to the ampulla of Vater. Apparent increased risk in patients with choledochal cysts, ulcerative colitis, chronic biliary infection with *Opisthorchis sinensis* and *Giardia lamblia*.

MORPHOLOGY. Most are adenocarcinomas; uncommonly, squamous metaplasia gives rise to squamous cell carcinomas or adenosquamous carcinomas. May take form of papillary fungating masses, intraductal nodules, or diffuse infiltrative lesions of the duct walls. Tumors arising at the confluence of the right and left hepatic bile ducts are called *Klatskin tumors,* notable for slow growth, sclerosing behavior, and infrequency of distant metastasis.

CLINICAL FEATURES. Symptoms similar to those of cholelithiasis. Progressive obstruction, may wax and wane as necrosis of the tumor re-establishes the ductal lumen. Most have invaded adjacent structures at the time of diagnosis, and the prognosis is only fair.

MISCELLANEOUS DISORDERS OF
THE BILIARY TREE (p. 893)

CHOLESTEROLOSIS. Focal accumulation of lipid-laden macrophages within tips of mucosal folds; red mucosa studded with yellow flecks (*strawberry gallbladder*). Of no clinical significance.

HYDROPS OR MUCOCELE. Distention of the gallbladder by a clear, watery, mucinous secretion in an obstructed gallbladder.

IATROGENIC INJURY TO THE BILIARY TREE. Needle injuries may lead to bile leaks of gallbladder, and thus *bile peritonitis*. *Surgical injury to the biliary tree* may lead to *biliary stricture*.

PANCREAS

THE EXOCRINE PANCREAS
CONGENITAL ANOMALIES (p. 899)

- *Agenesis:* Associated with other severe congenital malformations, usually incompatible with life.
- *Hypoplasia:* Persistence as dorsal and ventral pancreas.
- *Annular pancreas:* The pancreatic head encircles the duodenum, with attendant risk of obstruction.
- *Pancreas divisum:* Persistence of two separate pancreatic ducts from dorsal and ventral pancreas; predisposes to recurrent pancreatitis.

Aberrant (or ectopic) *pancreas* is found in 2% of all routine postmortem examinations. Located in stomach, duodenum, jejunum, Meckel's diverticulum, ileum. Single or multiple firm, yellow-gray nests of pancreatic substance, 1 mm to 3–4 cm in diameter in wall of gut, typically submucosal.

PANCREATITIS
Acute Pancreatitis (p. 899)

An acute condition, typically presenting with abdominal pain, associated with raised levels of pancreatic enzymes (amylase and lipase) in blood or urine. Caused by inflammation and necrosis of pancreatic tissue, with edema (*interstitial pancreatitis*). *Acute hemorrhagic pancreatitis* (*necrotizing pancreatitis*) exhibits extensive fat necrosis in and around the pancreas and in other fatty depots in the abdominal cavity, and hemorrhage into the parenchyma of the pancreas.

ASSOCIATED CONDITIONS. See Table 17–8.

PATHOGENESIS. Pancreas secretes 22 enzymes (15 proteases, 3–6 amylases, lipase, phospholipase), most secreted as proenzymes, requiring trypsin cleavage before activation. *Features of pancreatitis: Proteolysis, lipolysis, and hemorrhage, resulting from the destructive effect of pancreatic enzymes released from acinar cells.* Locally, activated trypsin converts other proenzymes to active enzymes, prekallikrein to kallikrein, activating kinin system and clotting, leading to local inflammation and thrombosis, and systemic clotting derangement.

Proposed mechanisms for activation of pancreatic enzymes:

- *Cholelithiasis* with impaction in ampulla of Vater can cause pancreatic obstruction and increased ductal pressure.
- *Alcohol:* Chronic alcohol ingestion causes secretion of a protein-rich pancreatic fluid, predisposing to inspissation of calcified protein plugs.
- *Acinar cell injury:* Direct toxicity as from alcohol, viruses, endotoxin, drugs, ischemia, trauma. Mis-sorting of normally secreted pancreatic enzymes may occur with alcohol.

MORPHOLOGY. Pancreatic tissue undergoes proteolytic destruction, with necrosis of blood vessels and hemorrhage; necrosis of fat (local and regional) by lipolytic enzymes—fatty soaps precipitate as radiopaque calcium salts; and inflammatory reaction, especially with neutrophils. *Gross:* Gray-white necrosis of parenchyma, hemorrhage, chalky white fat necrosis. Peritoneal fluid is serous, slightly turbid, and brown-tinged, with globules of oil. Resolution leaves diffuse or focal parenchymal fibrosis, calcification, and irregular ductal dilatation. Commonly, pancreatic secretions accumulate as a *pseudocyst*. Pancreatic liquefaction leads to sterile *pancreatic abscesses*.

Table 17–8. Conditions and Etiologic Agents Associated with Pancreatitis

CHOLELITHIASIS
ALCOHOLISM
IDIOPATHIC
OTHER CAUSES
Abdominal operations
Endoscopic pancreatic duct injection
Infection: bacterial, viral, and parasitic
Ischemia or vasculitis
Drugs
Trauma
Extension from adjacent inflamed tissues
Mass lesions
Endocrine/metabolic: hereditary hyperlipidemias, hypercalcemia, hemochromatosis, uremia, diabetic ketoacidosis, hypothermia

From Cotran, R. S., Kumar, V., and Robbins, S. L.: Robbins Pathologic Basis of Disease. 5th ed. Philadelphia, W. B. Saunders Co., 1994, p. 899.

Pancreatitis may appear as *acute hemorrhagic pancreatitis:* variegated pattern of blue-black hemorrhages and gray-white necrotic softening alternating with sprinkled foci of yellow-white, chalky fat necrosis.

CLINICAL FEATURES. Full blown, acute pancreatitis is a medical emergency: acute abdomen, constant and intense abdominal pain with upper back radiation, peripheral vascular collapse, and shock. Death from shock, adult respiratory distress syndrome (ARDS), or acute renal failure.

Chronic Pancreatitis (p. 902)

Better termed *chronic relapsing pancreatitis:* progressive destruction by repeated flare-ups of mild or subclinical pancreatitis. Etiology: alcoholism, biliary tract disease. Less common: hypercalcemia, hyperlipidemia, pancreas divisum, familial tendency, protein-deficient malnutrition. Postulated inciting events: *ductal obstruction by concretions,* and/or *interstitial fat necrosis and hemorrhage.*

MORPHOLOGY. Irregularly distributed fibrosis, reduced number and size of acini with relative sparing of the islets of Langerhans, and variable obstruction of pancreatic ducts. Hard pancreas with foci of calcification; fully developed calculi may be present (*chronic calcifying pancreatitis*) in alcoholics. *Chronic obstructive pancreatitis* with impacted ampullary stones is centered around ducts and irregular in its glandular distribution. Pseudocyst formation is common, especially in alcoholics.

CLINICAL FEATURES. Silent, or recurrent attacks of pain at scattered intervals. Attacks precipitated by alcohol abuse, overeating, drug use. Late complications: diarrhea (malabsorption), steatorrhea, diabetes, pseudocyst.

TUMORS

Non-neoplastic Cysts (p. 904)

Congenital cysts: anomalous development of the pancreatic ducts; frequently coexist with kidney and liver cysts in *congenital polycystic disease. Von Hippel–Lindau disease:* pancreatic cysts and angiomas of the central nervous system.

Pseudocysts (p. 904)

Localized collections of fluid representing pancreatic secretions, almost always arising following bouts of acute or chronic pancreatitis. Do not possess an epithelial lining, but instead a fibrosed inflammatory tissue wall. They are usually unilocular.

Neoplasms

Cystic Tumors (p. 904)

Five per cent of pancreatic neoplasms.

- Painless, slow-growing tumors, multiloculated, mucin-secreting (benign *mucinous cystadenoma* or malignant *mucinous cystadenocarcinoma*).
- *Microcystic adenoma:* Cystic tumor with serous secretions.
- *Solid-cystic tumor:* Rare papillary-cystic tumor of young women.

Carcinoma of the Pancreas (p. 905)

Refers to carcinomas of the exocrine pancreas, almost always arising from ductal epithelial cells.

EPIDEMIOLOGY. Five per cent of all cancer deaths in United States. Incidence increasing (?smoking, diet, ?chemical carcinogens). Occur in sixth to eighth decade, blacks more than whites, males more than females, diabetics more than nondiabetics.
MORPHOLOGY. *Distribution:* Head (60%); body (15% to 20%); tail (5%); diffuse or widely spread (20%). May be small and ill-defined or large (8–10 cm), with extensive local invasion and regional metastasis. *Microscopic:* More or less differentiated glandular patterns (*adenocarcinoma*) arising from ductal epithelium; mucus or non–mucus secreting. Rare histologic variants: *adenosquamous carcinoma, anaplastic carcinoma* with giant cell formation, or arising from acinar cells with abundant eosinophilic cytoplasm (*acinar cell carcinoma*). *Periampullary carcinomas* refer to pancreatic carcinomas in the immediate vicinity of the ampulla of Vater, as well as tumors of the most distal common bile duct and ampulla itself.
CLINICAL FEATURES. Insidious growth over years, unresectable at presentation, dismal outlook: first-year mortality exceeds 80%. Obstructive jaundice for tumors in the head or periampullary region. Weight loss, pain, massive metastasis to the liver (via splenic vein invasion) are features of tumors of body and tail. Migratory thrombophlebitis (*Trousseau's sign*): characteristic of pancreatic and pulmonary neoplasms, also other visceral cancers.

THE ENDOCRINE PANCREAS

DIABETES MELLITUS (p. 909)

A group of disorders exhibiting a defective or deficient insulin secretory response, glucose underutilization, and hyperglycemia.
CLASSIFICATION AND INCIDENCE (Table 17–9)
Primary Diabetes

- *Type I Diabetes Mellitus* (IDDM—insulin-dependent DM, juvenile-onset DM, ketosis-prone DM): 10% to 20% of cases.
- *Type II Diabetes Mellitus* (NIDDM—non–insulin-dependent DM, adult-onset DM). Also includes a third rare form, *maturity-onset diabetes of the young* (MODY), transmitted as an autosomal dominant trait, with mild hyperglycemia.

For both types, long-term complications affect the *blood vessels, kidneys, eyes,* and *nerves;* annual U.S. death toll of 144,000.
Secondary Diabetes. Hyperglycemia associated with identifiable causes of islet destruction: inflammatory pancreatic disease (pancreatitis), surgery (pancreatectomy), tumors (pheochromocytoma, pituitary tumors), drugs (corticosteroids), iron overload (hemochromatosis), some genetic disorders (e.g., lipodystrophy).
PATHOGENESIS
Type I Diabetes Mellitus. A severe, absolute lack of insulin caused by a reduction in the beta-cell mass; insulin necessary for survival. Interlocking mechanisms:

- *Genetic susceptibility* to altered immune regulation, related to HLA class II inheritance (alleles frequently seen in type I DM: *HLA-DQ3.2* and *HLA-DR3*).
- *Autoimmunity* to islet beta-cells, with lymphocytic *"insulitis"* (CD4+ and CD8+); 10% coincidence of Graves' disease, Addison's disease, thyroiditis, and pernicious anemia.
- Triggering of autoimmunity by *an environmental insult.* Marked variability between world populations. *Viruses* are suspected as initiators.

Table 17–9. Type I Versus Type II Diabetes

	IDDM (Type I)	NIDDM (Type II)
Clinical	Onset <20 years	Onset >30 years
	Normal weight	Obese
	Decreased blood insulin	Normal or increased blood insulin
	Islet cell antibodies	No islet cell antibodies
	Ketoacidosis common	Ketoacidosis rare
Genetics	50% concordance in twins	90% to 100% concordance in twins
	HLA-D linked	No HLA association
Pathogenesis	Autoimmunity Immunopathologic mechanisms	Insulin resistance
	Severe insulin deficiency	Relative insulin deficiency
Islet cells	Insulitis early	No insulitis
	Marked atrophy and fibrosis	Focal atrophy and amyloid
	Beta-cell depletion	Mild beta-cell depletion

IDDM: Insulin-dependent diabetes mellitus.
NIDDM: Non–insulin-dependent diabetes mellitus.
From Cotran, R. S., Kumar, V., and Robbins, S. L.: Robbins Pathologic Basis of Disease. 5th ed. Philadelphia, W. B. Saunders Co., 1994, p. 909.

Postulated scenario: mild environmental (?viral) beta-cell injury, followed by autoimmune reaction against altered beta-cells in persons with HLA-linked susceptibility. *Chemical toxins* (streptozotocin, alloxan, pentamidine) may act directly on islet cells or may trigger autoimmunity. *Molecular mimicry* following development of antibodies to the bovine serum albumin found in *cow's milk* also may trigger autoimmunity.

Type II Diabetes Mellitus. By far the more common type, but much less is known—*multifactorial*. Metabolic defects: *deranged insulin secretion; insulin resistance* of peripheral tissues.

- *Genetic predisposition:* Not linked to HLA locus, but >90% concordance in twins; a subgroup have polymorphic alleles for *glycogen synthase*. Exception is *autosomal dominant* maturity-onset diabetes of the young (MODY): mutated gene for glucokinase (chromosome 7) leads to altered glucose-sensing mechanism.
- *Insulin deficiency* is due in part to loss of GLUT-2 (glucose) transporters in beta-cells. *Obesity* causes hyperinsulinemia and is common. Regardless of body weight, a deficiency of insulin develops in type II, milder than in type I diabetes. Cause of deficiency is unclear. A role is postulated for *amylin*: 37-amino acid peptide normally produced by beta-cells and cosecreted with insulin. In type II diabetes, amylin accumulates around beta-cells.

- *Insulin resistance:* A major factor in type II DM; also seen in pregnancy and *obesity;* is based on *a decrease in peripheral insulin receptors,* and *postreceptor defects* including *impaired postreceptor signaling.* Insulin resistance produces *excessive stress on beta-cells,* which may fail in the face of sustained stimulation.

PATHOGENESIS OF METABOLIC DERANGEMENTS. Insulin is a major anabolic hormone; deranged insulin function affects glucose, fat, and protein metabolism. Counter-regulatory hormones (e.g., growth hormone, epinephrine) are secreted unopposed; peripheral tissues cannot accumulate glucose. Excess glycosuria induces osmotic diuresis and *polyuria,* with profound loss of water and electrolytes. Intense thirst (*polydipsia*) develops, with increased appetite (*polyphagia*), completing the classic diabetic triad.

Diabetic Ketoacidosis. Occurs exclusively in type I diabetes due to severe insulin deficiency and absolute or relative increases in glucagon: excessive release of free fatty acids from adipose tissue; hepatic oxidation generates ketone bodies (butyric acid and acetoacetic acid). Ketonemia and ketonuria, with dehydration, generate life-threatening *systemic metabolic ketoacidosis.*

Nonketotic Hyperosmolar Coma. Can develop in type II diabetics in the setting of severe dehydration (from sustained hyperglycemic diuresis) and an inability to drink water.

PATHOGENESIS OF COMPLICATIONS. *Microangiopathy, retinopathy, nephropathy, neuropathy.* These late systemic complications are the major causes of morbidity and mortality of diabetes; onset and severity are extremely variable.

Nonenzymatic Glycosylation. Glucose chemically attaches to amino groups of proteins, reflected in *glycosylated hemoglobin* (HbA_{1c}) blood levels. With glycosylation of collagens and other long-lived proteins, *irreversible advanced glycosylation end products (AGE)* accumulate over the lifetime of blood vessel walls. AGE formation of proteins, lipids, nucleic acids leads to protein cross-linking, trapping plasma lipoproteins (among others) in vessel walls; reduction in normal proteolysis; AGE binding to cell receptors, inducing a variety of (undesired) biologic activities.

Intracellular Hyperglycemia with Disturbances in Polyol Pathways. Some tissues (nerve, lens, kidney, blood vessels) that do not require insulin develop increased intracellular glucose, which is metabolized to *sorbitol* and thence *fructose.* The osmotic load leads to influx of water and osmotic cell injury. Sorbitol decreases phosphoinositide metabolism and signal transduction.

MORPHOLOGY OF DIABETES AND ITS LATE COMPLICATIONS

Islet Changes (Variable). Reduction in size and number of islets (especially type I DM); increase in size and number of islets in infants of diabetic mothers; beta-cell degranulation; fibrosis of islets. Other findings: amyloid (amylin) replacement of islets; leukocytic infiltrations, especially *insulitis* (a heavy lymphocytic infiltrate within and about islets) in newly symptomatic type I diabetics.

Diabetic Microangiopathy. Diffuse thickening of basement membranes, most evident in capillaries of the skin, skeletal muscles, retina, renal glomeruli, and renal medulla. May affect nonvascular structures such as renal tubules, Bowman's capsule, peripheral nerves, and placenta. Seen in all patients; related to hyperglycemia and AGEs. Capillaries are actually more leaky than normal to plasma proteins.

Hyaline Arteriolosclerosis. The vascular lesion associated with hypertension is more prevalent and more severe in diabetics.
Atherosclerosis. Begins within a few years of onset of type I or type II diabetes. Numerous and florid complicated lesions (ulceration, calcification, and superimposed thromboses) lead to coronary artery narrowing and occlusion, ischemia, aneurysmal dilatation (e.g., of aorta, with rupture), narrowing of mesenteric arteries. Large vessel disease leads to myocardial infarction, cerebral stroke, and gangrene of the lower extremities.

Contributing Influences to the Development of Atherosclerosis

- *Hyperlipidemia* with *reduction in high-density lipoprotein (HDL) levels* in type II diabetics.
- *Nonenzymatic glycosylation* of low-density lipoprotein (LDL), rendering it more recognizable by the LDL receptor.
- *LDL cross-linking to collagen,* retarding efflux of cholesterol from vascular wall.
- *Increased platelet adhesiveness;* obesity and hypertension.

Diabetic Nephropathy. Kidneys are the most severely damaged organ in diabetics, and renal failure is a major cause of mortality. *Glomerular involvement:* Diffuse glomerulosclerosis, nodular glomerulosclerosis, and/or exudative lesions, resulting in progressive proteinuria and chronic renal failure. *Vascular:* Arteriosclerosis, including benign nephrosclerosis with hypertension. *Infection:* Bacterial urinary tract infection, with *pyelonephritis,* and sometimes *necrotizing papillitis.*
Diabetic Ocular Complications. Visual impairment due to *diabetic retinopathy, cataract formation,* or *glaucoma;* affects virtually all diabetics. Nonproliferative retinopathy consists of intraretinal and preretinal hemorrhages, exudates, edema, thickening of retinal capillaries, microaneurysms.
Diabetic Neuropathy. A *symmetric peripheral neuropathy* affecting motor and sensory nerves of the lower extremities: Schwann cell injury, myelin degeneration, axonal damage. *Autonomic neuropathy* may lead to sexual impotence and bowel and bladder dysfunction. Focal neurologic impairment (*diabetic mononeuropathy*) most likely due to microangiopathy.

CLINICAL FEATURES

Type I Diabetes Mellitus. Begins by age 20 years, dominated by signs of altered metabolism: polyuria, polydipsia, polyphagia. Chemical indices: ketoacidosis, low or absent plasma insulin, elevated plasma glucose. Metabolic derangement and insulin need are directly related to physiologic stress: deviations from normal dietary intake, increased physical activity, infections, surgery.
Type II Diabetes Mellitus. Patients usually older than age 40 years, polydipsia and polyuria, often (but not necessarily) obesity. Metabolic derangements are usually mild and controllable.
Complications of Both Types. Atherosclerotic events: myocardial infarction (a major cause of death), cerebrovascular accidents, gangrene of the lower extremity, renal insufficiency. Diabetic microangiopathy: blindness, peripheral neuropathy. Increased susceptibility to infection.

ISLET CELL TUMORS (p. 922)

Rare compared with tumors of exocrine pancreas: hormonally functional or nonfunctional, single or multiple, benign or malignant.

Beta-Cell Tumors (Insulinoma) (p. 922)

Most common islet cell tumor. May elaborate sufficient insulin to cause hypoglycemia; symptomatic attacks with serum glucose below 50 mg/dl. *Symptoms:* Confusion, stupor, loss of consciousness; attacks promptly relieved by glucose feeding or infusion.
MORPHOLOGY. Seventy per cent are solitary adenomas, 10% are multiple adenomas, 10% are metastasizing carcinomas; the remainder are diffuse islet hyperplasia and adenomas in ectopic pancreatic tissue. Minute to over 1500-gm lesions, usually encapsulated, firm, yellow-brown nodules composed of cords and nests of well-differentiated beta-cells, with typical beta-cell granules seen by EM. Malignant tumors are not anaplastic; diagnosis of malignancy depends on evidence of invasion or spread.

Diffuse islet cell hyperplasia is characteristic of infants born to diabetic mothers and subjected to sustained hyperglycemia *in utero.*

Zollinger-Ellison Syndrome (Gastrinoma) (p. 923)

Triad of recalcitrant peptic ulcer disease, gastric hypersecretion, and pancreatic islet cell tumor elaborating gastrin.
MORPHOLOGY. Sixty per cent of gastrinomas are malignant, with spread to lymph nodes and metastasis, 40% are benign. Most common in the pancreas, but 10% to 15% arise in duodenum. Histologic and ultrastructural features similar to normal intestinal and gastric G cells. Peptic ulcers in the usual sites in the stomach or duodenum (75% of cases), abnormally located ulcers in stomach or first and second portion of duodenum in 25%. Stomach shows hyperplasia of parietal cells.
CLINICAL FEATURES. Striking gastric hypersecretion with intractable ulcers; severe diarrhea, with fluid and electrolyte imbalance and malabsorption. Surgical removal extraordinarily difficult, with postsurgical recurrence of symptoms common.

Other Rare Islet Cell Tumors (p. 924)

Elaboration of multiple hormones occasionally seen (*multihormonal tumors*): insulin, glucagon, gastrin, ACTH, MSH, vasopressin, norepinephrine, serotonin. Differentiation among these tumors depends on identification of a secretory product.
ALPHA-CELL TUMORS (GLUCAGONOMAS). Extremely high plasma glucagon levels, mild features of diabetes mellitus, migratory necrotizing skin erythema, anemia. Seen in peri- and postmenopausal women.
DELTA-CELL TUMORS (SOMATOSTATINOMAS). High plasma somatostatin levels. Features of diabetes mellitus, cholelithiasis, steatorrhea, hypochlorhydria.
VIP-OMA (DIARRHEOGENIC ISLET CELL TUMOR). Watery diarrhea, hypokalemia, achlorhydria; associated with neural crest tumors.
PANCREATIC CARCINOID TUMORS. Serotonin-producing—rare.
PANCREATIC POLYPEPTIDE-SECRETING ISLET CELL TUMORS. Rare, asymptomatic.

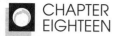
Urinary Tract

KIDNEY

Renal diseases are traditionally divided into four categories, based on the four basic anatomic compartments: glomeruli, tubules, interstitium, and blood vessels. However, the anatomic interdependence of these compartments means that damage to one will secondarily affect the others.

Whatever the origin, then, there is a tendency for all forms of chronic renal disease ultimately to destroy all four components of the kidney, culminating in chronic renal failure and end-stage kidneys.

The functional reserve of the kidney is large, and much damage may occur before there is evident functional impairment.

CLINICAL MANIFESTATIONS OF RENAL DISEASES (p. 932)

- *Acute nephritic syndrome.* Acute onset of usually grossly visible hematuria, mild to moderate proteinuria, and hypertension.
- *Nephrotic syndrome.* Heavy proteinuria (over 3.5 gm per day), hypoalbuminemia, severe edema, hyperlipidemia, and lipiduria (oval fat bodies in urine).
- *Asymptomatic hematuria and/or proteinuria.* Usually a manifestation of subtle or mild glomerular abnormalities.
- *Acute renal failure.* Recent onset of azotemia with oliguria or anuria resulting from severe injury to glomeruli, tubules, interstitium, or blood vessels.
- *Chronic renal failure.* Prolonged uremia, the end result of all chronic renal diseases.
- *Renal tubular defects.* Dominated by polyuria, nocturia, and electrolyte disorders (e.g., metabolic acidosis).
- *Urinary tract infection.* Bacteriuria and/or pyuria affecting the kidney (pyelonephritis) or bladder (cystitis).
- *Nephrolithiasis.* Renal stones causing renal colic and/or hematuria.

RENAL FAILURE (p. 932)

- *Azotemia* refers to an elevation of the blood urea nitrogen (BUN) and creatinine levels and is largely related to decreased glomerular filtration rate (GFR).

  - *Prerenal azotemia* occurs with hypoperfusion of the kidneys, as poccurs with congestive heart failure, shock, volume depletion, and hemorrhage.

- *Postrenal azotemia* occurs with urinary outflow obstruction below the level of the kidney.
- *Uremia* is characterized by azotemia associated with a constellation of clinical signs and symptoms and is the sine qua non of chronic renal failure.

Stages of progression in renal disease:
- Diminished renal reserve (~50% of normal GFR).
- Renal insufficiency (20%–50% of normal GFR).
- Renal failure (<20%–25% of normal GFR).
- End-stage renal disease (<5% of normal GFR).

Complications of Chronic Renal Failure (p. 933)

The major systemic abnormalities occurring in renal failure with uremia are listed in Table 18–1.

CONGENITAL ANOMALIES (p. 933)

About 10% of newborns have potentially significant malformations of the urinary system. Renal dysplasias and hypoplasias

Table 18–1. Principal Systemic Manifestations of Chronic Renal Failure and Uremia

Fluid and Electrolytes
  Dehydration
  Edema
  Hyperkalemia
  Metabolic acidosis
Calcium Phosphate and Bone
  Hyperphosphatemia
  Hypocalcemia
  Secondary hyperparathyroidism
  Renal osteodystrophy
Hematologic
  Anemia
  Bleeding diathesis
Cardiopulmonary
  Hypertension
  Congestive heart failure
  Pulmonary edema
  Uremic pericarditis
Gastrointestinal
  Nausea and vomiting
  Bleeding
  Esophagitis, gastritis, colitis
Neuromuscular
  Myopathy
  Peripheral neuropathy
  Encephalopathy
Dermatologic
  Sallow color
  Pruritus
  Dermatitis

From Cotran, R. S., Kumar, V., and Robbins, S. L.: Robbins Pathologic Basis of Disease. 5th ed. Philadelphia, W. B. Saunders Co., 1994, p. 933.

account for 20% of chronic renal failure in children. Most arise from developmental defects rather than inherited genes.

- *Renal agenesis. Bilateral* absence of renal development is incompatible with life. *Unilateral* agenesis is associated with compensatory hypertrophy of the remaining kidney, which in later life may develop progressive glomerulosclerosis and renal failure.
- *Hypoplasia.* Failure of kidneys to develop to normal size, usually unilateral. A truly hypoplastic kidney should show no scars and should possess a reduced number of renal lobes and pyramids (six or fewer).
- *Ectopic kidneys.* Lie either just above the pelvic brim or sometimes within the pelvis; kinking or tortuosity of the ureters may cause urinary obstruction, predisposing to bacterial infection.
- *Horseshoe kidney.* Fusion of the upper (10%) or lower (90%) poles produces a horseshoe-shaped structure continuous across the midline anterior to the great vessels.

CYSTIC DISEASES OF THE KIDNEY (p. 934)

Cystic Renal Dysplasia (p. 934)

Sporadic, nonfamilial disease resulting from abnormal metanephric differentiation. Frequently associated with obstructive abnormalities of the ureter and lower urinary tract. May be unilateral or bilateral. Affected kidneys are enlarged and multicystic. Histologically, kidneys show immature ducts surrounded by undifferentiated mesenchyme, often with focal cartilage formation.

Autosomal Dominant (Adult) Polycystic Kidney Disease (p. 935)

Affects 1 in every 1000 persons and accounts for about 10% of cases of chronic renal failure. Ninety percent of cases are due to defect in APKD1 gene on chromosome 16. The genes responsible for the remaining 10%, which have a later onset, have not been identified.

- Polycystic changes are always bilateral and present from early childhood to as late as 80 years of age. Patients have pain, hematuria, hypertension, proteinuria, progressive renal failure, and/or bilateral abdominal masses.
- The kidneys are enlarged, achieving massive size, and are composed of a mass of cysts up to 3 to 4 cm in diameter. Cysts arise anywhere along the nephron and compress adjacent parenchyma.
- Forty per cent of patients have scattered liver cysts (polycystic liver disease) and 10% to 30% have cerebral berry aneurysms, which may cause death from subarachnoid hemorrhage.
- About one-third die of renal failure, another one-third from hypertension, and the remainder from unrelated causes.

Autosomal Recessive (Childhood) Polycystic Kidney Disease (p. 936)

Rare bilateral anomaly presenting at perinatal, neonatal, infantile, and juvenile periods. Infants usually succumb rapidly to renal failure.

Kidneys are enlarged by multiple, cylindrically dilated collecting ducts, which are oriented at right angles to the cortex and fill both the cortex and medulla. The liver almost always has cysts and proliferating bile ducts, which in the infantile and juvenile forms give rise to the condition *congenital hepatic fibrosis*.

Medullary Sponge Kidney (p. 937)

A term that should be restricted to lesions consisting of multiple cystic dilatations in the collecting ducts of the medulla, usually presenting in adults. Most frequently an innocuous lesion discovered radiographically, it may predispose to renal calculi.

Nephronophthisis—Uremic Medullary Cystic Disease (UMCD) Complex (p. 937)

A family of progressive renal disorders, usually beginning in childhood, characterized by small cysts in the medulla (especially the corticomedullary area) associated with cortical tubular atrophy and interstitial fibrosis.

There are four variants: (1) sporadic (20%), (2) familial (recessive) juvenile nephronophthisis (50%), (3) renal-retinal (recessive) dysplasia (15%), and (4) adult-onset (dominant) medullary cystic disease (15%). Diagnosis of these disorders should be strongly considered in children or adolescents with otherwise unexplained chronic renal failure, a positive family history, and chronic tubulointerstitial nephritis on biopsy.

Acquired (Dialysis-Associated) Cystic Disease (p. 937)

The end stage kidneys of patients undergoing prolonged renal dialysis may develop multiple cortical and medullary cysts. The cysts are often lined by atypical, hyperplastic epithelium that can undergo malignant transformation to renal cell carcinoma.

Simple Cysts (p. 937)

Commonly encountered, single or multiple cysts of the cortex (rarely medulla) lined by low cuboidal epithelium and usually 2 to 5 cm in diameter, but up to 10 cm. They show smooth walls and are filled with clear serous fluid, but on occasion hemorrhage and stromal reaction may cause flank pain and irregular contours, thus mimicking renal carcinoma.

GLOMERULAR DISEASES (p. 938)

Glomerular injury is a major cause of renal disease. In *primary glomerulonephritis* the kidney is the principal organ involved, whereas in *secondary glomerular diseases* the kidney is one of many organ systems damaged by a systemic disease (Table 18–2).

Chronic glomerulonephritis is the most common cause of chronic renal failure in humans.

Some glomerular diseases cause mainly the nephritic syndrome, others cause mainly a nephrotic syndrome, and some may cause mixtures of both.

Pathogenesis of Glomerular Injury (p. 939)

There are two basic mechanisms of glomerular injury: immune and nonimmune.

Table 18-2. Glomerular Diseases

Primary Glomerulopathies
  Acute diffuse proliferative glomerulonephritis (GN)
    Poststreptococcal
    Nonpoststreptococcal
  Rapidly progressive (crescentic) glomerulonephritis
  Membranous glomerulopathy
  Lipoid nephrosis (minimal change disease)
  Focal segmental glomerulosclerosis
  Membranoproliferative glomerulonephritis
  IgA nephropathy
  Focal proliferative glomerulonephritis
  Chronic glomerulonephritis

Systemic Diseases
  Systemic lupus erythematosus
  Diabetes mellitus
  Amyloidosis
  Goodpasture's syndrome
  Polyarteritis nodosa
  Wegener's granulomatosis
  Henoch-Schönlein purpura
  Bacterial endocarditis

Hereditary Disorders
  Alport's syndrome
  Fabry's disease

From Cotran, R. S., Kumar, V., and Robbins, S. L.: Robbins Pathologic Basis of Disease. 5th ed. Philadelphia, W. B. Saunders Co., 1994, p. 939.

IMMUNE MECHANISMS. The deposition of antigen-antibody complexes in glomeruli is a major mechanism of glomerular injury, whether they are formed in situ with glomerular antigens or are trapped circulating complexes (Table 18-3).

In in situ immune mechanisms, antibodies can be directed against

- Fixed intrinsic antigens, e.g., the glomerular basement membrane (anti-GBM disease), the Heymann antigen of epithelial cells (membranous GN), or mesangial antigens.
- Exogenous or endogenous antigens planted in the glomerulus because of some affinity to glomerular structures.

With the circulating immune complexes, the antigens may be endogenous (e.g., thyroglobulin) or exogenous (e.g., infectious agents).

In human GN, the inciting endogenous or exogenous antigens are frequently unknown.

The immune complexes can be visualized by immunofluorescence microscopy either in a *linear pattern* in anti-GBM nephritis or in a *granular pattern* in all other types.

Once immune complexes are deposited in glomeruli, injury is induced by both cellular and soluble mediators, including

- *Neutrophils,* which release proteases, oxygen free radicals, and arachidonic acid metabolites in response to activated complement.
- *Monocytes, macrophages, and lymphocytes,* which release cytokines, cytotoxic cell mediators, and growth factors.

Table 18–3. Immune Mechanisms of Glomerular Injury

I. Antibody-mediated injury
   A. *In situ* immune complex deposition
      1. Fixed intrinsic tissue antigens
         a. Goodpasture's antigen (anti-GBM nephritis)
         b. Heymann's antigen (membranous GN)
         c. Mesangial antigens
         d. Others
      2. Planted antigens
         a. Exogenous (drugs, lectins, infectious agents)
         b. Endogenous (DNA, immunoglobulins, immune complexes, IgA)
   B. Circulating immune complex deposition
      1. Endogenous antigens (e.g., DNA, tumor antigens)
      2. Exogenous antigens (e.g., infectious products)
   C. Cytotoxic antibodies
II. Cell-mediated injury
III Activation of alternative complement pathway

From Cotran, R. S., Kumar, V., and Robbins, S. L.: Robbins Pathologic Basis of Disease. 5th ed. Philadelphia, W. B. Saunders Co., 1994, p. 940.

- *Platelets,* which aggregate and release eicosanoids and growth factors.
- *Resident glomerular cells, particularly mesangial cells,* which can initiate inflammatory responses by releasing cytokines, oxygen-free radicals, eicosanoids, and endothelin.
- *C5b-C9,* the terminal membrane attack complex of complement, which causes cell lysis.
- *Coagulation proteins,* especially fibrin, which may stimulate crescent formation in crescentic GN.
- *Hemodynamic regulators,* e.g., eicosanoids, nitric oxide, endothelin.
- *Cytokines,* e.g., IL-1, TNF.
- *Growth factors,* e.g., PDGF, TGF-β (the latter being important for ECM deposition in glomerulosclerosis).

NONIMMUNE MECHANISMS. Once any renal disease, glomerular or otherwise, destroys sufficient functioning nephrons to reduce the GFR to about 30% to 50% of normal, progression to end-stage glomerulosclerosis and renal failure follows inexorably (although at variable rates). Adaptive changes in glomeruli to the increased workload (hypertrophy and glomerular capillary hypertension along with systemic hypertension) cause epithelial and endothelial injury and resultant proteinuria. The mesangial response, involving mesangial cell proliferation and matrix deposition, and intraglomerular coagulation cause the glomerulosclerosis. The glomerular damage results in further loss of functioning nephrons and a vicious circle of progressive glomerulosclerosis (*renal ablation glomerulopathy*).

Acute Poststreptococcal (Proliferative) Glomerulonephritis (GN) (p. 945)

Acute nephritic syndrome (hematuria, red cell casts, and usually moderate proteinuria and edema) presents 1 to 2 weeks after a streptococcal infection of the throat or less commonly the skin (but other bacterial, viral, and parasitic infections can produce the same disease picture). Serum complement levels are low and antistreptococcal exoenzyme (ASO) titers are elevated.

- Biopsy shows *diffuse* GN (all glomeruli involved and *global* hypercellularity) resulting from proliferation of endothelial, mesangial, and epithelial cells, and from *exudation* of neutrophils and monocytes.
- Immunofluorescence shows a granular, "starry-sky" pattern of IgG, IgM, and C3, and electron microscopy (EM) shows subepithelial, "hump-like" deposits, supporting the belief that the mechanism is immune complex deposition.
- Clinically, over 95% of children recover. A few develop a rapidly progressive form of the disease, and the remainder progress to chronic renal failure. In adults, the epidemic form has a good prognosis, but only 60% recover after the sporadic form; the remainder develop rapidly progressive disease, chronic renal failure, or delayed but eventual resolution.

Crescentic (Rapidly Progressive) Glomerulonephritis (RPGN) (p. 947)

A syndrome characterized by the accumulation of cells in Bowman's space in the form of "crescents" accompanied by a rapid, progressive decline in renal function. Most glomeruli demonstrate crescents. RPGN may occur in the course of three broad disease groups:

- Postinfectious RPGN, complicating acute GN (see above).
- Systemic diseases:

  - Systemic lupus erythematosus (SLE)
  - Goodpasture's syndrome
  - Vasculitis (polyarteritis nodosa)
  - Wegener's granulomatosis
  - Henoch-Schönlein purpura
  - Essential cryoglobulinemia

- Idiopathic RPGN.

GOODPASTURE'S SYNDROME. *This autoimmune disease consists of pulmonary hemorrhage and acute GN, usually RPGN type.* The pulmonary hemorrhage occurs most often in smokers, usually precedes GN, and causes most morbidity and mortality. Note: renal/pulmonary syndromes can also be caused by SLE, Wegener's, scleroderma, and systemic vasculitis.

Goodpasture's disease is the result of autoantibodies reacting with the Goodpasture antigen, which resides in the noncollagenous portion of the $\alpha 3$ chain of collagen type IV. Because the antigen is present in both GBM and alveolar basement membranes, immunofluorescence shows *continuous linear staining of these structures for IgG*. Serum tests specific for these antibodies can help in diagnosing the disease.

The crescents result from parietal epithelial cell proliferation and monocyte infiltration in Bowman's space. Fibrin is universally present within the crescents, having leaked through focal disruptions of the GBM. Although dramatic remissions may follow intensive plasmapheresis, most patients eventually develop chronic renal failure.

IDIOPATHIC RPGN. About half the cases of RPGN present without a history of infection or the presence of systemic disease. Of these, half again show histologic features of crescentic GN with little or no immune complex deposition (*pauci-immune* *crescentic GN*); almost all these patients have circulating antineu-trophil cytoplasmic antibodies (*ANCA*), which may be patho-genic. Linear immunofluorescence patterns are seen in one-fourth of patients with idiopathic RPGN, suggesting anti-GBM disease. The remainder show granular immune complexes.

The prognosis is bleak, with most patients progressing to chronic renal failure.

NEPHROTIC SYNDROME (NS) (p. 948)

Results from excessive permeability of the glomerular capillary wall to plasma proteins with proteinuria greater than 3.5 gm per day. Depending on the severity of basement membrane damage, this may be highly selective proteinuria, mostly of low-molecular-weight proteins (albumin and transferrin); with more severe injury, poorly selective proteinuria appears of higher-molecular-weight proteins as well as albumin. *Patients with NS also have sodium and water retention, hyperlipidemia, lipiduria, vulnerability to infection, and thrombotic complications.* The diseases causing the nephrotic syndrome in children and adults are shown in Table 18–4.

Membranous Glomerulonephritis (MGN) (p. 949)

Major cause of nephrotic syndrome in adults; characterized by immunoglobulin-containing electron-dense deposits along the subepithelial side of the GBM. *In situ* formation or deposition of circulating immune complexes, involving intrinsic glomerular antigens or endogenous and exogenous or planted antigens, is

Table 18–4. Causes of Nephrotic Syndrome

	Prevalence[*] %	
	Children	*Adults*
Primary Glomerular Disease		
Membranous GN	5	40
Lipoid nephrosis	65	15
Focal segmental glomerulosclerosis	10	15
Membranoproliferative GN	10	7
Other proliferative GN (focal, "pure mesangial," IgA nephropathy)	10	23
Systemic Diseases		
Diabetes mellitus		
Amyloidosis		
Systemic lupus erythematosus		
Drugs (gold, penicillamine, "street heroin")		
Infections (malaria, syphilis, hepatitis B, AIDS)		
Malignancy (carcinoma, melanoma)		
Miscellaneous (bee-sting allergy, hereditary nephritis)		

[*]Approximate prevalence of primary disease = 95% in children, 60% in adults. Approximate prevalence of systemic disease = 5% in children, 40% in adults.

From Cotran, R. S., Kumar, V., and Robbins, S. L.: Robbins Pathologic Basis of Disease. 5th ed. Philadelphia, W. B. Saunders Co., 1994, p. 949.

postulated to account for the subepithelial electron-dense deposits.

By light microscopy, there is diffuse thickening of the capillary wall, hence the term "membranous." Immunofluorescence studies show immunoglobulins and complement in a *diffuse granular pattern* along the GBM.

The disease is idiopathic in 85% of patients; the remainder have secondary disease associated with various types of carcinoma, SLE, exposure to gold or mercury, drugs (penicillamine, captopril), infections (hepatitis B, syphilis, schistosomiasis, malaria), and metabolic disorders (thyroiditis).

The condition usually starts as insidious onset of NS or subnephrotic-range proteinuria. Up to 40% of cases progress to renal insufficiency over an unpredictable time span of 2 to 20 years. It is necessary in any patient with MGN to first rule out the secondary causes described above.

Minimal Change Disease (MCD) (Lipoid Nephrosis) (p. 950)

Major cause of NS in children; *characterized by normal glomeruli on light microscopy but uniform and diffuse effacement of the foot processes of visceral epithelial cells on EM.* Immunofluorescence shows no immune deposits. The most characteristic feature of this condition is the dramatic response to corticosteroid therapy.

Proteinuria is usually selective and is associated with loss of glomerular polyanion (negative charge) and a hyperpermeable capillary wall. How this occurs is unknown. One hypothesis implicates dysfunction of T-cell immunity and elaboration of a lymphokine-like circulating substance that increases glomerular permeability.

The long-term prognosis is excellent for children and adults, even those with steroid-dependent disease.

Focal Segmental Glomerulosclerosis (FSG) (p. 952)

A cause of NS or heavy proteinuria, this lesion is characterized by *sclerosis of some, but not all, glomeruli (thus, it is focal), and in the affected glomeruli only a portion of the capillary tuft is involved (segmental).* FSG can be

- Idiopathic.
- Superimposed on another primary glomerular disease (e.g., IgA nephropathy).
- Associated with loss of renal mass (renal ablation FSG) as the result of chronic reflux, analgesic abuse, or unilateral renal agenesis.
- Secondary to other known disorders (e.g., heroin abuse, HIV infection).

The primary lesion is *epithelial damage* in affected glomerular segments. Unlike minimal change disease, the proteinuria is relatively nonselective, and there is progressive segmental sclerosis (with associated IgM and C3 deposition). In addition, patients with FSG are more likely to suffer hematuria, reduced GFR, and hypertension. Idiopathic FSG responds poorly to steroids, and progression to chronic renal failure is common. Recurrences are seen in 25% to 50% of patients receiving allografts.

Membranoproliferative GN (MPGN) (p. 954)

The name implies both thickened capillary loops and proliferation of glomerular cells. It accounts for 5% to 10% of NS in children and adults, but some patients have hematuria or proteinuria and others demonstrate a combined *nephritic-nephrotic* picture.

Glomeruli have a "lobular" appearance due to mesangial proliferation, and the capillary wall has a "double-contour" or "tramtrack" appearance. The latter is caused by extension of the mesangium around the inside of the capillary loop, so-called "mesangial interposition," accounting for the alternative name "mesangiocapillary" GN.

There are two major types of MPGN, I and II.

Type I shows subendothelial electron-dense deposits and occasional subepithelial and mesangial deposits of C3, early complement components (C1q and C4), and immunoglobulins in a granular manner. Type I changes can occur in patients with SLE, hepatitis B, hepatitis C with cryoglobulinemia, infected ventriculoatrial shunts, schistosomiasis, alpha$_1$-antitrypsin deficiency, chronic liver disease, and certain malignancies.

Type II (dense-deposit disease) shows the GBM to contain very electron-dense material in a ribbon-like fashion. Subepithelial "hump-like" deposits are also found occasionally. C3 is present but there are no early complement components.

Type I disease appears related to immune complexes, whereas type II exhibits evidence of alternate complement pathway activation (decreased serum C3, properdin, and factor B). Most type II patients have *C3 nephritic factor* in the serum, an autoantibody against C3 convertase that stabilizes the C3 convertase activity.

Although steroids may slow the progression of MPGN, about 50% of patients develop chronic renal failure within 10 years. There is a high recurrence rate in transplant recipients, particularly those with type II disease.

IgA Nephropathy (Berger's Disease) (p. 956)

A major cause of recurrent glomerular hematuria, characterized by mesangial proliferation and *IgA deposition* by immunofluorescence microscopy.

The exclusive mesangial deposition of IgA suggests entrapment of circulating IgA aggregates. Defects in regulation of IgA synthesis, secretion, or clearance have been postulated in the pathogenesis. Similar IgA deposits are seen in *Henoch-Schönlein purpura* in children.

The hematuria typically lasts for several days and then subsides, only to recur every few months. Although most patients have an initial benign course, chronic renal failure develops in up to 50% over a period of 20 years. Onset in old age, heavy proteinuria, hypertension, crescents, and vascular sclerosis portend a poorer prognosis.

Focal Proliferative GN (p. 958)

Focal GN is a histologic entity marked by glomerular proliferation and/or damage restricted to segments of individual glomeruli (segmental) and involving only some glomeruli (focal). There are three circumstances in which this picture may be observed; in each case the histology may change with the extent and progression of the underlying disease:

- An early or mild manifestation of a systemic disease that might otherwise involve all segments (global) of all glomeruli (diffuse), such as SLE, polyarteritis nodosa, Henoch-Schönlein purpura, Goodpasture's disease, subacute bacterial endocarditis, and Wegener's granulomatosis.
- A component of a known glomerular disease (e.g., IgA nephropathy).
- A form of primary idiopathic focal GN, a diagnosis made by excluding other potential causes.

Chronic Glomerulonephritis (p. 958)

An end-stage pool of glomerular diseases fed by a number of different glomerulonephritides. Some contributors and the percentage of cases progressing to chronic GN are listed:

- Poststreptococcal GN (1% to 2%).
- RPGN (90%).
- Membranous GN (40%).
- Focal glomerulosclerosis (50% to 80%).
- Membranoproliferative GN (50%).
- IgA nephropathy (30% to 50%).

However, about 20% of cases arise mysteriously with no history of any well-recognized form of early GN. Because glomeruli in chronic GN are totally replaced by hyalinized connective tissue, it may be difficult to know the nature of the antecedent lesion.

GLOMERULAR LESIONS ASSOCIATED WITH SYSTEMIC DISEASE (p. 959)

- *SLE.* Covered in detail in Chapter 6.
- *Henoch-Schönlein purpura.* Purpuric skin lesions (leukocytoclastic vasculitis), abdominal symptoms (pain, vomiting, bleeding), arthralgia, and GN. GN lesions vary from focal mesangial proliferation to crescentic GN, but are always associated with mesangial IgA deposition. Usually occurs in children, and the course is variable. For most children resolution of the lesions is the rule. However, chronic renal failure may ensue, especially in those with diffuse lesions or the nephrotic syndrome. There is progressive renal failure in those with crescents.
- *Bacterial endocarditis.* Variably severe, immune complex–mediated GN showing a morphologic continuum from focal necrotizing GN to diffuse GN, sometimes with crescents. Not "embolic" as previously thought.
- *Diabetic glomerulosclerosis.* Produces proteinuria (sometimes in the nephrotic range) in 55% of juvenile-onset and 30% of adult-onset diabetics. Usually discovered 12 to 22 years after diabetes appears, and heralds the onset of end-stage renal disease 4 to 5 years later in about 30% of juvenile diabetics. Morphologic changes in glomeruli include capillary basement membrane thickening, diffuse diabetic glomerulosclerosis, and nodular glomerulosclerosis (the latter also known as Kimmelstiel-Wilson disease). Diabetes and renal changes are further discussed on *page 920.*
- *Amyloidosis.* Amyloid deposited in glomeruli and in vessel walls in either primary or secondary forms, producing heavy proteinuria. Eventually end-stage renal disease occurs, but the

kidneys tend to be of normal size or slightly enlarged (*see* p. 236).

- *Miscellaneous.* Goodpasture's syndrome, polyarteritis nodosa, allergic vasculitis, and Wegener's granulomatosis all produce a similar form of GN ranging from focal segmental necrotizing GN to crescentic GN. Essential mixed cryoglobulinemia can induce cutaneous vasculitis, synovitis, and GN. Plasma cell dyscrasias can be associated with amyloidosis, monoclonal cryoglobulinemia, and a peculiar nodular GN (granular dense deposits) ascribed to the deposition of nonfibrillar light chains usually of the kappa type, known as *light-chain disease.*

HEREDITARY NEPHRITIS (p. 963)

A heterogeneous group of hereditary renal diseases manifesting primarily as GN, usually presenting with hematuria, and sometimes progressing to renal failure. *The best characterized, Alport's syndrome, has GN associated with nerve deafness, lens dislocation, cataracts, and corneal dystrophy.* In some patients, electron microscopy demonstrates irregular thickening of the GBM, with pronounced splitting of the lamina densa. The X-linked form of the disease, in which males are most severely affected, is due to mutations in the $\alpha 5$ chain of collagen type IV.

ACUTE RENAL FAILURE (ARF)

Acute renal failure signifies acute suppression of renal function, often with a fall in urine output to less than 400 ml in 24 hr. ARF is caused by

- Organic vascular obstruction.
- Severe glomerular disease.
- Acute tubulointerstitial nephritis.
- Massive infection, especially with papillary necrosis.
- Disseminated intravascular coagulation (DIC).
- Acute tubular necrosis (the most common cause).

ACUTE TUBULAR NECROSIS (ATN) (p. 964)

ATN is characterized by destruction of renal tubular epithelial cells either from *ischemia* or *nephrotoxins.*

- *Ischemic ATN* occurs after shock produced by sepsis, burns, crush injury, or circulatory collapse (ATN is uncommon after hemorrhagic shock).
- *Nephrotoxic ATN* is caused by a wide variety of drugs (e.g., gentamicin, cephalosporin, methoxyflurane, cyclosporine, contrast media) and toxins (e.g., mercury, lead, arsenic, methyl alcohol, ethylene glycol, and certain mushrooms, insecticides, and herbicides). ATN may also follow massive hemoglobinuria or myoglobinuria (from rhabdomyolysis), usually associated with dehydration and hypoxia.

Although the morphologic abnormalities may be very subtle by light microscopy, careful studies reveal that:

Ischemic ATN shows patchy tubular necrosis mostly in the straight segments of the proximal tubules and ascending limbs of Henle's loops.

Nephrotoxic ATN shows extensive tubular necrosis mostly in proximal tubules, although other tubular segments can be affected.

In both types the distal tubules and collecting ducts contain casts. The recovery phase shows epithelial regeneration (i.e., flattened tubular cells and mitotic figures).

Although the exact pathogenesis of ARF in ATN is debated, tubular damage likely leads to

- Arteriolar vasoconstriction, probably involving the renin-angiotensin mechanism.
- Cast formation and tubular obstruction.
- Back-leak of tubular fluids.
- Altered glomerular ultrafiltration.

The clinical course of ATN proceeds through

- *An initiating stage* (dominated by the inciting event).
- *A maintenance stage* (dominated by persistent renal failure and hyperkalemia).
- *A recovery stage* (dominated by polyuria and perhaps hypokalemia).

The prognosis depends on the cause: very good for nephrotoxic ATN, poor for ATN secondary to overwhelming sepsis.

PYELONEPHRITIS (PN) AND URINARY TRACT INFECTION (p. 967)

Urinary tract infection (UTI) implies involvement of the bladder (cystitis, see *p. 995*), or the kidneys (PN), or both. UTI may be clinically silent (asymptomatic bacteriuria) but more often causes dysuria and frequency, and (in PN) flank pain and fever. UTI is much more common in females, perhaps due to a shorter urethra and hormonal changes affecting mucosal adherence of bacteria. Other risk factors for UTI include long-term catheterization, pregnancy, diabetes mellitus, immunosuppression, and lower urinary tract obstruction due to congenital defects, benign prostatic hypertrophy, tumors, or calculi.

- PN is most commonly the result of *ascending infection,* the consequence of *vesicoureteral reflux* (VUR) through an incompetent vesicoureteral orifice.
- VUR is most often due to congenital defects in the intravesicular portion of the ureter and may be accentuated by cystitis, allowing retrograde seeding of the renal pelvis and renal papillae (intrarenal reflux). *E. coli, Proteus,* and *Enterobacter* are the most frequent culprits.
- *Hematogenous seeding of kidneys* occurs most often in the setting of septicemia or infective endocarditis, is frequently due to *Staphylococcus* or *E. coli,* and is enhanced by urinary obstruction.

Acute Pyelonephritis (p. 969)

Acute infection of the kidney is marked by patchy, interstitial, suppurative inflammation; tubular necrosis; and neutrophilic casts. More advanced changes include abscesses, necrotizing papillitis (especially in diabetics and in those with obstruction), pyonephrosis (pelvis filled with pus), perinephric abscesses, and eventually renal scars with fibrotic deformation of the cortex and underlying calyx and pelvis (see Chronic Pyelonephritis, next).

Chronic Pyelonephritis (CPN) and Reflux Nephropathy (p. 971)

CPN is a disorder in which *tubulointerstitial inflammation causes discrete, corticomedullary scars overlying dilated, blunted, and deformed calyces.* CPN is the cause of 11% to 20% of cases of chronic renal failure.

It can be divided into two forms:

- *Obstructive CPN.* Chronic obstruction predisposes the kidney to infections, and multiple recurrences over time produce CPN. Usually caused by enteric bacteria.
- *Reflux nephropathy–associated CPN.* Most common cause of CPN. Begins in childhood, as a result of infection superimposed on congenital vesicoureteral reflux and intrarenal reflux. Whether sterile reflux can cause CPN is controversial. Reflux nephropathy may have a silent, insidious onset, often with hypertension and polyuria.
- *Xanthogranulomatous PN* is an uncommon form of CPN associated with *Proteus* infections, in which a mixed inflammatory infiltrate with abundant foamy macrophages produces large, yellow-orange nodules that can clinically and radiologically mimic renal cell carcinoma.

ACUTE DRUG-INDUCED INTERSTITIAL NEPHRITIS (p. 972)

Occurs most frequently 2 to 40 days after exposure to a variety of drugs (methicillin, ampicillin, rifampicin, thiazides, various nonsteroidal anti-inflammatory agents, phenindione, cimetidine, etc.). Withdrawal of drug is followed by recovery in most patients.

The syndrome is variably characterized by fever, eosinophilia, skin rash, hematuria, mild proteinuria, sterile pyuria, azotemia, and even ARF.

Biopsy shows edema, patchy tubular necrosis, and tubulointerstitial infiltrates, with variable combinations of lymphocytes, histiocytes, eosinophils, neutrophils, plasma cells, and occasionally well-formed granulomas.

ANALGESIC ABUSE NEPHROPATHY (p. 973)

Caused by excessive intake of analgesic mixtures and characterized by chronic tubulointerstitial nephritis with papillary necrosis. Although the condition was initially ascribed to phenacetin, *most patients consume phenacetin-containing mixtures, and cases ascribed to aspirin, phenacetin, or acetaminophen alone are uncommon.* The drugs act synergistically to cause papillary necrosis first; the tubulointerstitial nephritis is secondary.

Patients may have polyuria, headaches, anemia, GI symptoms, pyuria, UTIs, and hypertension. Chronic renal failure may result, but drug withdrawal often stabilizes renal function. Unfortunately, these patients have an increased incidence of transitional cell carcinoma of the renal pelvis.

OTHER TUBULOINTERSTITIAL DISEASES (p. 974)

- *Urate nephropathy.* Can cause acute renal failure (ARF) or chronic renal failure (CRF), depending on the time course of uric acid crystal deposition. The former is particularly apt to occur in patients with hematolymphoid malignancies who are undergoing chemotherapy; the latter in patients with gout. Patients with increased exposure to lead may develop gout and also become nephrotic.

- *Hypercalcemia.* From whatever cause, hypercalcemia can cause stones (nephrolithiasis) or deposition within the kidney (nephrocalcinosis). Both may lead to renal insufficiency.
- *Multiple myeloma.* Renal insufficiency occurs in about 50% of patients, the direct result of Bence Jones (light-chain) proteinuria. Bence Jones proteins are directly toxic to tubular epithelial cells, and combine with Tamm-Horsfall protein to form obstructive and inflammatory casts. Both CRF and ARF can result, the latter often in patients with dehydration, hypercalcemia, or infection or who are receiving nephrotoxic antibiotics.

DISEASES OF BLOOD VESSELS (p. 976)

Nearly all diseases of the kidney and many systemic diseases secondarily affects the blood vessels of the kidney. In particular, hypertension has marked effects on the renal vessels and, conversely, the vascular changes augment the hypertension. The two principal renovascular lesions are benign nephrosclerosis and malignant nephrosclerosis.

BENIGN NEPHROSCLEROSIS (BNS) (p. 976)

BNS is the term used for abnormalities of the kidney induced by benign hypertension, with associated *hyaline arteriolosclerosis*. The latter is characterized by narrowing of the lumina of the arterioles, caused by thickening and hyalinization of the walls. Larger muscular arteries show *fibroelastic hyperplasia*. The changes are more severe in patients with essential hypertension and/or diabetes mellitus. *The vascular lesions cause diffuse ischemic atrophy of nephrons, hence the small kidneys and granular surfaces encountered in benign nephrosclerosis.*

BNS rarely causes renal failure, but mild proteinuria can occur and up to 5% of patients develop CRF, usually after development of *malignant hypertension.*

MALIGNANT PHASE OF HYPERTENSION (MALIGNANT NEPHROSCLEROSIS) (p. 977)

Malignant nephrosclerosis is the kidney disease associated with an accelerated phase of hypertension. Although occasionally developing in previously normotensive people, most cases are superimposed on pre-existing benign essential hypertension, chronic renal disease (particularly GN or reflux nephropathy), or scleroderma.

The condition occurs in 1% to 5% of patients with hypertension, and in pure form is most frequent in black males.

Pathologic changes include *fibrinoid necrosis of arterioles (necrotizing arteriolitis), hyperplastic arteriolosclerosis (onion-skinning), and necrotizing glomerulitis, often associated with a thrombotic microangiopathy.* Onset of diffuse intravascular coagulation may trigger malignant hypertension, and there is markedly increased renin, angiotensin, and aldosterone.

Patients have a diastolic pressure greater than 130 mm Hg, marked proteinuria, hematuria, papilledema, encephalopathy, cardiovascular abnormalities, and eventually renal failure. Currently, 50% of patients with treatment survive 5 years.

RENAL ARTERY STENOSIS (p. 978)

Unilateral renal artery stenosis accounts for 2% to 5% of renal hypertension, resulting from excessive renin secretion by the involved kidney. Seventy per cent of stenoses are caused by obstructive *atheromatous plaque* at the origin of the renal artery, the remainder by *fibromuscular dysplasia.* Before arteriolosclerosis develops in the opposite kidney, surgery cures about 80% in fibromuscular dysplasia and 60% in atherosclerotic stenosis.

THROMBOTIC MICROANGIOPATHIES (p. 979)

A group of diseases with overlapping clinical manifestations (e.g., microangiopathic hemolytic anemia, thrombocytopenia, renal failure, and manifestations of intravascular coagulation) are all characterized morphologically by thrombosis in the interlobular arteries, afferent arterioles, and glomeruli, together with necrosis and thickening of the vessel walls.

The morphologic changes are similar to those in malignant hypertension, but in this group the changes may precede the development of hypertension or be seen in its absence. The diseases include

- Childhood and adult hemolytic uremic syndromes (HUS).
- Thrombotic thrombocytopenic purpura.
- Scleroderma.

Although these diseases may have diverse causes, endothelial injury and intravascular coagulation appear to be shared pathogenetic mechanisms.

Classic (Childhood) Hemolytic-Uremic Syndrome

Produces acute renal failure, usually after a GI or flu-like prodrome of hematemesis and/or melena, oliguria, hematuria, microangiopathic hemolytic anemia, and (in some patients) neurologic signs. Up to 75% of patients are infected with verocytotoxin-producing *E. coli*. Kidneys show renal cortical necrosis, glomerular capillary wall thickening (due to deposits of fibrin-related materials), and arteriolar changes (fibrinoid necrosis, intimal hyperplasia, and thrombi).

Adult Hemolytic-Uremic Syndrome (HUS)

A syndrome similar to that in children arises in adults under a variety of settings:

- *In association with infection,* such as typhoid fever, *E. coli* septicemia, viral infections, and shigellosis.
- In women with *pregnancy complications,* or in postpartum women after an uneventful pregnancy (*postpartum renal failure*).
- *Secondary HUS,* associated with other vascular renal disease (SLE, scleroderma, malignant hypertension), or drug therapy (mitomycin, cyclosporine).
- *Hereditary HUS,* with recurrent attacks, similar to that in children.

Thrombotic Thrombocytopenic Purpura (TTP)

This entity differs from HUS in that CNS involvement is the dominant feature, whereas renal involvement occurs in only 50%. Platelet/fibrin thrombi are present in the terminal interlobular arteries, afferent arterioles, and glomerular capillaries.

ATHEROEMBOLIC RENAL DISEASE (p. 981)

Cholesterol crystals and debris embolize from atheromatous plaques after manipulation of severely diseased aortas, usually for repair of aortic aneurysms or during intra-aortic cannulization. They lodge in intrarenal vessels, causing arterial narrowing and focal ischemic injury. Rarely, renal function becomes compromised.

RENAL INFARCTS (p. 982)

Kidneys are favored sites of infarction since they receive 25% of cardiac output. Infarcts usually develop in a clinical setting of atrial fibrillation or myocardial infarction complicated by mural thrombosis. Most renal infarcts are asymptomatic but may cause pain and hematuria. Large infarcts of one kidney can cause hypertension.

URINARY TRACT OBSTRUCTION (OBSTRUCTIVE UROPATHY) (p. 982)

Obstruction increases susceptibility to infection and to stone formation, and unrelieved obstruction almost always leads to permanent renal atrophy. *Hydronephrosis is the term used to describe dilatation of the renal pelvis and calyces associated with progressive atrophy of the kidney due to obstruction of the outflow of urine.*
    Causes of urinary tract obstruction include

- Congenital anomalies (urethral valves, urethral strictures, meatal stenosis, bladder neck obstruction, ureteropelvic junction narrowing or obstruction, severe vesicoureteral reflux).
- Urinary calculi.
- Prostatic hypertrophy.
- Tumors.
- Inflammation (prostatitis, ureteritis, urethritis, retroperitoneal fibrosis).
- Sloughed papillae or blood clots.
- Normal pregnancy.
- Functional disorders (neurogenic bladder).

    When obstruction is sudden and complete, the reduction of GFR usually leads to only mild dilatation of the pelvis and calyces but sometimes to atrophy of the renal parenchyma. When subtotal or intermittent, GFR is not suppressed and progressive dilatation ensues.
    Unilateral (complete or partial) obstruction may remain silent for long periods, since the unaffected kidney can maintain adequate renal function. In bilateral partial obstruction the earliest manifestations are inability to concentrate the urine, reflected by polyuria and sometimes acquired distal tubular acidosis, salt wasting, renal calculi, tubulointerstitial nephritis, atrophy, and hypertension.

UROLITHIASIS (RENAL CALCULI, STONES)

(p. 984)

Renal stones can arise at any level in the urinary tract, frequently causing clinical symptoms: obstruction, ulceration, bleeding, and pain (known as renal colic). They also predispose to renal infection.

There are four types of calculi:

1. About 75% of stones are *calcium containing*, composed of calcium oxalate or calcium oxalate mixed with calcium phosphate.
2. About 15% are so-called "triple stones" or struvite stones composed of magnesium ammonium phosphate.
3. Six per cent are uric acid stones.
4. One per cent to 2% are made up of cystine.

An organic matrix of mucoprotein, making up 1% to 5% of the stone by weight, is present in all calculi.

Calcium-containing stones are usually associated with hypercalcemia and hypercalciuria (about 60%); hyperoxaluria and hyperuricosuria are associated in others. However, in about 25% there is no demonstrable metabolic abnormality.

Struvite stones are associated with infection by urea-splitting bacteria that convert urea to ammonia. So-called "staghorn" calculi are almost always associated with infection.

Uric acid stones may or may not form in the presence of hyperuricemia or hyperuricosuria.

Increased concentrations of stone constituents, changes in urinary pH, decreased urine volume, and bacteria all play a role in stone formation, but many calculi occur in the absence of these factors. Some authors have postulated that urinary mucoproteins or inhibitors of crystal formation are important in the pathogenesis of some stones.

TUMORS OF THE KIDNEY (p. 985)

BENIGN TUMORS

CORTICAL ADENOMA. Small, discrete (usually yellow) tumors *less than 3 cm in diameter.* They are common, occurring in 7% to 22% of autopsies. Histologically, most consist of vacuolated epithelial cells forming tubules; they may be histologically indistinguishable from renal cell carcinoma. The size of the tumor is a useful diagnostic feature. Tumors over 3 cm in diameter are much more likely to metastasize than those less than 3 cm.

RENAL FIBROMA OR HAMARTOMA. Small (less than 1 cm) nodule of fibroblast-like cells and collagen found in the medulla; completely benign.

ANGIOMYOLIPOMA. Often associated with tuberous sclerosis and considered a hamartomatous malformation.

ONCOCYTOMAS. Epithelial tumors composed of eosinophilic epithelial cells. On EM the cells are packed with mitochondria. They may be large (up to 12 cm) but almost never metastasize.

MALIGNANT TUMORS

Renal Cell Carcinoma (Hypernephroma or Adenocarcinoma of Kidney) (p. 986)

Represents 1% to 3% of visceral cancers and 90% of renal cancers in adults. They are most common in the sixth to seventh decades of life. Males predominate 3:1. Nearly two-thirds of patients with von Hippel–Lindau syndrome develop renal cell carcinomas; frequently bilateral.

Grossly, they present as rounded masses 3 to 15 cm in diameter, composed of yellow to gray-white tissue with focal hemorrhages, necrosis, and cyst formation. Often they invade the renal vein and extend into the inferior vena cava.

Histologically, they are composed of clear cells (from glycogen and lipid) and/or granular cells (from numerous mitochondria) that show mild-to-marked cytologic variation, often within the same tumor. Anaplastic sarcomatoid variants may mimic a primary sarcoma.

Clinically, patients may show hematuria (90%), fever, constitutional symptoms, and/or a paraneoplastic syndrome (polycythemia, hypercalcemia, hypertension, feminization or masculinization, Cushing's syndrome, eosinophilia, leukemoid reaction, and amyloidosis).

Prognosis is dependent on tumor size and the extent of spread (either local or distant) at diagnosis. Renal cell carcinoma has a tendency to metastasize widely before giving rise to any local symptoms; indeed, in 25% of new patients there is radiographic evidence of metastases at presentation.

The time course of disease can be variable, but the average 5-year survival is about 45%, and up to 70% in the absence of distant metastasis at diagnosis.

Urothelial Carcinomas of Renal Pelvis (p. 987)

About 5% to 10% of renal tumors occur in the pelvis, where they present early because of obstruction. Their histology exactly mimics urothelial tumors in the bladder, ranging from well-differentiated papillary lesions to anaplastic, invasive carcinomas. They are often multifocal, and in 50% of cases there is a synchronous or metachronous bladder tumor. Despite these observations, recent evidence suggests that they are clonal in origin. Five-year survivals vary from 70% for low-grade superficial tumors to 10% for high-grade infiltrating tumors.

URETERS

CONGENITAL ANOMALIES (p. 992)

Occur in 2% to 3% of autopsies, and for the most part of only incidental interest without clinical relevance. However, *ureteropelvic junction narrowing or obstruction* can cause hydronephrosis. They may be congenital or acquired; the latter are ascribed to disorganized smooth muscle at the junction, excess stromal deposition of collagen, or rarely extrinsic compression by aberrant renal vessels.

TUMORS (p. 992)

Can be urothelial or connective tissue in origin, and reflect features analogous to tumors in the renal pelvis and bladder.

OBSTRUCTIVE LESIONS (p. 993)

The major causes of ureteral obstruction are listed in Table 18–5.

Table 18–5. Major Causes of Ureteral Obstruction

Intrinsic	
Calculi	Of renal origin, rarely over 5 mm in diameter
	Larger renal stones cannot enter ureters
	Impact at loci of ureteral narrowing—ureteropelvic junction, where ureters cross iliac vessels, and where they enter bladder—and cause excruciating "renal colic"
Strictures	Congenital or acquired (inflammations, sclerosing retroperitoneal fibrosis)
Tumorous masses	Transitional cell carcinomas arising in ureters
	Rarely, benign tumors or fibroepithelial polyps
Blood clots	Massive hematuria from renal calculi, tumors, or papillary necrosis
Neurogenic causes	Interruption of the neural pathways to the bladder
Extrinsic	
Pregnancy	Physiologic relaxation of smooth muscle or pressure on ureters at pelvic brim from enlarging fundus
Periureteral inflammation	Salpingitis, diverticulitis, peritonitis, sclerosing retroperitoneal fibrosis
Endometriosis	With pelvic lesions, followed by scarring
Tumors	Cancers of the rectum, bladder, prostate, ovaries, uterus, cervix, lymphomas, sarcomas. Ureteral obstruction is one of the major causes of death from cervical carcinoma

From Cotran, R. S., Kumar, V., and Robbins, S. L.: Robbins Pathologic Basis of Disease. 5th ed. Philadelphia, W. B. Saunders Co., 1994, p. 993.

SCLEROSING RETROPERITONITIS (RETROPERITONEAL FIBROMATOSIS) (p. 993)

An uncommon cause of hydronephrosis. It is characterized by ill-defined fibrous masses that begin over the sacral promontory, encircle the lower abdominal aorta, and extend laterally through the retroperitoneum to enclose and encroach on the ureters. Microscopically, the fibrosis is marked by a prominent inflammatory infiltrate of lymphocytes, often with germinal centers, plasma cells, and eosinophils. Sometimes, foci of fat necrosis and granulomatous inflammation are present. The cause is unclear. Some cases are associated with methysergide therapy for migraine headache.

URINARY BLADDER

CONGENITAL ANOMALIES (p. 994)

DIVERTICULA (p. 994)

May arise as congenital defects but more commonly are acquired lesions from persistent urethral obstruction. They are the sites of urinary stasis, and predispose to infection and the formation of bladder calculi. They also predispose to vesicoureteric reflux, and rarely carcinomas may arise within them.

EXSTROPHY (p. 995)

Exstrophy of the bladder is due to a defect in the anterior abdomen, wherein the bladder communicates directly through a large defect with the body surface, or lies as an exposed sac. Chronic infections supervene and there is an increased incidence of carcinoma, mostly adenocarcinoma.

INFLAMMATIONS (p. 995)
ACUTE AND CHRONIC CYSTITIS (p. 995)

Lower UTIs have already been discussed, but in addition to the common causal agents of infectious cystitis (*E. coli, Proteus, Klebsiella,* and *Enterobacter*), *tuberculous cystitis* can be a sequel to renal tuberculosis. *Candida* and *Cryptococcus* can cause cystitis in immunosuppressed patients or those receiving long-term antibiotics. *Schistosomiasis* is common in Middle Eastern countries, notably Egypt. *Adenovirus, Chlamydia,* and *Mycoplasma* can cause cystitis. *Radiation cystitis* can also occur, and the *antitumor agents* cyclophosphamide and busulfan can cause hemorrhagic cystitis.

Often the cystitis associated with long-term indwelling catheters results in mucosal bulges into the lumen, forming polyps (polypoid cystitis), a lesion that should not be mistaken for papillary carcinoma.

The symptoms caused by cystitis include urinary frequency, lower abdominal pain, and pain or burning on urination (dysuria).

SPECIAL FORMS OF CYSTITIS (p. 996)

ULCERATIVE INTERSTITIAL CYSTITIS (HUNNER'S ULCER). Chronic cystitis, usually in women, and associated with localized ulceration with inflammation and fibrosis of all layers of the bladder wall.

MALAKOPLAKIA. Chronic cystitis characterized by soft, yellow, slightly raised mucosal plaques, 3 to 4 cm in diameter. The plaques consist of lymphocytes and foamy histiocytes, the latter containing PAS-positive granules and "targetoid" intracellular structures called Michaelis-Gutmann bodies. The intracellular material represents incompletely digested bacterial substances. Identical lesions occur in the colon, lungs, bones, kidney, prostate, and epididymis and are sometimes associated with immunosuppression.

METAPLASIAS (p. 997)

GLANDULAR METAPLASIA (INTESTINAL METAPLASIA). May occur in the presence or absence of chronic inflammation and is marked by the formation of cystic infoldings of the urothelium (cystitis cystica), lined by columnar cells. When extensive and long-standing, it is associated with an increased risk for adenocarcinoma.

NEPHROGENIC METAPLASIA. An uncommon lesion consisting

of discrete mucosal projections formed of benign-appearing tubules that must be distinguished from adenocarcinoma.

SQUAMOUS METAPLASIA. May result from chronic inflammation, bladder exstrophy, calculi, or schistosomal infections and may predispose to squamous cell carcinoma of the bladder.

NEOPLASMS (p. 997)

Transitional Cell Tumors

Comprise 95% of bladder neoplasms; the remainder are of connective tissue origin. Transitional cell tumors include

Exophytic (benign) papilloma, a rare lesion composed of finger-like papillae that contain a central fibrovascular core and are covered by normal-appearing transitional cells *seven or fewer layers in thickness.* These growths are prone to recur but very rarely progress to carcinoma.

Inverted papilloma, in which downward growth of papillae forms a smooth-surfaced, benign nodule.

Carcinoma, of which 90% are transitional, 5% are squamous, and 5% are mixed. Adenocarcinomas of the bladder are rare.

Transitional cell carcinoma (TCC) presents most often between the ages of 50 and 80 years, and the male:female ratio is 3:1. Established risk factors for TCC include

• Industrial exposure to arylamines.
• Cigarette smoking.
• *Schistosoma haematobium* infection, a major cause of bladder cancer in Egypt and most often associated with squamous morphology.
• Analgesic abuse.
• Cyclophosphamide therapy.

TCC ranges from low-grade (grades I to II) papillary tumors that are usually noninvasive to high-grade tumors (grade III) that are papillary, nodular, or flat and are associated with invasion of the bladder wall (muscularis) and metastasis. The majority of tumors are low grade, and though they often recur, progression to invasion is uncommon; deletions in chromosome 9q are frequent in low-grade tumors. High-grade TCC tends to be aneuploid and is associated with alterations in p53.

Carcinoma in situ (CIS) is a flat, noninvasive form of high-grade TCC, often seen adjacent to high-grade papillary lesions. In half of patients diagnosed with CIS, the tumor will become invasive.

Clinically, TCC presents with painless hematuria, frequency, urgency, and/or dysuria. The prognosis is dependent primarily on stage and grade at first diagnosis. Five-year survivals drop significantly from 95% for noninvasive grade I papillary TCC to 10% for deeply invasive grade III TCC.

URETHRA (p. 1004)

Urethritis can be caused by gonococci and nongonococci. The nongonococcal forms can be caused by *E. coli*, other enteric organisms, *Chlamydia,* and *Mycoplasma.*

The *caruncle* is an inflammatory tumor, 1 to 1.5 cm in diameter, of the external urethral meatus in women; excision is curative.

Malignant tumors are rare, usually squamous cell carcinoma.

CHAPTER NINETEEN

Male Genital System

PENIS

CONGENITAL ANOMALIES (p. 1007)

- Include a variety of abnormalities in size and form, including aplasia/hypoplasia, hypertrophy, duplication, and, more commonly, *hypospadias, epispadias,* and *phimosis.*
- Malformations of the urethral groove and canal may produce abnormal urethral orifices involving the *ventral* or *dorsal* aspects of the penis, designated *hypospadias* and *epispadias,* respectively. These may be associated with other urogenital malformations, including *undescended testes,* and may produce lower urinary tract *obstruction* and *sterility.*
- *Phimosis* designates an abnormally small orifice in the prepuce; it may arise as a primary developmental defect or occur secondary to inflammation. Phimosis predisposes to secondary *infections* and *carcinoma,* owing to chronic accumulation of secretions and other debris under the foreskin. *Paraphimosis* refers to abnormal, painful swelling of the glans penis after forcible retraction of a phimotic prepuce; it may cause urethral obstruction.

INFLAMMATIONS (p. 1008)

- Characteristically involve both the glans penis and the prepuce.
- Include *nonspecific* inflammatory processes and specific *sexually transmitted diseases* (e.g., syphilis, gonorrhea, chancroid, lymphopathia venereum, genital herpes, granuloma inguinale).
- *Balanoposthitis* refers to nonspecific infection of the glans penis and prepuce, generally associated with *phimosis* or a *redundant prepuce,* and resultant chronic accumulation of smegma; it may be caused by a wide variety of bacteria, fungi, mycoplasmas, and chlamydiae.

TUMORS

Benign Tumors

Condyloma Acuminatum (p. 1008)

- A benign epithelial proliferation caused by *human papilloma virus* (HPV), especially types 6 and 11.
- May involve mucocutaneous genital surfaces of either sex; *sexual contact* is the most likely mode of transmission. It is most common after puberty; its presence in a prepubertal child should arouse suspicion of sexual abuse.
- Gross morphology is that of a sessile or pedunculated papillary

excrescence, often involving the coronal sulcus or inner surface of the prepuce.

- Characterized histologically by branching stromal papillae covered by hyperplastic stratified squamous epithelium, often associated with prominent hyperkeratosis. Vacuolation of superficial epithelial cells (*koilocytosis*) is common. Maturation of epithelial cells is orderly, in contrast to carcinoma *in situ*.
- Most lesions remain benign; they may recur owing to persistence of HPV infection.

Giant Condyloma (Buschke-Löwenstein Tumor, Verrucous Carcinoma)

- Presents as a solitary, exophytic lesion that may destroy much of the penis; it is generally larger than condyloma acuminatum.
- Associated with HPV 6 and 11 infection.
- Locally invasive and recurrent; metastases rare.
- Histologic appearance characterized by exophytic, well-differentiated papillary squamous projections with koilocytosis comparable with condyloma acuminatum, and broad, bulbous projections extending into subjacent stroma; cytologic atypia most often seen at invasive margin.

Carcinoma *in Situ* (p. 1009)

- Indicates cytologic evidence of malignancy confined to epithelium (i.e., no invasion of underlying connective tissue). Variants include Bowen's disease, erythroplasia of Queyrat, and bowenoid papulosis.

BOWEN'S DISEASE. May occur in the genital region in both males and females, generally those over the age of 35. In males, presents most commonly as a thickened, gray-white plaque over the shaft of the penis. Microscopic features include marked epithelial atypia with complete loss of normal surface maturation, but *no invasion* of underlying stroma. Transition to invasive squamous cell carcinoma is estimated to occur in approximately 10% to 20% of cases; there is a possible association with *visceral malignancies*.

ERYTHROPLASIA OF QUEYRAT. Presents as a single or multiple shiny red, sometimes velvety plaque on the glans and prepuce; histologic features and evolution are comparable to those of Bowen's disease; there is no association with visceral malignancy.

BOWENOID PAPULOSIS. Presents as multiple, pigmented papular lesions on external genitalia; may mimic condyloma acuminatum grossly. Histologically indistinguishable from Bowen's disease. E6 and E7 portions of HPV type 16 DNA are present in most patients.

Malignant Tumor

Squamous Cell Carcinoma (p. 1010)

- Accounts for 1% of cancers in males in the United States; prevalence is higher in regions where circumcision is not routinely practiced. Most cases are seen between ages 40 and 70 years.
- Potential etiologies include *carcinogens* within smegma accumulating under the foreskin, and *HPV* types 16 and 18.
- Typically presents as epithelial thickening on the glans or inner surface of the prepuce, progressing to ulceroinfiltrative or exophytic growth eroding the penile tip and/or shaft.
- Histologic appearance is identical to squamous cell carcinomas involving other cutaneous sites.

- Clinical course is characterized by slow growth, with metastases to regional (inguinal and iliac) lymph nodes; distant metastases are uncommon. The 5-year survival rate is 66% for lesions confined to the penis, 27% with regional node involvement.

TESTIS AND EPIDIDYMIS

CONGENITAL ANOMALIES (p. 1011)

Anomalies include cryptorchidism, aplasia, fusion (synorchism), and a variety of developmental cysts.

Cryptorchidism (p. 1011)

- Affects 0.3% to 0.8% of the male population.
- Represents *failure of descent;* testes may be found anywhere along the normal path of descent, from the abdominal cavity to the inguinal canal.
- Most cases are idiopathic; other causes include
  1. Genetic abnormalities (e.g., trisomy 13).
  2. Hormonal abnormalities (e.g., deficiency of luteinizing hormone-releasing hormone).
- Most cases are unilateral; 25% are bilateral.
- Histologic changes may be apparent as early as 2 years of age, including *decreased germ cell development, thickening* and *hyalinization* of seminiferous tubular basement membrane, interstitial *fibrosis,* and relative sparing of Leydig cells. Regressive changes may also occur in contralateral descended testis.
- Clinical significance is related to high prevalence of *inguinal hernias, sterility,* and a 7- to 11-fold increased incidence of *testicular neoplasms;* surgical correction (orchiopexy) decreases the likelihood of sterility if performed early, but does *not* decrease the risk of neoplasia, which may occur in either testis.

ATROPHY (p. 1013)

- May be secondary to cryptorchidism, vascular disease, inflammatory disorders, hypopituitarism, malnutrition, obstruction of outflow of semen, elevated levels of female sex hormones (endogenous or exogenous), persistently elevated levels of follicle-stimulating hormone, radiation, and chemotherapy.
- May also be encountered as a *primary developmental abnormality* in patients with Klinefelter's syndrome.
- Morphologic alterations identical to those in cryptoorchidism.

INFLAMMATIONS (p. 1013)

Inflammatory conditions are generally more common in the epididymis than in the testis; however, some infections, notably syphilis, may begin in the testis with secondary involvement of the epididymis. Inflammatory diseases include *nonspecific* epididymitis and orchitis, *granulomatous (autoimmune)* orchitis, and several *specific* infectious diseases (e.g., gonorrhea, mumps, tuberculosis, syphilis).

Nonspecific Epididymitis and Orchitis

- Often associated with infection of the *urinary tract,* with secondary infection of the epididymis via the vas deferens or lymphatics of the spermatic cord.

- Causes vary with the age of the patient and include

  - Gram-negative rods associated with genitourinary malformations in pediatric patients.
  - *Chlamydia trachomatis* and *Neisseria gonorrhoeae* in sexually active males under the age of 35.
  - *E. coli* and *Pseudomonas* species in older males.

- Nonspecific interstitial congestion, edema, and neutrophilic infiltrates in the early stages, with subsequent involvement of tubules; severe cases may progress to generalized suppuration of the entire epididymis. Inflammation may extend to the testis via efferent ductules or local lymphatic channels. Scarring of the testis and epididymis may occur with resultant *infertility*. Leydig cells are less severely affected and sexual activity generally is not disturbed.

Granulomatous (Autoimmune) Orchitis

- An uncommon cause of *unilateral testicular enlargement* in middle-aged men. Possible *autoimmune* origin.
- Most cases present with sudden onset of a tender testicular mass, sometimes associated with fever; it may be painless in some patients and difficult to distinguish from testicular neoplasia.
- *Granulomas* within testicular tubules and adjacent connective tissue, accompanied by occasional plasma cells and neutrophils. Lesions must be differentiated from granulomas of tuberculosis.

Specific Inflammations (p. 1013)

GONORRHEA

- Most cases represent *retrograde extension* of infection from the posterior urethra to the prostate, seminal vesicles, and epididymis.
- The inflammatory pattern is identical to that seen in nonspecific epididymitis and orchitis (discussed above); infection may extend to the testis and produce suppurative orchitis in untreated cases.

MUMPS

- Orchitis is uncommon in children; develops in 20% to 30% of postpubertal males with mumps.
- Orchitis typically develops about 1 week after onset of parotid inflammation; it may precede parotitis, or occur in the absence of parotitis in a minority of patients. Testicular involvement is *unilateral* in approximately 70% of cases.
- There are interstitial edema and mononuclear inflammatory cells (lymphocytes, plasma cells, and macrophages); neutrophils usually are not conspicuous, but may be prominent in severe cases. Orchitis is not usually associated with sterility, owing to unilateral testicular involvement and the patchy, predominantly interstitial pattern of inflammation.

TUBERCULOSIS

- Almost always begins in the *epididymis*, with secondary involvement of the testis.
- There is granulomatous inflammation associated with caseous necrosis, identical to active tuberculosis in other sites.

SYPHILIS

- Virtually always begins as *orchitis*, with secondary involvement of the epididymis; may present as isolated orchitis, without involvement of adnexal structures. May occur in both congenital and acquired syphilis.
- May produce nodular *gummas* or *diffuse interstitial inflammation*. Interstitial changes include edema, lymphoplasmacytic inflammatory cells, and typical obliterative endarteritis.

VASCULAR DISTURBANCES (TORSION) (p. 1014)

- These occur secondary to twisting of the spermatic cord, with resultant *venous obstruction;* arteries may also be occluded, but often remain patent because of thicker walls.
- Typically occur in patients with preexisting structural lesions, such as incompletely descended testicles, absence of scrotal ligaments, or testicular atrophy. Torsion is generally precipitated by trauma or other violent movement.
- Changes range from congestion and interstitial hemorrhage to extensive hemorrhagic necrosis, depending on the duration and severity of the process.

TESTICULAR TUMORS (p. 1015)

A wide range of histologic types are recognized, giving rise to many different classification schemes. Can be divided into two major groups: *germ cell tumors* (accounting for approximately 95% of cases) and *nongerminal tumors* (stromal or sex cord tumors). Most germ cell tumors are aggressive lesions, although outlook has improved considerably with current therapy.

Germ Cell Tumors

Incidence approximately 2 per 100,000 males annually, with peak incidence between 15 and 34 years. Account for 10% of cancer deaths in this group.

CLASSIFICATION AND HISTOGENESIS. Diverse classification schemes, based on a wide spectrum of morphologic patterns and variable concepts of histogenesis. Testicular germ cell neoplasms may contain a *single* histologic pattern (40% of cases) or a *mixture* of patterns (60% of cases). Histogenesis may be related to the ability of a neoplastic germ cell to give rise to *seminoma,* or to transform into a *totipotential* neoplastic cell (embryonal carcinoma) capable of further differentiation. Germ cell neoplasms, accordingly, may be divided broadly into *seminomas* and *nonseminomatous tumors.* The *WHO classification* of testicular neoplasms (Table 19–1) is the most widely used classification scheme in the U.S.

PATHOGENESIS. Important risk factors include

1. *Cryptorchidism.* Associated with 10% of testicular tumors.
2. *Genetic factors.* Higher risk of testicular neoplasia among siblings of patients with testicular tumors; some familial clustering reported. Significant racial differences also exist (rare in African blacks).
3. *Testicular dysgenesis.* Includes testicular feminization and Klinefelter's syndrome.

Cytogenetic abnormalities involving *chromosomes 12* and *1* are common; *i(12p)* present in 90% of testicular germ cell tumors.

Table 19–1. WHO Pathologic Classification of Testicular Tumors

---

Germ Cell Tumors
Tumors of one histologic pattern
  Seminoma
  Spermatocytic seminoma
  Embryonal carcinoma
  Yolk sac tumor (embryonal carcinoma, infantile type)
  Polyembryoma choriocarcinoma
  Teratomas
    Mature
    Immature
    With malignant transformation
Tumors showing more than one histologic pattern
  Embryonal carcinoma plus teratoma (teratocarcinoma)
  Choriocarcinoma and any other types (specify types)
  Other combinations (specify)

Sex Cord–Stromal Tumors
Well-differentiated forms
  Leydig cell tumor
  Sertoli cell tumor
  Granulosa cell tumor
Mixed forms (specify)
Incompletely differentiated forms

From Cotran, R. S., Kumar, V., and Robbins, S. L.: Robbins Pathologic Basis of Disease. 5th ed. Philadelphia, W. B. Saunders Co., 1994, p. 1015.

Nonrandom gains of chromosomes 1, 7, 9, 12, 17, 21, 22, or X present in 70% of cases.

Seminoma (p. 1016)

- Accounts for 30% of all testicular germ cell tumors; the most likely germ cell neoplasm to present with a single histologic pattern.
- Peak incidence in the fourth decade.
- Variants include

  - Classic seminoma (85% of seminomas).
  - Anaplastic seminoma (5% to 10%).
  - Spermatocytic seminoma (4% to 6%) (discussed below).

- A homogeneous, lobulated, gray-white mass, generally devoid of hemorrhage or necrosis; the tunica albuginea usually remains intact. Microscopically, composed of large polyhedral "seminoma cells" containing abundant clear cytoplasm, large nuclei, and prominent nucleoli; cytoplasmic glycogen is typically present. A fibrous stroma of variable density divides the neoplastic cells into irregular *lobules;* an accompanying *lymphocytic infiltrate* (usually T-cell) is present in most cases; granulomas may also be present. Neoplastic giant cells, and syncytial cells resembling placental syncytiotrophoblast, may be seen in some cases; human chorionic gonadotropin (HCG) is present in such cells and presumably accounts for the elevated serum HCG levels demonstrable in some patients with pure seminoma. The tumor cells contain placental alkaline phosphatase. Classic seminoma cells do not contain alpha-fetoprotein (AFP). *Anaplastic seminomas* are distinguished from classic seminomas by greater nuclear atypia and a higher mitotic rate.

• Histologically identical tumors may occur in the ovary (dysgerminomas) and central nervous system (germinomas).

Spermatocytic Seminoma (p. 1017)

• Uncommon neoplasms, occurring in *patients older* than those with classic seminoma.

• *Indolent* growths, with virtually no tendency to metastasize.

• Lesions tend to be larger than those of classic seminoma; composed of a *mixed* population of cells, including smaller (6 to 8 μm) cells resembling secondary spermatocytes (hence the "spermatocytic" designation), medium-sized (15 to 18 μm) cells, and scattered giant cells.

Embryonal Carcinoma (p. 1017)

• Peak incidence in 20- to 30-year age group; more *aggressive* than seminoma, although recent developments in chemotherapy have improved the prognosis considerably.

• Lesions may be small and confined to the testis; most examples are poorly demarcated, gray-white masses punctuated by foci of hemorrhage and/or necrosis. They may extend through the tunica albuginea into the epididymis or spermatic cord. Microscopically, they are composed of primitive epithelial cells with indistinct cell borders, forming irregular sheets, tubules, alveoli, and papillary structures. Mitotic figures and neoplastic giant cells are common; syncytial cells containing HCG and/or cells containing AFP may be seen, and when present indicate a *mixed germ cell tumor* with concomitant trophoblastic or yolk sac differentiation, respectively.

Yolk Sac Tumor (p. 1018)

• The most common testicular neoplasm in infants and young children; synonyms include *infantile embryonal carcinoma* and *endodermal sinus tumor;* prognosis good in children up to 3 years of age.

• Most adult cases occur as a component of a *mixed* germ cell neoplasm.

• Pure forms present as infiltrative, homogeneous, yellow-white mucinous lesions. Microscopically, they are composed of cuboidal neoplastic cells arrayed in a lace-like (reticular) network; solid areas and papillae may also be seen. Structures resembling primitive glomeruli, so-called *endodermal sinuses,* are seen in 50% of cases. Eosinophilic, hyalin globules containing immunoreactive *AFP* and *alpha₁-antitrypsin* are present within and around the neoplastic cells.

Choriocarcinoma (p. 1018)

• A highly malignant neoplasm composed of both cytotrophoblastic and syncytiotrophoblastic elements.

• Similar neoplasms may occur in the ovary, placenta, or ectopic pluripotential germ cell rests in other sites (e.g., mediastinum, abdomen). This neoplasm is rare in pure form within the testis; it is more often encountered as a component of a *mixed germ cell neoplasm.*

• The primary testicular neoplasm is often quite small, even in the presence of widespread systemic metastases. The gross appearance ranges from a bulky, hemorrhagic mass to an inconspicuous lesion replaced by a fibrous scar. Histologically, it is composed of polygonal, comparatively uniform cytotrophoblastic cells growing in sheets and cords, admixed with multinucleated syncytiotrophoblastic cells; well-developed villi are not seen. HCG is readily demonstrable within the cytoplasm of the syncytiotrophoblastic elements.

Teratoma (p. 1019)

- A group of neoplasms exhibiting evidence of simultaneous differentiation along endodermal, mesodermal, and ectodermal lines. They may occur at any age.
- Variants include
  1. *Mature teratomas,* composed of a haphazard array of *differentiated* mesodermal (e.g., muscle, cartilage, adipose tissue), ectodermal (e.g., neural tissue, skin), and endodermal (e.g., gut, bronchial epithelium) elements. Mature teratomas are more common in infants and children; diagnosis of pure testicular teratoma should be made with extreme caution in adults, owing to the likelihood of concomitant malignant germ cell elements elsewhere in the neoplasm.
  2. *Immature teratomas,* containing elements of three germ layers in incomplete stages of differentiation. They should be regarded as malignant, even though cytologic features of malignancy may be inconspicuous.
  3. *Teratoma with malignant transformation.* Characterized by malignancy, generally in the form of a carcinoma (e.g., squamous cell carcinoma or adenocarcinoma) developing within a mature teratoma.

Mixed Tumors (p. 1020)

- Account in aggregate for approximately 60% of germ cell neoplasms.
- Histologic patterns are variable; the most common includes a mixture of teratoma, embryonal carcinoma, yolk sac tumor, and HCG-containing giant cells. *Teratocarcinoma* designates neoplasms containing both teratoma and embryonal carcinoma. Metastases from such lesions may contain virtually any germ cell element, including elements not present in the primary tumor.

Clinical Features of Germ Cell Neoplasms

- Most cases present with *painless enlargement of the testis;* neoplasia should be considered in the differential diagnosis of *all* testicular masses. However, clinical evaluation does not reliably distinguish between the various types of germ cell tumors.
- *Lymphatic* metastases are most common in *retroperitoneal paraaortic* nodes, but may occur in more distant sites (e.g., mediastinal and supraclavicular nodes); the *lungs* are the most common site for *hematogenous* metastases, followed by liver, brain, and bone. The histologic appearance of metastases may be identical to that of primary tumor, or may contain other germ cell elements (e.g., teratomatous metastases in a patient with a primary embryonal carcinoma).
- The biologic behavior of nonseminomatous germ cell tumors (NSGCTs) is, in general, more aggressive than that of seminomas. Roughly 70% of seminomas present with localized (clinical stage I) disease; in contrast, 60% of NSGCTs present with advanced (stage II or III) disease. Extensive metastases may be present even with small primary lesions, particularly in the case of choriocarcinoma.

- *Clinical staging* is accomplished via physical examination, radiographic imaging of the retroperitoneum and chest, and assay of various tumor markers (see below). Clinical stages include

  - Stage I. Tumor confined to the testis.
  - Stage II. Metastases limited to retroperitoneal nodes below the diaphragm.
  - Stage III. Metastases outside the retroperitoneal nodes or above the diaphragm.

- Several peptides may be produced by germ cell neoplasms and can be detected in body fluids by sensitive assays; AFP and HCG are the most commonly assayed. Serum markers are of value in

  - The *evaluation* of testicular masses;
  - The *staging* of germ cell tumors; and
  - Monitoring the response of a germ cell tumor to therapy.

- Treatment includes radiation and chemotherapy, depending on the histologic type of the neoplasm (seminoma versus NSGCT) and the stage of disease; chemotherapy, in particular, has dramatically improved the prognosis of patients with NSGCT.

Tumors of Sex Cord–Gonadal Stroma (p. 1022)

Classification is based on differentiation into Leydig or Sertoli cells.

Leydig (Interstitial) Cell Tumors

- Relatively uncommon neoplasms, accounting for 2% of all testicular tumors; most occur between the ages of 20 and 60 years, but they may be found at any age.
- May elaborate androgens or mixtures of androgens and other steroids (estrogens, corticosteroids).
- Clinical manifestations include a *testicular mass* and changes referable to *hormonal abnormalities* (e.g., gynecomastia, sexual precocity in prepubertal males).
- Grossly circumscribed nodules with a homogeneous, golden brown cut surface. Microscopically, they are composed of polygonal cells with abundant granular, eosinophilic cytoplasm and indistinct cell borders. Lipochrome pigment, lipid droplets, and eosinophilic Reinke crystalloids are commonly present. Ten per cent invade and/or metastasize.

Sertoli Cell Tumors (Androblastoma)

- Uncommon neoplasms, composed of Sertoli cells or a mixture of Sertoli and granulosa cells.
- May elaborate androgens or estrogens, but rarely in sufficient quantity to produce feminization or precocious masculinization.
- Homogeneous gray-white to yellow masses of variable size. The microscopic picture is dominated by cells with tall, columnar cytoplasm, often forming cords reminiscent of immature seminiferous tubules. Most are benign; 10% demonstrate invasion and/or metastases.

Testicular Lymphomas (p. 1022)

- Account for 5% of all testicular neoplasms; the most common testicular neoplasm in patients over the age of 60 years.
- Most are diffuse, large cell, non-Hodgkin's lymphomas and disseminate widely; the prognosis is accordingly poor.

MISCELLANEOUS LESIONS OF
TUNICA VAGINALIS (p. 1022)

Conditions include

1. *Hydrocele.* Accumulation of serous fluid within the tunica vaginalis, either secondary to generalized edema or due to incomplete closure of the processus vaginalis. May become secondarily infected.
2. *Hematocele.* Accumulation of blood within the tunica vaginalis secondary to trauma, torsion, hemorrhage; a generalized bleeding diathesis; or, rarely, invasion of the tunica by neoplasms.
3. *Chylocele.* Accumulation of lymphatic fluid within the tunica vaginalis, secondary to lymphatic obstruction (e.g., in patients with elephantiasis).
4. *Spermatocele.* Local accumulation of semen in the spermatic cord, generally within a dilated duct in the head of the epididymis.
5. *Varicocele.* Local accumulation of blood within a dilated vein in the spermatic cord; more appropriately designated "cystic venous varix."

PROSTATE

Major disorders of the prostate include inflammations (prostatitis), nodular hyperplasia, and carcinoma.

INFLAMMATIONS (p. 1023)

Conditions include *acute bacterial prostatitis, chronic bacterial prostatitis,* and *chronic abacterial prostatitis.* Diagnosis is based on microscopic examination and culture of fractionated urine specimens and prostatic secretions expressed by prostatic massage. Diagnosis of prostatitis is based on the presence of more than 15 leukocytes per high-power field in a urine fraction containing expressed prostatic secretions. In *bacterial* prostatitis, cultures of prostatic secretions are positive, and bacterial counts are significantly higher (>1 log) than in cultures of urethral and bladder urine.

Acute Bacterial Prostatitis (p. 1024)

- Most cases are caused by organisms associated with urinary tract infections (UTIs) (e.g., *Escherichia coli* and other gram-negative rods), *Enterococcus,* or *Staphyococcus aureus.*
- Organisms reach the prostate via *direct extension* from the urethra or urinary bladder, or by *lymphatic* or *hematogenous seeding* from more distant sites. This may follow *surgical manipulation* of the urethra or prostate.
- Presents with fever, chills, dysuria, and a boggy, markedly tender prostate. Diagnosis is based on clinical features and urine culture.

Chronic Bacterial Prostatitis (p. 1024)

- May be asymptomatic or associated with low back pain, suprapubic and perineal discomfort, and dysuria; frequently associated with a history of *recurrent UTIs* caused by the same organism.
- *Diagnosis* is established by demonstration of leukocytes in

expressed prostatic secretions (discussed above) and positive bacterial cultures in prostatic secretions and urine; most cases are caused by organisms similar to those responsible for acute prostatitis.

- Most cases appear *insidiously,* without a history of acute prostatitis.

Chronic Abacterial Prostatitis (p. 1024)

- The most common form of prostatitis; typically affects sexually active males.
- Manifestations similar to those of chronic bacterial prostatitis, but *without* a history of recurrent UTIs.
- Expressed prostatic secretions contain more than 15 leukocytes per high-power field; cultures are uniformly *negative.*
- Etiology is uncertain; potential pathogens include *Ureaplasma urealyticum* and *Chlamydia trachomatis.*

MORPHOLOGY

- *Acute* cases are associated with variable degrees of edema, congestion, and neutrophilic infiltration of parenchyma; neutrophils may also be present in glandular lumina. Severe cases are associated with a variable degree of parenchymal necrosis and abscess formation.
- *Chronic* cases are manifested histologically by aggregates of macrophages, lymphocytes, plasma cells, and neutrophils within prostatic parenchyma. Diagnosis should *not* be based solely on the presence of lymphocytes within the prostatic stroma, because isolated lymphoid aggregates may be encountered in otherwise normal glands in elderly patients.

NODULAR HYPERPLASIA (BENIGN PROSTATIC HYPERPLASIA) (p. 1025)

- Present in approximately 20% of males at age 40 years, increasing to 70% by age 60 years, and to 90% by the eighth decade.
- Asymptomatic in most patients; a minority require surgical intervention.
- Etiology is uncertain, but likely related to effects of *androgens;* dihydrotestosterone (DHT), derived from testosterone via 5α-reductase activity, probably mediates prostatic growth. Estrogen (estradiol) may further sensitize the prostate to the effects of DHT.

MORPHOLOGY

- The gland is enlarged by nodules of variable size arising in the *inner* (periurethral) portion. Nodules arising lateral to the urethra may compress the urethral lumen to a slitlike orifice; those arising more medially may project directly into the floor of the proximal urethra, contributing to obstruction. In other cases, nodules project into the lumen of the bladder and produce a ball-valve obstruction at the mouth of the urethra. Cut surface demonstrates well-demarcated nodules involving the inner portion of the prostate.
- Microscopically, nodules are composed of variable mixtures of proliferating *glands* and *fibromuscular stroma;* cystic dilatation of glandular elements is common and contributes further to nodularity. Hyperplastic glandular epithelium may form irregular papillae, but retains two cell layers characteristic of normal

prostatic glands. Other changes include areas of *squamous metaplasia* and *infarcts.*

CLINICAL FEATURES

- Produces symptoms in 50% of men beyond the age of 60 years.
- Manifestations related to *urinary tract obstruction,* including

  - Urinary frequency, nocturia, and difficulty starting and stopping the stream of urine.
  - Acute urinary retention.
  - Chronic urinary stasis with resultant bacterial overgrowth and UTI.

- Chronic obstruction may result in a variety of secondary structural alterations, including hypertrophy of the urinary bladder, urinary bladder diverticula, and hydronephrosis.
- *No relationship* has been established between nodular hyperplasia of the prostate and prostatic carcinoma.

CARCINOMA OF PROSTATE (p. 1026)

- The *most common* form of cancer in men; currently the second leading cause of cancer death. Approximately 200,000 new cases detected annually; 20% prove fatal. Postmortem and surgical biopsy material indicate an even larger number of *incidental* (occult) prostatic carcinomas.
- Occurs predominantly in males over the age of 50 years. Incidence is 4.8 cases per 100,000 population in the 45- to 49-year age group, increasing to 513 per 100,000 between the ages of 70 and 75.
- Rare in Asians; more common in blacks than in whites.
- The *etiology* remains unknown; clinical and epidemiologic data suggest that advancing age, race, *hormonal influences,* genetic factors, and environmental factors (e.g., diet) all play a role in its development. A role for *hormonal influences,* in particular, is suggested by the retardation of the growth of some prostatic carcinomas by castration or estrogen administration, and by the presence of androgen receptors on both normal and neoplastic prostatic epithelium.

MORPHOLOGY

- Most cases (70%) arise in the *peripheral* part of the prostate, particularly in the *posterior* region, facilitating palpation during rectal examination.
- Primary lesions characteristically are poorly demarcated, firm, gritty foci, often somewhat yellower than the adjacent non-neoplastic parenchyma. Locally advanced cases may infiltrate the seminal vesicles and urinary bladder; invasion of the rectum may occur but is uncommon. *Lymphatic metastases* occur initially in obturator nodes, followed by spread to perivesical, hypogastric, iliac, presacral, and para-aortic nodes. *Hematogenous dissemination* occurs primarily to bone, most often in the form of *osteoblastic* metastases.
- Microscopically, the vast majority of prostatic carcinomas are *adenocarcinomas,* ranging from well-differentiated lesions to poorly differentiated neoplastic cells forming sheets and cords. Well-differentiated lesions may be difficult to distinguish from nodular hyperplasia in some cases, but contain acini that are smaller and more *closely spaced* ("back to back") than those encountered in hyperplasia, and lined by a *single layer* of

epithelial cells. Invasion of vascular channels and perineural spaces aids in the diagnosis of malignancy.
- Dysplastic change (prostatic intraepithelial neoplasia) is common in the epithelium of adjacent ducts, and presumably represents the precursor of invasive carcinoma.

GRADING AND STAGING

- *Grading* systems attempt to define histologic criteria (degree of differentiation, nuclear atypia, growth pattern) that predict the biologic behavior of a carcinoma. Several available systems (e.g., the Gleason) provide a good correlation between the histologic appearance of a carcinoma and the clinical stage and prognosis of the neoplasm.
- Staging of disease is also important in the selection of therapy and determination of prognosis (Fig. 19–1).
- DNA ploidy of tumor cells provides additional prognostic information (prognosis is worse for aneuploid and tetraploid tumors than for diploid tumors).

CLINICAL FEATURES

- A minority of cases are diagnosed in *asymptomatic* patients (stage A); the prognosis is generally favorable for stage A_1 cases (carcinoma identified in <5% of tissue resected); more ominous for A_2 lesions.
- Five to 10% of patients present with a *palpable prostatic nodule* (stage B); most progress to locally aggressive disease and distant dissemination if untreated.
- *Locally advanced* or *disseminated* disease is present in over 75% of patients at the time of diagnosis, manifested by signs

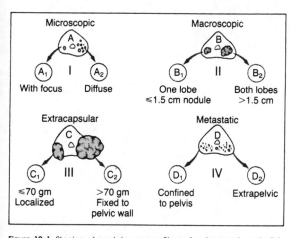

Figure 19–1. Staging of prostate cancer. Stage A: microscopic, not clinically palpable tumor (A_1, with focus in less than 5% of tissue examined, low grade; A_2, with multiple areas (more than 5%) or Gleason grade higher than 4). Stage B: palpable, macroscopic tumor. Stage C: tumor with extracapsular extension but still clinically localized. Stage D: demonstrated metastatic tumor. The tumor, node, and metastasis (TNM) staging for local tumors is indicated by Roman numerals I through IV. (Redrawn and adapted from Gittes, R. F.: Carcinoma of the prostate. N. Engl. J. Med. 1991, Volume 324, Page 240. Copyright 1991. Massachusetts Medical Society. All rights reserved.)

and symptoms of *urinary obstruction, local pain,* or *bone pain.* Urinary obstruction does not occur in the early stages of the disease, owing to the origin of most carcinomas in the periphery of the prostate. *Osteoblastic metastases* in elderly males are virtually diagnostic of metastatic prostatic carcinoma.

- Rectal digital examination, supplemented by transrectal sonography or transperineal needle biopsy, is the most useful method of diagnosing early prostatic carcinoma. *Lymphatic metastases* may be diagnosed by a variety of methods, including lymphangiography, CT scan, and histologic examination of lymphadenectomy specimens during staging procedures. Skeletal surveys and bone scans are useful in the diagnosis of *skeletal metastases.*

- Serum *prostatic acid phosphatase* measurements are useful in the diagnosis and staging of patients with prostatic carcinoma; elevations indicate that the carcinoma has *extended beyond the prostatic capsule, or has metastasized.* Serum acid phosphatase activity is also of value in monitoring the *progression* of disease; increasing levels indicate the progression of the carcinoma.

- Serum *prostate-specific antigen* (PSA) levels are elevated in patients with both localized and advanced carcinoma; lesser elevations may be seen in prostatic hyperplasia. Monitoring PSA levels may be particularly useful in assessing response to therapy or progression of disease.

- The treatment and prognosis of prostatic carcinoma are influenced primarily by the stage of the disease. Localized (stage A or B) disease is treated primarily with *surgery and/or radiotherapy,* with a 15-year survival rate of 90%. *Hormonal* treatment includes orchiectomy, or the administration of estrogens or synthetic analogs of luteinizing hormone–releasing hormone; it is used primarily in patients with advanced disease. Ten-year survival rates for patients with advanced disease range from 10% to 40%.

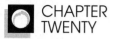

Female Genital Tract and Breast

VULVA

BARTHOLIN'S CYST (p. 1039)

Results from inflammatory occlusion of the main ducts of Bartholin's vulvovaginal glands. Gonorrheal and other infections may have caused the inflammatory obstruction, which also occasionally produces abscesses that must be drained. Uninflamed cysts are lined by transitional or flattened epithelium.

VESTIBULAR ADENITIS

This is a poorly understood inflammatory condition of the minor vestibular glands, resulting in exquisitely painful ulcerative lesions.

VULVAR DYSTROPHY (p. 1039)

Refers to benign mucosal alterations of the vulva, which should be differentiated from the more ominous dysplasias and cancer (*see p. 1041*). There are two main varieties of dystrophy:

- *Lichen sclerosus,* which consists of yellowish-blue papules or macules that eventually coalesce into thin, gray, parchment-like areas. Microscopically, there is epithelial thinning and subepithelial fibrosis (occasionally marked hyperkeratosis) and mononuclear perivascular reaction. The cause is unknown.
- *Squamous hyperplasia (hyperplastic dystrophy),* characterized by thickened hyperplastic epithelium, hyperkeratosis, and leukocytic dermal inflammation. The lesions appear as white plaques, clinically called *leukoplakia.*

Clinically, leukoplakia can denote a benign condition (e.g., vitiligo, chronic dermatitis) or an atypical and malignant lesion. Biopsy is therefore indicated in all such lesions. Neither lichen sclerosus nor hyperplasia is considered premalignant *per se.* However, both are often found in association with vulvar carcinoma. The reason for this is unknown.

TUMORS (p. 1041)

Condyloma Acuminatum (p. 1041)

This wart-like, verrucous lesion occurs on the vulva, perineum, vagina, and (rarely) cervix. The lesions are sexually transmitted and induced by human papilloma virus (HPV), mostly types 6 and 11.

Histologically, they consist of a treelike proliferation of stratified squamous epithelium with a peculiar perinuclear vacuolization of squamous cells called *koilocytosis* attributed to a viral effect. The lesions are benign but are often multiple.

Papillary Hidradenoma (p. 1041)

A benign tumor arising from modified apocrine sweat glands, presenting as a sharply circumscribed nodule, consisting of tubular ducts lined by nonciliated columnar cells underlain by a layer of flattened myoepithelial cells.

Vulvar Intraepithelial Neoplasia and Carcinoma (p. 1041)

Vulvar dysplasia, or vulvar intraepithelial neoplasia (VIN), presents as multicentric mucosal, sometimes raised, lesions characterized histologically by nuclear and epithelial atypia, increased mitoses, and lack of surface differentiation. The degree of epithelial atypia may vary, and in its most severe form is called *carcinoma in situ* (VIN III, Bowen's disease). HPV, mostly type 16, is present in 80% to 90% of cases of VIN and may play some causal role. Untreated, the lesions may progress to invasive carcinoma, particularly in older (over 40 years) or immunosuppressed patients.

Invasive vulvar carcinomas usually occur in women over age 60 years and may arise from HPV-associated VIN lesions (one-third) or as HPV-negative, well-differentiated carcinomas, the latter in association with hyperplasia, lichen sclerosus, or normal mucosa. Tumors metastasizing to regional lymph nodes indicate a poor prognosis.

Extramammary Paget's Disease (p. 1043)

Appears as a red, crusted, sharply demarcated, maplike area, mostly on the labia majora. It is characterized histologically by large, anaplastic, sometimes vacuolated tumor cells lying singly or in small clusters *within the epidermis and its appendages.* The tumor cells are mucin positive. Most lesions are confined to the epidermis.

Unlike Paget's disease of the nipple (see p. 1105), in which 100% of cases have an underlying ductal breast carcinoma, an underlying or adjacent sweat gland adenocarcinoma in the vulva is uncommon in vulvar Paget's disease.

Other vulvar carcinomas include basal cell carcinoma, adenocarcinoma arising in Bartholin's glands or sweat glands, and malignant melanoma; the latter has a poor prognosis.

VAGINA

CARCINOMA (p. 1044)

Primary carcinoma of the vagina is rare. The most common type is *squamous cell carcinoma,* accounting for 95% of cases. The peak incidence is between 60 and 70 years of age. From 1%

to 2% of women with cervical carcinoma will develop a vaginal carcinoma.

Grossly, the lesions are either plaquelike or occasionally fungating. They invade the cervix and perivaginal structures, such as the urethra, urinary bladder, and rectum.

Vaginal adenocarcinomas are rare but important because of the *increased frequency of clear cell adenocarcinoma in young women whose mothers were treated with diethylstilbestrol (DES) during pregnancy (for a threatened abortion).* Fortunately, only 0.14% of DES-exposed young women develop adenocarcinoma.

The tumors are discovered in patients between the ages of 15 and 20 years and are composed of glands lined by vacuolated, glycogen-containing clear cells. Early detection through careful follow-up of daughters of DES-exposed women is mandatory.

EMBRYONAL RHABDOMYOSARCOMA (p. 1045)

An uncommon, highly malignant vaginal tumor, consisting of embryonal rhabdomyoblasts, in infants and children. The tumors are polypoid, bulky masses with grapelike clusters that may protrude from the vagina. The tumor cells are small, have oval nuclei, and have small protrusions of cytoplasm from one end ("tennis-racket" cells).

PELVIC INFLAMMATORY DISEASE (PID) (p. 1038)

Refers to *an ascending infection that begins in the vulva or vaginal glands but usually spreads upward through the entire genital tract*, potentially involving all the structures of the female genital system.

There are at least three known causes of PID:

- The *gonococcus*, the most common, as part of a gonorrheal infection.
- Postabortal and postpartum PID, usually caused by staphylococci, streptococci, coliform bacteria, or *Clostridium perfringens.*
- Chlamydial infection.

Gonococcal inflammation begins in Bartholin's glands, in Skene's ducts and periurethral glands, or sometimes in the endocervical glands. The organisms then spread upward over the mucosal surfaces, eventually to involve fallopian tubes and tubo-ovarian regions.

Gonococcal disease is characterized by an acute suppurative reaction, largely confined to the superficial mucosa and underlying submucosa.

Acute suppurative salpingitis is the most significant pathologic lesion. This may lead to salpingo-oophoritis, pyosalpinx (pus in the distended tubes), and tubo-ovarian abscesses. Untreated or poorly treated infection results in chronic salpingitis, with tubo-ovarian adhesions, and fibrosis of the fallopian tube, occlusion of its lumen, and resultant infertility.

In *postabortal and postpartum PID,* caused by a variety of organisms, infection spreads through the uterine wall to involve the serosa and peritoneum. Bacteremia is a frequent complication of this type of PID.

Other complications of PID include (1) peritonitis, (2) intestinal obstruction, (3) infertility, and (4) ectopic tubal pregnancy.

CERVIX

INFLAMMATIONS (p. 1045)

Acute and Chronic Cervicitis

Can be caused either by specific infections such as gonococci, chlamydia, *Trichomonas vaginalis, Candida,* and *Mycoplasma,* or by endogenous vaginal aerobes and anaerobes: streptococci, enterococci, *E. coli,* and staphylococci (nonspecific cervicitis).

Acute cervicitis is most commonly encountered postpartally and is characterized by acute infiltration of neutrophils beneath the lining mucosa.

Chronic cervicitis is far more common and, although it may be caused by one of the pathogens previously mentioned, is often of unknown etiology. Inflammation may lead to stenosis of cervical gland ducts and the formation of *nabothian cysts* lined by columnar epithelium. There may also be squamous metaplasia of endocervical glands.

Chronic cervicitis is benign and is present to some degree in every cervix during the reproductive years. If the epithelial response to inflammation is exuberant (*reactive atypia*), cervical intraepithelial neoplasia must be excluded.

TUMORS (p. 1047)

Benign tumors include

- *Endocervical polyps,* made up of connective tissue stroma harboring dilated glands and covered by endocervical epithelium.

Intraepithelial and Invasive Squamous Cell Neoplasia (p. 1047)

One of the most common tumors in women. Its peak incidence is at 40 to 45 years for invasive cancer. Cervical carcinoma is usually preceded by *cervical dysplasia* (also called cervical intraepithelial neoplasia [CIN]).The peak incidence of CIN III (carcinoma *in situ*) is 30 years.

The *epidemiology* of increased risk for cervical cancer and precancerous dysplasia is first intercourse at an early age, multiple sex partners, and high-risk male sex partners; the high incidence in married women and rarity in virgins and nuns suggests sexual transmission of an oncogenic agent from male to female at an early age.

Currently, human papilloma virus is being implicated as a *promoter* of cervical carcinoma. HPV infection with types 6 and 11 and other low-risk HPV predominate in condylomas and very low-grade dysplasias (CIN I). Higher-grade dysplasias (CIN II and III) predominately contain high-risk HPV types (16,31,33, 35,39, etc.). Cofactors could be other viruses, such as herpes type II, bacteria, tobacco, other environmental agents, or host factors. **MORPHOLOGY.** These cancers arise from precursor lesions. Precancerous lesions are classified according to the degree of epithelial maturation and the distribution of cytologic atypia:

- CIN I (including condyloma), in which the atypia is predominately in the superficial cell layers (koilocytosis), with preservation of epithelial maturation.

- CIN II, in which the atypia is conspicuous in both the superficial and basal cell layers, but with decreasing maturation.
- CIN III, in which the atypia is in all cell layers, but with minimal or no maturation (carcinoma *in situ*).

Risk of progression to malignancy is proportional to the grade of CIN, but the rates of progression are not uniform. Carcinoma *in situ* is clearly a precursor of invasive carcinoma, the latter developing in up to 70% of women followed without treatment after a diagnosis of carcinoma *in situ*.

Invasive cervical carcinoma manifests itself in three gross morphologic patterns: exophytic or fungating, ulcerating, and infiltrative. Histologically, 65% of tumors are large cell, nonkeratinizing, and moderately well differentiated. Some 25% are large and keratinizing, and the rest are composed of small, undifferentiated squamous cells.

Stages of cervical cancer:

- Stage 0. Carcinoma in situ.
- Stage I. Carcinoma confined to the cervix.

  - IA. Preclinical carcinoma diagnosed only by microscopy.
  - IB. Histologically invasive carcinoma greater than 5 mm in depth.

- Stage II. Carcinoma extends beyond the cervix but not into the pelvic wall; into the vagina but not the lower third.
- Stage III. Carcinoma extends to the pelvic wall or lower third of the vagina.
- Stage IV. Carcinoma has extended beyond the pelvis.

The prognosis of squamous cell carcinoma depends on the stage: 100% cure for stage 0; 80% to 90% for stage I; 75% for stage II; 35% for stage III; and 10% to 15% for stage IV.

Of cervical carcinomas, 25% consist of adenocarcinomas, adenosquamous carcinomas, and undifferentiated carcinomas.

BODY OF UTERUS AND ENDOMETRIUM

INFLAMMATIONS (p. 1053)

Chronic endometritis occurs in

- Patients suffering from chronic PID.
- Tuberculosis of the female genital tract.
- Postabortal or postpartal endometrial cavities, usually due to retained gestational tissue.
- Patients with intrauterine contraceptive devices.

In about 15% of patients, there is no predisposing condition and the cause is unknown. Chronic endometritis is associated clinically with abnormal endometrial bleeding and histologically with infiltration of plasma cells and macrophages into the endometrium.

ADENOMYOSIS (p. 1054)

Refers to nests of endometrium in the myometrium of the uterine wall. The condition causes uterine enlargement and irregular thickening of the uterine wall, and is diagnosed histologically by the finding of endometrial stroma and glands in the myometrium.

ENDOMETRIOSIS (p. 1054)

Describes the presence of endometrial glands or stroma in abnormal locations *outside* the uterus. This condition involves the ovaries, uterine ligaments, rectovaginal septum, pelvic peritoneum, and laparotomy scars, and rarely the umbilicus, vagina, vulva, or appendix.

Endometriosis presents clinically as severe dysmenorrhea and pelvic pain, *and is a common cause of female infertility.*

Endometrial foci are under the influence of ovarian hormones and therefore undergo cyclic menstrual changes with periodic bleeding.

A definite histologic diagnosis requires two of the three following features: endometrial glands, stroma, and hemosiderin pigment in the ectopic lesions.

FUNCTIONAL MENSTRUAL DISORDERS (DYSFUNCTIONAL UTERINE BLEEDING) (p. 1055)

The most common gynecologic problem in women, during active reproductive life, is excessive bleeding during or between menstrual periods. The causes of abnormal bleeding are many, and vary among women of different age groups (Table 20–1). In some instances, bleeding is a result of a well-defined organic lesion such as a leiomyoma, carcinoma, or polyp, but the largest single group is so-called *dysfunctional uterine bleeding,* defined as abnormal bleeding in the absence of an organic lesion.

An important cause of dysfunctional uterine bleeding is lack of ovulation, called *anovulatory cycles,* which occur as a result of

- An endocrine disorder, such as thyroid or adrenal disease, or pituitary tumors.

Table 20–1. Causes of Abnormal Uterine Bleeding by Age Group

Age Group	Cause(s)
Prepuberty	Precocious puberty (hypothalamic, pituitary, or ovarian origin)
Adolescence	Anovulatory cycle
Reproductive age	Complications of pregnancy (abortion, trophoblastic disease, ectopic pregnancy)
	Organic lesions (leiomyomas, adenomyosis, polyps, endometrial hyperplasia, carcinoma)
	Anovulatory cycle
	Ovulatory dysfunctional bleeding (e.g., inadequate luteal phase)
Perimenopause	Anovulatory cycle
	Irregular shedding
	Organic lesions (carcinoma, hyperplasia, polyps)
Postmenopause	Organic lesions (carcinoma, hyperplasia, polyps)
	Endometrial atrophy

From Cotran, R. S., Kumar, V., and Robbins, S. L.: Robbins Pathologic Basis of Disease. 5th ed. Philadelphia, W. B. Saunders Co., 1994, p. 1056.

- A primary lesion of the ovary, such as a functioning estrogenic ovarian tumor or polycystic ovaries.
- A generalized metabolic disturbance, such as obesity or malnutrition.
- Unexplained causes.

Morphologically, in all these circumstances the endometrium reveals a persistent proliferative pattern with possibly mild hyperplasia.

ENDOMETRIAL HYPERPLASIA (p. 1057)

An important cause of abnormal uterine bleeding, a result of a variety of disordered glandular and stromal growth patterns. *Although endometrial hyperplasia per se is benign, hyperplasias in which there are atypical changes in cells (cellular atypia) are precancerous lesions.* Like endometrial adenocarcinoma (*see p. 1060*), hyperplasia is associated with hyperestrogenism.

Histologically, there are two general categories of hyperplasia. Low-grade hyperplasias include

- *Simple hyperplasia without atypia* (also known as cystic or mild hyperplasia) in which benign hyperplastic glands become cystically dilated.
- *Complex hyperplasia* in which glands of varying size are crowded together into clusters ("back to back"), but there is no cellular atypia.

High-grade hyperplasias include

- *Atypical hyperplasia* in which the glandular complexity is accompanied by *cellular atypia* of the hyperplastic epithelium.

All these types produce abnormal uterine bleeding, but *only atypical hyperplasia is associated with a significant frequency of progression to carcinoma.*

TUMORS (p. 1058)

Leiomyoma (p. 1059)

The most common tumors in women; composed of benign masses of smooth muscle cells. They are most common in women in active reproductive life and are related to estrogenic stimulation.
MORPHOLOGY. Sharply circumscribed, discrete, round, firm, gray-white nodules that occur within the myometrium (intramural), beneath the serosa (subserosal), or immediately beneath the endometrium (submucosal). They may undergo cystic degeneration and calcification.

Leiomyomas may be asymptomatic or may be associated with abnormal uterine bleeding, pain, urinary bladder disorders, and impaired fertility. Malignant transformation is extremely rare.

Carcinoma of Endometrium (p. 1060)

Accounts for 7% of all invasive cancers in women. The peak age incidence is 55 to 65 years.

An increased incidence is associated with

- Obesity.
- Diabetes.
- Hypertension.
- Infertility.

There is compelling evidence that prolonged estrogen stimulation plays some causal role.

MORPHOLOGY. Grossly, endometrial carcinoma presents either as a localized polypoid tumor or as a diffuse spreading lesion involving the entire endometrial surface.

Histologically, most endometrial carcinomas are adenocarcinomas. Biologically, the less aggressive tumors include well-differentiated carcinomas closely resembling normal endometrial glands (endometrioid), with *squamous, secretory,* or *mucinous* differentiation. More aggressive neoplasms are poorly differentiated carcinomas, including *clear cell carcinomas* and *papillary serous carcinomas.*

The patient usually presents with abnormal bleeding. The prognosis depends on the state of the disease and is excellent in patients in whom the carcinoma is confined to the corpus uteri itself.

Mesenchymal Tumors (p. 1062)

Malignant mixed mesodermal (mixed müllerian) tumors are relatively rare tumors derived from primitive stromal cells, originally derived from müllerian mesoderm. They consist of malignant glandular and stromal elements; the stromal sarcomatous elements may show muscle, cartilage, and osteoid differentiation. Grossly, the tumors protrude into the endometrial cavity and vagina, and are bulky and polypoid.

Clinically, the tumors occur in postmenopausal women and are associated with postmenopausal bleeding. They are highly malignant and have a 5-year survival rate of 25%.

Endometrial stromal tumors are varied and include

- *Benign stromal nodules:* nodules of stromal cells within the myometrium.
- *Low-grade stromal sarcoma or endolymphatic stromal myosis:* masses of well-differentiated endometrial stroma that penetrate lymphatic channels.
- *Endometrial stromal sarcoma:* an overtly cancerous counterpart in which the cells display atypia and mitoses. These tumors are capable of widespread metastases.

Leiomyosarcomas (p. 1062)

Uncommon malignancies that form bulky, fleshy masses in the uterine wall. They are differentiated from benign leiomyomas by the presence of (1) more than ten mitoses per ten high-power fields (HPFs), with or without cellular atypia; or (2) five to ten mitoses per HPF with cellular atypism.

These tumors disseminate throughout the abdominal cavity and metastasize. The 5-year survival rate is 40%.

FALLOPIAN TUBES

INFLAMMATIONS (p. 1063)

Suppurative salpingitis is due to infection with pyogenic organisms, including streptococci, staphylococci, and gonococci, and is a part of PID. *Tuberculous salpingitis* is due to hematogenous spread of tuberculosis into the tubes and is sometimes associated with tuberculosis of the endometrium and peritoneum. Both forms of salpingitis are associated with infertility.

TUMORS

Rare. The most common is an *adenocarcinoma,* which resembles serous adenocarcinoma of the ovary.

OVARIES

NON-NEOPLASTIC CYSTS (p. 1064)

Follicular and luteal cysts are very common, measure 1 to 8 cm in diameter, and are lined by follicular or luteinized cells. They may be asymptomatic or may rupture, causing a peritoneal reaction and pain.

Polycystic ovarian syndrome (the Stein-Leventhal syndrome) is a disorder of young women and is associated with oligomenorrhea, infertility, hirsutism, sometimes obesity, persistent anovulation, and fibrotic cystic ovaries.

Patients exhibit excessive production of androgens, increased conversion of androgen to estrogen, and inappropriate gonadotropin production by the pituitary.

The ovaries are large, white, studded with subcortical cysts 0.5 to 1 cm in diameter, and covered by a thickened, fibrosed outer tunica. The pathogenesis is unknown, but this is an important cause of infertility.

TUMORS (p. 1065)

Ovarian tumors are common forms of neoplasia in women and arise from either the surface epithelium, germ cells, or sex cord-stroma (Tables 20–2 and 20–3). The malignant tumors collectively account for about 6% of all cancers in women. Risk factors include nulliparity and family history.

Tumors of Surface Epithelium

Serous Tumors (p. 1067)

The most common cystic neoplasms. Cysts are lined by tall, columnar, ciliated epithelial cells, and filled with serous fluid. *Serous tumors are either benign (60%), frankly malignant (25%), or of low malignant potential (also called borderline) (15%).* They present grossly as large (up to 40 cm in diameter) spherical or ovoid masses. The benign cystadenomas have a smooth and glistening inner lining. The *cystadenocarcinomas* often have small, mural, solid nodularities; papillary projections; and capillary invasion.

- Twenty per cent of benign tumors, 30% of borderline tumors, and two-thirds of malignant forms are bilateral.
- In the benign tumors, the lining epithelium is composed of a single layer of tall, columnar, ciliated epithelial cells with small, microscopic papillae.
- Frankly malignant cystadenocarcinomas have multilayered epithelium with many papillary areas and the formation of large, solid epithelial masses with atypical cells in places invading the stroma.
- Tumors of low malignant potential show epithelial atypia and solid areas but no obvious invasion of the stroma.

Mucinous Tumors (p. 1068)

In contrast to serous neoplasms, 80% of mucinous tumors are benign and only 5% to 10% are malignant.

Table 20-2. Ovarian Neoplasms
(1993 WHO Classification)*

1. Surface epithelial-stromal tumors
     Serous tumors
         Benign (cystadenoma)
         Of borderline malignancy
         Malignant (serous cystadenocarcinoma)
     Mucinous tumors, endocervical-like and intestinal-type
         Benign
         Of borderline malignancy
         Malignant
     Endometrioid tumors
         Benign
         Of borderline malignancy
         Malignant
         Epithelial—stromal
             Adenosarcoma
             Mesodermal (müllerian) mixed tumor
     Clear cell tumors
         Benign
         Of borderline malignancy
         Malignant
     Transitional cell tumors
         Brenner tumor
         Brenner tumor of borderline malignancy
         Malignant Brenner tumor
         Transitional cell carcinoma (non–Brenner-type)
2. Sex cord–stromal tumors
     Granulosa-stromal cell tumors
         Granulosa cell tumors
         Tumors of the thecoma-fibroma group
     Sertoli-stromal cell tumors; androblastomas
     Sex-cord tumor with annular tubules
     Gynandroblastoma
     Steroid (lipid) cell tumors
3. Germ cell tumors
     Teratoma
         Immature
         Mature (adult)
             Solid
             Cystic (dermoid cyst)
         Monodermal (e.g., struma ovarii, carcinoid)
     Dysgerminoma
     Yolk sac tumor (endodermal sinus tumor)
     Mixed germ cell tumors
4. Malignant, NOS
5. Metastatic nonovarian cancer (from nonovarian primary)

NOS = Not otherwise specified.
*Modified.
From Cotran, R. S., Kumar, V., and Robbins, S. L.: Robbins Pathologic Basis of Disease. 5th ed. Philadelphia, W. B. Saunders Co. 1994, p. 1065.

- Grossly, they tend to produce large cystic masses (exceeding the size of serous tumors), often multiloculated, and filled with sticky, gelatinous fluid. Five per cent of benign tumors and 20% of carcinomas are bilateral.
- Histologically, the tumors are lined by tall, columnar epithelium showing apical mucinous vacuolation. In cystadenocarci-

Table 20–3. Certain Frequency Data for Major
Ovarian Tumors

Type	Percentage of Malignant Ovarian Tumors	Percentage That Are Bilateral
Serous	40	
Benign (60%)		25
Borderline (15%)		30
Malignant (25%)		65
Mucinous	10	
Benign (80%)		5
Borderline (10%)		10
Malignant (10%)		20
Endometrioid carcinoma	20	40
Undifferentiated carcinoma	10	—
Clear cell carcinoma	6	40
Granuloma cell tumor	5	5
Teratoma		
Benign (96%)		15
Malignant (4%)	1	Rare
Metastatic	5	>50
Others	3	—

From Cotran, R. S., Kumar, V., and Robbins, S. L.: Robbins Pathologic
Basis of Disease. 5th ed. Philadelphia, W. B. Saunders Co., 1994, p. 1066.

nomas, the papillary projections are more numerous, mural
nodules are present, and epithelial cells show atypia and invade
the capsule.
- Borderline tumors have similar atypia but are noninvasive.
- Malignant and borderline mucinous tumors can seed the peritoneal cavity with multiple implants, filling it with mucinous
secretions to produce *pseudomyxoma peritonei.*

Endometrioid Tumors (p. 1070)

Account for 20% of all ovarian cancers, and distinguished from
serous and mucinous tumors by the close resemblance of tubular
glands to benign or malignant endometrium. In 15% to 30% of
endometrioid carcinomas, independent endometrial carcinomas
appear.
Grossly, the ovarian lesions are a combination of solid and
cystic masses. Forty per cent are bilateral, and histologically the
glandular patterns bear a strong resemblance to endometrial
adenocarcinoma.

Brenner's Tumor (p. 1070)

These usually small, solid tumors are characterized by dense
fibrous stroma and nests of transitional cells resembling urinary
transitional or rarely columnar epithelium. They are occasionally
encountered in the wall of mucinous cystadenomas and are
usually unilateral; the vast majority are benign.

Clinical Course of Surface Epithelial Tumors
(p. 1070)

All large epithelial tumors cause similar symptoms, including
lower abdominal pain, abdominal enlargement, and GI and uri-

nary complaints. Benign tumors are resected with cure. Carcinomas in time extend through the capsule and seed the peritoneal cavity, occasionally causing massive ascites.

Carcinomas grow slowly and unfortunately usually are first seen when the lesions are no longer confined to the ovary. They thus have a relatively poor prognosis. Metastases occur to the other ovary, to lymph nodes, and eventually to distant organs.

Germ Cell Tumors

Represent 15% to 20% of all ovarian tumors. They are similar to germ cell tumors in males and are presumed to arise from totipotential germ cells capable of differentiating into the three germ cell layers.

Teratomas (p. 1072)

Divided into (1) mature (benign), (2) immature (malignant), and (3) monodermal (specialized) teratomas.

MATURE (BENIGN) TERATOMAS. Most are cystic, relatively small, and known as *dermoid cysts.* They are lined by skin with adnexal structures and filled with hair-bearing sebaceous secretion. The tumors are bilateral in 10% to 15% of cases and histologically reveal epidermis, hair follicles and other skin adnexae, and tooth structures. Cartilage, bone, thyroid tissue, and other organ formations can also be found.

- Dermoid cysts are clinically benign and are cured by resection. About 1% undergo malignant transformation of any of the component elements, but most commonly develop into squamous cell carcinoma.

IMMATURE (MALIGNANT) TERATOMAS. These rare tumors differ from benign teratomas in that embryonic (rather than adult) elements derived from more than one of the three germ layers are usually present. These tumors are most common in adolescents and young women.

- *Grossly,* the tumors are bulky and predominantly solid with areas of necrosis and hemorrhage.
- *Microscopically,* there are varied amounts of immature tissue differentiating toward cartilage, glands, bone, muscle, nerve, and others. Extraovarian spread of immature teratomas depends primarily on the degree of immaturity of the tissues and the presence of *neuroepithelium.* Most are malignant, grow rapidly, and metastasize widely. However, they can be cured with chemotherapy if treated early.

MONODERMAL OR SPECIALIZED TERATOMAS. These consist of teratomas that differentiate along the line of a single abnormal tissue. The most common is struma ovarii, composed entirely of mature thyroid tissue. Another example is the ovarian carcinoid, similar to carcinoids elsewhere.

Dysgerminoma (p. 1073)

The ovarian counterpart of testicular seminoma. The tumors are uncommon and may occur in childhood or in the second and third decades of life. Most are nonfunctional.

Eighty per cent to 90% are unilateral. The tumors are solid, yellowish-white to gray-pink, and fleshy. Histologically, they consist of sheets and cords of large vesicular cells separated by scant fibrous stroma.

All dysgerminomas are malignant, but only about one-third

are highly aggressive. They are also radiosensitive and chemosensitive and thus have a relatively good prognosis if treated early.

Endodermal Sinus Tumor (p. 1074)

This rare tumor is thought to be derived from multipotential embryonal carcinoma cells differentiating toward yolk sac structures. The tumor consists histologically of cystic spaces into which protrude papillary projections with central blood vessels enveloped by immature epithelium (glomeruloid). Intracellular and extracellular hyalin droplets are characteristic, some of which can be shown to be alpha-fetoprotein.

The tumors occur in children and young women and grow rapidly and aggressively.

Choriocarcinoma (p. 1074)

Arises in the ovary from the teratogenous development of germ cells. Most such tumors exist in combination with other germ cell tumors. Histologically, they are identical to the more common placental lesions and, like gestational choriocarcinoma, elaborate chorionic gonadotropins (*see p. 1084*). Ovarian choriocarcinomas are highly malignant, metastasize widely, and are much more resistant to chemotherapy than their placental counterparts.

Sex Cord–Stromal Tumors (p. 1074)

Originate either from the sex cords of the embryonic gonad or from the stroma of the ovary. The tumors are frequently functional and mostly have feminizing effects.

GRANULOSA–THECA CELL TUMORS. Composed of various combinations of granulosa and theca cells. Two-thirds occur in postmenopausal women.

- The tumors are usually unilateral and solid and have a white-yellow coloration. The granulosa cell component consists of small cuboidal to polygonal cells growing in cords, sheets, or strands; the thecal cell components are composed of sheets of plump spindle cells closely resembling those of a fibroma. Thecal cells contain lipid droplets.
- Granulosa-theca cell tumors have the potential of elaborating large amounts of estrogen and thus produce precocious sexual development and endometrial hyperplasia and predispose to endometrial carcinoma.
- All granulosa cell tumors are potentially malignant, clinical malignancy occurring in 5% to 25%. However, they are slow growing, and the 10-year survival rate is almost 85%. Pure thecomas are benign.

FIBROMAS. Common forms of ovarian neoplasms. They are usually unilateral, solid, hard, gray-white masses made up histologically of well-differentiated fibroblasts. Curiously, 40% are associated with hydrothorax (usually right-sided) and ascites (Meigs' syndrome).

SERTOLI–LEYDIG CELL TUMORS. These tumors recapitulate the cells of the testes and commonly produce masculinization or defeminization. They are usually unilateral and consist histologically of tubules composed of tubular Sertoli cells or Leydig cells interspersed with stroma.

Metastatic Tumors (p. 1077)

Metastases of abdominal and breast tumors to the ovary are common. *Krukenberg tumor* refers to metastatic ovarian cancer (usually bilateral) composed of mucin-producing signet cells that metastasize from the GI tract, mostly the stomach.

GESTATIONAL AND PLACENTAL DISORDERS

PLACENTAL INFLAMMATIONS AND INFECTIONS (p. 1077)

Placental infection occurs by two pathways:

- Ascending through the birth canal.
- Hematogenous (transplacental infection).

Ascending infections are the most common. They are most often bacterial and associated with premature rupture of membranes. Bacterial infection results in chorioamnionitis characterized by a neutrophilic infiltration of the chorion and amnion, and acute vasculitis in the umbilical cord.

ECTOPIC PREGNANCY (p. 1079)

Denotes implantation of the embryo in any site other than the uterus—most commonly the fallopian tubes (90%), but also rarely in the ovary or abdominal cavity. Predisposing factors include PID with chronic salpingitis and peritubular adhesions, but 50% occur in apparently normal tubes.

Tubal pregnancy has one of four outcomes:

- Intratubal hemorrhage with the formation of hematosalpinx.
- Tubal rupture with intraperitoneal hemorrhage.
- Spontaneous regression with resorption of the products of conception.
- Extrusion into the abdominal cavity (tubal abortion).

Tubal rupture is a medical emergency characterized by an acute abdomen and shock. Early diagnosis is critical and can be suggested by high chorionic gonadotropin levels, the ultrasonographic findings, and an endometrial biopsy showing decidual changes and absent chorionic villi.

TOXEMIA OF PREGNANCY (p. 1079)

Refers to a symptom complex characterized by hypertension, proteinuria, and edema (pre-eclampsia). Eclampsia is the severe form associated with convulsions and coma. Toxemia occurs in 6% of pregnancies, usually in the last trimester, and is most common in primiparas.

PATHOGENESIS. Unclear. It is thought, however, that primary causes such as immune or genetic factors cause mechanical or functional obstruction of uterine spiral arterioles. A recent theory proposes that inadequate implantation results in decreased uteroplacental perfusion and placental ischemia. This results in increased production of vasoconstrictors (e.g., thromboxane, angiotensin) and decreased vasodilators (e.g., PGI_2, PGE_2), leading to arterial vasoconstriction and systemic hypertension.

- Placental ischemia also results in endothelial injury and activation of disseminated intravascular coagulation (DIC), accounting for the decreased GFR and proteinuria, CNS disturbances, abnormal liver function tests, and fibrin thrombi and ischemia in most other organs.
- *Clinically,* pre-eclampsia usually occurs after the 32nd week of pregnancy and is characterized by hypertension, edema, proteinuria, headaches, and visual disturbances. Mild toxemia

can be controlled by bed rest, diet, and antihypertensive agents, but induction of delivery is the only definitive treatment for established pre-eclampsia and eclampsia.

GESTATIONAL TROPHOBLASTIC DISEASE (GTD) (p. 1081)

A spectrum of tumors and tumor-like conditions of progressive malignant potential, characterized by proliferation of trophoblastic tissue. The lesions include hydatidiform mole (complete and partial), invasive mole, and choriocarcinoma.

Hydatidiform Mole (HM) (p. 1082)

Characterized by cystic swelling of the chorionic villi, accompanied by variable trophoblastic proliferation; this is a common precursor of choriocarcinoma.

Moles present in the fourth or fifth month of pregnancy with vaginal bleeding. *There are two types of benign noninvasive moles, complete and partial, that can be differentiated by histologic, cytogenetic, and flow cytometric studies* (Table 20–4).

- *Grossly,* moles consist of masses of thin-walled, translucent, cystic, grapelike structures. Fetal parts are rarely seen in complete moles and are more common in partial moles.
- *Microscopically,* complete moles show hydropic swelling of villi, inadequate vascularization of villi, and significant trophoblastic proliferation. Partial moles show only focal edema and focal and slight trophoblastic proliferation. Most complete moles have diploid karyotypes, whereas partial moles are usually triploid.
- Moles can be diagnosed by ultrasound examination and by quantitative analysis of serum hCG, revealing levels exceeding those produced by a normal pregnancy of similar age. *Once curetted, 80% to 90% give no further difficulty, 10% develop into invasive moles, and 2.5% develop into choriocarcinoma.* Follow-up with periodic determination of hCG is essential in these patients.

Invasive Mole (p. 1084)

A mole that penetrates and may even perforate the uterine wall, marked by active proliferation of both cyto- and syncytiotropho-

Table 20–4. Features of Complete Versus Partial Hydatidiform Mole

Feature	Complete Mole	Partial Mole
Karyotype	46, XX(46,XY)	Triploid
Villous edema	All villi	Some villi
Trophoblast proliferation	Diffuse; circumferential	Focal; slight
Atypia	Often present	Absent
Serum hCG	Elevated	Less elevated
hCG in tissue	+ + + +	+
Behavior	2% choriocarcinoma	Rare choriocarcinoma

hCG = Human chorionic gonadotropin.
From Cotran, R. S., Kumar, V., and Robbins, S. L.: Robbins Pathologic Basis of Disease. 5th ed. Philadelphia, W. B. Saunders Co., 1994, p. 1083.

blasts. It does not metastasize. It is associated with a persistent elevated hCG level and varying degrees of luteinization of the ovaries. The tumor responds well to chemotherapy.

Choriocarcinoma (p. 1084)

A malignant tumor arising in one in 20,000 to 30,000 pregnancies in the United States but is much more common in some Asian and African countries. *Fifty per cent arise in HM, 25% in previous abortions, 22% in normal pregnancies, and the rest in ectopic pregnancies.*

- *Grossly,* the tumor is large, soft, yellowish-white, and fleshy with areas of necrosis and hemorrhage.
- *Histologically,* it consists of abnormal proliferations of both cyto- and syncytiotrophoblasts. The tumor invades the underlying endometrium, penetrates blood vessels and lymphatics, and metastasizes to the lungs, bone marrow, liver, and other organs.
- Clinically, choriocarcinomas are manifested by vaginal bleeding and discharge that may appear in the course of an apparently normal pregnancy, after a miscarriage, or following a curettage. hCG titers are elevated to levels above those seen in HM. When the condition is first discovered, widespread metastases may have already occurred.
- *Gestational choriocarcinomas are highly sensitive to chemotherapy,* and cures can be achieved even in patients with metastatic disease.

Placental Site Trophoblastic Tumor (p. 1086)

A rare tumor composed of proliferating *intermediate trophoblasts* that are larger than cytotrophoblasts, but mononuclear rather than syncytial. The lesion differs from that of choriocarcinoma by the absence of cytotrophoblastic elements and low levels of hCG production. Most are locally invasive only. Malignant variants are distinguished by a high mitotic index, extensive necrosis, and local spread. About 10% result in metastases and death.

BREAST (p. 1089)

The preponderance of breast lesions occur in women. In men the rudimentary breast appears to be resistant to pathogenetic stimuli, although breast lesions, including carcinoma, can occur. Most breast lesions in women present as palpable, sometimes painful, nodules or masses. When biopsied about 40% prove to be fibrocystic changes, 10% cancer, 7% fibroadenoma, 13% miscellaneous benign lesions, and 30% with little or no significant pathology.

CONGENITAL ANOMALIES (p. 1091)

- *Supernumerary nipples* or breast tissue occur along the milk line and may rarely be sites of origin of breast carcinoma. They undergo hyperplasia during pregnancy.
- *Inversion of nipple* may mimic carcinomatous inversion and hinder normal nursing.

INFLAMMATIONS (p. 1091)

- *Acute mastitis and breast abscess* follow the development of cracks or fissures of the nipple resulting from nursing, or dermatitis involving the nipple. Healing may leave a scar that may mimic carcinoma grossly.
- *Mammary duct ectasia* (plasma cell or periductal mastitis) is characterized by inspissation of secretions, duct dilatation, and periductal inflammation (granulomatous, lymphoid, and plasmocellular). It affects multiparous women in the fifth or sixth decade. The lesion affects major excretory ducts and may mimic carcinoma grossly.
- *Fat necrosis,* almost always traumatic, but sometimes appearing after radiation therapy, is followed by inflammation and fibrosis that may present as a hard mass grossly resembling cancer.

FIBROCYSTIC CHANGE (FIBROCYSTIC DISEASE) (FCD) (p. 1093)

These terms refer to a heterogeneous group of morphologic patterns within the breast showing various combinations of cyst formation, epithelial hyperplasias, and/or fibrous stromal overgrowth. These alterations commonly produce palpable lumps, but may be so mild as to be clinically silent.

In unselected autopsies, significant FCD was present in about 29% of individuals, minimal FCD in an additional 24%. FCD accounts for about one half of breast operations. It is unusual before adolescence, is most common between the ages of 20 and 40 years, peaks in perimenopausal years, and rarely develops after menopause.

The pathogenesis remains obscure. Relative or absolute estrogen excess and progesterone deficiency appears important, but abnormal end-organ responses to hormones may also be contributory.

There are three dominant morphologic patterns of FCD:

- *Cysts and fibrosis without epithelial cell hyperplasia* (simple fibrocystic changes) are the most common and are not known to be associated with an increased risk of subsequent development of carcinoma.

  Morphologically, the changes may largely consist of increased collagenous density in a focal area, compressing glands or ducts, or may also include micro- to macrocysts lined by a single layer of epithelium, sometimes flattened by compression.

- *Epithelial cell hyperplasia* (proliferative fibrocystic change) is frequently accompanied by cysts and fibrosis.

  Morphologically, either the cystic changes (usually 0.2 to 3.0 cm in diameter) may predominate or the hyperplastic changes, with papillary infoldings of the ductal or lobular epithelium. The hyperplasias are associated with an increased risk of invasive carcinoma (1.5 to 2 times the general population), and so when sufficiently atypical (*either ductal or lobular*) as to approach carcinoma *in situ,* they are known as *atypical hyperplasias.* Atypical hyperplasia is associated with a four- to fivefold increased risk of carcinoma.

  A family history of breast carcinoma increases the risk of subsequent invasive carcinoma in all histologic categories.

- *Sclerosing adenosis* is characterized by intralobular fibrosis and a proliferation of small epithelial ductules and myoepithelial cells. The lesion can be mistaken for invasive carcinoma, but its tendency to maintain the juxtaposition of epithelial and myoepithelial cells and a lobular growth pattern are key to its recognition as benign. It slightly increases the risk of subsequent cancer.

TUMORS (p. 1097)

Fibroadenoma (p. 1097)

The most common benign tumor of the female breast, occurring most often during the reproductive period.

Grossly, it appears as a solitary, discrete, yellow-white, freely movable nodule from 1 to 10 cm in diameter. Histologically, it consists of various degrees and patterns of benign proliferations of ducts, acini, and stroma. It requires excision for verification of its benign nature.

Similar benign tumors include tubular adenoma, lactating adenoma, and myoepithelioma.

Phyllodes Tumor (p. 1098)

Previously known as "cystosarcoma phyllodes," this neoplasm is a bulky, fibroadenoma-like tumor (i.e., made up of proliferative ducts and stroma) having on cross section numerous clefts and slits creating leaflike patterns of intervening tumor. Phyllodes tumors can be very large, causing breast distortion and pressure necrosis of overlying skin.

- These lesions can be either malignant (uncommon) or benign (common). Changes suggesting malignant potential include increased cellularity, anaplasia, high mitotic activity, and overgrowth of the *stromal component.*
- Malignant phyllodes tumors may metastasize hematogenously, usually to the lungs, demonstrating only the stromal component in the metastases, and may be lethal.

Intraductal Papilloma (p. 1099)

A papillary growth (both epithelial and fibrovascular) within a duct, usually in a lactiferous duct. *Nipple adenoma* and *florid papillomatosis of the nipple* are terms used to describe tumors of the nipple exhibiting papillary hyperplasia of the duct epithelium, intermixed with fibrosis.

The lesion presents clinically either with serous or bloody nipple discharge, or as a small subareolar tumor a few millimeters in diameter. Although benign, papillomas are associated with an increased risk of the development of invasive breast carcinoma (1.5 to 2 times), particularly when they are multiple or involve the nipple.

Carcinoma of Breast (p. 1099)

The unqualified term "breast cancer" implies carcinoma arising in the ductal and glandular structures of the breast. Currently, about one in ten women develops breast cancer during her lifetime, and breast carcinoma causes some 20% of cancer deaths among women.

INCIDENCE/EPIDEMIOLOGY. Rarely develops before the age of 25 years, with a peak incidence during perimenopausal years.

- More common in patients with a family history of breast

carcinoma; the risk increases in proportion to the number of first-degree relatives with cancer.
- Greater risk in women who have an early menarche and late menopause (long reproductive life).
- More frequent in nulliparous than in multiparous women.
- Obesity associated with increased risk attributed to synthesis of estrogens in fat depots.
- Exogenous estrogens for menopausal symptoms associated with moderately increased risk of breast carcinoma.
- Oral contraceptives present no clear-cut increased risk.
- Proliferative fibrocystic changes, especially those with atypical hyperplasias, associated with increased risks.
- Previous carcinoma of the opposite breast, endometrium, or ovary associated with increased risk.

ETIOLOGY AND PATHOGENESIS. Although the cause remains unknown, the following influences appear important:

- Genetic factors. Their role is supported by the high incidence in first-degree relatives of carcinoma patients. Germ line mutations in p53 tumor suppressor gene account for cases with the rare familial *Li-Fraumeni syndrome.* The BRCA-1 gene, on chromosome 17q21, accounts for a large percentage of familial cancer occurring at an early age.
- Hormone imbalances: (1) endogenous estrogen excess, whether from abnormally high levels produced by functioning ovarian tumors in postmenopausal women or from prolonged exposure (e.g., prolonged reproductive life), appears to increase the risk of breast carcinoma; (2) breast carcinomas frequently contain estrogen and progesterone receptors; (3) certain carcinoma-associated growth factors (i.e., transforming growth factors alpha and beta) secreted by breast carcinoma cells appear to be estrogen dependent; (4) interactions between circulating hormones, hormone receptors in cancer cells, and autocrine growth factors made by tumor cells play a role in breast cancer progression.
- Environmental influences: high dietary fat and moderate alcohol consumption have been reported in some studies to increase the risk of breast carcinoma.
- Viruses: mouse mammary tumor virus (MMTV) can cause breast cancer in suckling mice, but a similar oncogenic virus in humans has *not* yet been demonstrated.
- Oncogenes: amplification of the proto-oncogene *erb* β2/*neu,* int 2, c-*ras* and c-*myc* genes, and somatic mutations of p53 and Rb suppressor genes occur in up to 50% of breast cancers.

DISTRIBUTION AND CLASSIFICATION. Of breast carcinomas, about 50% arise in the upper outer quadrant, 10% in each of the remaining quadrants, and 20% in the central or subareolar region.

Lesions are multifocal (i.e., occurring in quadrants other than the main tumor mass) in about one third of patients and not infrequently bilateral, especially in the lobular variant of breast carcinoma.

Most breast carcinomas arise within the terminal duct units (exceptions being Paget's disease and lobular carcinomas), and the distinctions between the various types, which have distinctive clinicopathologic features, are based on individual cytologic and architectural features.

The current classification of the major types of breast carcinoma is as follows:

A. *Noninvasive* (noninfiltrating)
    1a. Intraductal carcinoma
    1b. Intraductal carcinoma with Paget's disease
    2. Lobular carcinoma *in situ*
B. *Invasive* (infiltrating)
    1a. Invasive ductal carcinoma—not otherwise specified (NOS)
    1b. Invasive ductal carcinoma with Paget's disease
    2. Invasive lobular carcinoma
    3. Medullary carcinoma
    4. Colloid carcinoma (mucinous carcinoma)
    5. Tubular carcinoma
    6. Adenoid cystic carcinoma
    7. Apocrine carcinoma
    8. Invasive papillary carcinoma

Most tumors are invasive at detection, but with increasing patient awareness, careful physical examination, and screening mammography, the percentage of total cases that are *in situ* tumors is increasing, now 25% in some series. The relative frequencies of various invasive tumors are as follows:

• Invasive duct carcinomas	
Pure	52.6%
Combined with other types	22.0%
• Colloid carcinoma	2.4%
• Paget's disease	2.3%
• Medullary carcinoma	1.0%
• Other pure types	2.0%
• Other combined types	1.6%
• Infiltrating lobular carcinoma	4.9%
• Combined lobular and ductal	6.0%
• Unclassified	5.2%

Common Types of Carcinoma (p. 1102)

INTRADUCTAL CARCINOMA. Characterized by relatively large and/or pleomorphic carcinoma cells that grow, fill, and plug the ducts and ductules with carcinoma cells but remain confined within the basement membrane. Various patterns are present: solid, cribriform, papillary, micropapillary, and comedocarcinoma variants.

• *Poorly differentiated, pleomorphic,* in situ *tumors* often show central necrosis. This necrotic substance can be readily extruded on slight pressure, hence the designation *comedocarcinoma. In situ* comedocarcinomas are more aggressive, with recurrence or invasion in up to 40% of cases after lumpectomy.
• *Well-differentiated variants* exhibit very little necrosis within ducts. When treated by biopsy alone, recurrence or invasion occurs in 0% to 10% of cases.

LOBULAR CARCINOMA IN SITU. Characterized by a proliferation of small, uniform cells within ductules or acini that fill, distend, or distort at least 50% of the acinar units of a single lobule. Isolated LCIS cells frequently extend out into larger ducts in a pagetoid fashion. These *in situ* cancers appear to be a marker for subsequent development of invasive breast carcinoma.

Invasive carcinoma develops in about 30% of cases of LCIS if untreated with mastectomy. *The invasive cancer develops with equal frequency in the same or contralateral breast and can be either ductal or lobular in histologic type.*

INFILTRATING (INVASIVE) DUCT CARCINOMA. The most common type of breast cancer, occurring as an irregular, hard nodule averaging 1 to 2 cm. Histologically, the tumor is composed of malignant ductal cells disposed in cords, solid cell nests, tubules, anastomosing sheets, and various mixtures of all these. These cells are dispersed in a dense stromal reaction responsible for the hard consistency of the tumor (scirrhous carcinoma). Tumors are graded according to the degree of nuclear atypia and histologic (tubule) differentiation.

MEDULLARY CARCINOMA. Accounts for 1% of breast carcinomas. It presents as a relatively large, soft, well-circumscribed tumor averaging 2 to 3 cm in diameter. Histologically, medullary carcinoma shows (1) absence of desmoplasia, (2) a moderately dense lymphoplasmacytic infiltrate, and (3) large, pleomorphic tumor cells growing in solid, syncytium-like, anastomosing masses. Only when the tumor has all these features does it follow a less malignant course than the typical infiltrating duct carcinoma (NOS).

COLLOID OR MUCINOUS CARCINOMA. Accounts for about 2% to 3% of breast carcinomas, is slow growing, occurs most commonly in older women, and has a good prognosis when it is a pure mucinous carcinoma, occupying over 75% of the tumor mass. Morphologically, it appears as soft, gelatinous masses composed of lakes of lightly staining mucin, within which are floating small islands of well-differentiated tumor cells.

PAGET'S DISEASE. A form of duct carcinoma that arises within the large excretory ducts and extends to involve the skin of the nipple and areola. The duct carcinoma cells appear as large, pale, somewhat vacuolated cells located *within* the overlying keratinizing squamous epithelium. The nipple often shows eczematoid changes. An *in situ* or invasive duct carcinoma is invariably present in the underlying breast tissue.

INVASIVE LOBULAR CARCINOMA. Accounts for 5% of invasive carcinomas, but tends to be more frequently multifocal and bilateral compared with other breast carcinomas of duct origin. It has about the same prognosis as invasive duct carcinoma but tends to be bilateral (20%) or multicentric.

It appears as a rubbery, often poorly circumscribed mass. Occasionally, tumors are scirrhous. Histologically, the tumor is composed of small, uniform cells forming strands of infiltrating tumor cells, sometimes arranged concentrically about ducts. Differentiation from duct carcinomas can be difficult in some cases, and breast carcinomas sharing features of both lobular and duct carcinoma are not rare.

Features Common to All Invasive Carcinomas

Local invasion into adjacent structures produces tumor fixation, retraction of the nipple, and dimpling of the skin. Lymphatic invasion correlates with lymph nodal metastases and, when extensive in the skin, results in lymphedema, causing the breast skin to resemble orange peel (peau d'orange or inflammatory carcinoma). Microcalcifications detected by mammography within or associated with carcinoma are noted in about 60% of cases. Unfortunately, many benign lesions also show microcalcifications.

About two-thirds of breast carcinomas present with lymph nodal metastases. Although any breast cancer can metastasize to axillary, supraclavicular, and/or internal mammary nodes, tumors in the outer quadrant tend to metastasize to axillary nodes, whereas tumors in the inner quadrants and center of the breast tend to metastasize to internal mammary nodes. Other favored sites of spread are skin, bones, lung, liver, and adrenals.

CLINICAL FEATURES. Although most breast carcinomas are discovered by the patients and at an advanced stage (average size 4 cm and two thirds with lymph nodal spread), mammography has been found to be a highly useful technique for detecting early, small carcinomas (so-called minimal cancers less than 1 cm and/or *in situ*), which have a much better prognosis.

Factors influencing the prognosis in breast cancer include

- Tumor size—the larger the tumor, the worse the prognosis.
- Lymph nodal spread and the number of positive nodes: 80% 5-year survival for node-negative patients, 50% for patients with one to three positive nodes, and 21% for patients with four or more positive nodes.
- The histologic grade of the tumor, including nuclear characteristics and degree of differentiation.
- Three prognostic categories based on histologic *type* of breast carcinoma: (1) *nonmetastasizing:* in situ carcinoma; (2) *uncommonly metastasizing:* pure colloid carcinoma, medullary carcinoma, tubular carcinoma, infiltrating papillary carcinoma, and adenoid cystic carcinoma; (3) *moderate to highly metastasizing:* all other types.
- Estrogen/progesterone receptor status. Seventy per cent of tumors containing estrogen receptors regress after hormonal manipulation, whereas only 5% of those that are negative respond.
- A relatively high proliferative rate as measured by flow cytometry suggests poor prognosis.

The presence of amplified or activated oncogenes (e.g., c-*erb2*) has been shown to correlate with unfavorable outcome, as has the degree of angiogenesis in the tumor.

MALE BREAST (p. 1109)

Gynecomastia, or enlargement of the male breast, is of chief importance as an indicator of hyperestrinism, suggesting the possible existence of a functioning testicular tumor or cirrhosis of the liver. Histologically, there is proliferation of both epithelial and stromal components.

Carcinoma of the male breast is very rare. Histologically, it most resembles infiltrating duct carcinoma of the female breast.

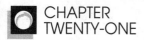

CHAPTER
TWENTY-ONE

The Endocrine System

INTRODUCTION (p. 1113)

Cellular homeostasis is regulated by the nervous system and endocrine system. These systems are closely integrated, particularly in the *hypothalamus,* which modulates pituitary function, and in the widely dispersed *neuroendocrine cells* (formerly designated the Amine Precursor Uptake and Decarboxylation, or *APUD,* system). Hormones elaborated by endocrine glands interact with cell receptors specific for a given hormone:

- *Peptide* and *amine* hormones interact with receptors on the *cell surface,* usually resulting in activation of a *second messenger,* such as cyclic AMP (cAMP).
- *Steroid* hormones penetrate the lipid-rich cell membranes to interact with *cytoplasmic* or *intranuclear* receptors. Hormone-receptor complexes, in turn, bind to DNA, resulting in activation of specific genes, transcription, and translation of new proteins, which mediate the steroid hormone's effects.
- *Thyroid hormones* bind to sites on the cell surface and are internalized to interact with receptors *within the cytoplasm* or, more commonly, *within the nucleus.* The hormone-receptor complex, in turn, activates the transcription of specific genes.

The *activity* of some endocrine organs, e.g., the pituitary, is controlled by the presence of stimulatory or inhibitory hormones produced in the hypothalamus. In other sites, such as the adrenal cortex, hormones produced by the gland inhibit the synthesis of tropic hormones released by the hypothalamus and pituitary, a process known as *feedback inhibition.* In general, diseases of the endocrine system (endocrinopathies) are characterized by either *overproduction* or *underproduction* of hormones, with the clinical appearance of a hypofunctional or hyperfunctional state. Such disorders are invariably associated with disturbances of normal feedback mechanisms.

PITUITARY GLAND

Diseases of the pituitary may involve the *anterior* lobe, *posterior* lobe, or *both regions* of the gland. They may produce:

1. *Endocrine abnormalities,* due to increased or decreased production of tropic hormones. Abnormally increased production of tropic hormones (*hyperpituitarism*) is usually caused by a functioning anterior lobe *neoplasm,* but may also result from

hypothalamic abnormalities or loss of normal feedback inhibition. Decreased production of tropic hormones (*hypopituitarism*) is usually associated with *destruction* of >75% of the anterior lobe; rarely, hypothalamic disturbances are responsible.

2. *Local (mass) effects,* including radiographic evidence of enlargement of the sella turcica, visual disturbances, and evidence of increased intracranial pressure.

HYPERPITUITARISM—ANTERIOR PITUITARY NEOPLASMS (p. 1116)

- Generally caused by an *adenoma* of the anterior pituitary; less commonly due to primary hypothalamic disorders. Carcinomas of the anterior pituitary are exceedingly *rare.*
- Hormones most commonly produced by functional adenomas include prolactin (*Prl*), growth hormone (*GH*), and adrenocorticotropic hormone (*ACTH*). Thyroid stimulating hormone (TSH)- and gonadotropin (FSH/LH)-secreting adenomas are *rare.* Some adenomas may secrete more than one hormone, most commonly *GH* and *Prl.* Such pleurihormonal tumors may contain a *mixture* of cell types, or a *single* cell type, presumably a progenitor cell, that secretes both hormones. Approximately 25% of adenomas are *nonfunctional* and may produce *hypopituitarism* because of compression of normal gland.

The great majority of adenomas, including pleurihormonal tumors, appear to be monoclonal.

General Morphology

- Hypophyseal adenomas can be divided into *microadenomas* (<10 mm in diameter) and *macroadenomas* (>10 mm in diameter). Adenomas are usually solitary and, in early stages, form discrete masses within the sella. Larger lesions may compress or infiltrate adjacent structures (e.g., cavernous sinus, base of brain, sphenoid bone).
- Microscopically, adenomas are generally composed of *monomorphous* cells, in contrast to the normal anterior pituitary. The neoplastic cells may be arrayed in sheets, cords, nests, or papillae and have only a *scanty reticulin network.* Nuclear atypia may be present but does not imply malignancy. Necrosis and hemorrhage may be seen; extensive hemorrhage is sometimes referred to as *pituitary apoplexy* and may cause a rapid increase in the size of the tumor. Ultrastructurally, variable numbers of membrane-bound *secretory granules* are present in the cytoplasm of most cells.
- In addition to adenomas, multiple microscopic foci of *hyperplasia* also may produce excessive secretion of pituitary hormones. The distinction between multifocal hyperplasia and multiple adenomas is cloudy at best.

Somatotropic Adenomas (p. 1117)

- Responsible for the vast majority of examples of *excess GH,* with associated acromegaly or gigantism. Only rare cases of acromegaly/gigantism associated with somatotroph cell hyperplasia or hypothalamic disorder.
- *Acromegaly* appears when GH excess appears in adults (following closure of epiphyses in long bones). Features include enlargement of head, hands, feet, jaw, tongue, and soft tissues.

Changes usually develop subtly over decades, and responsible adenomas may be quite large at the time of diagnosis. *Gigantism* is rare and appears when GH excess occurs prior to closure of epiphyses.

- About half of somatotropic adenomas are composed of *densely granulated*, mature cells that stain strongly for GH. The cytoplasm of such cells is generally strongly eosinophilic ("acidophilic"). Remaining tumors are more sparsely granulated and react more weakly with immunostains for GH. About one-third of GH-producing adenomas are bihormonal and elaborate *both GH and Prl*. Bihormonal tumors may contain *two distinct cell populations* (mixed GH-Prl adenomas) or may be *monomorphous* (mammosomatotroph and acidophil stem cell adenomas).

Prolactinomas (p. 1117)

- *Most common* functional pituitary tumor. Most are *macroadenomas,* composed of *sparsely granulated* acidophilic or chromophobic cells. Immunostaining for Prl is required to demonstrate secretory product in histologic sections.
- *Clinical manifestations* include *hypogonadism* in males and females and *galactorrhea* in females. Note that hyperprolactinemia often results from conditions *other* than a Prl-secreting tumor, including hypothalamic disorders, drugs that impair dopaminergic transmission, and estrogen therapy. Any lesion that disturbs the normal anatomic relationship between the hypothalamus and pituitary may also cause hyperprolactinemia. Prolactin-cell hyperplasia is rare.

Corticotroph Tumors (p. 1117)

- Most are small, *basophilic microadenomas;* others may be *chromophobic.* Chromophobic tumors are often larger and produce symptoms from local mass effects. Immunostaining for ACTH yields a strong reaction in basophilic adenomas. *Crooke's hyaline change* may be seen in the cytoplasm of corticotroph cells, including those in the non-neoplastic surrounding gland.
- Clinical manifestations are those of *Cushing's syndrome,* due to excessive production of ACTH and resultant hypersecretion of cortisol (see adrenal section, later in this chapter).
- Infrequently, excessive production of ACTH may be caused by corticotroph cell *hyperplasia.*

Other Functioning Adenomas

- *Gonadotroph adenomas* (6% of pituitary tumors) are usually associated with increased levels of FSH and overproduction of the beta subunit of FSH; evidence of LH production is less common. Most common presenting manifestation is *hypogonadism.*
- *Thyrotroph adenomas* are uncommon but may cause hyperthyroidism. Tumors elaborate the glycoprotein thyrotropin-releasing hormone.

Carcinoma

- *Exceedingly* rare; generally nonfunctional.
- Diagnosis requires the demonstration of *metastases.*

HYPOPITUITARISM (p. 1118)

- May result from hypothalamic or primary pituitary disturbances.
- *Hypothalamic* lesions that produce hypopituitarism are rare, and include craniopharyngioma, glioma, germinoma (see below).
- Primary *pituitary* disorders underlie about 90% of cases; the three most common causes include nonsecretory adenomas, Sheehan's syndrome, and empty sella syndrome. Less common causes include radiation, surgical ablation, metastatic carcinoma, pituitary apoplexy, ischemic injury, and inflammatory lesions.
- Generally not manifest until more than 75% of the gland is ablated.
- Clinical manifestations are *variable. GH deficiency* in the adult is virtually undetectable except by assay of GH levels. In the prepubertal child, GH deficiency results in *pituitary dwarfism* and is often accompanied by retarded sexual development. Manifestations of *hypogonadotropism* include amenorrhea, atrophy of gonads, loss of pubic and axillary hair, sterility and, in men, recession of the hairline. Deficiencies of *TSH* and *ACTH* may result in hypothyroidism and hypoadrenalism, respectively. Hypopituitarism must be distinguished from primary end-organ failure.

Nonsecretory Chromophobe Pituitary Adenomas (p. 1119)

- Present as space-occupying lesions, with clinical symptoms referable to local *mass effect,* including visual disturbances, headache, and hypofunction of target organs normally under pituitary control.
- Grossly indistinguishable from functioning adenomas. Lesions are generally *large* by the time of diagnosis.
- Microscopic appearance is variable and includes sparsely granulated, *chromophobic* adenomas and mitochondria-rich, eosinophilic (*"oncocytic"*) tumors, designated oncocytomas.

Sheehan's Syndrome (p. 1120)

- Usually caused by *infarction* of the anterior pituitary; classically associated with obstetric hemorrhage/shock. Enlargement of the gland during pregnancy, combined with low-pressure portal blood supply, renders the adenohypophysis vulnerable to ischemic injury. The syndrome may also occur in males and nonpregnant females (trauma, sickle cell anemia, disseminated intravascular coagulation [DIC], vascular accidents).
- Generally associated with destruction of 90% to 95% of the gland.
- Common initial manifestations include gonadal failure and inability to lactate. Concomitant deficiency of TSH and ACTH may induce hypothyroidism and adrenocortical insufficiency. Onset of symptoms may be delayed.
- Infarcted organ appears soft, pale, and sometimes hemorrhagic in early stages. Over time, ischemic areas replaced by dense fibrous tissue, resulting in a firm, shrunken gland.

Empty Sella Syndrome (p. 1120)

- Includes *primary* lesions, related to herniation of the arachnoid and CSF through a defect in the diaphragma sellae, with resultant compression of the pituitary.

- *Secondary* lesions following destruction of normal gland via ischemic injury, infarction of adenoma, or radiation/surgical ablation of the gland.
- Most cases are *not* associated with clinically significant hypopituitarism; enlargement of the sella may be mistaken radiographically for a pituitary neoplasm.

HYPOTHALAMIC SUPRASELLAR NEOPLASMS (p. 1120)

- Include craniopharyngioma, germinoma, primary glial neoplasms, others.
- May present with hyper- or hypopituitarism of anterior pituitary, or diabetes insipidus (discussed below).

Craniopharyngioma (p. 1120)

- Five per cent of intracranial neoplasms; most are found in patients during the second to third decades.
- Characteristically cystic; calcification is present in 75%; they may encroach on the hypothalamus, third ventricle, optic chiasm.
- *Microscopically,* composed of a mixture of squamous epithelial elements and delicate reticular stroma, recapitulating the appearance of the enamel organ of a developing tooth; gliosis is common at the periphery; rupture of cyst contents may provoke a vigorous inflammatory reaction. Malignancy is *rare*.

POSTERIOR PITUITARY SYNDROMES (p. 1121)

- Most are caused by suprasellar/hypothalamic lesions or extra-CNS disorders.
- Manifestations are referable to excessive or deficient *antidiuretic hormone (ADH)* secretion; no defined syndromes are referable to abnormal oxytocin release.

ADH Deficiency (Diabetes Insipidus)

- Inability to concentrate urine, with resultant polyuria, excessive thirst (polydipsia), and hypernatremia.
- *Causes* include

  - Inflammatory and infiltrative disorders of the hypothalamus and pituitary region.
  - Hypothalamic radiation or surgery.
  - Head injury.
  - Idiopathic (sporadic or hereditary) causes.
  - Regressive changes in hypothalamic ganglion cells.

Inappropriate ADH Secretion

- Characterized by persistently high levels of ADH, with abnormal resorption of water, expansion of the extracellular fluid compartment, hyponatremia, and inability to excrete dilute urine.
- Causes include

  - Secretion of ectopic ADH by nonendocrine neoplasms (especially small cell carcinoma of the lung).

- Non-neoplastic pulmonary disease (e.g., pulmonary tuberculosis, pneumonia).
- Primary CNS disorders (e.g., intracranial hemorrhage, meningitis, cerebral infarcts).

THYROID GLAND

Thyroid abnormalities are relatively *common* in the general population. Manifestations of thyroid disease include *hyperthyroidism, hypothyroidism,* and focal or diffuse *enlargement* of the gland.

THYROTOXICOSIS (HYPERTHYROIDISM)

(p. 1122)

- A *hypermetabolic state* caused by increased levels of circulating triiodothyronine (T_3) and thyroxine (T_4).
- Clinical manifestations include *nervousness, weight loss* despite increased appetite, *warm, moist, flushed skin* secondary to peripheral vasodilatation and hypermetabolic state, tremor, and variable enlargement of the thyroid gland. *Eye changes* are often striking and include wide-eyed gaze, lid lag, and, in Graves' disease, proptosis. *Cardiac manifestations* include tachycardia, palpitations, atrial arrhythmias, and cardiomegaly. The origin of the cardiomegaly is obscure; cardiac failure is uncommon in young patients.
- *Morphologic* changes in nonthyroidal tissues include patchy lymphocytic infiltrates, lymphoid hyperplasia, skeletal muscle atrophy, osteoporosis, and mild, fatty change in liver.
- Most commonly associated with diffuse hyperplasia (*Graves' disease*), toxic *multinodular goiter,* or toxic *adenoma* (in order given). Less common etiologies include thyroiditis, gestational trophoblastic disease, (choriocarcinoma and hydatidiform moles), struma ovarii, TSH-secreting pituitary adenoma, excessive TRH release, administration of thyroid hormone supplements, and excess iodine ingestion in patients with pre-existing thyroid disease (Jodbasedow disease).

HYPOTHYROIDISM (p. 1124)

- A *hypometabolic* state caused by deficiency of thyroid hormones.
- *Manifestations* include *cretinism* if thyroid deficiency develops during the perinatal period or infancy, and *myxedema* in older children and adults.
- *Cretinism* may occur in both *endemic* form, associated with dietary iodine deficiency and endemic goiter, and *sporadic* form, often associated with a biosynthetic defect in hormone synthesis. Characterized by retardation of physical and intellectual growth. Manifestations include dry, rough skin; wideset eyes; periorbital puffiness; enlarged tongue; and, depending on age at onset, variable degrees of retarded skeletal and brain development.
- *Myxedema* is manifested by an insidious slowing of physical and mental activity, associated with fatigue, cold intolerance, and apathy. *Signs* include periorbital edema, coarsening of skin and facial features, cardiomegaly, pericardial effusion, hair

loss, and accumulation of mucopolysaccharide-rich ground substance within the dermis ("myxedema") and other tissues.
- General causes of hypothyroidism include

  - *Agenesis* or *ablation* of thyroid.
  - Interference with *thyroid hormone synthesis,* due to idiopathic primary hypothyroidism (?immune blockage of TSH receptors), hereditary enzymatic defects, iodine deficiency, certain drugs, and Hashimoto's thyroiditis.
  - *Suprathyroidal disorders,* including pituitary and hypothalamic lesions.

THYROIDITIS (p. 1125)

Includes infectious thyroiditis, Riedel's fibrosing thyroiditis, and, more commonly, Hashimoto's disease, subacute granulomatous thyroiditis, and lymphocytic thyroiditis.

Infectious Thyroiditis (p. 1125)

- *Agents* include *Staphylococcus aureus,* streptococci, *Salmonella, Enterobacter,* mycobacteria, and fungi. *Viral* infection has been implicated in some forms of thyroiditis (e.g., subacute granulomatous thyroiditis.).
- Generally hematogenous in origin.
- Manifestations include painful enlargement of gland.

Riedel's Fibrosing Thyroiditis (p. 1125)

- An uncommon *fibrosing* process of unknown etiology associated with replacement of thyroid parenchyma by dense fibrous tissue penetrating the capsule and extending into *contiguous neck structures.*
- Manifestations include glandular atrophy and hypothyroidism. May be mistaken for infiltrating neoplasm. May be associated with idiopathic fibrosis in other sites.

Hashimoto's Thyroiditis (p. 1126)

An *autoimmune* inflammatory disorder that includes both *classic* (*goitrous*) and *atrophic* variants.

- Represents most common cause of *goitrous hypothyroidism* in regions where dietary iodine is adequate;
- Major cause of *nonendemic goiter in children;*
- Archetypic example of *organ-specific autoimmune disease;*
- *Female* predominance (5:1); incidence increases with age.

PATHOGENESIS

- Probably related to defect in function of thyroid-specific suppressor T cells, resulting in the emergence of CD4 + *helper T cells* directed at thyroid, and the production of *autoantibodies* to various components of thyroid (thyroid peroxidase, thyroglobulin, TSH receptor, and others). Uncertain whether cell-mediated injury, humoral mechanisms, or both cause injury to thyroid.
- Etiology uncertain but may have a *genetic* component; goitrous form associated with HLA-DR5 and atrophic form with HLA-DR3.
- Associated with *other autoimmune diseases,* including SLE, Sjögren's syndrome, rheumatoid arthritis, pernicious anemia, type II diabetes, and Graves' disease.

MORPHOLOGY

- *Goitrous form* characterized by enlarged, often asymmetric gland with an intact capsule; the parenchyma is generally paler than the normal gland. Microscopic changes include an exuberant infiltrate of lymphocytes, plasma cells, and macrophages, often associated with germinal centers; abundant eosinophilic granular cytoplasm in residual follicular cells ("Hürthle" cells or "oncocytes"); and delicate fibrosis.
- *Atrophic variant* associated with more extensive fibrosis and less inflammation; size of gland is often reduced.

CLINICAL COURSE

- Characterized by *hypothyroidism,* usually associated with painless enlargement of the gland; thyromegaly is absent in atrophic (fibrosing) variant.
- *Hyperthyroidism* ("hashitoxicosis") may be seen early in course of disease, associated with presence of anti-TSH receptor antibodies, but is transient.

Subacute Granulomatous (De Quervain's) Thyroiditis (p. 1127)

- A self-limited form of thyroiditis, also referred to as *giant cell* or *granulomatous* thyroiditis.
- Peak incidence second to fifth decades with female predominance (3:1); associated with *HLA-B35.*
- Etiology uncertain, but evidence implicates *viral infection* (mumps, measles, influenza, adenovirus, coxsackievirus, echovirus). *Antibodies* to viruses demonstrable in half of cases.

MORPHOLOGY. Variable enlargement of the gland; early lesions include *disruption of thyroid follicles* with a *neutrophilic* infiltrate; cellular aggregates, possibly representing *macrophages* or *altered follicular epithelial* cells, appear subsequently, and form *multinucleate giant cells* surrounding colloid fragments.

CLINICAL COURSE. Presentation varies considerably and includes

- Acute, systemic febrile illness associated with elevated erythrocyte sedimentation rate.
- Sudden, painful enlargement of the thyroid.
- Less painful enlargement accompanied by transient hyperthyroidism.

Condition is self-limited, with recovery usual in 6 to 8 weeks.

Subacute Lymphocytic Thyroiditis (p. 1128)

- Uncommon cause of goitrous hyperthyroidism.
- An inflammatory disorder of unknown etiology defined histologically by *nonspecific lymphoid infiltration* of the thyroid parenchyma; there is no germinal center formation or significant plasma cell infiltrate.
- *No* clear association with viral infection, subacute granulomatous thyroiditis, Hashimoto's disease, or primary idiopathic myxedema.
- Most common in women in postpartum period; may be associated with painless enlargement of the gland and/or hyperthyroidism. Self-limited; may be followed by *hypo*thyroidism.

GRAVES' DISEASE (p. 1129)

- Characterized by *hyperthyroidism* due to a hyperfunctioning *diffuse goiter*, infiltrative *ophthalmopathy* and, in 10% to 5% of cases, an edematous *dermopathy* ("localized myxedema").
- *Female* predominance (10:1); occurs in 1.5% to 2% of women in U.S.
- Associated with *HLA-DR3* and with *other autoimmune disorders,* including Hashimoto's disease, pernicious anemia, and rheumatoid arthritis.

PATHOGENESIS

- *Autoimmune* process, initiated by IgG antibodies against portions of the *TSH receptor.* Anti-TSH antibodies include

  - *Thyroid-stimulating antibody* (TSAb), also designated thyroid-stimulating immunoglobulin, which stimulates increased adenylate cyclase activity, elevated cAMP levels, and increased activity of thyroid epithelial cells.
  - *Thyrotropin-binding inhibitor immunoglobulin* (TBII), which binds to the TSH receptor and may either mimic the action of TSH or inhibit thyroid cell activity.

- Origin of autoantibody production uncertain, but may involve defect in thyroid-specific suppressor T-cell function comparable to that proposed for Hashimoto's thyroiditis.
- *Infiltrative ophthalmopathy* is also probably autoimmune in origin.

MORPHOLOGY. The gland is mildly and *symmetrically enlarged,* with an intact capsule and soft parenchyma. Microscopic changes include widespread *hypertrophy and hyperplasia* of follicular epithelium, manifested by crowding of columnar cells into irregular papillary folds. Colloid is substantially decreased. Interfollicular parenchyma contains *hyperplastic lymphoid tissue* and increased numbers of blood vessels.

- Preoperative therapy influences the histologic appearance: *thiouracil* exaggerates hyperplasia, while *iodine* promotes devascularization, colloid accumulation, and follicular involution.
- Orbital soft tissues contain increased fluid, mucopolysaccharides, collagen, and lymphocytic infiltrates.
- Generalized lymphoid hyperplasia is present in other sites.

CLINICAL FEATURES. Include thyrotoxicosis, thyromegaly, exophthalmos, and infiltrative dermopathy. Ophthalmopathy may be self-limited or may progress to severe proptosis despite control of thyrotoxicosis. Laboratory values include elevated T_3 and T_4 levels, decreased TSH levels, and elevated radioactive iodine uptake. Decreased TSH levels are the most important test.

DIFFUSE NONTOXIC GOITER AND MULTINODULAR GOITER (p. 1131)

- Most cases begin as *diffuse* enlargement, with nodularity developing at a later stage; hence, the two entities represent a continuum.
- Most cases represent *compensatory hypertrophy and hyperplasia* of follicular epithelium secondary to impaired production of thyroid hormones.

DIFFUSE NONTOXIC (SIMPLE) GOITER (p. 1131)

- The gland is diffusely and uniformly enlarged, with no evidence of hyper- or hypothyroidism in most cases.
- Occurs in *endemic* and *sporadic* forms.
- *Endemic goiter* is most prevalent in areas with dietary iodine deficiency (e.g., Alps, Andes, Himalayas, central Africa); prevalence in the United States has declined secondarily to use of iodized salt. Dietary *goitrogens* (e.g., calcium, fluorides, thiocyanates) may also contribute to endemic goiter. Decreased production of thyroid hormone produces a *compensatory increase in TSH* with resultant hyperplasia and hypertrophy of the gland, and establishment of a *euthyroid* state. Female predominance; generally appears around puberty.
- *Sporadic goiter* is less common than endemic goiter. There is female predominance (8:1), with a peak incidence in puberty or young adult life. The mechanisms are not well understood in most cases; TSH levels are elevated in some but not all patients. *Biosynthetic defects* in thyroid hormone synthesis underlie some cases, including defective iodine transport, organification, dehalogenation, and iodotyrosine coupling.

MORPHOLOGY. The gland is modestly enlarged in early stages; initial histologic changes include *hypertrophy and hyperplasia* of follicular epithelium with *scant colloid.* Later changes include accumulation of colloid and variable atrophy of follicular epithelium. Marked enlargement of the gland secondary to massive accumulation of colloid is designated *colloid goiter.*

CLINICAL FEATURES. Most manifestations related to enlargement of the gland; most patients remain *euthyroid.* Hypothyroidism is more common in children with underlying biosynthetic defects.

MULTINODULAR GOITER (p. 1132)

- Preceded by *diffuse goiter.*
- May be *nontoxic* or associated with *hyperthyroidism* (toxic multinodular goiter or Plummer's disease); there is no associated ophthalmopathy or dermopathy, in contrast to Graves' disease.

MORPHOLOGY. Irregular *nodularity* of the gland associated with focal hemorrhage, fibrosis, calcification, and cystic change; histologic changes include a variable degree of *colloid* accumulation, follicular *epithelial hyperplasia,* and follicular *involution* with focal intervening areas of scarring, hemorrhage, etc. Glands may become massively enlarged (>2000 gm) and extend behind the sternum, trachea, and esophagus.

CLINICAL FEATURES. Include (1) signs and symptoms referable to *mass effect,* and (2) occasionally, abnormal thyroid function due to hyperactivity of a focal nodule with resultant *thyrotoxicosis* (rarely associated with hypothyroidism). Problems related to *mass effect* include cosmetic deformity, esophageal compression with dysphagia, tracheal compression, and, occasionally, obstruction of the superior vena cava. Hemorrhage into goiter may cause pain and contribute to mass effect. *Thyrotoxicosis* occurs in fewer than one half of patients; infiltrative ophthalmopathy and dermopathy are *not* seen in the absence of concomitant Graves' disease. *Cardiovascular* manifestations (tachycardia, atrial fibrillation, congestive heart failure) may be prominent. Laboratory findings include variable elevations in T_3, T_4, and radioactive iodine uptake; scintiscans reveal irregular functional activity with patchy or focal accumulations of radioiodine. Distinction between multinodular goiter and neoplasm may be difficult, especially in patients with a dominant mass.

NEOPLASMS (p. 1133)

- Solitary thyroid nodules present in 2% to 4% of U.S. population; higher frequency in areas of endemic goiter.
- Most solitary nodules are *non-neoplastic* (cysts, multinodular goiter, Hashimoto's thyroiditis).
- Among thyroid neoplasms, >90% prove to be *adenomas.*
- Certain clinical features may help in the evaluation of non-neoplastic nodules:

  - *Solitary* nodules are more likely to be neoplastic.
  - *Functioning* ("hot") nodules on scintiscans are more likely benign than malignant.
  - Nodules in younger *patients* (<40) and in *males* are more likely to be neoplastic than those in older patients.

- *Fine-needle aspiration* biopsy is often useful in the evaluation of thyroid nodules.

ADENOMAS (p. 1134)

- Multiple histologic variants are recognized, all representing *follicular* neoplasms.
- *Gross* appearance is of well-demarcated, solitary lesions, occasionally accompanied by fibrosis, hemorrhage, or calcification.
- *Microscopic* features include

  - *Sharp demarcation* from adjacent parenchyma by a fibrous "capsule."
  - *Architecture distinct* from that of the adjacent gland.
  - *Compression* of the surrounding gland by adenoma.
  - *Absence of multinodularity* in the remaining gland.

- Histologic patterns range from closely-apposed nests and trabeculae reminiscent of developing (embryonal) thyroid to well-developed follicles containing abundant colloid. *Hürthle cell* adenomas feature granular, eosinophilic cells containing abundant mitochondria.

CLINICAL FEATURES. A *focal mass,* which must be differentiated from carcinoma; may enlarge progressively or remain stable. *Hemorrhage* into adenoma may produce rapid, painful enlargement of the mass. Most are "cold" (nonfunctioning) on scans; *rarely* associated with hyperthyroidism.

MALIGNANT NEOPLASMS (p. 1136)

- Uncommon in U.S. (account for <1% of cancer deaths).
- *Female* predominance (2:1 to 3:1) in lesions occurring during middle age.
- Almost all are *carcinomas.*
- *Morphologic variants* and their frequencies include

  - Papillary carcinoma, 75% to 85%
  - Follicular carcinoma, 10% to 20%
  - Medullary carcinoma, 5%
  - Anaplastic carcinoma, rare

- Most (90% to 95%) are *well-differentiated* lesions.
- *Pathogenesis* of some carcinomas related to head and neck *irradiation* during first two decades of life; *Hashimoto's thyroiditis* is associated with increased risk of *lymphoma* (and possibly carcinoma). Relationship between adenomas or nontoxic nodular goiter and malignancy remains unclear.
- *Oncogenes* have been implicated in the genesis of certain forms of thyroid cancer, including the *PTC oncogene* (in papillary thyroid carcinoma) and the *RET proto-oncogene* (in medullary carcinoma in patients with MEN syndrome IIa, discussed below).

Papillary Carcinoma (p. 1137)

- *Most common* form of thyroid cancer; peak incidence in third to fifth decades; female predominance (2:1 to 3:1).
- Often appear as *multifocal* tumors, due to propensity for lymphatic invasion.
- Involves *regional nodes* in 50% of cases at time of diagnosis; distant metastases uncommon at presentation (5%).
- *Gross appearance* is usually that of an infiltrative lesion, sometimes associated with calcification or cystic change.
- *Microscopic appearance* ranges from lesions that are predominantly *papillary* in architecture to those with a predominance of *follicular* elements (follicular variant of papillary carcinoma); mixtures of papillary and follicular elements are common. Other features include

  - Hypochromatic empty nuclei devoid of nucleoli ("Orphan Annie eyes").
  - Nuclear grooves.
  - Eosinophilic intranuclear inclusions (cytoplasmic invaginations).
  - Psammoma bodies.

- Histologic variants of papillary carcinoma include

  - *Encapsulated variant* (designated "papillary adenoma" in past).
  - *Follicular variant* (should be distinguished from true follicular carcinoma, which carries a worse prognosis).
  - *Tall cell variant* (occurs in older individuals; associated with poorer prognosis than other papillary carcinomas).

- *Prognosis* generally excellent (90% survival at 20 years); favorable factors include

  - Female sex.
  - Age less than 20 years.
  - Confinement of lesion to thyroid.
  - Well-differentiated histology.

Follicular Carcinoma (p. 1138)

- Account for *10% to 20%* of thyroid cancers; peak incidence fifth to sixth decades with female predominance (3:1).
- Increased prevalence noted in areas of dietary *iodine deficiency*, suggesting that multinodular goiter may predispose to follicular carcinoma.
- *Gross features* include apparent encapsulation in many cases, rendering distinction from adenoma difficult in some instances; others may infiltrate extensively.
- *Microscopically,* architecture may vary considerably; the nu-

clear features noted in papillary carcinomas (described above) are absent. Most contain a microfollicular pattern, with relatively uniform, colloid-filled follicles reminiscent of normal thyroid. Other patterns include a trabecular and sheetlike architecture. Some variants contain large numbers of eosinophilic cells resembling Hürthle cells.

- Presence of capsular and vascular invasion increases likelihood of metastases; majority of metastases are *hematogenous* (bone, lungs, liver).
- *Prognosis* is influenced by size of lesion, presence or absence of capsular or vascular invasion, presence of metastases, and the degree of histologic anaplasia. Better-differentiated lesions may take up *radioactive iodine,* which may be used to identify and palliate metastatic lesions.

Anaplastic Carcinoma (p. 1140)

- Accounts for less than 5% of thyroid carcinomas; most common in elderly patients, particularly in areas of endemic goiter.
- *Histological patterns* include

  - Spindle cell carcinomas.
  - Giant cell carcinomas.
  - Small cell carcinomas (may be difficult to distinguish from lymphoma or metastatic small cell carcinoma).

- *Dismal prognosis;* dissemination is common, but death is usually attributable to aggressive local growth.

Medullary Thyroid Carcinoma (p. 1140)

- Represent *neuroendocrine* neoplasms originating from parafollicular (C) cells, in contrast to other thyroid carcinomas.
- *Distinctive features* include

  - Secretion of calcitonin in most cases (other secretory products may be elaborated as well).
  - Amyloid stroma in many cases.
  - Association with MEN syndromes IIa and IIb in 20% to 25% of cases (may also occur in other familial patterns).

- *Peak incidence* 5th–6th decade for sporadic cases; 3rd–4th decade for MEN-associated cases. Isolated familial cases occur in elderly patients.
- Pathogenesis of MEN IIa-associated cases related to germ-line mutation in *RET proto-oncogene.*
- *Gross patterns* include

  1. Discrete tumors in one lobe.
  2. Numerous nodules, usually involving both lobes; *sporadic* cases tend to originate in one lobe, whereas *familial* cases are usually bilateral and multicentric.

- *Microscopic features* include polygonal to spindle-shaped cells arrayed in organoid nests, trabeculae, and, occasionally, follicles. Some tumors resemble gastrointestinal carcinoids. *Amyloid deposits,* probably derived from calcitonin molecules, occur in about half of cases.
- Foci of *C-cell hyperplasia* are often present in familial cases but are typically absent in sporadic cases.
- *Clinical features* vary, depending upon whether case is sporadic or familial. *Sporadic cases* usually present as a thyroid mass, sometimes associated with dysphagia, hoarseness, or cough;

occasional cases may present with manifestations related to the secretion of a peptide product (e.g., diarrhea due to calcitonin or vasoactive intestinal polyptide). *Familial* cases usually detected through screening of asymptomatic relatives of affected patients with calcitonin levels.

- *Prognosis variable;* sporadic lesions, and those associated with MEN IIb are often aggressive. Lesions arising in patients with isolated familial medullary carcinoma syndrome are more often indolent.

MISCELLANEOUS LESIONS (p. 1142)
Thyroglossal Duct (Cyst)

- Most common clinically significant congenital anomaly.
- May present at any age, as midline mass anterior to trachea.
- *Histologic features* include squamous epithelium in segments occurring high in neck, thyroidal acinar epithelium in lesions arising more inferiorly. Lymphocytic infiltrates are often conspicuous.
- May become infected; rarely may give rise to carcinoma.

PARATHYROID GLANDS

PRIMARY HYPERPARATHYROIDISM (PHPT)

- Represents an *autonomous hypersecretion of parathormone* (PTH), resulting in

  1. Increased bone resorption and calcium mobilization from the skeleton.
  2. Increased renal tubular reabsorption and retention of calcium.
  3. Increased renal synthesis of $1,25\text{-}(OH)_2D_3$ with enhanced absorption of calcium by the GI tract.
  4. Resultant *hypercalcemia.*

- Over 90% of cases of hypercalcemia are related to *PHPT* or to *malignancy.* Hypercalcemia associated with malignancy may be caused by the elaboration of cytokines or other factors by metastatic deposits, producing local osteolysis. In other nonendocrine malignancies, PTH-related peptide elaborated by neoplastic cells may interact with PTH receptors in a fashion similar to normal PTH.

- *Causes of PHPT* include

  - Parathyroid adenoma (75% to 80% of cases).
  - Primary hyperplasia (diffuse or nodular) (10% to 15% of cases).
  - Parathyroid carcinoma (<5%).

- *Incidence of PHTP* is roughly 25 cases per 100,000 annually in U.S. and Europe; most cases occur during sixth decade and beyond, with a female predominance (3:1).

- Most cases of PHPT in the past diagnosed by symptoms referable to hypercalciuria and renal stone formation, often associated with bone disease. *Routine serum calcium determinations* in medical evaluations have resulted in the diagnosis of most cases of PHPT at an earlier stage; kidney stones and bone disease are correspondingly less frequent (10% of patients).

- Most cases of PHPT occur *sporadically;* may occur in association with *MEN syndrome I* or *IIa* (usually due to parathyroid hyperplasia in MEN syndromes). Pathogenesis of familial cases and occasional sporadic cases may be related to homozygous loss of suppressor gene activity on chromosome 11q11-13.

MORPHOLOGY. *Parathyroid adenomas.*

- Usually *solitary,* averaging 0.5 to 5.0 gm; if more than one lesion is present, nodular *hyperplasia* must be excluded. Features of adenomas include

  - Presence of a "capsule," associated with compression of adjacent gland.
  - Minimal stromal fat in adenomas.
  - Monoclonality.

- Most common in *inferior glands;* may also be found in *ectopic* sites (e.g., thymus, thyroid, pericardium, retroesophageal area). *Grossly,* most are well-encapsulated, soft, tan to red.
- Usually composed predominantly of *chief cells* arrayed in sheets, trabeculae, or follicles; oxyphil cells may be present.

MORPHOLOGY. *Primary hyperplasia.*

- May occur sporadically, or in association with MEN syndromes I and IIa.
- Usually involves *all glands* histologically, although *asymmetric* involvement may be seen, particularly in cases of nodular hyperplasia; combined weight rarely exceeds 1.0 gm.
- *Microscopic patterns* include diffuse and nodular variants. Usually composed of chief cells, although water clear cells may predominate; nodules of oxyphil cells are common. Cells may form solid sheets, trabeculae, nests, or follicles; fat cells are usually interspersed.
- Hyperplasia may be difficult to distinguish from adenoma.

MORPHOLOGY. *Parathyroid carcinoma.*

- Usually presents as masses involving one gland; may be difficult to distinguish from adenoma, both grossly and microscopically.
- Diagnosis of malignancy is based on the presence of *local invasion and/or metastases.*

CLINICAL FEATURES

- *Multiple systems* affected, including

  - Renal (nephrolithiasis, nephrocalcinosis).
  - Skeletal (osteitis fibrosa cystica, osteoporosis).
  - Gastrointestinal (nausea, vomiting, peptic ulcers, pancreatitis).
  - Central nervous system (headaches, lethargy, memory loss, depression, seizures).
  - Miscellaneous (muscle weakness, skin and eye changes).

- Most cases are *asymptomatic* or *minimally symptomatic* at the time of diagnosis.

SECONDARY HYPERPARATHYROIDISM

- Encountered most commonly in patients with *renal failure;* may also be seen in severe vitamin D deficiency or osteomalacia and, rarely, in pseudohypoparathyroidism.
- *Pathogenesis in renal failure* related to phosphate retention and hypocalcemia, with compensatory hypersecretion of PTH. Impaired GI calcium absorption due to reduced $1,25\text{-}(OH)_2D_3$

synthesis, and skeletal resistance to the effects of PTH and vitamin D also may contribute.

- *Morphology* of parathyroid glands is identical to that of primary hyperplasia. Skeletal changes, including osteitis fibrosa cystica and osteomalacia, are present (renal osteodystrophy).
- Condition may remit with correction of underlying renal failure; occasionally, an *autonomous adenoma* may develop ("tertiary" hyperparathyroidism).

HYPOPARATHYROIDISM (p. 1147)

- Largely a functional disorder, with few distinctive anatomic changes.
- *Multiple etiologies,* including

  - Inadvertent surgical removal of all parathyroid glands.
  - Congenital absence of glands (e.g., DiGeorge's syndrome).
  - Autoimmune destruction.
  - Rare familial autosomal syndromes and metabolic disorders (hypomagnesemia).

- *Clinical features* include

  - Increased neuromuscular excitability due to hypocalcemia, associated in severe cases with tetany, muscle cramps, carpopedal spasms, laryngeal stridor, and convulsions.
  - Mental changes (irritability, psychosis).
  - Intracranial abnormalities (calcification of basal ganglia, parkinsonism, elevated intracranial pressure with papilledema).
  - Calcification of lens.
  - Cardiac conduction abnormalities.

PSEUDOHYPOPARATHYROIDISM

- *Rare.*
- Pathogenesis of pseudohypoparathyroidism related to *abnormality in PTH receptor complex* and loss of responsiveness to PTH, with resultant hypocalcemia, compensatory parathyroid hyperfunction, and a variety of skeletal and developmental abnormalities (short stature, round face, short neck, short metacarpals and metatarsals).

ADRENAL CORTEX

HYPERFUNCTION OF ADRENAL CORTEX (HYPERADRENALISM) (p. 1150)

Includes three basic syndromes referable to excessive secretion of adrenal cortical hormones:

- Cushing's syndrome (excess cortisol).
- Hyperaldosteronism.
- Adrenogenital syndromes (excess androgens).

CUSHING'S SYNDROME (p. 1150)

Multiple etiologies, including

- Administration of exogenous glucocorticoids, the most common cause.

- Pituitary hypersecretion of ACTH.
- Ectopic production of ACTH or corticotropin-releasing factor (CRF) by a nonendocrine neoplasm.
- Autonomous hypersecretion of cortisol by an adrenal adenoma, carcinoma, or ACTH-independent adrenal cortical hyperplasia.

Pituitary hypersecretion of ACTH (also called **Cushing's disease**)

- Accounts for 65% to 70% of cases of *endogenous* hypercortisolism.
- Most cases associated with *pituitary adenoma* (may be basophilic or sparsely granulated "chromophobic" neoplasm); *corticotroph hyperplasia* accounts for 15% of cases.
- Adrenals are bilaterally hyperplastic, and elevated serum ACTH is usually readily detectable.
- Encountered most commonly in young adult life; female predominance (8:1).

Ectopic ACTH secretion by nonpituitary tumors.

- Accounts for 10% to 15% of cases of endogenous Cushing's syndrome. Differentiation from pituitary disease may be difficult.
- Most commonly associated with *small cell carcinoma of lung,* carcinoids of bronchus or pancreas, malignant thymoma, pheochromocytoma, medullary carcinoma of the thyroid, and gastrinomas.
- May rarely be associated with *ectopic secretion of CRF,* with resultant overproduction of ACTH.
- Adrenals are bilaterally hyperplastic.
- Most common in men during the fifth to sixth decades of life.

Adrenal adenoma, carcinoma, and primary cortical hyperplasia.

- Account, in aggregate, for 20% to 25% of cases of endogenous Cushing's syndrome.
- Lesion is independent of ACTH.
- Adenomas and carcinomas equally common in adults; carcinomas predominate in children. Hypercortisolism is usually more marked with carcinomas than with adenomas or hyperplasia.
- In patients with a unilateral neoplasm, native adrenal cortex is usually atrophic due to *ACTH suppression* and low levels of ACTH.

MORPHOLOGY

- Pituitary changes include *Crooke's hyaline change* within pituitary basophils, caused by the presence of elevated cortisol levels. In primary pituitary disease, as noted, a basophilic microadenoma, basophilic macroadenoma, chromophobic adenoma, or diffuse corticotroph hyperplasia may be present.
- *Diffuse adrenal cortical hyperplasia* is present in 60% to 70% of cases of Cushing's syndrome; glands are affected bilaterally. *Nodular adrenal cortical hyperplasia* is present in 15% to 20% of cases; the appearance of the cortex between nodules is identical to that in diffuse hyperplasia, suggesting that nodular hyperplasia probably evolves from the latter. *ACTH levels are elevated* in most cases of hyperplasia.
- *Adrenal cortical adenomas and carcinomas* resemble nonfunctional cortical neoplasms (described below). Lesions occur most commonly in fourth to sixth decades, with a female predominance. Adenomas are generally small and well circum-

scribed; carcinomas tend to be larger and unencapsulated. The zona reticularis and fasciculata of the adjacent residual cortex and the contralateral gland are *atrophic;* the zona glomerulosa is intact.

Clinical features of Cushing's syndrome include

- Central obesity (85% to 90%).
- Moon facies (85%).
- Weakness and fatigability (85%).
- Hirsutism (75%).
- Hypertension (75%).
- Plethora (75%).
- Glucose intolerance/diabetes (75%/20%).
- Osteoporosis (75%).
- Neuropsychiatric abnormalities (75% to 80%).
- Menstrual abnormalities (70%).
- Cutaneous striae (50%).
- Delayed wound healing/bruisability.

Laboratory evaluation, especially ACTH levels and the ability of high doses of dexamethasone to suppress ACTH levels, coupled with imaging of pituitary and adrenals, is necessary to characterize Cushing's syndrome, fully. *Prognosis* is favorable in cases of surgically correctable disease.

PRIMARY HYPERALDOSTERONISM (p. 1153)

Uncommon syndromes, characterized by chronic, excessive secretion of aldosterone independently of the renin-angiotensin system.

- *Features* include suppression of plasma renin activity, hypokalemia, sodium retention, and hypertension.
- *Common causes* include
  - A solitary aldosterone-secreting adenoma in 65% of cases (Conn's syndrome).
  - Bilateral idiopathic adrenal hyperplasia (30% of cases).
- Uncommon causes include
  - Glucocorticoid-suppressible hyperaldosteronism.
  - Adrenal cortical carcinoma.
  - Familial non–glucocorticoid-suppressible variant.
  - Others.

MORPHOLOGY. *Aldosterone-producing adenomas.*

- Usually *solitary, small, encapsulated lesions;* more common on left side.
- *Peak incidence* in fourth to fifth decades; female predominance.
- May be buried within the adrenal and not apparent externally; cut surface is usually bright yellow, reflecting high lipid content.
- Constituent lipid-laden cells more often resemble cells of zona fasciculata than zona glomerulosa.

MORPHOLOGY. *Bilateral idiopathic hyperplasia.*

- Characterized by hyperplasia of cells resembling normal zona glomerulosa, interspersed with nodules resembling zona fasciculata.
- Source of cortical stimulation is unknown; a non-ACTH pituitary glycoprotein has been implicated.

CONGENITAL ADRENAL HYPERPLASIA; ADRENOGENITAL SYNDROMES (p. 1154)

- *Variable manifestations,* including hermaphroditism, pseudo-hermaphroditism, virilization in the female, and precocious puberty in the male.
- *Adrenogenital syndrome* (adrenal virilism) may be caused by (1) androgen-secreting adrenal cortical neoplasms, or (2) congenital metabolic defects in corticosteroid biosynthesis, leading to decreased cortisol production, a compensatory increase in ACTH secretion, adrenal hyperplasia, and increased production of other cortical steroids, including androgens. Certain enzymatic defects may also be associated with *"salt-wasting"* due to impaired aldosterone production.
- *21-Hydroxylase deficiency* accounts for 85% to 90% of cases of congenital adrenal hyperplasia; variants include

  - *Salt-wasting adrenogenitalism,* associated with a complete absence of hydroxylase activity and resultant mineralocorticoid and cortisol deficiency; syndrome usually recognized after birth, with virilization in females, salt-wasting, hyponatremia, hyperkalemia, and cardiovascular collapse.
  - *Simple virilizing adrenogenital syndrome without salt wasting,* associated with incomplete loss of hydroxylase activity.
  - *Nonclassic adrenal virilism,* often asymptomatic or only mildly symptomatic; diagnosis based on demonstration of biosynthetic defects and genetic studies. More common than "classic" patterns.

- All adrenogenital syndromes are autosomal recessive disorders; the 21-hydroxylase deficiency is transmitted by a single gene located in chromosome 6p21.3. Multiple alleles exist, providing an explanation for the variable clinical manifestations of the disorder.
- Morphologic changes include substantial, bilateral adrenal enlargement; cortex is widened, brown, and lipid-depleted.

HYPOFUNCTION OF ADRENAL CORTEX (HYPOADRENALISM) (p. 1157)

May be caused by any lesion of the adrenal cortex that impairs corticosteroid production, or may be secondary to ACTH deficiency. Patterns include

1. Primary acute adrenocortical insufficiency (adrenal crisis).
2. Primary chronic adrenocortical insufficiency (Addison's disease).
3. Secondary adrenocortical insufficiency.

PRIMARY ACUTE ADRENOCORTICAL INSUFFICIENCY

May occur in a variety of settings, including

- A *sudden increase in glucocorticoid requirements* in patients with chronic adrenocortical insufficiency.
- *Rapid withdrawal of steroids* from patients with adrenal suppression secondary to long-term glucocorticoid therapy, or *failure to increase steroid doses* in adrenalectomized patients during episodes of stress.

- *Massive destruction* of the adrenals (e.g., neonatal adrenal hemorrhage, postsurgical disseminated intravascular coagulation, Waterhouse-Friderichsen syndrome).

Waterhouse-Friderichsen Syndrome

- Characterized by

  - Overwhelming septicemic infection usually caused by *meningococci*, less often by other virulent bacteria (pneumococci, gonococci, staphylococci).
  - Rapidly progressive hypotension and shock.
  - Disseminated intravascular coagulation.
  - Massive adrenal hemorrhage with adrenal insufficiency.

- Most common in *children* but may occur at any age.
- *Morphologic changes* are those of *massive, bilateral adrenal hemorrhage,* which begins in the medulla; genesis of hemorrhage unclear but may involve direct bacterial seeding of adrenal vessels, DIC, endotoxin-induced vasculitis, or a hypersensitivity vasculitis.

PRIMARY CHRONIC ADRENOCORTICAL INSUFFICIENCY (ADDISON'S DISEASE)

An uncommon condition, occurring most often in adults; requires destruction of at least 90% of the adrenal cortex.

- *Multiple etiologies,* including

  - Autoimmune adrenalitis.
  - Infectious processes (tuberculosis, histoplasmosis, other fungi).
  - Metastatic cancer.

- *Autoimmune adrenalitis* accounts for 60% to 70% of cases of Addison's disease. Adrenal may be *sole target,* or adrenal destruction may be part of a *polyglandular process:*

  - *Type I* includes adrenal insufficiency, candidiasis, and hypoparathyroidism.
  - *Type II* includes adrenal insufficiency and thyroid disease (Schmidt's syndrome), sometimes with insulin-dependent diabetes mellitus.
  - *Type III* is polyglandular disease without adrenal involvement.
  - Circulating antibodies are present in 50% of cases; basis of immune attack unclear but may involve genetic mechanisms (increased incidence of HLA-B8 and DR3); female predominance in type III disease (3:1).
  - *Tuberculous adrenalitis* accounts for 10% to 25% of cases; usually always associated with disseminated disease (other infectious etiologies include histoplasmosis, coccidioidomycosis, and blastomycosis). Destruction of *medulla and cortex* results in combined deficiency of glucocorticoids, mineralocorticoids, and catecholamines.
  - *Metastatic cancer* is an uncommon cause of adrenal insufficiency. Common primary tumors include carcinomas of the lung, stomach, and breast, as well as melanoma and lymphoma.
  - *Morphologic features* vary, depending on cause of adrenalitis (e.g., metastatic neoplasm, tuberculous granulomas). *Autoimmune adrenalitis* usually produces small glands, lipid deple-

tion of adrenal cortex, and mixed lymphocytic, plasmacytic, and histiocytic infiltrate in cortex. Medulla is spared.

- *Clinical features* of Addison's disease include weakness, fatigue, anorexia, hypotension, nausea, vomiting, and cutaneous hyperpigmentation. Laboratory values include hyperkalemia, and low sodium, chloride, bicarbonate, and glucose. Serum *ACTH levels are elevated* in primary adrenocortical insufficiency.

SECONDARY ADRENOCORTICAL INSUFFICIENCY

May be caused by any disorder of the hypothalamus or pituitary associated with *decreased production of ACTH*.

Distinguished from primary hypoadrenalism by

- Absence of hyperpigmentation (ACTH and precursor peptides with melanocyte-stimulating activity are not elevated in secondary cases).
- Normal or near-normal aldosterone levels (aldosterone production is independent of ACTH; severe hyponatremia and hyperkalemia are *not* features of secondary adrenocortical insufficiency).

ACTH deficiency may be isolated or associated with decreased levels of other pituitary hormones (panhypopituitarism).

Morphologically, characterized by variable degrees of atrophy of the adrenal cortex, with *sparing of the zona glomerulosa and medulla.*

NONFUNCTIONAL CORTICAL NEOPLASMS

In addition to hyperplasias and neoplasms associated with steroid production, nonfunctional adrenal cortical neoplasms also may occur.

Adrenal Adenomas

- Typically poorly encapsulated, yellow-orange lesions; may lie within cortex or protrude into medulla or subcapsular region.
- Larger lesions may contain areas of hemorrhage, cystic change, and calcification.
- Adjacent adrenal cortex is of normal thickness (in contrast to atrophic changes seen adjacent to functional adenomas).

Adrenal Cortical Carcinomas

- Highly malignant neoplasms, usually of large size at the time of diagnosis.
- Predominantly yellow on cut surface but usually contain areas of hemorrhage, cystic change, and necrosis.
- Histologically, cells range from well-differentiated to markedly anaplastic; may be difficult to differentiate from metastatic carcinoma (e.g., metastatic bronchogenic carcinoma).
- Commonly invade vascular channels, with metastases to regional and periaortic lymph nodes, and to viscera, especially lung.

ADRENAL MEDULLA

Most adrenomedullary disorders are *neoplasms,* the most significant of which are pheochromocytoma, neuroblastoma, and ganglioneuroma. Neuroblastomas and ganglioneuromas are discussed elsewhere.

PHEOCHROMOCYTOMA (p. 1162)

- A relatively uncommon neoplasm associated with *catecholamine production* and *hypertension* (accounts for 0.1% to 0.3% of all cases of hypertension). May occasionally produce biogenic steroids or peptides, with resultant Cushing's syndrome or other endocrine disorder.
- *Eighty-five per cent arise within adrenal medulla;* remainder may occur anywhere within extra-adrenal paraganglion system; chromaffin-negative, extra-adrenal tumors are often designated *paragangliomas.*
- May occur *sporadically* (90%), or in association with *familial syndromes* (usually autosomal dominant), including

  - *MEN II or IIa* (pheochromocytomas and adrenal medullary hyperplasia, medullary carcinomas and C-cell hyperplasia of thyroid, parathyroid hyperplasia).
  - *MEN III or IIb* (pheochromocytomas and medullary thyroid hyperplasia, medullary carcinomas and C-cell hyperplasia of thyroid, mucosal neuromas, marfanoid features).
  - *von Hippel–Lindau* (visceral cysts, renal cell carcinomas, pheochromocytomas, angiomatosis, cerebellar hemangioblastoma).
  - *von Recklinghausen* (neurofibromatosis, cafè au lait spots, schwannomas, meningiomas, gliomas, pheochromocytomas).
  - Sturge-Weber (cavernous hemangiomas in trigeminal nerve distribution, pheochromocytomas).

- Most *sporadic lesions* occur in adulthood (40 to 60 years) with slight female predominance; *familial lesions* may arise in childhood, with strong *male predominance.*
- *Bilateral lesions* in 10% to 15% of sporadic cases, and in 70% of familial cases.
- *Malignancy* in 2% to 10% of adrenal lesions, and in 20% to 40% of extra-adrenal tumors.

MORPHOLOGY. Vary widely in size (1 gm to 4 kg); cut surface is usually pale gray or brown, often associated with hemorrhage, necrosis, or cystic change. Usually highly vascular. Fixation of tumor in a dichromate fixative (e.g., Zenker's), tumor turns brown-black due to oxidation of catecholamines (hence the term "chromaffin").

- *Microscopically,* composed of mature medullary-type cells containing basophilic cytoplasmic granules, arrayed in trabeculae or small nests; some tumors may be composed of predominantly spindle cells or small cells. Cellular and nuclear pleomorphism are common. *There are no reliable histologic predictors of malignancy:* pleomorphism, mitotic activity, and intravascular neoplastic cells may be seen in benign neoplasms. The only reliable criterion of malignancy is metastasis, most commonly to lymph nodes, liver, lungs, and bones.

CLINICAL FEATURES. Manifested by *hypertension* (sustained or intermittent) that may be associated with other organ dysfunction, including congestive heart failure, myocardial infarcts, cardiac arrhythmias, and cerebral hemorrhage. Cardiac complications attributed to ischemic myocardial damage (focal areas of myocytolysis, myofiber necrosis, scarring, and mononuclear infiltrates) secondary to catecholamine-induced vasoconstriction ("catecholamine cardiomyopathy"). Paroxysmal release of catecholamines may also be associated with episodic headache, anxiety, sweating, tremor, visual disturbances, abdominal pain, and nausea.

- Preoperative diagnosis is based on laboratory evaluation, including measurement of urinary catecholamines and their metabolites, plasma catecholamine assays, and radiographic imaging studies (CT, MRI, ultrasound).

TUMORS OF EXTRA-ADRENAL PARAGANGLIA (p. 1165)

- Uncommon neoplasms; most common in second to third decades. *Multicentric* in 15% to 25% of cases.
- Terminology unsettled. Related terms include *extra-adrenal pheochromocytoma* for functional (i.e., catecholamine-producing) tumors, and *chemodectoma* for lesions arising in carotid and jugulotympanic bodies.
- *Malignant* in 10% to 40% of cases; 10% metastasize widely.

MORPHOLOGY. Usually firm, 1- to 6-cm lesions, often densely adherent to adjacent tissues. Composed of well-differentiated neuroendocrine cells arrayed in nests (*Zellballen*) or cords, separated by prominent fibrovascular stroma. May contain mitotic figures and may exhibit substantial pleomorphism.

THYMUS

DEVELOPMENTAL DISORDERS (p. 1166)

- *Thymic hypoplasia* or *aplasia.*

  - Seen in *DiGeorge's syndrome,* accompanied by parathyroid hypoplasia/aplasia.
  - Characterized by absence or severe lack of *cell-mediated immunity* and *hypoparathyroidism.*
  - May be accompanied by developmental defects involving heart and great vessels.

- *Thymic cysts.*

  - Uncommon lesions, usually discovered incidentally.
  - Probably congenital.
  - Lined by columnar or stratified squamous epithelium.
  - Usually not clinically significant.

THYMIC HYPERPLASIA (p. 1166)

- Refers to the presence of *lymphoid follicles* distributed *diffusely* within the thymus.
- Gland may be of normal size.
- Morphology of follicles is identical to that in lymph nodes, with germinal centers containing B cells and dendritic reticular cells.
- Encountered most frequently (65% to 75% of cases) in association with *myasthenia gravis,* where B-cell hyperplasia may

contribute to the development of autoantibodies to acetylcholine receptors in skeletal muscle; similar thymic changes may be encountered in Graves' disease, SLE, systemic sclerosis, rheumatoid arthritis, and other autoimmune disorders.

THYMOMAS (p. 1167)

- Designates a neoplasm of *thymic epithelial cells;* should not be used to designate other neoplasms arising in thymus (e.g., Hodgkin's disease, non-Hodgkin's lymphoma, germ cell tumors, carcinoids, and others). Basic subtypes include

  - *Benign thymoma*—cytologically and biologically benign.
  - *Malignant thymoma:*
    Type I—cytologically benign but biologically aggressive
    Type II—cytologically and biologically malignant

- Most common in adults older than 40 years; males and females affected equally.
- Most occur in anterior or superior mediastinum; may occur in neck, thyroid, pulmonary hilus.

MORPHOLOGY

- *Grossly,* appear as lobulated, firm, gray-white masses; may measure up to 15 to 20 cm. Calcification and cystic change may be present. Twenty per cent to 25% demonstrate locally *infiltrative* growth.
- *Microscopically,* composed of a variable mixture of neoplastic epithelial cells and non-neoplastic lymphocytes. *Benign thymomas* are composed of elongated or spindle-shaped cells similar to normal thymic medullary cells ("medullary thymoma"), sometimes admixed with plumper, cortical-type cells ("mixed thymoma"). *Malignant thymoma type I* (20% to 25% of all thymomas) may be similar to benign variants; the distinction from benign thymoma is based on penetration of the capsule of the tumor and invasion of adjacent structures. *Malignant thymoma type II,* or *thymic carcinomas* (5% of all thymomas) are obviously invasive. Most are squamous cell carcinomas of varying differentiation; other patterns include sarcomatoid, basaloid, clear cell, and "lymphoepithelioma" variants, the latter associated with Epstein-Barr virus genome.

PINEAL GLAND

Pineal region neoplasms account for less than 1% of brain tumors; they include both *germ cell* tumors and neoplasms of *pineal parenchymal* origin.

PINEALOMAS (p. 1169)

- Classified as *pineoblastomas* or *pineocytomas,* depending on the level of differentiation.
- *Pineoblastomas* occur predominantly in the pediatric population and are composed of *primitive neuroectodermal cells* reminiscent of cerebellar medulloblastoma. They may *invade* local structures and *metastasize* via CSF pathways. Most patients die within 1 to 2 years.
- *Pineocytomas* are more common in adults and are composed

of a variable mixture of *glial* and *neuronal* elements, recapitulating the structure of the mature pineal gland. Prolonged survival (average 7 years).

MULTIPLE ENDOCRINE NEOPLASIA (p. 1169)

Usually *autosomal dominant* syndromes characterized by hyperplasia or tumors of several endocrine glands simultaneously. Variants include

MEN I (Wermer's) Syndrome

- Involvement of parathyroid, pancreas, and pituitary.
- *Parathyroid hyperplasia* or *multiple adenomas* are seen in 90% to 95% of cases, causing hypercalcemia and renal stones.
- *Pancreatic islet cell lesions,* including adenomas, carcinomas, and hyperplasia, are seen in a third of patients, and account for most deaths. Secretory products include gastrin (Zollinger-Ellison syndrome), insulin (hypoglycemia), serotonin, vasoactive intestinal polypeptide.
- *Pituitary adenomas* are present in 10% to 15% of cases, usually nonfunctional.
- Etiology may involve mutation in chromosome 11q11-q13, with loss of tumor suppressor gene on chromosome 11.

MEN II (Sipple's) Syndrome (MEN IIa)

- Genetically distinct from MEN I; sometimes designated "medullary thyroid carcinoma–pheochromocytoma" syndrome.
- *Medullary thyroid carcinomas* are usually multifocal and usually dominate the syndrome; C-cell hyperplasia may also be present. In addition to *calcitonin,* medullary carcinomas may elaborate other biologically active peptides. Most pursue a malignant course.
- *Pheochromocytomas* are present in 50% of patients; often bilateral and extra-adrenal. Most lesions are benign.
- *Parathyroid hyperplasia* or *adenoma* occurs in 10% of cases.
- Etiology likely involves germ line mutations of the *RET proto-oncogene* on chromosome 10q11.2, identifiable in medullary carcinomas and pheochromocytomas of MEN II (not in parathyroid lesions).
- Mean survival six to seven decades.

MEN IIb or III

- Similar to *MEN IIa,* with additional feature of *neuromas* or *ganglioneuromas* involving lips, oral cavity, eyes, respiratory tract, GI tract, urinary bladder, and other sites.
- May be accompanied by marfanoid body habitus and parathyroid hyperplasia.
- Presenting clinical manifestations often referable to neuromas; mean survival shorter than MEN IIa (three to four decades).
- Etiology of familial cases likely related to *RET* proto-oncogene mutation, different from that in MEN IIa; 50% of cases are *sporadic.*

CHAPTER TWENTY-TWO

The Skin

DEFINITION OF TERMS

Macroscopic

Macule Flat, circumscribed area distinguished from surrounding skin by coloration.

Papule Elevated solid area ≤ 5 mm.

Nodule Elevated solid area > 5 mm.

Plaque Elevated flat-topped lesion > 5 mm.

Vesicle Elevated fluid-filled lesion ≤ 5 mm.

Bulla Elevated fluid-filled lesion > 5 mm.

Blister Common term for vesicle or bulla.

Pustule Discrete, pus-filled raised area.

Wheal Pruritic, erythematous elevated area resulting from dermal edema.

Scale Dry, plate-like excrescence resulting from aberrant cornification.

Lichenification Thick, rough skin with prominent skin markings, usually secondary to repeated rubbing.

Excoriation Linear, traumatic lesion resulting in epidermal breakage (i.e., a deep scratch).

Onycholysis Loss of nail substance.

Microscopic

Hyperkeratosis Stratum cornea hyperplasia, often with aberrant keratinization.

Parakeratosis Retention of nuclei in stratum corneum; normal on mucous membranes.

Acanthosis Epidermal hyperplasia.

Dyskeratosis Abnormal keratinization below the stratum granulosum.

Acantholysis Loss of intercellular connections between keratinocytes.

Papillomatosis Elongation or widening of the dermal papillae.

Lentiginous Linear pattern of melanocyte proliferation within the epidermal basal cell layer; may be reactive or neoplastic.

Spongiosis Epidermal intercellular edema.

Exocytosis Inflammatory cells infiltrating the epidermis.

Erosion Focal, incomplete loss of epidermis.

Ulceration Focal complete loss of epidermis; may include dermis and subcutaneous fat.

Vacuolization Vacuoles within or adjacent to cells.

DISORDERS OF PIGMENTATION AND MELANOCYTES (p. 1175)

VITILIGO

A common disorder presenting as irregular, well-demarcated macules (few to many centimeters) devoid of pigmentation. It occurs in all races but is most apparent in darkly pigmented individuals. It often involves the wrists, axilla, and perioral, periorbital, and anogenital regions.

Pathogenetic theories include (1) autoimmunity (best supported by the data, including melanocyte autoantibodies and T-cell abnormalities); (2) neurohumoral factors; and (3) toxic intermediates in melanin synthesis.

Histologically, loss of melanocytes is seen on electron microscopy (EM). This contrasts with some forms of *albinism* in which melanocytes are present but nonfunctional.

FRECKLE (EPHELIS) (p. 1176)

Common pigmented lesions of childhood; tan-red to brown macules, 1 to 10 mm, occurring after sun exposure, fading and recurring with subsequent cycles of winter and summer.

Histologically, there is a normal melanocyte number (? slight hypertrophy) but increased melanin within basal keratinocytes.

MELASMA (p. 1176)

Masklike facial hyperpigmentation, typically seen in hyperestrogenic states such as pregnancy. It presents as blotchy, irregular, ill-defined macules. Sunlight accentuates the pigmentation, which usually fades postpartum. It is caused by enhanced melanin transfer from melanocytes to other cell types with subsequent accumulation.

Histologically, characterized by either

- Increased melanin deposition in basal layers (*epidermal type*) or
- Papillary dermal macrophage phagocytosis of melanin released from the epidermis: i.e., pigment incontinence (*dermal type*).

LENTIGO (p. 1176)

Common, benign, hyperpigmented macules (5 to 10 mm) in skin and mucous membranes, most often in infancy and childhood; in contrast to freckles, they do not darken with sun exposure. The etiology and pathogenesis are unknown.

Histologically, there is linear basal hyperpigmentation due to melanocyte hyperplasia, often with elongation and thinning of rete ridges.

NEVOCELLULAR NEVUS (PIGMENTED NEVUS, MOLE) (p. 1176)

Nevus denotes any congenital skin lesion; *nevocellular nevus specifically refers to a group of congenital or acquired melanocyte neoplasms* having different histologic characteristics. Clinically, common acquired nevocellular nevi are well-demarcated, uniformly tan-brown papules ≤ 6 mm; features of common variants are described in Table 22–1.

Table 22-1. Variant Forms of Nevocellular Nevi

Nevus Variant	Diagnostic Architectural Features	Diagnostic Cytologic Features	Clinical Significance
Congenital nevus	Deep dermal and sometimes subcutaneous growth around adnexae, neurovascular bundles, and blood vessel walls	Identical to ordinary acquired nevi	Present at birth; large variants have increased melanoma risk
Blue nevus	Non-nested dermal infiltration, often with associated fibrosis	Highly dendritic, heavily pigmented nevus cells	Black-blue nodule; often confused with melanoma clinically
Spindle and epithelioid cell nevus (Spitz's nevus)	Fascicular growth	Large, plump cells with pink-blue cytoplasm; fusiform cells	Common in children; red-pink nodule; often confused with hemangioma clinically
Halo nevus	Lymphocytic infiltration surrounding nevus cells	Identical to ordinary acquired nevi	Host immune response against nevus cells and surrounding normal melanocytes
Dysplastic nevus	Large, coalescent intraepidermal nests	Cytologic atypia	Potential precursor of malignant melanoma

From Cotran, R. S., Kumar, V., and Robbins, S. L.: Robbins Pathologic Basis of Disease. 5th ed. Philadelphia, W. B. Saunders Co., 1994, p. 1178.

The melanocytes of nevocellular nevi derive from basal dendritic cells that differentiate into round-to-oval cells with uniform nuclei and prominent nucleoli.

NATURAL HISTORY

- Begin as well-defined nests along the dermoepidermal (DE) junction: *junctional nevi.* A lentigo-like (lentiginous) melanocyte proliferation may also be present.
- With time, extension of melanocytes forms nests within both dermis and epidermis: *compound nevi.*
- Eventually, the epidermal component is lost, resulting in *dermal nevi.*
- With progressive dermal downgrowth, the *nevus cells undergo maturation* to resemble neural tissue.

Benign nevi can be distinguished from malignant melanoma on the basis of this normal maturation sequence.

DYSPLASTIC NEVI (p. 1177)

Found in persons with an autosomal dominant (susceptibility gene on chromosome 1) predisposition to develop acquired nevi; these may evolve into malignant melanoma (50% of affected individuals by age 59 years). May also occur as isolated sporadic lesions with a low risk of malignant transformation.

Typically, these are larger than acquired nevi (>5 mm) and may occur as hundreds of irregular macules/plaques with pigment variegation on both sun-exposed and nonexposed skin (unlike typical moles).

The risk of developing melanoma (*heritable melanoma syndrome*) is increased for unaffected skin as well as for areas with pre-existing nevi; however, most dysplastic nevi are clinically stable.

Histologically, there is cytologic and architectural atypia, with enlarged and fused epidermal nevus cell nests, lentiginous hyperplasia, linear dermoepidermal junction fibrosis, and pigment incontinence.

MALIGNANT MELANOMA (p. 1179)

A relatively common neoplasm, currently increasing in incidence; sun exposure is an important pathogenic factor, and lightly pigmented individuals are at greater risk than darkly pigmented persons. Hereditary substrates (e.g., dysplastic nevus syndrome) also increase the risk.

These are pruritic, variegated, irregular maculopapular lesions most commonly on skin, but occasionally involving the mucosa, conjunctiva, orbit (see below), nail beds, esophagus, and leptomeninges.

Diagnostically important is a change in coloration. Typically, a melanoma initially extends horizontally within the epidermis and superficial dermis (*radial growth phase*) during which it does not metastasize. Specific types of radial growth phase melanomas (e.g., *lentigo maligna* and *superficial spreading*) are defined by architectural and cytologic features and exhibit different biologic behaviors. Eventually a *vertical growth phase* evolves, with extension into the deep dermis, loss of cellular maturation, and development of the capacity to metastasize. The clinical behavior (e.g., *probability of metastasis*) is determined by the characteristics and measured depth of invasion of the vertical growth; prediction of the clinical outcome may be further refined

by determination of mitotic rates and the degree of lymphocytic infiltrate.

Histologically, melanoma cells are larger than nevus cells, with
irregular nuclei and prominent eosinophilic nucleoli; they grow
as loose nests lacking the typical features of melanocyte maturation.

MELANOMA OF THE EYE. Represents about 5% of all melanomas, arising most commonly in melanocytes of the uvea (iris,
ciliary body, and choroid). These are composed of either cohesive
spindle cells or poorly cohesive *epithelioid cells,* or a mixture
thereof. Lesions predominated by spindle cells have a good
prognosis (15-year survival of 75%); epithelioid lesions are aggressive and frequently metastasize despite early enucleation
(15-year survival of 35%).

BENIGN EPITHELIAL TUMORS (p. 1181)

Common, generally biologically inconsequential lesions derived
from keratinocytes or skin appendages.

SEBORRHEIC KERATOSES (p. 1181)

Spontaneous lesions, most often in middle-aged and older individuals, and most numerous on the trunk. Similar smaller facial
lesions in blacks are called *dermatosis papulosa nigra.*

They may occur spontaneously in large numbers as part of a
paraneoplastic syndrome (*sign of Leser-Trélat*), ? due to tumor
elaboration of growth factors (e.g., transforming growth factor-
alpha).

Macroscopically, they are uniform, tan-brown, velvety/granu-
lar, round plaques millimeters to several centimeters in diameter;
keratin-filled plugs may be evident.

Histologically, they are sharply demarcated, exophytic lesions
with hyperplasia of variably pigmented basaloid cells and *hyperkeratosis;* there are occasional keratin-filled "horn cysts."

ACANTHOSIS NIGRICANS (p. 1182)

Thickened, hyperpigmented zones, typically in flexural areas (axilla, groin, neck, anogenital region), associated with benign and
malignant conditions elsewhere in the body.

The *benign* type makes up 80% of all cases; it develops
gradually, usually arising in childhood through puberty, and occurs

- As an autosomal dominant trait with variable penetrance.
- In association with obesity or endocrine disorders (especially
  diabetes and pituitary or pineal tumors).
- As part of a number of rare congenital disorders.

The *malignant* type arises in middle-aged and older individuals, often in association with an occult adenocarcinoma (? tumor
elaboration of epidermal growth factors).

Histologically, both types are characterized by hyperkeratosis,
with prominent rete ridges and basal hyperpigmentation (without
melanocyte hyperplasia).

FIBROEPITHELIAL POLYP (p. 1182)

Also called *acrochordon, squamous papilloma,* or *skin tag,* this
is an exceptionally common benign lesion in middle-aged and

older individuals, found on the neck, trunk, face, or intertriginous zones. It is a soft, flesh-colored tumor attached by a slender stalk, with a fibrovascular core covered by benign epidermis.

It may be associated with pregnancy, diabetes, or intestinal polyposis.

EPITHELIAL CYST (WEN) (p. 1182)

Common lesions presenting as well-circumscribed, firm, subcutaneous nodules; formed by downgrowth and cystic expansion of the epidermal or follicular epithelium.

Histologically, they are subdivided on the basis of the cyst wall characteristics. All are filled with keratin and variable amounts of lipid and debris from sebaceous secretions.

- *Epidermal inclusion cysts.* The wall is almost identical to normal epidermis.
- *Pilar (trichilemmal) cysts.* The wall resembles follicular epithelium (i.e., without a granular cell layer).
- *Dermoid cysts.* The wall is much like epidermis but with multiple skin appendages, especially hair follicles.
- *Steatocystoma multiplex.* The wall resembles sebaceous gland ductal epithelium with numerous compressed sebaceous lobules; frequently of dominant inheritance.

KERATOACANTHOMA (p. 1183)

A self-limited, *spontaneously healing,* rapidly growing lesion, typically in sun-exposed skin of Caucasians 50 years of age and older, in men more often than in women.

Macroscopically, they are flesh-colored, superficial lesions of several centimeters with central keratin-filled craters, often on the face or hands.

Histologically, they are cup-shaped epithelial proliferations, often with atypical cells, enclosing a central keratin-filled plug. The pattern of keratinization recapitulates the normal hair follicle (no granular cell layer), suggesting a follicular epithelium origin. Minimal inflammation is present during the rapid proliferative phase, but as the lesion evolves there is a dermal inflammatory and fibrotic reaction, and eventual regression and disappearance.

ADNEXAL (APPENDAGE) TUMORS (p. 1183)

A large family of benign neoplasms (although malignant variants do exist). Some have mendelian patterns of inheritance; others may indicate visceral malignancy (e.g., multiple trichilemmomas and breast cancer: *Cowden's syndrome*).

Most are single or multiple nondescript papules and nodules. Occasionally there is a site predilection (e.g., *eccrine poromas* on palms and soles).

Cylindromas typically occur as multiple coalescing nodules on the forehead and scalp. They may be dominantly inherited and appear early in life. *Histologically,* they display apocrine differentiation with islands of basaloid cells within a fibrous matrix.

Syringomas usually occur as multiple, small, tan papules near the lower eyelids. *Microscopically,* they are composed of tadpole-shaped islands of basaloid epithelium with focal eccrine differentiation.

Trichoepitheliomas, which may be dominantly inherited, usually present as multiple semitransparent papules on the face, scalp, neck, and upper trunk, composed of proliferations of basaloid cells forming hair follicle–like structures.

Trichilemmomas are proliferations of cells resembling hair follicle infundibulum.

Malignant variants of adnexal tumors also exist, e.g., *sebaceous carcinoma* arising in meibomian glands of the eyelid.

PREMALIGNANT AND MALIGNANT EPIDERMAL TUMORS

ACTINIC KERATOSIS (p. 1185)

A premalignant dysplastic lesion associated with chronic sun exposure, especially in light-skinned individuals. Ionizing radiation, hydrocarbons, and arsenicals may induce similar lesions.

Macroscopically, these are less than 1 cm, tan-brown, red, or flesh-colored, with a rough consistency. Hyperkeratosis may produce cutaneous horns.

Histologically, there is cytologic atypia in the lower epidermis, frequently with basal cell hyperplasia and dyskeratosis. Intercellular bridges are present. *Hyperkeratosis* and *parakeratosis* may be present, or there may be epidermal atrophy. The dermis contains thickened, blue-gray elastic fibers (*elastosis*), due to aberrant synthesis by sun-damaged fibroblasts.

Since many undergo malignant transformation, local eradication is indicated.

SQUAMOUS CELL CARCINOMA (p. 1186)

The most common tumor of sun-exposed skin of older individuals; it is more frequent in men than in women with the exception of lower leg lesions.

Sunlight (specifically ultraviolet [UV] irradiation) is the most commonly accepted predisposing factor. It directly causes DNA damage and also exerts an immunosuppressive effect by injuring antigen-presenting Langerhans' cells in the epidermis. Other predisposing factors include industrial carcinogens, chronic skin ulcers, old burn scars, draining osteomyelitis, ionizing radiation, and (for oral mucosa) tobacco or betel nut chewing. Immunosuppression (as a consequence of chemotherapy or tissue transplantation) and xeroderma pigmentosum (an inherited defect in DNA repair, *see Chapter 7*) also increase the risk of tumor. Human papilloma virus (HPV 36) occasionally may play a role as well.

Grossly, in situ squamous cell carcinoma appears as well-demarcated, red, scaling plaques. *Invasive lesions* are nodular, variably hyperkeratotic, and prone to ulceration. Mucosal involvement is manifested as white thickening called *leukoplakia.* Most tumors remain localized. Less than 5% have metastasized to regional nodes at the time of resection.

Microscopically, in situ carcinoma has full-thickness epidermal atypia (versus actinic keratosis which has only basal atypia). Invasive tumors vary from well differentiated (with prominent keratinization) to highly anaplastic with necrosis and abortive keratinization.

BASAL CELL CARCINOMA (p. 1187)

Common, slow-growing tumors, typically in sun-exposed skin; *they rarely metastasize.* Immunosuppression and xeroderma pigmentosum increase the incidence.

Basal cell nevus syndrome is a rare, dominantly inherited trait with numerous basal cell carcinomas in early life, as well as bone, nervous system, eye, and reproductive organ anomalies.

Grossly, basal cell carcinomas appear as pearly papules or expanding plaques; some are melanin pigmented. Advanced lesions ulcerate and there is extensive local invasion, hence the term *"rodent ulcer."*

Microscopically, there is basal cell proliferation, either as *multifocal superficial growths* over a large area (several centimeters) of skin or as *nodules* extending deeply into the dermis.

MERKEL CELL CARCINOMA (p. 1187)

A rare neoplasm of epidermal, neural crest–derived *Merkel cells,* involved in tactile sensation in lower animals. These potentially lethal tumors are composed of small, round malignant cells containing neurosecretory-type cytoplasmic granules and closely resemble small cell carcinoma in the lung.

TUMORS OF DERMIS

BENIGN FIBROUS HISTIOCYTOMA (p. 1188)

A heterogeneous group of benign, indolent neoplasms of dermal fibroblasts and histiocytes. Usually seen in adults and frequently on the legs of young to middle-aged women. The histogenesis is unknown, although antecedent trauma and aberrant healing are often implicated. Should not be confused with clinically aggressive malignant fibrous histiocytoma, arising in skin and extracutaneous cells.

Grossly, these are tan-brown, firm papules, sometimes tender, that may achieve several centimeters in diameter. Lateral compression causes these to dimple inward.

Histologically, the most common form is the *dermatofibroma* composed of spindle-shaped fibroblasts in a well-defined though nonencapsulated mass in the mid-dermis, frequently extending into the subcutaneous fat. Other variants have conspicuous foamy histiocytes with fewer fibroblasts, or have numerous blood vessels and hemosiderin deposits (*sclerosing hemangioma*).

DERMATOFIBROSARCOMA PROTUBERANS (p. 1189)

A well-differentiated, slow-growing fibrosarcoma of the skin that is locally aggressive but rarely metastasizes.

Grossly, these are firm solid nodules arising as protuberant, occasionally ulcerated aggregates within an indurated plaque, typically on the trunk.

Microscopically, these are cellular neoplasms composed of radially oriented (storiform) fibroblasts; mitoses are not as numerous as in fibrosarcoma. The overlying epidermis is thinned and there often is microscopic extension into subcutaneous fat.

XANTHOMAS (p. 1189)

Not true neoplasms, but rather focal accumulations of foamy histiocytes. They may be idiopathic or associated with familial or acquired hyperlipidemias, or lymphoproliferative disorders. They may be subdivided on the basis of the gross appearance and an associated form of hyperlidemia:

ERUPTIVE XANTHOMA. Sudden showers of yellow papules that wax and wane with plasma triglyceride and lipid levels; they occur on the buttocks, posterior thighs, knees, and elbows (*hyperlipidemia types I, IIB, III, IV, and V*).

TUBEROUS XANTHOMA. Yellow, flat-to-round nodules over the joints, especially knees and elbows (*types IIA and III*).

TENDINOUS XANTHOMA. Yellow nodules over the Achilles tendon and finger extensor tendons (*types IIA and III*).

PLANE XANTHOMA. Linear yellow lesions in skin folds, especially palmar creases (*type III*). Occasionally associated with primary biliary cirrhosis (*type IIA*).

Xanthelasma. Soft yellow plaques on the eyelids (*types IIA and III, or without lipid abnormality*).

All are characterized by variably cellular dermal aggregates of macrophages with vacuolated cytoplasm containing cholesterol, phospholipids, and triglycerides.

DERMAL VASCULAR TUMORS (p. 1189)

Hemangiomas and malignant vascular tumors, Kaposi's sarcoma, and bacillary angiomatosis are discussed in *Chapter 11.*

TUMORS OF CELLULAR IMMIGRANTS TO THE SKIN (p. 1190)

Proliferative disorders of cells arising elsewhere but which have homed to the skin.

HISTIOCYTOSIS X (p. 1190)

The systemic pattern is discussed in *Chapter 14.* The *cutaneous form* may present as solitary or multiple papules or nodules or may occur as scaling erythematous plaques resembling seborrheic dermatitis.

Histologic lesions frequently include variable numbers of eosinophils and may show different patterns:

- Diffuse dermal infiltrates of mononuclear cells with bland, indented nuclei.
- Similar cells clustered to resemble granulomas.
- Dermal infiltrates composed of mononuclear cells with foamy cytoplasm.

Ultrastructural demonstration of Birbeck granules and immunohistochemical documentation of CD1 antigens on the infiltrating cells confirms their Langerhans' cell derivation.

MYCOSIS FUNGOIDES (CUTANEOUS T-CELL LYMPHOMA) (p. 1190)

Occurs in various patterns including (1) *mycosis fungoides (MF)*; (2) a nodular eruptive variant, *mycosis fungoides d'emblée*; and (3) a form with an aggressive course called *adult T-cell leukemia* or *lymphoma* (attributed to HTLV-1).

MF is a lymphoproliferative disorder that arises primarily in the skin, but may eventually seed the blood (*Sézary's syndrome*) and evolve into a more generalized T-cell leukemia or lymphoma.

Grossly, MF initially presents as eczema-like lesions, evolving into scaly, red-brown patches or plaques, and eventually into nodules (up to 10 cm) on the trunk, extremities, face, and scalp. Nodular cutaneous growth correlates with deep dermal invasion and the onset of lymph node and visceral involvement.

The *histologic hallmark* of MF is the *Sezary-Lutzner cell,* a malignant CD4-positive (T-helper) cell with a hyperconvoluted or "cerebriform" nucleus. These typically form bandlike dermal infiltrates with invasion of single cells or small clusters into the epidermis (*Pautrier's microabscesses*).

MASTOCYTOSIS (p. 1192)

A family of rare disorders characterized by cutaneous (and occasionally visceral) mast cell proliferation. Symptoms reflect the consequences of mast cell degranulation, with release of histamine and heparin.

- Pruritus and flushing, triggered by specific foods, temperature changes, alcohol, or certain drugs.
- Rhinorrhea.
- Dermal edema and erythema (*wheal*) when lesional skin (*Darier's sign*) or normal skin (*dermatographism*) is rubbed.
- Rarely epistaxis or gastrointestinal bleeding secondary to the effects of heparin release.

Urticaria pigmentosa (50% of all cases) is an exclusively cutaneous form, with a generally favorable prognosis, occurring mainly in children. In 10% of patients, usually adults, there is systemic mastocytosis, which carries a much poorer prognosis.

Grossly, skin lesions of urticaria pigmentosa and systemic mastocytosis are multiple, round-to-oval, nonscaling, red-brown papules and plaques. *Microscopically,* there are variable dermal fibrosis, edema, eosinophils, and mast cells, the latter distinguishable by special metachromatic stains.

ACUTE INFLAMMATORY DERMATOSES
(p. 1192)

A large family of conditions characterized by short-lived lesions (days to weeks), marked by mononuclear cell infiltrates with associated edema and occasionally local tissue damage.

URTICARIA (HIVES) (p. 1192)

A common disorder characterized by focal mast cell degranulation, with histamine-mediated dermal pruritus, edema, and wheal. It typically occurs in young adults. Individual lesions develop and regress within hours, but sequential lesions may appear for months. *Angioedema* is related but is characterized by dermal and *subcutaneous fat* edema.

Microscopically, there is a sparse mononuclear perivascular infiltrate with edema, but no evidence of increased mast cell numbers.

Most lesions are mediated by antigen-specific IgE, but *IgE-independent urticaria* can occur by direct chemical-induced mast cell degranulation in sensitive patients, or by suppression of prostaglandin synthesis (i.e., with aspirin). Persistent urticaria may reflect an inability to clear the inciting antigen or may announce cryptic collagen-vascular disorders or Hodgkin's disease.

Hereditary angioneurotic edema consists of recurrent attacks of angioedema with GI tract and laryngeal involvement. It is due to deficient C1 esterase inhibitor and unregulated activation of the early complement components.

ACUTE ECZEMATOUS DERMATITIS (p. 1193)

A variety of pathogenetically different conditions, all with similar histologic features. Five primary types of *eczema* are described in Table 22–2. Many forms constitute a cutaneous delayed-type hypersensitivity response, with pathogenesis attributed to cytokine release and nonspecific recruitment of the bulk of the inflammatory cells.

Grossly, all types of acute eczema are pruritic, red, papulovesicular to blistered, oozing, and subsequently crusted lesions (e.g., contact hypersensitivity to poison ivy). With chronic exposure, lesions may evolve into psoriasis-like scaling plaques.

Histologically, there is initially *spongiosis;* with progressive

Table 22–2. Classification of Eczematous Dermatitis

Type	Cause or Pathogenesis	Histology°	Clinical Features
Contact dermatitis	Topically applied chemicals Pathogenesis: delayed hypersensitivity	Spongiotic dermatitis	Marked itching or burning or both; requires antecedent exposure
Atopic dermatitis	Unknown, may be heritable	Spongiotic dermatitis	Erythematous plaques in flexural areas; family history of eczema, hay fever, or asthma
Drug-related eczematous dermatitis	Systemically administered (e.g., penicillin)	Spongiotic dermatitis; eosinophils often present in infiltrate; deeper infiltrate	Eruption occurs with administration of drug; remits when drug is discontinued
Photo-eczematous eruption	Ultraviolet light	Spongiotic dermatitis; deeper infiltrate	Occurs on sun-exposed skin; phototesting may help in diagnosis
Primary irritant dermatitis	Repeated trauma (rubbing)	Spongiotic dermatitis in early stages	Localized to site of trauma

°All types, with time, may develop chronic changes.
From Cotran, R. S., Kumar, V., and Robbins, S. L.: Robbins Pathologic Basis of Disease. 5th ed. Philadelphia, W. B. Saunders Co., 1994, p. 1194.

fluid accumulation, intraepidermal vesicles are formed. There is also a dermal perivascular lymphocytic infiltrate with mast cell degranulation and papillary dermal edema. Lesions due to drug hypersensitivity may have eosinophils. In chronic lesions, the vesicular phase is replaced with progressive *acanthosis* and *hyperkeratosis.*

ERYTHEMA MULTIFORME (p. 1195)

An uncommon, self-limited hypersensitivity response to certain drugs or infections, or to systemic disorders (malignancy or collagen vascular diseases), characterized by extensive epidermal degeneration and necrosis. It is presumably due to cell-mediated (CD8 + cytotoxic T cells) immune injury.

Grossly, lesions are "multiform" and include macules, papules, vesicles, and bullae, as well as characteristic "targets" consisting of red maculopapular lesions with central vesicular or eroded pallor. There is frequent symmetric involvement of the extremities.

A severe, febrile form typically occurring in children is called *Stevens-Johnson syndrome;* it is marked by erosions and hemorrhagic crusting of lips, oral mucosa, conjunctiva, urethra, and anogenital regions. Bacterial superinfection may be life threatening.

Toxic epidermal necrolysis is another variant, characterized by diffuse mucocutaneous epithelial necrosis and sloughing; it is clinically analogous to extensive third-degree burns.

Microscopically, early lesions of erythema multiforme show dermoepidermal junction and superficial perivascular lymphocytic infiltrates with dermal edema, and focal basal keratinocyte degeneration and necrosis. *Exocytosis* is associated with epidermal necrosis, blistering, and shallow erosions. *Target lesions* show central epidermal necrosis with a surrounding perivenular inflammation.

ERYTHEMA NODOSUM AND ERYTHEMA INDURATUM (p. 1196)

Both are forms of *panniculitis* or inflammation of subcutaneous fat, occurring often in the legs. Panniculitis may principally affect (1) connective tissue septa (erythema nodosum) or (2) fat lobules (erythema induratum) and may be acute or chronic.

Erythema nodosum is the most common form, typically with an acute onset, and may be idiopathic or occur in association with specific drugs, infections, sarcoidosis, inflammatory bowel disease, or visceral malignancy. Ill-defined, exquisitely tender erythematous nodules are noted, occasionally with fever and malaise. With time, old lesions flatten and become ecchymotic without scarring, while new lesions develop.

Deep-wedge biopsy shows distinctive early septal widening (edema, fibrin deposition, and neutrophil infiltration), followed by lymphohistiocytic infiltration (occasionally with giant cells and eosinophils) without vasculitis.

Erythema induratum is an uncommon form of panniculitis of unknown cause, typically affecting adolescents and menopausal women. It is believed to represent a primary vasculitis of subcutaneous fat with subsequent inflammation and necrosis of adipose tissue. It presents as an erythematous, slightly tender nodule that eventually ulcerates and scars.

Early lesions show necrotizing vasculitis in small- to medium-sized vessels in deep dermis and subcutis. Eventually, the fat lobules develop granulomatous inflammation and necrosis.

A rare form of panniculitis, *Weber-Christian disease* (*relapsing febrile nodular panniculitis*) seen as crops of erythematous plaques or nodules, mainly on the legs, associated with deep lymphohistiocytic infiltrates and occasional giant cells.

Factitial panniculitis (from self-administered foreign substances), deep mycotic infections in immunocompromised hosts, and occasionally disorders such as SLE may mimic the clinical and histologic appearance of primary panniculitis.

CHRONIC INFLAMMATORY DERMATOSES

(p. 1196)

Persistent inflammatory disorders (over months to years) characterized by scaling and shedding (*desquamation*); to be distinguished from *noninflammatory* scaling lesions, such as *hereditary ichthyosis* with fishlike scales secondary to a defect in stratum corneum adhesiveness.

PSORIASIS (p. 1197)

A common (1%–2% of all people in the U.S.) disorder. An association with certain HLA types suggests a genetic component; the genesis of new lesions at sites of trauma (*Koebner's phenomenon*) suggests a role for exogenous stimuli. Damage to the stratum corneum may induce the deposition of complement-fixing antibodies with secondary complement-mediated injury. Alternatively, psoriatic endothelium may be especially sensitive to cytokine-induced expression of adhesion molecules, with a subsequent enhanced neutrophil recruitment.

Psoriasis may be associated with other diseases, including myopathies, enteropathies, AIDS, or mild or deforming arthritis (resembling rheumatoid arthritis).

Grossly, the lesions are typically well-demarcated salmon pink plaques with silvery scaling; they usually occur on the elbows, knees, scalp, lumbosacral area, intergluteal cleft, and glans penis. *Annular, linear, gyrate,* or *serpiginous* variations occur.

- Psoriasis may also present as total body scaling and erythema: *erythroderma.*
- Nail changes (discoloration, pitting, onycholysis) occur in 30% of patients.
- *Pustular psoriasis* is a rare variant, which when generalized may be life threatening.

Microscopically, there is marked acanthosis with rete elongation and mitoses well above the basal layer. The stratum granulosum is thinned or absent, with extensive overlying parakeratosis.

Epidermis overlying dermal papillae is thinned; dilated vessels in these papillae yield pinpoint bleeds when the overlying scale is removed (*Auspitz sign*).

Aggregates of neutrophils in epidermis occur within small spongiotic foci in the stratum spinosum (*spongiform pustules*) or within the parakeratotic stratum corneum (*Munro's microabscesses*). Larger, abscess-like accumulations may also occur in pustular psoriasis.

LICHEN PLANUS (p. 1198)

A self-limited disease that after 1 to 2 years generally leaves only postinflammatory hyperpigmentation. Oral lesions may persist longer and occasionally become malignant.

The *pathogenesis* is unknown, but cell-mediated immune injury to basal cells is suspected. Koebner's phenomenon occurs in lichen planus.

Grossly, lesions are *pruritic, purple, polygonal papules* that may coalesce into plaques. They are often highlighted by white dots or lines called *Wickham's striae.*

Lesions are typically multiple and symmetrically distributed, often on the wrists and elbows, and on the glans penis; oral mucosal lesions are generally white and reticulated. A form with preferential involvement of hair follicle epithelium is called *lichen planopilaris.*

Histologically, there is a dense, band-like dermoepidermal junction lymphocytic infiltrate with basal cell degeneration and necrosis, and jagged rete "saw-toothing."

Necrotic basal cells may be sloughed into inflamed papillary dermis, forming *colloid* or *Civatte bodies.* Lesions are also typified by chronic changes, including acanthosis, hyperkeratosis, and thickening of the granular cell layer.

LUPUS ERYTHEMATOSUS (p. 1199)

Systemic lupus erythematosus (SLE) is detailed elsewhere (*see Chapter 6*). Discoid lupus erythematosus (*DLE*) *is a localized cutaneous form without systemic manifestations.* However, one-third of patients with SLE develop DLE-like skin pathology, so that evaluation of the cutaneous lesions *alone* does not distinguish the two entities.

The *pathogenesis* of DLE involves immune complex—mediated, and to a lesser extent cell-mediated injury to pigment-containing basal cells (*see also Chapter 6*). Sun exposure exacerbates the cutaneous lesions.

Grossly, skin lesions of both SLE and DLE include an ill-defined malar erythema (more characteristic of SLE) or sharply demarcated "discoid" erythematous scaling plaques with zones of irregular pigmentation and small keratotic plugs in hair follicles.

Microscopically, DLE is marked by dermoepidermal junction, perivascular, and periappendageal lymphocytic infiltrates. Preferential infiltration of subcutaneous fat is called *lupus profundus.* There are also basal cell vacuolization, epidermal atrophy, and variable hyperkeratosis.

By immunofluorescence, there is a *granular* band of immunoglobulin and complement along the dermoepidermal and dermal-follicular junctions (*lupus band test*).

ACNE VULGARIS (p. 1200)

A common, chronic, inflammatory dermatosis affecting hair follicles, typically in the middle to late teens, in males more often than in females, presumably secondary to hormonal changes and alterations in hair follicle maturation.

It may be induced or exacerbated by sex hormones, corticosteroids, occupational exposure (coal tars), or occlusive conditions (heavy clothes). There may be a heritable component.

The *pathogenesis* is speculative but may involve bacterial (*Propionibacterium acnes*) lipase degradation of sebaceous oils to highly irritating fatty acids. Antibiotics (e.g., tetracyclines) may be effective by inhibiting the lipase activity. The vitamin A derivative 13-cis-retinoic acid has also shown efficacy.

Grossly, noninflammatory acne is characterized by *open comedones* (follicular papules with central black keratin plugs) and *closed comedones* (follicular papules with central plugs trapped beneath the epidermis and therefore not visible). The latter may rupture with inflammation. *Inflammatory acne* shows erythematous papules, nodules, and pustules.

Histologically, comedones are composed of expanding vessels of lipid and keratin at the midportion of hair follicles, with follicular dilation and epithelial and sebaceous gland atrophy.

There is a variable lymphohistiocytic infiltrate, but with rupture, there is extensive acute and chronic inflammation, occasionally with ensuing scar formation.

BLISTERING (BULLOUS DISEASES) (p. 1201)

Primary blistering disorders, as opposed to vesicles and bullae that occur as a secondary phenomenon in a variety of unrelated conditions. Level of blister involvement within the skin is critical in diagnosis (Fig. 22–1).

PEMPHIGUS (p. 1201)

A rare, autoimmune disorder, typically in the fourth to sixth decades, with no sex predilection. Patients have circulating antibodies to keratinocyte intercellular cement components that bind and trigger release of plasminogen activator by keratinocytes.

There are four clinical and pathologic variants:

PEMPHIGUS VULGARIS. Accounts for 80% of pemphigus. Involves the oral mucosa, scalp, face, intertriginous zones, trunk, and pressure points. Lesions are superficial, easily ruptured blisters that leave shallow, crusted erosions. If untreated, it is almost uniformly fatal.

PEMPHIGUS VEGETANS. A rare form presenting with large, moist verrucous plaques studded with pustules, typically in flexural and intertriginous zones.

PEMPHIGUS FOLIACEUS. A more benign form occurring epidemically in South America and sporadically elsewhere. Lesions occur mainly on the face, scalp, and upper trunk. Bullae are extremely superficial, leaving only slight erythema and crusting after rupture.

PEMPHIGUS ERYTHEMATOSUS. A localized, milder variant of pemphigus foliaceus, typically involving only the malar zone on the face.

Microscopically, all variants are characterized by *acantholysis* leading to intercellular clefting and eventually broad-based, *intraepithelial* blisters. For *pemphigus vulgaris* and *vegetans,* the separation occurs immediately above the basal layer (suprabasal blister); in the foliaceus variant, only the stratum granulosum is involved.

With anti-immunoglobulin or anticomplement immunofluorescence, staining may be seen around each keratinocyte.

BULLOUS PEMPHIGOID (p. 1202)

A relatively common autoimmune vesiculobullous disease of skin and mucosa typically affecting elderly individuals, caused by

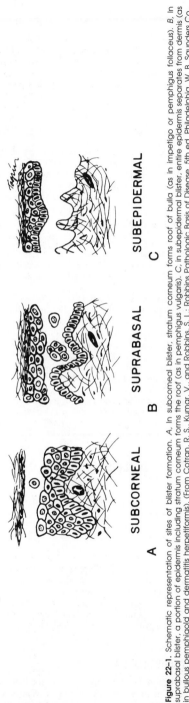

A. SUBCORNEAL

B. SUPRABASAL

C. SUBEPIDERMAL

Figure 22–1. Schematic representation of sites of blister formation. *A*, In subcorneal blister, stratum corneum forms roof of bulla (as in impetigo or pemphigus foliaceus). *B*, In suprabasal blister, a portion of epidermis including stratum corneum forms the roof (as in pemphigus vulgaris). *C*, In subepidermal blister, entire epidermis separates from dermis (as in bullous pemphigoid and dermatitis herpetiformis). (From Cotran, R. S., Kumar, V., and Robbins, S. L.: Robbins Pathologic Basis of Disease. 5th ed. Philadelphia, W. B. Saunders Co., 1994, p. 1202.)

473

circulating antibodies (with secondary complement activation and granulocyte recruitment) to an antigen of the *lamina lucida* in the epidermal basal membrane. Occasionally it may herald an underlying lymphoreticular neoplasm.

Macroscopically, there are tense bullae (up to 4 to 8 cm in diameter, containing clear fluid), typically on the inner thigh, forearm flexor surfaces, lower abdomen, and intertriginous zones; oral mucosa is involved in one third of patients. The blisters do not rupture as easily as those in pemphigus and, if uninfected, heal without scarring.

Microscopically, there is a *subepidermal nonacantholytic blister* with *linear* dermoepidermal junction staining for immunoglobulin and complement. There is a variable, mostly superficial, perivascular infiltrate of lymphocytes, eosinophils, and neutrophils.

DERMATITIS HERPETIFORMIS (p. 1203)

A rare disorder, typically in the third to fourth decades, in males more often than in females.

It is associated with specific HLA types and with celiac disease (*see Chapter 16*). Both cutaneous and GI lesions respond to a gluten-free diet.

Dermatitis herpetiformis is presumably mediated either by immune complex deposition in the skin or by antigliadin (gliadin is a protein in gluten) antibodies cross-reacting with junction-anchoring components (e.g., reticulin). By direct immunofluorescence, there are granular IgA deposits at the dermal papillae tips.

Grossly, intensely pruritic, urticarial plaques and vesicles, characteristically symmetric, involve the extensor surfaces, upper back, and buttocks.

Microscopically, neutrophils and fibrin accumulate in the tips of dermal papillae ("microabscesses") with overlying basal vacuolization and microscopic blisters coalescing to large *subepidermal* blisters.

NONINFLAMMATORY BLISTERING DISEASES
(p. 1205)

Primary disorders with vesicles and bullae not mediated by inflammatory mechanisms.

PORPHYRIA (p. 1205)

A group of inborn or acquired disturbances of porphyrin metabolism (there are five major types). Porphyrins are the ring structures that bind the metal ions in hemoglobin, myoglobin, and cytochromes. The pathogenesis is unknown. The cutaneous lesions consist of urticaria and vesicles that are exacerbated by sun exposure and heal without scarring. Histologically, there are subepidermal vesicles with associated marked superficial dermal vascular thickening.

EPIDERMOLYSIS BULLOSA (p. 1205)

A pathogenetically unrelated group of disorders that have in common blistering at pressure sites or trauma. The *junctional type* shows blistering at the lamina lucida in otherwise histologically normal skin. The scarring *dystrophic type* shows blistering beneath the lamina densa that presumably is due to defective anchoring fibrils. The *simplex type* results from epidermal basal cell degeneration.

INFECTION AND INFESTATION (p. 1205)

A representative sampling follows of common entities with primary clinical manifestations in the skin.

VERRUCAE (WARTS) (p. 1205)

Common, spontaneously regressing (in 6 months to 2 years) lesions, typically in children and adolescents. Caused by papilloma viruses, transmitted by direct contact.

They are subdivided on the basis of clinical morphology and anatomic location. Certain lesions are typically caused by particular papilloma virus types. For example, types 6, 11, 16, and 18 are associated with anogenital warts. Type 16 is associated with anogenital wart dysplasia and in situ squamous cell carcinoma of the genitalia.

VERRUCA VULGARIS. The most common type of wart, most frequently on the dorsum of the hand. *Grossly,* gray-white to tan, flat to convex, 0.1- to 1-cm papules with a rough pebbly surface.

VERRUCA PLANA (FLAT WART). Usually on the face or dorsum of the hand; grossly, flat, smooth, tan papules smaller than those of verruca vulgaris.

VERRUCA PLANTARIS (SOLES) OR PALMARIS (PALMS). Rough, scaly lesions 1 to 2 cm in diameter that may coalesce and be confused with calluses.

CONDYLOMA ACUMINATUM (ANOGENITAL AND VENEREAL WARTS). Soft, tan, cauliflower-like masses up to many centimeters in diameter.

Microscopically, all variants have undulant (verrucous) epidermal hyperplasia and superficial keratinocyte perinuclear vacuolization (*koilocytosis*). EM reveals numerous viral particles within nuclei.

MOLLUSCUM CONTAGIOSUM (p. 1206)

A common, self-limited disease caused by a poxvirus, transmitted by direct contact.

Grossly, firm, pruritic, pink to skin-colored, umbilicated papules 0.2 to 2 cm are seen typically on the trunk or anogenital regions. Cheesy material containing diagnostic *molluscum bodies* can be expressed from the central umbilications.

Microscopically, there is cuplike verrucous epidermal hyperplasia with pathognomonic *molluscum bodies*—large (35-μm) eosinophilic cytoplasmic inclusions in the stratum granulosum or stratum corneum containing numerous virions.

IMPETIGO (p. 1207—*see also Chapter 8*)

Streptococcal or staphylococcal skin infection seen in normal children or sick adults, especially on the face and hands. It begins as an erythematous macule that progresses to small pustules and eventually to a shallow erosion with a honey-colored crust.

Microscopically, there are subcorneal pustules filled with neutrophils and gram-positive cocci, with accompanying dermal inflammation. Pustule rupture releases serum and necrotic debris to form the characteristic crust.

SUPERFICIAL FUNGAL INFECTIONS (p. 1207)

Typically caused by dermatophytes (fungi growing in soil and on animals) and *confined to the nonviable stratum corneum*.

TINEA CAPITIS. Typically noted in children. Involves the scalp, causing asymptomatic hairless patches, associated with mild erythema, crusting, and scale.

TINEA BARBAE. Uncommon dermatophytosis of the beard area in adult men.

TINEA CORPORIS. Common superficial dermatophytosis of the body, especially in children. Predisposing factors are excessive heat or humidity, exposure to infected animals, or chronic dermatophytosis of the feet or nails. Typically presents with an expanding erythematous plaque with an elevated scaling border ("ringworm").

TINEA CRURIS. Typically in the inguinal areas of obese men during warm weather. Occurs as moist red patches with raised scaling borders.

TINEA PEDIS (ATHLETE'S FOOT). Characterized by erythema and scaling, beginning in the webbed spaces. Most of the inflammation is due to secondary bacterial superinfection.

ONYCHOMYCOSIS. Nail dermatophytosis characterized by discoloration, thickening, and deformity of the nail plate.

TINEA VERSICOLOR. Due to *Malassezia furfur* and typically found on the upper trunk. Displays characteristic groups of various-sized hyper- or hypopigmented macules with a peripheral scale.

There is histologic variability, but basic reactive epidermal changes are similar to a mild eczematous dermatitis.

Fungal cell walls are revealed by special stains (silver or PAS). *The organisms are present in the stratum corneum,* and identification/cultures may be obtained by superficial scraping of affected areas.

ARTHROPOD-ASSOCIATED LESIONS (p. 1208)

Bites, stings, and infestations associated with arachnids (spiders, scorpions, ticks, mites), insects (lice, bees, fleas, flies, and mosquitos), and chylopods (centipedes). Reactions range from minimal to fatal. Gross bites range from urticarial lesions, to inflamed papules or nodules, to expanding, erythematous plaques (e.g., *erythema migrans* in the case of the bite from the tick vector for Lyme disease). Arthropod lesions include:

- *A direct irritant effect* of insect parts or secretions.
- *Immediate (IgE-mediated, including anaphylaxis) or delayed (cell-mediated) hypersensitivity responses* to body parts or secretions.
- *Specific effects of venom* (black widow spider venom causes pain and cramping; brown recluse spider venom produces significant tissue necrosis, often requiring radical surgical excision of involved areas).
- Lesions associated with secondary invaders (bacteria, rickettsiae, parasites).

SCABIES. A pruritic dermatosis caused by the mite *Sarcoptes scabiei*. The female burrows beneath the stratum corneum, producing linear, poorly defined furrows on the interdigital skin, palms, and wrists and on the periareolar skin in women and scrotal folds in men.

PEDICULOSIS. A pruritic dermatosis caused by the head, body, or crab louse. The insect or its eggs can usually be seen attached to hair shafts. Scalp pediculosis is complicated by impetigo and cervical lymphadenopathy, especially in children. Body lice may be accompanied by excoriations and hyperpigmentation.

Although arthropod bites have a variable histologic pattern, there is classically a *wedge-shaped dermal perivascular lympho-histiocytic and eosinophilic infiltrate.* There may be a highly focal central zone of epidermal necrosis with birefringent insect mouth parts delineating the bite site.

In some lesions there is an urticaria-like response; in others there is a florid inflammatory infiltrate or spongiosis resulting in intraepidermal blisters.

CHAPTER TWENTY-THREE

Skeletal System and Soft Tissue Tumors

BONES

DEVELOPMENTAL ABNORMALITIES (p. 1217)

MALFORMATIONS (p. 1218)

Achondroplasia

A derangement in epiphyseal cartilaginous growth resulting in dwarfism. Some cases are familial, but most are acquired mutations.

- Anatomically, retarded endochondral bone formation; results in abnormally short long bones but because appositional growth is not affected they are of normal width. The spine is of normal length, and the skull appears large.
- Heterozygotes have normal longevity with easily recognizable disease, because head and body are too large for the markedly shortened extremities. Mental, sexual, and reproductive development is normal.
- Homozygous disease with its constricted thoracic cage causes death soon after birth.

DISEASES ASSOCIATED WITH ABNORMAL MATRIX

OSTEOGENESIS IMPERFECTA (OI) OR BRITTLE BONES (p. 1218)

A group of closely related genetic disorders caused by qualitative or quantitative abnormal synthesis of type I collagen (constitutes about 90% of the matrix of bone).

- Based on specific biosynthetic abnormality, four major subsets of OI have been segregated; some have well-defined modes of inheritance and phenotypic changes, others are less well characterized.
- Syndromes range from one variant (type II) that is uniformly fatal in the perinatal period (from multiple bone fractures) to other variants marked by increased predisposition to fracture but compatible with survival.
- *Morphologically, the basic change in all is osteopenia (reduced bone), with marked thinning of the cortices and rarefaction of the trabeculae.*

MUCOPOLYSACCHARIDOSES (p. 1219)

A group of lysosomal storage diseases caused by deficiencies in enzymes that degrade the various mucopolysaccharides (e.g., dermatan sulfate, heparan sulfate, others). Chondrocytes play a role in metabolism of mucopolysaccharides, and therefore in these disorders there are abnormalities in hyaline cartilage, including growth plates, costal cartilages, and articular surfaces. Patients are frequently of short stature and have malformed bones as well as other cartilage abnormalities.

OSTEOPOROSIS (p. 1219)

A reduction in bone mass owing to small but incremental losses incurred in the constant turnover of bone. A very common condition seen most often in the elderly of both sexes but more pronounced in postmenopausal women. May occur as a primary disorder of obscure origin or as a secondary complication of a large variety of diseases (Table 23–1). Osteoporosis becomes clinically significant when it induces vertebral instability with back pain and increased vulnerability to fractures of hips, wrists, vertebral bodies.

MORPHOLOGY. In postmenopausal and senile osteoporosis, the entire skeleton is involved, but patients may have localized disease with immobilization or paralysis of an extremity.

- Cortex and trabeculae are thinned and haversian systems widened.
- Such bone as remains is of normal composition.

Table 23–1. Categories of Generalized Osteoporosis

Primary	**Gastrointestinal**
Postmenopausal	Malnutrition
Senile	Malabsorption
Idiopathic juvenile	Subtotal gastrectomy
Idiopathic middle	Hepatic insufficiency
adulthood	Vitamin C, D deficiencies
Secondary	**Rheumatologic Disease**
Endocrine Disorders	**Drugs**
Hyperparathyroidism	Anticoagulants
Hyperthyroidism	Chemotherapy
Hypothyroidism	Corticosteroids
Hypogonadism	Anticonvulsants
Acromegaly	Lithium
Cushing's syndrome	Alcohol
Prolactinoma	*Miscellaneous*
Diabetes, type I	Osteogenesis imperfecta
Addison's disease	Immobilization
Neoplasia	Pulmonary disease
Multiple myeloma	Chronic obstructive pulmonary
Carcinomatosis	disease
Mast cell disease	Homocystinuria
	Gaucher's disease
	Anemia

From Cotran, R. S., Kumar, V., and Robbins, S. L.: Robbins Pathologic Basis of Disease. 5th ed. Philadelphia, W. B. Saunders Co., 1994, p. 1220.

PATHOGENESIS. Cause is largely unknown, but many factors probably contribute to slow loss of bone mass, as indicated in Figure 23–1. In essence, it is proposed that genetic factors determine the size of the bone mass achieved in young adulthood. Thereafter, aging-related slowing of osteoblastic function and increased osteoclastic activity induced by endocrine influences, particularly decreased serum estrogen levels, perhaps acting through IL-1, result in a net negative balance in the continued turnover of bone. Accumulating evidence that estrogen replacement therapy coupled with calcium supplementation, when begun during or soon after the onset of the menopause, can slow or prevent the abnormal loss of bone.

CLINICAL FEATURES. Osteoporosis causes bone pain owing to microfractures, loss in height and stability of the vertebral column, and particularly predisposes to fractures of femoral necks, wrists, and vertebrae. Condition is difficult to diagnose because

- It remains asymptomatic until skeletal fragility is well advanced.
- There is no easy way to determine the severity of the bone loss (radiographs unreliable with <30% to 40% bone loss); most reliable are absorptiometry and quantitive CT.
- It is only one of a group of osteopenic disorders, difficult to differentiate from each other (e.g., osteomalacia, osteogenesis imperfecta, and osteitis fibrosa [hyperparathyroidism]).

DISEASES CAUSED BY OSTEOCLAST DYSFUNCTION

OSTEOPETROSIS (p. 1222)

A group of rare hereditary diseases characterized by overgrowth and sclerosis of bone, with marked thickening of the cortex and narrowing or filling of the medullary cavity (impairs hematopoiesis). Despite "too much bone," it is brittle and fractures like chalk.

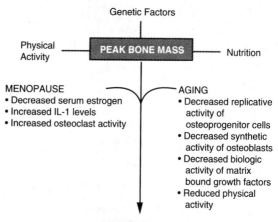

Figure 23–1. Pathophysiology of postmenopausal and senile osteoporosis. (From Cotran, R. S., Kumar, V., and Robbins, S. L.: Robbins Pathologic Basis of Disease. 5th ed. Philadelphia, W. B. Saunders Co., 1994, p.1221.)

- Autosomal recessive form evident at birth, with anemia, neutropenia, infections, and eventual death.
- Autosomal dominant form is benign, but predisposes to fractures.
- *Common to all forms is a hereditary defect in osteoclast function resulting in reduced bone resorption and enhanced net bone overgrowth.*
- Nature of the genetic defect unknown but may involve osteoclast bone-solubilizing enzymes.

PAGET'S DISEASE (OSTEITIS DEFORMANS) (p. 1223)

Monostotic in about 15% of cases and polyostotic in the remainder, with variation in the stage of the process from one site to another. Paget's disease can be divided into

1. An initial *osteolytic stage,* followed by
2. A mixed *osteolytic-osteoblastic stage,* evolving ultimately into
3. A burnt-out, *quiescent osteosclerotic stage.*

PATHOGENESIS

- Currently considered a slow virus infection of osteoblasts and then osteoclasts by paramyxovirus. Virus identified in osteoclasts by *in situ* hybridization but cannot be isolated.

MORPHOLOGY

- The *osteolytic phase* marked by resorption by numerous, overly large osteoclasts (some containing more than 100 nuclei).
- *The mixed phase* shows, in addition, disordered neo-osteogenesis of predominantly woven bone (but some lamellar) that produces *a tilelike or mosaic pattern pathognomonic of Paget's disease.* Adjacent marrow is fibrotic.
- Eventually, after many years, there is the *burnt-out phase,* marked predominantly by bone formation and osteosclerosis.
- Because the new bone formation in active disease is disordered and poorly mineralized, it is soft and porous, lacks structural stability, and is vulnerable to fracture or deformation under stress.

CLINICAL FEATURES

- Patients may demonstrate fractures, nerve compression, osteoarthritis, and skeletal deformities (e.g., tibial bowing, skull enlargement).
- Any bone can be involved, and coarsening of the facial bones *may produce* leontiasis ossea (lionlike facies). Less commonly, the vascularity of polyostotic lesions can cause high-output heart failure, and sometimes secondary sarcoma develops (in about 1% of patients).

DISEASES ASSOCIATED WITH ABNORMAL MINERAL HOMEOSTASIS

RICKETS AND OSTEOMALACIA (p. 1225)

Rickets in growing children and osteomalacia in adults are *caused by either vitamin D deficiency or phosphate depletion* resulting in defective matrix mineralization. The causes of vitamin D deficiency include

1. Dietary deficiency.
2. Inadequate exposure to sunlight.

3. Malabsorption: vitamin D, calcium, or phosphate.

4. Derangements in conversion of vitamin D to active metabolites (e.g., in renal disease).

5. End-organ resistance.

6. Rare hereditary or acquired disorders of vitamin D metabolism.

MORPHOLOGY. *The fundamental defect in osteomalacia or rickets is failure in bone mineralization, resulting in excess unmineralized matrix and abnormally wide osteoid seams.*

CLINICAL FEATURES. In the growing child, the skeleton is weak with bowing of legs and deformities of ribs, skull, and other bones. In adults after bone growth has ceased, it causes no skeletal deformities—only osteopenic osteomalacia.

HYPERPARATHYROIDISM (p. 1226)

Hyperparathyroidism, either primary or secondary (as occurs with renal failure), leads to

1. Demineralization, followed in time by

2. Increased osteoclastic activity with resorption of bone and peritrabecular fibrosis (osteitis fibrosa), evolving eventually to

3. Marrow fibrosis and more marked resorption, with formation of cysts within the marrow cavity (osteitis fibrosa cystica or *von Recklinghausen's disease of bone*). Now rare because parathyroid hyperfunction is detected earlier and controlled.

- Bone loss is particularly evident by x-ray as "moth-eaten," rarefied bones of the distal phalanges and clavicles and loss of the lamina dura about the tooth sockets.

- So-called "brown tumors" (resembling reparative giant cell granulomas) also can occur, and, paradoxically, soft tissue metastatic calcifications sometimes appear. The bone changes completely regress after control of hyperparathyroidism.

RENAL OSTEODYSTROPHY (p. 1227)

A complex set of bone changes appearing in most patients with chronic renal failure. Included are features of osteitis fibrosa cystica admixed with osteomalacia and sometimes, less prominently, areas of osteosclerosis.

- With protracted skeletal disease, metastatic calcifications may develop in the skin, eyes, and arterial walls and around joints.

- The pathogenesis is reviewed on *page 1227* of *Robbins Pathologic Basis of Disease.*

- Other factors that may contribute to the bone changes are metabolic acidosis and iron and aluminum deposition in bone (derived from dialysate, which interfere with mineralization of matrix).

FRACTURES (p. 1227)

Speed of healing and perfection of fracture repair depend on type of fracture and whether break has occurred in normal bone or in previously diseased bone (i.e., *pathologic fracture*).

- Incomplete (greenstick) and closed (intact skin) fractures heal most rapidly, with potentially complete reconstitution of the pre-existing architecture. Comminuted (splintered bone) and compound (open skin wound) fractures heal much more slowly, with poorer end results.

MORPHOLOGY

- Fracture healing is a continuous process that proceeds through three distinct stages:
  1. *Organization of hematoma* at the site, leading to a soft, organizing, weak *procallus.*
  2. Conversion of the procallus to a *fibrocartilaginous callus.*
  3. Replacement of the latter by an *osseous callus,* which is eventually remolded along lines of weightbearing to complete the repair.
- If the fracture has been well aligned and the original weight-bearing strains are restored, almost perfect repair is accomplished.
- Imperfect results are seen when there is malalignment, comminution, inadequate immobilization of fracture site, infection, and superimposed systemic abnormality (e.g., atherosclerosis, avitaminosis, dietary deficiency, osteoporosis).

OSTEONECROSIS (AVASCULAR NECROSIS)
(p. 1229)

Infarction of bone and marrow is relatively common and can occur in the medullary cavity of the metaphysis or diaphysis and the subchondral region of the epiphysis. The mechanisms leading to the local ischemia include

- Vascular interruption (fracture).
- Thrombosis and embolism (caisson disease).
- Vessel injury (vasculitis, radiation therapy, etc.).
- Vascular compression (possibly steroid-induced necrosis).
- Venous hypertension.

   Among the above, steroid-induced is most common.

MORPHOLOGY. A local geographic area of pale yellow infarction in marrow (cortex usually not affected because of its collateral blood flow). The focus is marked by death of osteocytes, empty lacunae, and necrotic fat cells. Creeping substitution occurs from margin. In subchondral infarcts the articular cartilage may collapse into the softened necrotic bone.

CLINICAL FEATURES. Patients may be asymptomatic, but subchondral lesions often cause joint pain and predispose to osteoarthritis later.

INFECTIONS

PYOGENIC OSTEOMYELITIS (p. 1230)

Results from bacterial seeding of bone by (1) hematogenous spread, (2) extension from a contiguous infection, or (3) open fracture or surgical procedure.

- Blood-borne infections are most common in developing countries, where *Staphylococcus aureus* (often penicillin-resistant) is most often implicated (other pathogens may be involved). Patients with sickle cell anemia prone, for obscure reasons, to salmonella.
- Extension of infection or traumatic inoculation is most common in developed countries, where mixed infections and/or anaerobes are most often responsible.

Basically, the suppurative reaction is associated with ischemic necrosis, fibrosis, and bony repair.

- Necrosis of a bone segment may produce a *sequestrum.*
- Subperiosteal new bone produces an *involucrum* that encloses and envelops the inflammatory focus.
- If new bone formation continues, focus becomes sclerotic: *Garré's sclerosing osteomyelitis.*
- Chronic cases may lead to bone deformity, sinus tracts, and secondary amyloidosis, but less severe cases may heal or be localized and walled off to create a *Brodie's abscess* (sometimes sterile).

Clinically, pyogenic osteomyelitis is an acute febrile illness with pain, tenderness, heat referable to local lesion. However, subtle lesions may present as unexplained fever in infants or localized pain without fever in adults. During the first 10 days, x-ray changes may be minimal, but radionuclide studies often will show localized uptake of tracers. Complications include fracture, amyloidosis, bacteremia with endocarditis, and development of squamous cell carcinoma in sinus tract.

TUBERCULOUS OSTEOMYELITIS (p. 1231)

Rare in developed countries but more common in developing nations where pulmonary and gastrointestinal TB is still common.

- Arises as an insidious infection, much more destructive and resistant to control than suppurative diseases.
- In the spine, known as *Pott's disease.*

SYPHILIS (p. 1232)

Although rare in the United States, syphilitic bone disease can occur in either congenital or acquired forms.

Congenital appears at birth and is marked by periostitis. Produces on x-ray a "crew haircut" appearance of new bone formation on cortex. *Saber shin* results when the tibia is involved.

Acquired appears in tertiary stage of disease. May be manifested as periostitis but more often by gummas in bone.

BONE TUMORS AND TUMOR-LIKE LESIONS
(p. 1232)

Great diversity of benign and malignant tumors of bone, as is evident in Table 23–2. Certain tumors tend to occur within certain age groups and at particular locations; thus, in the diagnosis of bone tumors the frequency of various lesions, the patients' age, the location of the neoplasm, and its radiologic appearance are all important.

BONE-FORMING TUMORS

Osteoma (p. 1233)

A bosselated, sessile tumor attached to a bone surface composed of densely sclerotic, well-formed bone (therefore an *osteoblastic tumor,* because it makes an osteoid matrix that may become mineralized).

- Osteomas protrude from cortical surfaces, most often the skull and facial bones.

Table 23–2. Classification of 8542 Primary Tumors of Bone in Mayo Clinic Patients

Histologic Type	Total Cases	Benign	Cases	Malignant	Cases
Hematopoietic	3401 (39.8%)			Myeloma	2932
				Malignant lymphoma	469
Chondrogenic	1822 (21.3%)	Osteochondroma	727	Primary chondrosarcoma	545
		Chondroma	245	Secondary chondrosarcoma	89
		Chondroblastoma	79	Dedifferentiated chondrosarcoma	79
		Chondromyxoid fibroma	39	Mesenchymal chondrosarcoma	19
Osteogenic	1638 (19.2%)	Osteoid osteoma	245	Osteosarcoma	1274
		Osteoblastoma	63	Parosteal osteosarcoma	56
Unknown origin	878 (10.3%)	Giant cell tumor	425	Ewing's tumor	402
				Malignant giant cell tumor	28
				Adamantinoma	23
Histiocytic origin	62 (0.7%)	Fibrous histiocytoma	10	Malignant (fibrous) histiocytoma	52
Fibrogenic	315 (3.7%)	Metaphyseal fibrous defect (fibroma)	99	Desmoplastic fibroma	9
				Fibrosarcoma	207
Notochordal	262 (3.1%)			Chordoma	262
Vascular	147 (1.7%)	Hemangioma	80	Hemangioendothelioma	60
				Hemangiopericytoma	7
Lipogenic	7 (0.1%)	Lipoma	6	Liposarcoma	1
Neurogenic	10 (0.1%)	Neurilemmoma	10		
Total	8542 (100%)		2028		6514

From Dahlin, D. C., and Unni, K. K.: Bone Tumors. 4th ed. Springfield, IL, Charles C Thomas, 1986, p. 8, by permission of Mayo Foundation.

- Of little clinical significance unless their location (e.g., the inner table of the skull) compromises local organ function, they are disturbing cosmetically, or they are associated with *Gardner's syndrome* (*see p. 814*).

Osteoid Osteoma and Osteoblastoma (p. 1234)

Osteoid osteoma is a small, benign neoplasm without malignant potential.

- Ninety per cent occur between the second and third decades of life; are usually about 1 cm in diameter, and are most often located near the ends of the tibia and femur (although all bones have been involved).
- They are very painful and appear by x-ray as a small radiolucent nidus within cortex surrounded by densely sclerotic bone.
- *Histologically, the radiolucent nidus consists of delicate trabeculae of woven bone rimmed by numerous osteoblasts and surrounded by highly vascular, spindled stroma, in turn enclosed by dense bone.*

The closely related *osteoblastoma* (giant osteoid osteoma) is usually a lytic tumor having the same histologic appearance as osteoma but without the surrounding sclerotic rim.

- Larger than osteoma (greater than 2 cm), it tends to be located in the vertebrae or long bones and does not cause much pain.
- Although it is considered benign, there are aggressive forms associated with repeated local recurrences; rarely, some transform to osteosarcoma.

Osteosarcoma ("Osteogenic" Sarcoma) (p. 1234)

Best defined as a tumor in which malignant cells directly form osteoid and/or bone *resulting in incorporation of anaplastic tumor cells within the lacunae of the osteoid matrix.*

- Excluding multiple myeloma, osteosarcoma is the most common form of primary bone cancer.
- Primary cases arise in the apparent absence of underlying bone disease, most in persons under 20 years old in the metaphyseal regions of long bones before the epiphyses have closed.
- Secondary osteosarcoma mostly in older people, in both flat and long bones, against a background of pre-existing bone pathology (e.g., Paget's disease, enchondromas, exostoses, osteomyelitis, fibrous dysplasia, infarcts, fractures) or exposure to oncogenic influences (previous irradiation).

PATHOGENESIS. Genetic, constitutional, and environmental influences important.

Patients with familial retinoblastoma have a greatly increased risk of osteosarcomas and have a hereditary mutation of the suppressor Rb gene on chromosome 13. Patients who survive hereditary retinoblastoma have continued risk of developing osteosarcoma, often in an irradiated area. Sporadic osteosarcomas not associated with Rb gene but often have mutations of the p53 suppressor gene on chromosome 17 (Li-Fraumeni syndrome).

Constitutional influences include the fact that it is during active bone growth that osteosarcoma develops, and favored locations are sites of greatest bone growth, e.g., at base of femoral growth plate.

Irradiation is the one environmental factor known to predispose to secondary osteosarcoma.

MORPHOLOGY. Eighty percent to ninety per cent of osteosarcomas arise in the medullary cavity of the metaphyseal ends of long bones (proximal tibia, distal/proximal femur, and proximal humerus), but any bone can be involved. After 25 years of age, the incidence in flat bones (jaws and pelvis) equals that in long bones and usually is superimposed on underlying bone disease.

- They present as gray-white, invasive, and destructive masses showing focal hemorrhages and necrosis.
- Some are largely fibroblastic, others largely osteoblastic, some chondroid, and others highly vascular (telangiectatic). *All form osteoid and/or bone incorporating malignant cells.*
- Cortical penetration of tumor with periosteal elevation causes "Codman's triangle," an x-ray finding in some patients. Tumor rarely penetrates the epiphyseal plate.
- Extraskeletal osteosarcoma also can occur.

CLINICAL FEATURES. Metastasize widely, usually to lung first but also to other organs and bones (lymph node metastases are rare).

- Present with local pain, tenderness, and swelling.
- Surgery alone results in 20% 5-year survivals, but surgery, radiation, and chemotherapy yield 60% 5-year survivals.
- Osteosarcomas of the jaw and the low-grade variants, parosteal (juxtacortical) and "intraosseous low grade" osteosarcoma, have a better prognosis than does classic osteosarcoma.

CARTILAGE-FORMING TUMORS

Osteochondroma (p. 1237)

Also known as an "exostosis," may occur as solitary sporadic lesions or in profusion in the autosomal dominant *multiple hereditary exostosis.* Are believed to result from displacement of the lateral portion of the growth plate, which then proliferates in a direction diagonal to the long axis of the bone and away from the nearby joint. Male-female ratio, 3:1.

- Occur most frequently on metaphysis of long bones. Occasionally the pelvis, scapula, and ribs are involved (rarely the small bones of the hands and feet).
- *Morphologically, are mushroom-shaped lateral protrusions, capped by hyaline cartilage, with outer, well-formed cortices and medullary cavities in continuity with the underlying marrow cavity.*
- Exostoses are usually discovered in late childhood or adolescence, often as chance x-ray findings.
- They are benign lesions, but, rarely in the hereditary condition, chondrosarcomas may arise from one or more.

Chondroma (p. 1238)

Benign tumors composed of mature hyaline cartilage.

- Those within the bone are called enchondromas, and, like exostoses, they are thought to arise from remnants of epiphyseal cartilage left behind.
- May be single or multiple. A nonfamilial multiple form is known as *enchrondromatosis* or *Ollier's disease,* and a familial

form with multiple chondromas associated with hemangiomas is known as *Maffucci's syndrome.*

Sarcomatous transformation of solitary sporadic chondromas is rare, but with the multiple tumors in the systemic syndromes sarcomatous transformation (usually chondrosarcoma) is frequent.

- Are usually asymptomatic but may cause bone deformity, pain, and fracture. Lesions of the hands and feet are almost always innocuous but may recur when incompletely removed. Those in long bones raise the differential diagnosis of well-differentiated chondrosarcoma.

Chondroblastoma (p. 1239)

An uncommon benign tumor almost invariably found in epiphyses of skeletally immature people (not to be confused with giant cell tumor or clear cell chondrosarcoma, both occurring in the same location but usually in older patients).

- Resembling embryonic chondroblasts, tumor cells are polygonal, arranged in sheets, and sometimes surrounded by a lacelike pattern of hyaline cartilage. Their nuclei are often deeply indented or longitudinally grooved.
- Multinucleated, osteoclast-like giant cells may be present and abundant enough to suggest giant cell tumor of bone.
- The great majority are benign, but rare examples have metastasized to lung as chondrosarcomas.

Chondromyxoid Fibroma (p. 1239)

An uncommon benign tumor composed of chondroid, fibrous, and myxoid tissues.

- Occurs in the metaphyses of the long bones about the knee, but any bone can be involved.
- There is a male preponderance, and most occur in the second and third decades.
- X-ray images show circumscribed lucency with scattered calcifications.
- Because focal atypia can be marked, these tumors can be misconstrued as sarcomas.
- They are adequately treated by curettage and despite possible recurrence pose no threat.

Chondrosarcoma (p. 1240)

Occurs about half as often as osteosarcoma.

- Seventy-five per cent arise de novo (primary); the remaining (secondary) chondrosarcomas arise from enchondromas, osteochondromas, and rarely chondroblastomas.
- Most occur in middle to later life, the primary lesions being in the central skeleton (ribs, shoulder, and pelvic girdle) and around the knee. Are rare beyond the ankles and wrists.
- *When transected, they appear as lobulated translucent tumors. Necrosis and spotty calcification may be present.*
- Distinction from enchondroma may be difficult in grade 1 (well-differentiated) tumors. Hyperchromatic nuclei, two or more cells per lacuna, multinucleate cells, and anaplasia point toward chondrosarcoma.
- Equally difficult may be the differentiation of chondrosarcoma

with ossification from osteosarcoma with chondroid differentiation. In chondrosarcomas, bone formation occurs within cartilage; osteosarcomas show bone arising out of a background of anaplastic, osteoblastic-fibroblastic cells.

- *X-ray images may be diagnostic. Classically, there is a localized area of bone destruction punctuated by mottled densities from calcification or ossification.*
- All require total removal, and 5-year survival rates for grades I, II, and III (increasing cytologic anaplasia) are 90%, 81%, and 43%, respectively. None of the grade I lesions and 70% of the grade III lesions disseminate.

FIBROUS AND FIBRO-OSSEOUS TUMORS

Fibrous Cortical Defect (Nonossifying Fibroma)
(p. 1241)

A non-neoplastic developmental lesion (sharply defined, radiolucent lesions of the metaphyseal cortex) in the femur, tibia, and fibula.

- Single (50%) or multiple and bilateral (50%).
- Does not transform to malignancy; generally asymptomatic but may (when large) lead to fracture; extremely common (reported in one-third of normal children); and disappears spontaneously.

Fibrous Dysplasia (p. 1242)

A localized, benign, progressive replacement of bone by a fibrous proliferation intermixed with poorly formed, haphazardly arranged trabeculae of woven bone. The latter are present in variable amounts, are not lined by osteoblasts, and form configurations likened to "Chinese figures." There are three, somewhat overlapping, presentations:

1. Involvement of a single bone (*monostotic*) (70%).
2. Involvement of several or many bones (*polyostotic*) (25%).
3. *Polyostotic disease associated with various endocrinopathies* (3% to 5%). When accompanied by irregular ("coast of Maine") skin pigmentation and precocious sexual development, is termed *McCune-Albright syndrome.*

- The monostotic form is often asymptomatic, whereas the polyostotic form is frequently associated with deformities and fractures, especially of the craniofacial bones.
- The clinical course of the polyostotic forms is unpredictable.
- Rarely, secondary sarcoma develops, sometimes after irradiation.

Fibrosarcoma and Malignant Fibrous Histiocytoma (MFH) (p. 1243)

These two lesions have overlapping clinical, radiographic, and pathologic features. Some deny the existence of MFH and reassign lesions.

- MFH more common in men but fibrosarcoma common in both sexes. Both gray-white masses, infiltrative.
- Usually arise *de novo* but some arise on a background of Paget's disease, bone infarcts, and prior radiation.

- Fibrosarcoma is composed of malignant fibroblasts in a herringbone pattern. More often, moderately well-differentiated but may be very anaplastic.
- MFH composed of spindled fibroblasts in a storiform (so-called) composed (starry) pattern admixed with bizarre multinucleated giant cells and neoplastic-appearing histiocytes (actually fibroblasts).
- MFH generally a high-grade pleomorphic tumor.
- May arise in soft tissues but also in the metaphyses of long bones and pelvis.

Prognosis depends on cytologic grade; anaplastic lesions yield a 20% 5-year survival.

MISCELLANEOUS TUMORS

Ewing's Sarcoma and Primitive Neuroectodermal Tumor (p. 1244)

Both neoplasms are composed of malignant small round cells and both are closely related, having an identical 11;22 chromosomal translocation. Major difference is Ewing's sarcoma is more undifferentiated, and neuroectodermal tumor often reveals neural differentiation, but the term *Ewing's sarcoma* is used here to represent both neoplasms.

- Ewing's arises most often in children 10 to 15 years old, and 80% are younger than 20 years.
- Males affected more often than females; blacks are rarely affected.
- Ewing's is second most common bone sarcoma in childhood.
- Arises in medullary cavity in the diaphysis of long tubular bones, especially femur and flat bones of the pelvis.
- Usually invades cortex and penetrates periostium to produce a soft tissue mass.
- Is composed of sheets of uniform small round cells that occasionally produce Homer-Wright pseudorosettes (tumor cells arrayed in a circle about a central fibrillary space).
- Cells have scant cytoplasm, which often contains glycogen.
- Generally there is little fibrous tissue but prominent necrosis in regions remote from vessels.

Clinically, Ewing's presents as a painful, enlarging mass often tender, warm, and swollen, suggesting an infection. The periosteal reaction produces layers of reactive bone deposited in an onionskin fashion. With combined radiation, chemotherapy, and surgery, there is now a 75% 5-year survival rate.

Giant Cell Tumor of Bone (p. 1245)

A locally aggressive neoplasm found most often in the epiphyseal ends of long bones in adults between 20 and 55 years of age. Over one-half occur about the knees, but virtually any bone can be involved.

- Rare in skeletally immature people and infrequent in the advanced years.

MORPHOLOGY

- The histologic pattern is one of uniformly distributed, osteoclast-like, multinucleated giant cells in a plump spindle cell background.
- *The neoplastic cell is the spindled stromal cell; the multinucleated cells are thought to arise from fusion of the spindle cells.*

- There may be foci of necrosis, hemorrhage, hemosiderin, and/ or osteoid.

CLINICAL FEATURES. *X-ray images are distinctive (not pathognomonic), revealing large, lytic, "soap-bubble" lesions. Absent are stippling and calcifications.*

- Histologic features do not allow prediction of which will recur or metastasize. A rare lesion is overtly malignant from the outset.
- This biologic unpredictability complicates clinical management. The majority of tumors are localized and can be eradicated by curettage or conservative resections; however, 40% to 60% recur locally, 1% to 2% develop deceptively benign looking metastases to the lungs, and about 10% develop obviously anaplastic metastases.

METASTATIC TUMORS TO THE SKELETON (p. 1246)

In adults, well over half of skeletal metastases originate from cancers of the prostate, breast, kidney, and lung. In children, there is secondary involvement of skeleton, most commonly from neuroblastoma, Wilms' tumor, osteosarcoma, Ewing's sarcoma, and rhabdomyosarcoma. Most metastases to bone are lytic. The tumor cells elaborate prostaglandins, interleukins, and parathyroid hormone–related protein that stimulate osteoclastic bone resorption. Osteosclerotic responses are most often induced by prostate and breast cancer by stimulating osteoblastic activity.

JOINTS

OSTEOARTHRITIS (OA) OR DEGENERATIVE JOINT DISEASE (DJD) (p. 1247)

Characterized by progressive deterioration and breakdown of articular cartilage, mainly in weightbearing joints, leading to subchondral bony thickening and bony overgrowths—osteophytes ("spurs")—about the joint margins. Also causes the bony, knobby protrusions at the margins of the distal interphalangeal joints, creating nontender, subcutaneous *Heberden's nodes.* Cause unknown but most likely related to metabolic and biochemical alterations.

DJD occurs in two clinical patterns:

1. *Primary DJD.* Occurs *de novo,* mostly in men in midlife, somewhat later in women. Frequency increases with age to about 80% of those over 70 years. Association between OA and aging is nonlinear, the prevalence increasing exponentially beyond the age of 50 years.

2. *Secondary DJD.* Appears at any age in a previously damaged or congenitally abnormal joint.

The relationship between age and previous injury suggests that "wear and tear" contributes to the genesis of this disease. Indeed, shoulder and elbow are often involved in baseball players and knees in basketball players. But usually knees and hands are more common in women and hips in men.

MORPHOLOGY

- Involvement usually is oligoarticular.
- Earliest changes are loss of proteoglycans and decreased meta-

chromasia of the articular cartilage, associated with focal loss of chondrocytes alternating with areas of chondrocyte proliferation ("cloning") and increased matrix basophilia.
* Next, fissuring, pitting, and flaking of the cartilage develop, followed by vertical clefts down to the subchondral bone.
* Flaking of the cartilage exposes underlying bone, which appears ivory-like (eburnation) as continued joint motion polishes the surface.
* Subchondral microcysts and fractures may develop.
* Synovium shows a mild chronic inflammatory infiltrate (nonspecific synovitis) and can develop osteocartilaginous metaplasia, fragments of which create osteocartilaginous loose bodies ("joint mice") within the joint space.

PATHOGENESIS. Remains unknown but is clearly related to aging and injury. Cause may well be multifactorial.

* With aging, capacity of chondrocytes to maintain cartilaginous matrix slows.
* Age-related changes include alterations in the proteoglycans and collagen within articular cartilage, which decrease resilience and increase vulnerability to injury.
* Under stresses of injury, chondrocytes elaborate IL-1, which initiates matrix breakdown.
* Secondary mediators such as TNF-α and TGF-β enhance release of lytic enzymes from chondrocytes while inhibiting matrix synthesis.
* However, precise signals inducing release of cytokines and enzymes are still unknown.

CLINICAL FEATURES. Although DJD may be asymptomatic, most patients experience morning stiffness in affected joints. There is usually no local heat or tenderness, but affected joints often show restricted range of motion, small effusions, and crepitus. Progressive reduction in mobility and increased painfulness with joint motion. Bone spurs and joint narrowing on x-rays.

* No known way of preventing or arresting DJD.

RHEUMATOID ARTHRITIS (RA) (p. 1249)

RA is basically a severe form of chronic synovitis that can lead to destruction and ankylosis of affected joints. Blood vessels, skin, heart, lungs, nerves, and eyes may also be affected.

* About 1% of the world's population suffers from RA; women affected three times more often than men; peak prevalence in the third to fourth decades of life.
* There is a familial association and a link with HLA-DR4, or DR1 or both.

MORPHOLOGY. RA generally first affects small, proximal joints of the hands and feet but then may involve, usually symmetrically, the wrists, elbows, ankles, and knees.

* Well-developed lesions show villous hypertrophy of the synovium, synoviocytic hyperplasia, and an intense lymphoplasmacytic and histiocytic synovial infiltrate. Exuberant synovium is known as a *pannus,* which eventually fills the joint space, encroaching upon the articular surfaces.
* Release of destructive enzymes (proteases and collagenases) and cytokines (particularly IL-1 and TNF-α) and pannus for-

mation destroy cartilage, leading to changes reminiscent of degenerative joint disease but with fibrous and bony ankylosis. Neutrophils (RA cells) can be present in synovial fluid.

- Other features include rheumatoid nodules in subcutaneous tissues (areas of necrosis surrounded by palisade of fibroblasts and white cells at pressure points such as elbows), acute vasculitis, and nonspecific, fibrosing inflammatory lesions of lungs, pleura, pericardium, myocardium, peripheral nerves, and eyes.

PATHOGENESIS. Although much remains uncertain, best hypothesis is this: *RA is initiated by an arthritogenic microbial agent in an immunogenetically susceptible host. After initial injury, a continuing autoimmune reaction ensues in which T cells (CD4 +) release cytokines and inflammatory mediators that ultimately destroy the joint.*

- Linkage to HLA-DR4 points to genetic susceptibility.
- Microbial trigger unknown but EBV a prime suspect. Other agents, such as retroviruses, mycobacteria, *Borrelia,* and *Mycoplasma,* also suspected.
- Once an inflammatory synovitis is initiated, an autoimmune reaction ensues; CD4 + cells are activated with release of many cytokines, particularly IL-1 and TNF-α. These cells within joints mediate lysis of articular cartilage and initiate the inflammatory synovitis.
- Autoantibodies are produced, some against autologous IgG.
- Autoantibody against the Fc portion of autologous IgG is called rheumatoid factor (RF) (is usually IgM, but sometimes IgG, IgA, or IgE).
- Rheumatoid factor does not contribute to pathogenesis, since about 20% of patients are RF negative, but may contribute to an Arthus-like reaction in blood vessels (acute vasculitis) and to the production of subcutaneous rheumatoid nodules and other extra-articular lesions.

CLINICAL FEATURES. Variable. Most patients experience a prodrome of malaise, fever, fatigue, and musculoskeletal pain before joint mobility reduced.

- The lucky patient experiences mild transient disease without sequelae, but most have fluctuating disease with the greatest progression during the initial 4 to 5 years. In a minority the onset is acute, with rapidly progressive limitation of motion and development of joint deformities.
- Characteristic deformities are radial deviation of the wrist with ulnar deviation of the fingers.
- Extra-articular manifestations (mentioned above), although infrequent, are rarely the presenting features of the disease and tend to develop in patients with high RF titers (? related to deposition of circulating immune complexes).
- Some of the total morbidity of RA is caused by GI bleeding from long-term aspirin therapy, infections from steroid use, or amyloidosis in long-term severe disease.
- Variants of RA include juvenile-onset RA, Felty's syndrome (features RA, splenomegaly, and neutropenia), arthritis associated with ulcerative colitis, and with Sjögren's syndrome.

SERONEGATIVE SPONDYLOARTHROPATHIES
(p. 1253)

These include ankylosing spondylitis, Reiter's syndrome, psoriatic arthritis, and enteropathic arthritis. All have similar clinical features and many are associated with HLA-B27, but all lack RF (hence seronegative).

- *Ankylosing spondyloarthritis (Marie-Strümpell disease)* is a chronic inflammatory joint disease of vertebrae and sacroiliac joints that usually occurs in males; begins in adolescence following some infection and is suspected to be of immunogenetic origin, with autoantibodies directed at joint elements. Follows a chronic progressive course, with extension to hips, knees, shoulders in one-third of patients and sometimes uveitis, aortitis, and amyloidosis.
- *Reiter's syndrome* comprises triad of arthritis, nongonococcal urethritis or cervicitis, and conjunctivitis. Men most often affected in the third to fourth decades of life, and most are positive for HLA-B27. Evidence suggests that disease is caused by an autoimmune reaction initiated by prior infection, usually gastrointestinal or genitourinary. Ankles, knees, and feet may be affected, but in chronic disease, the spine as well, indistinguishable from ankylosing spondylitis. Many extra-articular involvements of skin, eyes, heart, tendons, and muscles.
- *Psoriatic arthritis* appears in about 5% of patients with the skin disease. The arthritis usually affects small joints of the hands and feet but may also extend to ankles, knees, hips, and wrists. Spinal disease occurs in about one-quarter of the patients. Not as severe as rheumatoid arthritis. Less joint destruction.
- *Enteropathic arthritis* appears in 10% to 20% of patients with inflammatory bowel disease as a migratory oligoarthritis of the large joints and spine. May resemble ankylosing spondylitis but is generally less severe and remits spontaneously in a year or so.

INFECTIOUS ARTHRITIS (p. 1254)

Infectious arthritis is uncommon but can rapidly destroy a joint to produce permanent loss of motion. Any of a great variety of microorganisms can seed the joint hematogenously or, more rarely, by direct inoculation or spread from a nearby focus of infection.

- *Suppurative arthritis,* most commonly caused by gonococcus, staphylococcus, streptococcus, *H. influenzae,* and gram-negative coliforms. Individuals with sickle cell disease prone to infection with salmonella. *H. influenzae* predominates in children under 2 years of age; *S. aureus* in older children and adults; and the gonococcus in late adolescence and young adult life. In most instances a single joint is affected, usually the knee, followed in frequency by hip, shoulder, elbow, wrist, and sternoclavicular joint. Gonococcal arthritis is mostly oligoarticular and often associated with a skin rash and a genetic deficiency of C5, C6, or C7.
- *Tuberculous arthritis,* an insidious chronic arthritis from hematogenous spread or nearby tuberculous osteomyelitis. Most common site is the spine (Pott's disease) followed in frequency by hip, knee, elbow, wrist, ankle, and sacroiliac joints. Tends to be a more destructive process than suppurative arthritis.
- *Lyme arthritis,* as discussed in Chapter 8, follows several days or weeks after the initial skin infection. The arthritis tends to be remitting and migratory and primarily involves large joints, especially the knees, shoulders, elbows, and ankles. The articular involvement morphologically resembles rheumatoid arthri-

tis; in most cases it clears spontaneously or with therapy, but in about 10% of patients results in permanent deformities.

CRYSTAL ARTHROPATHIES

GOUT AND GOUTY ARTHRITIS (p. 1255)

A group of conditions that share

1. Hyperuricemia.
2. Attacks of acute arthritis triggered by crystallization of urates in joints.
3. Asymptomatic intervals.
4. Eventual development of chronic tophaceous gout and arthritis.

- Hyperuricemia is necessary for gout, but only a small fraction of hyperuricemic people develop gout. Most cases occur in men (after the third decade); women are almost never affected before menopause.

PATHOGENESIS. Primary and secondary forms exist:

1. *Primary (90% of all cases).* Overwhelming majority are idiopathic (>95%), are of multifactorial inheritance, and are associated with overproduction of uric acid with normal or increased excretion, or normal production of uric acid with underexcretion. Alcohol, obesity predispose. A very small percentage of primary cases are associated with specific enzyme defects (e.g., X-linked, partial deficiency of hypoxanthine-guanine phosphoribosyltransferase [HGPRT]).

2. *Secondary (10% of all cases).* Most are associated with increased nucleic acid turnover, which occurs with chronic hemolysis, polycythemia, leukemia, and lymphoma. Less commonly, drugs (especially diuretics, aspirin, nicotinic acid, and ethanol) or chronic renal disease lead to symptomatic hyperuricemia. Lead intoxication may induce "saturnine gout." Rarely, the specific enzyme defects causing von Gierke's disease (glycogen storage disease type I) and the Lesch-Nyhan syndrome (with a total lack of HGPRT seen only in males and associated with neurologic deficits) lead to gouty symptoms.

MORPHOLOGY. Acute arthritis represents an acute oligo- or monoarticular inflammatory synovitis initiated by urate crystal formation within joints.

- Needle-shaped crystals are birefringent with polarized light.
- The crystals activate Hageman factor, with the production of chemoattractants (e.g., C3a + 5a) and inflammatory mediators. Neutrophils and macrophages accumulate in joints and phagocytose crystals, leading to release of lysosomal enzymes, toxic free radicals, IL-1, IL-6, IL-8, and TNF-α, prostaglandins, and leukotrienes, which collectively produce acute synovitis.
- Chronic arthritis evolves from the progressive precipitation of urates into the synovial linings of joints after recurrent attacks of acute arthritis.
- The *tophus is the pathognomonic lesion of gout:* a mass of urates, crystalline or amorphous, surrounded by an intense inflammatory reaction, composed of macrophages, lymphocytes, fibroblasts, and foreign body giant cells. Tophi tend to occur on the ear, in the olecranon and patellar bursae, and in periarticular ligaments and connective tissue.

- Three types of renal disease result:
  1. Acute uric acid nephropathy (intratubular urate deposition).
  2. Nephrolithiasis.
  3. Chronic urate nephropathy (interstitial urate deposition).

CLINICAL CORRELATION. About 50% of the initial attacks of acute gouty arthritis involve the great toe, or less frequently the instep, ankle, or heel.

- Sometimes physical or emotional fatigue, an alcoholic spree, or dietary overindulgence precedes an attack.
- The initial attack subsides spontaneously or with therapy, usually recurring within several months to a few years.
- Other joints become involved, and multiple recurrences lead to chronic gouty arthritis.
- About 90% of patients with chronic arthritis develop some renal impairment.
- Therapy is very effective in controlling gout.

CALCIUM PYROPHOSPHATE
CRYSTAL DEPOSITION DISEASE (p. 1258)

Acute or chronic arthritis secondary to deposition of calcium pyrophosphate (chondrocalcinosis or pseudogout).

- Many of the clinicopathologic features of this disease are similar to those of gout.

   Pseudogout can be hereditary, sporadic, or associated with trauma or surgery. Calcium pyrophosphate crystals are frequently present in joint specimens from patients with DJD and in intervertebral disc material removed from patients with herniation of disc.

- The deposits appear as circular aggregates (pools) of basophilic-staining rhomboid crystals. Whether these deposits are causing the DJD or are a secondary phenomenon is unclear.
- In pseudogout almost any combination of joints as well as the intervertebral discs can be involved, but the knee is most frequently affected.
- Joint involvement may be transient, but about half the patients suffer significant joint damage.

TUMOROUS INVOLVEMENT OF JOINTS AND RELATED STRUCTURES
BURSITIS (p. 1259)

Inflammation of the bursa tends to be more common in men than in women, perhaps because of greater physical activity. It is

- Most common in the subdeltoid bursa, olecranon bursa, prepatellar bursa, and radiohumeral bursa, in order of frequency.
- Of unknown cause, and no precise initiating influence can be identified except possibly a history of excessive exercise.
- More painful than serious.

GANGLION AND SYNOVIAL CYST (p. 1260)

A ganglion is a small (1- to 1.5-cm) multiloculated, cavitated ("cystic") lesion found in connective tissues of joint capsules or tendon sheaths.

- It arises from focus of myxoid degeneration and softening of connective tissues. The cavities are not lined by epithelium, and they do not communicate with joint cavities.
- Favored location is the small joints of the wrist, where ganglions are palpated as a firm but yielding, pea-sized subcutaneous nodule.
- The lesions are easily treatable by surgical removal; occasionally they may erode underlying bone.

Herniations of a joint space may occur, particularly into the popliteal space from the knee joint when there is a marked increase of intra-articular fluid or exudate, as in rheumatoid or suppurative arthritis. The herniations of the knee joints are known as synovial or Baker's cysts.

- The anatomic changes are those of the underlying articular disease.

VILLONODULAR SYNOVITIS (p. 1260)

The term for a group of closely related lesions involving synovial membranes and tendons, usually of peripheral joints.

- Morphologically, synovial lesions are made up of fibroblasts, histiocytoid cells, and fibrohistiocytoid cells, often admixed with multinucleated, osteoclast-like cells; xanthoma cells; and pigmented macrophages.
- When the process is sharply localized, it is referred to as *nodular tenosynovitis* (or *giant cell tumor of tendons*); when it more diffusely involves the intra-articular synovial membrane (often with hemosiderin pigment), it is called *pigmented villonodular synovitis*.
- It is unclear whether these lesions are neoplasms (variants of benign fibrous histiocytoma) or reactive, inflammatory conditions (synovitis).
- They can recur, especially the poorly localized forms, and cause destruction of underlying bone.

SOFT TISSUE TUMORS AND TUMOR-LIKE LESIONS

Soft tissue tumors (STTs) are "mesenchymal proliferations that arise in the extraskeletal nonepithelial tissue of the body, exclusive of the viscera, coverings of the brain, and lymphoreticular system." May arise in any location, although about 40% occur in the lower extremity, especially thighs, 20% in the upper extremity, 10% in the head and neck, and 30% in the trunk and retroperitoneum. Critical to their clinical management are the following parameters:

- Size—the larger the mass, the poorer the outlook.
- Accurate histologic classification and grading (I–III based largely on the degree of differentiation), and an estimate of the rate of growth based on mitoses and extent of necrosis.
- Staging (*see Table 27–6, p. 1233, in Robbins Pathologic Basis of Disease*).
- Location of tumor—the more superficial, the better the prognosis.

FATTY TUMORS
LIPOMA AND LIPOSARCOMA (p. 1262)

Lipomas are the most frequent soft tissue tumors, arising in subcutaneous regions at any site but most commonly on the back, shoulder, and neck. They can also arise in the mediastinum, retroperitoneum, or bowel wall.

- Lipomas are delicately encapsulated, usually small tumors recapitulating normal, mature adipose tissue. Uncommonly, atypical examples occur in subcutaneous locations where they should not be mistaken for liposarcoma.

  Liposarcomas are much less common and tend to be bulky. They arise from primitive mesenchymal cells, some bearing lipid vacuoles that are requisite in at least some cells for the diagnosis of liposarcoma. Appear virtually anywhere in the body without regard to adipose tissue. Most arise in deep soft tissues and pursue a course closely dependent on their cytologic features.

- Well-differentiated (lipoma-like) liposarcoma and myxoid liposarcoma (with a nonspecific myxoid background) tend to be low-grade tumors, which are stubbornly recurrent, follow a more protracted course, and metastasize late.
- In contrast, round cell liposarcoma and pleomorphic liposarcoma are high-grade, aggressive sarcomas (85% to 90% metastasize).
- The myxoid variant (but not the others) has a characteristic balanced 12:16 translocation.

FIBROUS TUMORS AND TUMOR-LIKE LESIONS
REACTIVE PSEUDOSARCOMATOUS PROLIFERATIONS (p. 1263)
Nodular Fasciitis

A reactive, benign, fibroproliferative lesion, also known as *pseudosarcomatous fasciitis, is more commonly mistaken for a neoplasm than any other non-neoplastic condition.*

- The lesions appear as palpable nodules or small masses, most often in the extremities (but possibly elsewhere), in young and middle-aged adults of either sex.
- After a period of rapid growth, the tumors tend to plateau in size, indicating progressive maturation.
- *Morphologically, they are composed of spindled fibroblasts/myofibroblasts in a loose myxoid background resembling cultured fibroblasts.* Some of the more active cells are enlarged and have prominent nuclei and nucleoli; mitoses may be present.
- Recurrence after excision, even incomplete excision, is exceedingly rare and should lead to a reappraisal of the original diagnosis.

Myositis Ossificans (p. 1264)

A variant of fasciitis, sometimes preceded by trauma, occurring most often in skeletal muscle but sometimes in subcutaneous fat.

- Favored locations are the extremities, particularly the quadriceps or brachialis muscle.

- *Morphologically, they are circumscribed but unencapsulated masses composed of fibroblasts/myofibroblasts in a myxoid stroma, but, in addition, the periphery has a rim of woven, often mineralized bone. They should not be confused with osteogenic sarcoma.*
- Mature lesions are completely ossified.

Palmar, Plantar, and Penile Fibromatosis (p. 1264)

The *fibromatoses* encompass a group of fibroproliferative lesions with similar histopathologic features but variable clinical presentations.

- When on the palm, the process is known as *palmar fibromatosis* (*Dupuytren's contracture*); when on the foot, *plantar fibromatosis;* and when involving the penis, *penile fibromatosis* (*Peyronie's disease*). These lesions may recur after excision or spontaneously resolve in about 25% of patients.

Desmoid (Aggressive Fibromatosis) (p. 1265)

These curious lesions lie in the histologic interface between exuberant fibroproliferative lesions and low-grade fibrosarcomas.

- They present as infiltrative masses in abdominal (affecting mothers in the perinatal period), extra-abdominal (affecting men and women equally), and intra-abdominal (Gardner's syndrome) locations.
- They are composed of banal, "tame-looking" fibroblasts (actually myofibroblasts by electron microscopy) that do not metastasize.
- *Although curable by adequate excision, they stubbornly recur in the local site when incompletely removed.*

FIBROMA AND FIBROSARCOMA (p. 1265)

Fibromas are most common in the ovary but may occur around the teeth and at other body sites. They are well defined, usually small, gray-white tumors composed of sparse mature fibroblasts and collagenous tissue.

Fibrosarcomas occur in deep soft tissue, are gray, soft, "fish-flesh" masses with increased fibroblastic cellularity, anaplasia, high nuclear-to-cytoplasmic ratios, abundant mitotic figures, and *spindled growth in a "herringbone" pattern.*

- They often are large masses that appear deceptively encapsulated but are nonetheless infiltrative.
- Overall, 60% to 80% of patients survive 5 years with present methods of treatment.

FIBROHISTIOCYTIC TUMORS
Benign Fibrous Histiocytoma (p. 1266)

Distinctive unencapsulated but demarcated neoplasms composed of a mixture of cells resembling fibroblasts, myofibroblasts, histiocytes, primitive mesenchymal cells, and cells having intermediate or mixed features (fibrohistiocytoid cells).

- Benign and malignant giant cells and fat-laden foamy cells can also be found.
- Benign lesions predominantly occur in the skin and are most frequently referred to as dermatofibromas.

- Other variants may be very vascular—"sclerosing hemangioma."

TUMORS OF SKELETAL MUSCLE
RHABDOMYOSARCOMA (RMS) (p. 1267)

Cardiac rhabdomyomas (probably hemartomas) occur mostly in the setting of tuberous sclerosis. Extracardiac rhabdomyomas are divided into adult and fetal types based on the differentiation of cells (the degree to which they resemble myocytes). Are too rare for further description.

Rhabdomyosarcoma is more common, especially in children, in the head and neck and urogenital regions.

Are subdivided into four types based on morphologic features: (1) embryonal, (2) botryoid, (3) alveolar, and (4) pleomorphic. The botryoid pattern is basically a morphologic variant of the embryonal, which in submucosal locations projects into a cavity, e.g., vagina, bladder, as grapelike masses.

- The pleomorphic type (very rare) occurs in patients over 45 years; the other three in about 90% of cases occur before age 20 years. The pleomorphic variant has large, atypical tumor cells, some showing abundant cytoplasm with cross-striations characteristic of skeletal muscle differentiation.
- The other three variants are basically primitive, poorly differentiated tumors of small blue cells that have focal skeletal muscle differentiation (rhabdomyoblasts with abundant eosinophilic cytoplasm or cross-striations).
- Rhabdomyoblastic differentiation may be apparent only with electron microscopic or immunohistochemical techniques (ribosomal-myosin complexes or desmin/myoglobin immunoperoxidase positivity). The alveolar variant is characterized by a 2:13 chromosomal translocation.
- The embryonal, alveolar, and botryoid variants respond to surgery combined with radiation and chemotherapy (3-year median survivals). The pleomorphic variant has a poorer prognosis.

TUMORS OF SMOOTH MUSCLE
LEIOMYOMA AND LEIOMYOSARCOMA (p. 1268)

Both benign smooth muscle tumors occur predominantly in the female genital tract (*see p. 1059*), but they may also occur at other body sites where smooth muscle is well represented (e.g., scrotum, nipple, bowel wall).

Leiomyosarcomas are uncommon, more frequent in women than men.

- Most develop in skin and deep soft tissue.
- Are usually large, soft, gray masses of spindle cells with "cigar-shaped" nuclei.
- Variants may be myxoid or epithelioid.
- Superficial lesions often can be excised; deep tumors are invasive and rarely excisable.

SYNOVIAL SARCOMA (p. 1269)

These tumors occur around joints (but not in joint spaces), in the parapharyngeal region, in the abdominal wall, and less commonly at other body sites.

- *The highly distinctive feature of these infiltrative sarcomas (shared only by mesotheliomas and carcinosarcomas) is their biphasic pattern of cell growth: distinct epithelial components forming glands and papillary patterns, admixed with well-defined spindle cell components.*
- They range in behavior from aggressive lesions causing death within a few months to extremely indolent tumors permitting cure or long-term survival (5-year survivals are about 50%).
- Most have a reciprocal translocation between chromosomes X and 18 (p11.2;q11.2).

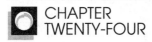

Peripheral Nerve and Skeletal Muscle

THE MOTOR UNIT (p. 1273)

NORMAL STRUCTURE (p. 1273)

Motor unit consists of (1) spinal anterior horn lower *motor neuron;* (2) *axon* of that neuron; and (3) *muscle fibers* it innervates.

Peripheral nerves are composed of intermingled *myelinated* (2 to 15 μm) and *unmyelinated* (0.2 to 3 μm) *axons* and their investing Schwann cells grouped into fascicles by connective tissue sheaths (epineurium—encloses the entire nerve; perineurium—encircles each fascicle; endoneurium—surrounds nerve; fibers). Single Schwann cells myelinate axonal segments (internodes) separated by nodes of Ranvier. Protein synthesis does not occur in the axon, and axoplasmic flow delivers proteins and other substances synthesized in the perikaryon down the axon; a retrograde transport system serves as a feedback to the cell body. The *perineurial barrier* is formed by the tight junctions between the perineurial cells, and endoneurial capillaries establish the *blood-nerve barrier (BNB)*.

Skeletal muscles (muscle fibers) are syncytial cells with multiple nuclei beneath the plasma membrane (*sarcolemma*) and contain identical repeating units (*sarcomeres*) of actin and myosin contractile proteins delimited by perpendicularly disposed Z bands (primarily α-actinin). In normal human muscle, there are two types of fibers with different functional characteristics and staining patterns (Table 24–1). All fibers of a motor unit are of the same type; they are randomly distributed across the cross-section of a muscle, giving a checkerboard pattern with special stains.

REACTIONS TO INJURY (p. 1277)

Nerve

- *Segmental demyelination:* Loss of myelin along discrete regions of axons from dysfunction of the Schwann cell and/or damage to the myelin sheath; no primary abnormality of the axon. With sequential episodes of demyelination and remyelination, tiers of Schwann cell processes accumulate around the axon (*onion bulbs*).
- *Axonal degeneration:* Primary destruction of the axon, with secondary disintegration of its myelin sheath. In the slowly evolving neuronopathies or axonopathies, evidence of myelin breakdown is scant because only few fibers degenerate at a time. *Wallerian degeneration* is the acute reaction distal to a

Table 24-1. Muscle Fiber Types

Characteristic	Type 1	Type 2
Action	Sustained force, weightbearing	Sudden movements, purposeful motion
Enzyme content	NADH: *dark staining* ATPase pH 4.2: *dark staining* ATPase pH 9.4: *light staining*	NADH: *light staining* ATPase pH 4.2: *light staining* ATPase pH 9.4: *dark staining*
Lipids	Abundant	Scant
Glycogen	Scant	Abundant
Ultrastructure	Many mitochondria Wide Z band	Few mitochondria Narrow Z band
Physiology	Slow twitch	Fast twitch
Color	Red	White
Prototype	Soleus (pigeon)	Pectoral (pigeon)

From Cotran, R. S., Kumar, V., and Robbins, S. L.: Robbins Pathologic Basis of Disease. 5th ed. Philadelphia, W. B. Saunders Co., 1994, p. 1276.

cut axon and consists of axonal and myelin breakdown with phagocytosis by macrophages.

Muscle

- *Denervation atrophy:* Down-regulation of myosin and actin synthesis and shrinkage of fibers to small, angulated shapes as a result of loss of innervation.
- *Reinnervation:* Occurs after nerve regeneration or, more commonly, when surviving axons sprout around denervated muscle cells and incorporate the fibers into their motor unit, imparting the same histochemical type to a group of contiguous fibers —*type grouping.*
- *Group atrophy:* Occurs when a type group becomes denervated.
- *Myopathic changes:* Varied patterns, including segmental necrosis (destruction of a portion of a myocyte), myophagocytosis, myocyte regeneration via satellite cells (large, internalized nuclei; prominent nucleoli; and the cytoplasm, laden with RNA, becomes basophilic), increased central nuclei, and variation in fiber size.

DISEASES OF PERIPHERAL NERVE (p. 1279)

INFLAMMATORY NEUROPATHIES (p. 1279)

ACUTE INFLAMMATORY DEMYELINATING POLYRADICULO-NEUROPATHY (GUILLAIN-BARRÉ SYNDROME; GBS)

- Life-threatening ascending paralysis, with weakness beginning in the distal limbs but rapidly advancing to affect proximal muscles.
- Annual incidence in the U.S. of 1 to 2 per 100,000.
- Nerve conduction velocity is slowed and CSF protein is elevated in the absence of increased cells.
- Pathologic features are segmental demyelination and chronic inflammatory cells involving the nerve roots.
- Appears to be an immunologically mediated disorder, often following a viral infection.

CHRONIC INFLAMMATORY DEMYELINATING POLYRADIC-ULONEUROPATHY (CIDP). A mixed sensorimotor polyneuropathy like GBS but follows a subacute or chronic course, usually with relapses and remissions. Peripheral nerves show recurrent demyelination and remyelination and onion bulbs.

INFECTIOUS POLYNEUROPATHIES (p. 1280)

- Direct infections of Schwann cells occur in leprosy (*p. 365*); the host response can either be limited (*lepromatous leprosy*) or vigorous (*tuberculoid leprosy*).
- Varicella-zoster virus (VZV) produces latent infection of neurons in the sensory ganglia of the spinal cord and brain stem following chickenpox, and its reactivation leads to a painful vesicular skin eruption in the distribution of sensory dermatomes (*shingles*), most frequently thoracic or trigeminal.
- In contrast to these direct infectious processes, diphtheritic neuropathy results from the effects of the diphtheria exotoxin. Begins clinically with paresthesias and weakness and is characterized pathologically by segmental demyelination.

HEREDITARY NEUROPATHIES (HN) (p. 1280)

Both strength and sensation are affected in the *hereditary motor and sensory neuropathies* (*HMSN*). In the *hereditary sensory and autonomic neuropathies* (*HSAN*), symptoms are usually limited to numbness, pain, and/or autonomic dysfunction such as orthostatic hypotension (Table 24–2). Some hereditary neuropathies are notable for the deposition of amyloid within the nerve; these *familial amyloid polyneuropathies* (*FAP*) have a clinical presentation similar to that of the HSAN. Some inborn errors of metabolism cause prominent peripheral nerve manifestations (Table 24–3).

ACQUIRED METABOLIC AND TOXIC NEUROPATHIES (p. 1282)
Adult-Onset Diabetes Mellitus

Three principal patterns of neuropathy:

- *Distal symmetric sensory or sensory-motor neuropathy* (most common: a chronic axonal neuropathy with dramatic reduction of small myelinated and unmyelinated fibers).
- *Autonomic neuropathy* (affects about 20% to 40% of diabetics with distal sensorimotor neuropathy).
- *Focal or multifocal asymmetric neuropathy* (mononeuropathy or multiple mononeuropathy; e.g., unilateral ocular nerve palsies, with sparing of reflexes).

Others

Neuropathies are encountered in patients with renal failure (prior to dialysis), chronic liver disease, chronic respiratory insufficiency, and hypothyroidism. Axonal neuropathies also occur with deficiencies of thiamine, vitamins B_{12} (cobalamin) and B_6 (pyridoxine), and E (alpha-tocopherol).

NEUROPATHIES ASSOCIATED WITH MALIGNANCY
(p. 1283)

1. Direct effects:
Infiltration or compression of peripheral nerves by tumor may cause a mononeuropathy, brachial plexopathy, cranial nerve palsy, or a polyradiculopathy involving the lower extremities when the cauda equina is involved by meningeal carcinomatosis.
2. Paraneoplastic syndromes:
   - Progressive sensorimotor neuropathy (less often a pure sensory neuropathy), most pronounced in the lower extremities, particularly with small cell lung carcinoma; loss of dorsal root ganglion cells, CD8+ T-cell infiltrates, and axonal loss in nerves and in the posterior columns of the spinal cord.
   - Peripheral neuropathy with deposition of light chain amyloid in peripheral nerves (AL type) in patients with plasma cell dyscrasias.

TOXIC NEUROPATHIES (p. 1284)

Peripheral neuropathies may occur following exposure to industrial or environmental chemicals, biologic toxins, heavy metals, or therapeutic drugs. Some examples are listed in Table 24–4.

TRAUMATIC NEUROPATHIES (p. 1285)

- *Lacerations:* May follow cutting injuries or bone fractures in which a sharp fragment of bone lacerates the nerve.
- *Avulsions:* Follow application of tension to a nerve, often as the result of a force applied to one of the limbs.
- *Traumatic neuroma:* Tangled nodule of axons and connective tissue from regenerating axonal sprouts of the proximal stump after nerve transection.
- *Compression neuropathy (entrapment neuropathy):* Most commonly seen with the median nerve at the level of the wrist within the compartment delimited by the transverse carpal ligament (*carpal tunnel syndrome*); observed with any condition that can cause decreased available space within the carpal tunnel, such as tissue edema, but predisposing factors include pregnancy, degenerative joint disease, hypothyroidism, amyloidosis (especially that related to β_2-microglobulin deposition in renal dialysis patients), and excessive usage of the wrist.

TUMORS OF PERIPHERAL NERVE (p. 1351)

These are discussed in association with tumors of the central nervous system (*see p. 537 in this volume*).

DISEASE OF SKELETAL MUSCLE (p. 1285)
MUSCULAR DYSTROPHIES (p. 1285)

A heterogeneous group of inherited disorders characterized by progressively severe muscular weakness and wasting, often beginning in childhood (Table 24–5).

Text continued on page 512

Table 24-2. Hereditary Neuropathies (HMSN and HSAN)

Disease	Inheritance	Clinical Findings	Pathologic Findings
HMSN I (Charcot-Marie-Tooth)—hypertrophic type	Autosomal dominant, gene on chromosome 17, myelin-specific protein gene, PMP-22 (type 1A), less often on chromosome 1 (type 1B), or neither (type 1C); less common X-linked forms	Onset in childhood or early adulthood; progressive calf muscle atrophy (peroneal muscular atrophy, enlarged nerves, pes cavus)	Some segmental demyelination, nerve fiber loss, and onion bulbs
HMSN II—neuronal type	Autosomal dominant (one locus on chromosome 1)	Similar to HMSN I, without nerve enlargement	Nerve fiber loss, no onion bulbs, loss of anterior horn cells in spinal cord
HMSN III (Déjérine-Sottas)—infantile type	Autosomal recessive (several separate loci)	Onset in early childhood, progressive upper and lower extremity weakness and muscle atrophy, greatly enlarged palpable nerves	Segmental demyelination, severe nerve fiber loss, and very prominent onion bulbs

HSAN I	Autosomal dominant	Predominantly sensory neuropathy, often presenting in young adults, with secondary consequences such as foot ulcers	Axonal degeneration (myelinated fibers affected more than unmyelinated)
HSAN II	Autosomal recessive (some cases are sporadic)	Predominantly sensory neuropathy, presenting in infancy or early childhood	Axonal degeneration (myelinated fibers affected more than unmyelinated); nerve biopsy may reveal complete absence of myelinated fibers
HSAN III (Riley-Day syndrome; familial dysautonomia)	Autosomal recessive (most often in Jewish children)	Predominantly autonomic neuropathy, often presenting in infancy with symptoms such as postural hypotension, absence of tears, and excessive sweating	Axonal degeneration (unmyelinated fibers affected more than myelinated); atropy and loss of sensory and autonomic ganglion cells

Table 24–3. Hereditary Neuropathies with Known Metabolic Cause

Disease	Metabolic Defect	Inheritance	Clinical Findings	Pathologic Findings
Adrenoleukodystrophy	Fatty acyl CoA ligase activity (peroxisomal enzyme) transporter	X-linked; 4% of female carriers are symptomatic	Mixed motor and sensory neuropathy, adrenal insufficiency, spastic paraplegia; onset between 10–20 years (a genetically distinct neonatal form also exists)	Axonal degeneration (myelinated and unmyelinated); segmental demyelination, with onion bulbs; EM; linear inclusions in Schwann cells
Familial amyloid polyneuropathies	Point mutations in transthyretin; rare pedigrees involve other molecules	Autosomal dominant	Sensory and autonomic dysfunction; age of onset is variable (depending on site of mutation)	Amyloid deposits in vessel walls and connective tissue with axonal degeneration
Porphyria (acute intermittent, coproporphyria, variegate)	Enzymes involved in heme synthesis	Autosomal dominant	Acute episodes of neurologic dysfunction, psychiatric disturbances, abdominal pain, seizures, proximal weakness, autonomic dysfunction; attacks may be precipitated by drugs	Acute and chronic axonal degeneration; regenerating clusters
Refsum disease	Phytanic acid α-hydroxylase (peroxisomal enzyme)	Autosomal recessive	Mixed motor and sensory neuropathy with palpable nerves; ataxia, night blindness, retinitis pigmentosa, ichthyosis; age of onset before 20 years (a genetically distinct infantile form also exists)	Severe onion bulb formation

From Cotran, R. S., Kumar, V., and Robbins, S. L.: Robbins Pathologic Basis of Disease. 5th ed. Philadelphia, W. B. Saunders Co., 1994, p. 1281.

Table 24-4. Toxic Neuropathies Due to Organic Compounds

Toxic Agent	Source of Exposure	Molecular Basis	Clinical Findings	Pathologic Findings
Ethanol	Alcoholic beverages	Probable superimposed nutritional deficiencies	Slowly progressive distal sensorimotor neuropathy	Axonal degeneration (myelinated and unmyelinated fibers)
Acrylamide	Industry (polymerizing agent used as flocculant and for grouting)	?	Numbness and sweating of hands and feet, progressing to distal sensorimotor neuropathy	Axonal degeneration, most pronounced in distal nerve (large-caliber fibers most affected)
Hexane	Industry (solvent) and inhalant abuse ("glue sniffing")	Protein alkylation; impaired intermediate filament transport	Distal symmetric sensorimotor polyneuropathy	Enlarged axons filled with neurofilaments; axonal degeneration predominantly affecting large-caliber axons
Organo-phosphorous esters	Industry and contaminated food products (used as pesticides, petroleum additives, and plasticizers)	Induction of esterase activity ("neurotoxic esterase"); altered protein phosphorylation	Rapidly progressive distal sensorimotor polyneuropathy after latent phase (7–21 days)	Axonal degeneration affecting long axons of the peripheral and central nervous systems
Vinca alkaloids	Therapy (vincristine used in therapy of certain malignancies)	Impaired assembly of microtubules	Diminished ankle jerk earliest sign; subsequent progression to sensorimotor neuropathy	Axonal degeneration; large intravenous doses may cause accumulation of filaments in cell bodies

From Cotran, R. S., Kumar, V., and Robbins, S. L.: Robbins Pathologic Basis of Disease. 5th ed. Philadelphia, W. B. Saunders Co., 1994, p. 1284.

Table 24-5. Muscular Dystrophies

Disease	Inheritance	Clinical Findings	Pathologic Findings
Duchenne's dystrophy	X-linked chromosome Xp21, 427 kDa protein, *dystrophin*	Onset in childhood (4–5 years), progressive proximal weakness, hypertrophic calves, elevated CK, cardiac involvement, death in second decade	Dystrophic myopathy: variation in fiber size, internalized nuclei, rounded/enlarged fibers, myophagocytosis and regeneration, increased endomysial connective tissue
Becker's dystrophy	X-linked chromosome Xp21, *dystrophin*	Milder form of muscular dystrophy, onset later, slower rate of progression	Dystrophic myopathy
Myotonic dystrophy	Autosomal dominant, chromosome 19q13.2–13.3 gene codes myotonin-protein kinase	Percussion myotonia, facial and distal extremity weakness, cataracts, frontal balding, gonadal atrophy, cardiac involvement, decreased plasma IgG	Dystrophic myopathy and striking internalized nuclei, ring fibers, type 1 fiber atrophy

Fascioscapulohumeral (FSH) muscular dystrophy	Autosomal dominant (gene localized to 4q35)	Variable age of onset (most commonly 10–30 years); weakness of muscles of face, neck, and shoulder girdle	Findings of dystrophic myopathy, but also often including inflammatory infiltrate of muscle
Oculopharyngeal muscular dystrophy	Autosomal dominant	Ptosis and weakness of extraocular muscles; difficulty swallowing; onset in mid-adult life	Findings of dystrophic myopathy, but often including rimmed vacuoles in type I fibers
Limb-girdle dystrophy (heterogeneous group)	Autosomal recessive and sporadic cases are common	Weakness of proximal muscles of upper and lower extremities; onset often at 10–30 years; usually slowly progressive, but prognosis is extremely variable	Variable findings of dystrophic myopathy

Modified from Cotran, R. S., Kumar, V., and Robbins, S. L.: Robbins Pathologic Basis of Disease. 5th ed. Philadelphia, W. B. Saunders Co., 1994, p. 1288.

CONGENITAL MYOPATHIES (p. 1288)

A group of muscle diseases characterized by onset in early life, nonprogressive or slowly progressive course, proximal or generalized muscle weakness, and hypotonia ("floppy babies") or severe joint contractures (*arthrogryposis*) (Table 24–6).

MYOPATHIES ASSOCIATED WITH INBORN ERRORS OF METABOLISM (p. 1288)

A wide variety of metabolic disorders may cause myopathy.

* *Glycogen synthesis and degradation:* Depending on the nature of the enzyme deficit, myopathy may or may not be a component of the disease (*see p. 146*); findings include abnormal amounts of glycogen and absence of relevant enzymes.
* *Lipid metabolism:* Deficiencies of carnitine (needed to shuttle fatty acids across mitochondrial membrane) or carnitine palmitoyl transferase (enzyme involve in process) lead to myopathy with increased lipid stores in muscle fibers.
* *Mitochondrial function:* Oxidative phosphorylation pathway abnormalities may cause myopathies (often involving extraocular muscles); genetic basis may be in either nuclear or mitochondrial genome; muscle fibers show "ragged red" appearance on trichrome staining and may have abnormal mitochondria by EM ("parking lot" inclusions).

TOXIC MYOPATHIES (p. 1291)

Thyrotoxic myopathy: Acute or chronic, proximal muscle weakness sometimes presenting prior to clinical thyroid dysfunction. In thyrotoxic periodic paralysis there is weakness and hypokalemia; periodic paralysis may also occur as a familial disease independent of thyroid dysfunction (with elevated, depressed, or normal serum potassium) and is associated with mutations in the muscle sodium channel.

Alcohol: "Binge" drinking can produce an acute toxic syndrome of rhabdomyolysis with accompanying myoglobinuria; may lead to renal failure.

Steroids: Proximal muscle weakness and atrophy may occur in Cushing's syndrome or during therapeutic administration of steroids; severity of clinical disability is variable and not directly related to the steroid level or the therapeutic regimen.

DISORDERS OF THE NEUROMUSCULAR JUNCTION (p. 1292)

Myasthenia gravis (MG): An autoimmune disease characterized clinically by easy fatigability, ptosis, and diplopia due to an immune-mediated injury which causes a decrease in the number of muscle acetylcholine receptors (AChRs).

* Morphologically, light microscopic examination of muscle is ordinarily unremarkable or may show disuse type 2 atrophy (rarely, aggregates of lymphocytes—lymphorrhages); ultrastructurally, junctional folds are greatly reduced or abolished at the neuromuscular junction.
* Antibodies to AChR are present in the serum of 85% to 90% of patients with MG. These antibodies accelerate degradation of the AChR.

Table 24–6. Congenital and Metabolic Myopathies

Disease	Inheritance	Clinical Findings	Pathologic Findings
Central core disease	Autosomal dominant	Early-onset hypotonia and nonprogressive weakness; associated skeletal deformities; may develop malignant hyperthermia	Cytoplasmic cores are lightly eosinophilic and distinct from surrounding sarcoplasm; only found in type 1 fibers, which usually predominate
Nemaline myopathy	Variable	Weakness, hypotonia, and delayed motor development; may also be seen in adults; usually nonprogressive; involves proximal limb muscle most severely; skeletal abnormalities may be present	Aggregates of subsarcolemmal spindle-shaped particles (*nemaline rods*); occur predominantly in type 1 fibers; derived from Z-band material (α-actinin)
Centronuclear myopathy	Autosomal recessive; rarer severe X-linked recessive; later-onset autosomal dominant; sporadic	Presents in infancy or early childhood with prominent involvement of extraocular and facial muscles; hypotonia; and slowly progressive limb muscle weakness	Abundance of centrally located nuclei involving the majority of muscle fibers; central nuclei are usually confined to type 1 fibers, which are small in diameter, but can occur in both fiber types
Lipid myopathy: CPT deficiency	Autosomal recessive; chromosome 1	Episodic acute myonecrosis (rhabdomyolysis) following exercise; often with myoglobinuria; may lead to renal failure	Accumulation of lipid droplets within myocytes; with acute exacerbations, myocyte necrosis is present
Mitochondrial myopathy	Maternal (when associated with mutations of mitochondrial genome)	Proximal muscle weakness, usually presenting in childhood; may predominantly affect extraocular muscles	Accumulation of abnormal mitochondria adjacent to plasma membrane ("ragged red" fibers); abnormal mitochondrial ultrastructure, including "parking lot" inclusions

Modified from Cotran, R. S., Kumar, V., and Robbins, S. L.: Robbins Pathologic Basis of Disease. 5th ed. Philadelphia, W. B. Saunders Co., 1994, p. 1258.

- About 15% of patients with MG have other autoimmune diseases, including autoimmune thyroid disease, RA, pernicious anemia, SLE, and other collagen-vascular disorders.
- Thymic hyperplasia is seen in about 65% to 75% of patients, and a thymoma is found in 15%.

Lambert-Eaton myasthenic syndrome: A paraneoplastic disorder of the neuromuscular junction, most commonly with small cell carcinoma of the lung (60% of cases); differs from MG in having increased contractions with repeated stimuli.

TUMORS OF SKELETAL MUSCLE (p. 1267)

These are discussed with soft tissue tumors.

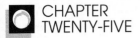

The Central Nervous System

Aspects of the central nervous system that are important for understanding pathologic processes include

- Localization of specific neurologic functions to distinct (often spatially clustered) groups of neurons.
- Inability to regenerate neurons (so focal destructive lesions can give rise to permanent clinical deficits).
- Selective vulnerability of certain neurons to injury based on differences in structure and function.
- Physical restrictions of the skull and spine.
- Cerebrospinal fluid (CSF) circulation, the lack of a lymphatic system, and a blood-brain barrier.
- Unique responses to injury and patterns of wound healing.

NORMAL CELLS AND THEIR REACTIONS TO INJURY (p. 1296)

NEURONS (p. 1296)

Vary in structure, functional interconnections, and biochemical properties. Pathologic changes include

- *Axonal reaction:* After the axon is cut or damaged, the cytoplasm around the nucleus becomes pale (chromatolysis) and swollen.
- *Acute cell injury (red neuron):* Intense eosinophilia of the perinuclear cytoplasm and pyknosis of the nucleus that follows acute anoxia or ischemia.
- *Atrophy and degeneration:* Loss of neurons without other recognized morphologic change (characteristic of slowly progressive neurologic diseases and system degenerations).
- *Intraneuronal deposits:* Occur in aging (lipofuscin), disorders of metabolism (storage material), viral diseases (inclusion bodies), or degenerative diseases (Alzheimer's neurofibrillary tangles, Lewy bodies of Parkinson's disease).

GLIA (p. 1296)

Glial cells provide supporting functions for neurons and their cellular processes; they also have a primary role in repair, fluid balance, and energy metabolism.

Astrocytes

Round/oval nucleus, finely stippled chromatin, branching cytoplasmic processes; contain the intermediate filament glial fibrillary acidic protein (GFAP). The processes are directed toward capillaries (end feet), neurons, and the subpial and subependymal surfaces. Important functions include

- Structural support, contribution to the blood-brain barrier (BBB), and action as metabolic buffers/detoxifiers.
- Principal cells responsible for repair and scar formation in the brain. In damaged brain they develop conspicuous eosinophilic cytoplasm (*gemistocytic astrocyte*); later they form a network of cellular processes, a process referred to as *gliosis*.

Additional pathologic reactions include

- *Rosenthal fibers:* Elongated, eosinophilic structures, containing αB-crystallin, within astrocytic processes and found in long-standing gliosis, pilocytic astrocytomas, and Alexander's disease.
- *Corpora amylacea:* Lamellated polyglucosan bodies occurring in increasing numbers with advancing age.
- *Alzheimer type II astrocytes:* Glia with an enlarged nucleus with pale chromatin, found in patients with hyperammonemia.

Oligodendrocytes

Lymphocyte-sized nucleus with densely packed chromatin and little cytoplasm visible with H&E stains. They produce and maintain CNS myelin.

Ependyma

Single layer of cuboidal cells that lines the ventricular system and rests on subependymal glia. After injury they do not regenerate, and the underlying subependymal glia proliferate, forming *ependymal granulations*.

Microglia

Bone marrow–derived, CD4+ mononuclear cells; bean-shaped nucleus and little cytoplasm visible with H&E stains. They respond to injury by developing elongated nuclei (rod cells), forming aggregates about small foci of tissue necrosis (microglial nodules), or congregating around portions of dying neurons (neuronophagia).

COMMON PATHOPHYSIOLOGIC COMPLICATIONS (p. 1298)

Three interrelated pathophysiologic phenomena of great significance are (1) *herniations,* (2) *cerebral edema,* and (3) *hydrocephalus.*

HERNIATIONS

The volume of the intracranial contents is fixed by the skull. As a result, the introduction of additional tissue or fluid (as may occur in a space-occupying lesion, cerebral edema, or hydrocephalus) raises intracranial pressure, which may lead to life-threatening herniation of the brain through openings of the dural partitions of the cranial cavity or across openings of the skull. The major herniations are

- *Subfalcine:* Cingulate gyrus herniates under the falx (may compromise the anterior cerebral artery).
- *Transtentorial:* Medial temporal lobe (uncus) passes over the free edge of the tentorium (may lead to distortion of the adjacent midbrain/pons and tearing of feeding vessels (*Duret hemorrhages*) or compress the posterior cerebral artery).
- *Tonsillar:* Cerebellar tonsils herniate through the foramen magnum (may result in compression of the medulla and compromise cardiorespiratory centers).

CEREBRAL EDEMA

The accumulation of extravascular fluid within the brain may cause life-threatening increased intracranial pressure since lymphatic drainage is essentially absent. The blood-brain barrier (BBB) closely regulates the movement of fluids and other substances in and out of the brain; *tight junctions between brain capillary endothelial cells constitute the cellular barrier.*

Three types of edema often occur in combination:

- *Vasogenic:* Accumulation of fluid outside the vascular compartment secondary to increased vascular permeability; commonly seen with cerebrovascular accidents, trauma, tumors, and infections. The brain is heavy, swollen, and softened; there is tissue vacuolation and preferential involvement of white matter.
- *Cytotoxic:* Secondary to altered cell regulation of fluid, seen in anoxia or toxic/metabolic disturbances. The fluid is intracellular and tends to involve the gray matter.
- *Interstitial:* Transudation of fluid from the ventricular system across the ependymal lining (characteristic of increased intraventricular pressure).

HYDROCEPHALUS

Obstruction of CSF flow leads to enlargement of the ventricles with an associated increase in the volume of CSF. Most often caused by congenital malformations and leptomeningeal or intraventricular tumors, hemorrhage, or infections.

Two principal forms of hydrocephalus:

- *Noncommunicating hydrocephalus:* Blockage anywhere along the ventricular system, most often the aqueduct or the foramina of Monro.
- *Communicating hydrocephalus:* Obstruction along the subarachnoid path of CSF flow, including the sites of its resorption.

In infants and children in whom fusion of the cranial bones has not yet occurred, hydrocephalus produces enlargement of the head. In adults, hydrocephalus may lead to increased intracranial pressure.

Normal pressure hydrocephalus is a clinical syndrome typically found in elderly people and characterized by mental slowness, incontinence, and gait disturbances associated with a slowly evolving hydrocephalus.

In diseases associated with extensive tissue loss, compensatory expansion of the entire CSF compartment results in *hydrocephalus ex vacuo.*

MALFORMATIONS AND DEVELOPMENTAL DISEASES (p. 1300)

Patterns of malformation and developmental lesions are determined by the gestational age of the fetus at the time of the injury. Etiologic environmental factors include maternal and fetal infections, drugs, anoxia, and ischemia.

Major categories of CNS malformations:

- *Neural tube defects* (NTD): Failure of closure or reopening of the caudal portions of the neural tube results in malformation of the vertebral arches (*spina bifida*) which may be associated with a disorganized segment of spinal cord and an overlying meningeal outpouching (myelomeningocele). Antenatal diagnosis can be made by imaging and maternal screening for α-fetoprotein. Folate deficiency during the initial weeks of gestation is a risk factor. *Anencephaly* is a malformation of the anterior end of the neural tube resulting in failure of development of the cerebrum. *Encephalocele* is a malformed diverticulum of CNS tissue extending through a defect in the cranium.
- *Forebrain abnormalities:* Include megalencephaly and micrencephaly (abnormally large or small brain volume), agyria and polymicrogyria (abnormally formed gyri), neuronal heterotopias (abnormal migration of neurons), holoprosencephaly (incomplete separation of the cerebral hemispheres), and agenesis of the corpus callosum.
- *Posterior fossa abnormalities:* Chiari II malformation (Arnold-Chiari malformation) consists of a small posterior fossa, a malformed midline cerebellum with extension of the vermis through the foramen magnum, hydrocephalus, and a lumbar myelomeningocele. *Dandy-Walker malformation* is characterized by an enlarged posterior fossa, absent cerebellar vermis, and a large midline cyst.
- *Hydromyelia/syringomyelia:* Segmental or continuous expansion of the central canal of the spinal cord or formation of a cleft-like cavity in the cord. Most occur in the cervical region. Symptoms are loss of pain and temperature sensation in the upper extremities, with retention of position sense and absence of motor deficits.

PERINATAL BRAIN INJURY (p. 1303)

Cerebral palsy is a nonprogressive neurologic motor deficit, with onset during the perinatal period, associated with several pathologic entities:

- *Intraparenchymal hemorrhage* within the germinal matrix, near the junction between the thalamus and caudate nucleus, sometimes extending into the ventricular system.
- *Ischemic infarcts* may occur focally in the periventricular white matter (*periventricular leukomalacia*) or develop throughout the hemispheres (*multicystic encephalopathy*). Ischemia and hemorrhage are seen in premature newborn infants.
- *Ulegyria* (thin, gliotic gyri) and *status marmoratus* (neuronal loss and gliosis associated with aberrant and irregular myelin formation in the basal ganglia and thalamus) are also related to ischemic injury. Choreoathetosis and related movement disorders are important clinical sequelae.

TRAUMA (p. 1304)

There are four categories of brain trauma: (1) skull fractures, (2) parenchymal injuries, (3) traumatic vascular injury, and (4) spinal cord injury.

SKULL FRACTURES (p. 1304)

Skull fractures may cross sutures (diastatic), resulting in bone displacement into the cranial cavity (displaced fracture). Their relative incidence among skull bones is related to the pattern of falls.

PARENCHYMAL INJURIES (p. 1304)

- *Concussion:* A transient neurologic syndrome occurring after trauma, with loss of consciousness, respiratory arrest, and loss of reflexes. Amnesia for the event persists. It is unassociated with permanent structural damage.
- *Contusions:* Bruises of the crests of gyri either at the site of impact (coup contusion) or at a point opposite (contrecoup contusion). Microscopically, there are foci of hemorrhagic brain. After resolution, a depressed, yellowish glial scar extends to the pial surface (plaque jaune).
- *Laceration:* A penetrating injury leading to tearing of tissue.
- *White matter injury:* Diffuse axonal injury (axonal swellings) and hemorrhages, in the corpus callosum and brain stem, in about 50% of patients who develop coma after trauma. Mechanical forces, including angular acceleration in the absence of impact, damage the axon.

TRAUMATIC VASCULAR INJURY (p. 1306)

Depending on the anatomic position of the ruptured vessel, trauma-related hemorrhages are *epidural, subdural, subarachnoid,* and *intraparenchymal.*

- *Epidural hematoma:* Arterial blood, usually from a fracture-related rupture of the middle meningeal artery, collects between the dura and the internal surface of the skull and compresses the brain. Patients are often lucid for several hours after the trauma. The lesion may expand rapidly, cause increased intracranial pressure/herniation, and requires drainage.
- *Subdural hematoma:* Venous blood from torn superficial bridging veins between the convexities and the dural venous sinuses collects in the space between the dura and the outer layer of the arachnoid. Chronic subdurals may occur in older individuals and alcoholics, sometimes after relatively minor trauma. The treatment is surgical drainage acutely and removal of the associated granulation tissue ("membranes") in long-standing lesions.
- *Traumatic subarachnoid hemorrhage and traumatic intraparenchymal hemorrhage:* Contusion of superficial cerebral tissue or, less frequently, cerebellar cortex, associated with disruption of small vessels within both the brain parenchyma and the overlying leptomeninges.

SPINAL CORD INJURY (p. 1308)

Most injuries that damage the cord are associated with displacement of the spinal column, either rapid and temporary or persistent. In the acute phase there is hemorrhage, necrosis, and white matter axonal swellings. Later the central necrotic lesion becomes cystic and gliotic, while the damaged ascending and descending white matter tracts undergo secondary degeneration.

CEREBROVASCULAR DISEASE (p. 1308)

Cerebrovascular disease is the most prevalent neurologic disorder in terms of both morbidity and mortality. The major categories are (1) hypoxia, ischemia, and infarction, (2) intracranial hemorrhage, and (3) hypertensive cerebrovascular disease.

HYPOXIA, ISCHEMIA, AND INFARCTION (p. 1308)

Brain oxygen deprivation causes either generalized (*ischemic or hypoxic encephalopathy*) or focal ischemic necrosis (*cerebral infarction*). Generalized hypoxia occurs with reduced blood oxygen content or with reduction of whole brain cerebral perfusion pressure, as with hypotension. *Watershed* or *border zone infarcts* occur with reduced perfusion in those regions of the brain and spinal cord that lie at the most distal fields of arterial irrigation, i.e., at the border zone between major vascular territories; that between the anterior and middle cerebral artery is most at risk. **MORPHOLOGY.** In the first 12 to 24 hours after ischemia, neurons show ischemic cell injury ("red neurons") and subsequently die. The most susceptible regions are the pyramidal neurons of Sommer's sector of the hippocampus, the Purkinje cell layer of the cerebellar cortex, and the pyramidal neurons in the neocortex (*pseudolaminar necrosis*). Healing is characterized by gliosis.

Cerebral infarction due to focal obstruction of blood flow may arise from either thrombotic or embolic arterial occlusion. These events are manifest as the *stroke syndrome*—the sudden onset of a neurologic deficit with clinical manifestations referable to the anatomic location of the lesion. The deficit evolves over time, and the outcome is either fatal or is characterized by some degree of slow improvement over a period of months. Venous infarcts are often hemorrhagic; they occur following thrombotic occlusion of the superior sagittal sinus or other sinuses or occlusion of the deep cerebral veins.

- *Thrombosis* most frequently affects the extracerebral carotid system and the basilar artery and usually is due to atherosclerosis.
- *Embolism* most commonly involves the intracerebral arteries (most often in middle cerebral artery distribution); emboli often originate from cardiac mural thrombi related to myocardial infarcts, valvular disease, and atrial fibrillation. Fragments of thrombotic material also may break off from arterial mural thrombi in neck vessels or occur as paradoxic emboli (particularly in children with cardiac anomalies).

MORPHOLOGY. *Nonhemorrhagic infarcts* ("*bland*" or *anemic infarcts*) are evident at 48 hours as pale, soft regions of edematous brain. The tissue then liquefies, and a fluid-filled cavity containing macrophages is lined by reactive glia. *Hemorrhagic infarcts*, characteristic of embolic occlusion with reperfusion injury, are manifest by blood extravasation, especially in the cerebral cortex.

NONTRAUMATIC INTRACRANIAL HEMORRHAGE

(p. 1311)

May be (1) intraparenchymal, (2) subarachnoid, or (3) mixed, as seen in vascular malformations.

Intraparenchymal Hemorrhage

The leading cause of death in stroke patients; *hypertension* is a predisposing factor in 80% of cases.

Hypertensive intracerebral hemorrhage is most commonly observed in the putamen, thalamus, pontine tegmentum, and cerebellar hemispheres. Vascular rupture is believed to be due to arteriolar injury with formation of microaneurysms (*Charcot-Bouchard aneurysms*). *Lobar hemorrhages* involve areas supplied by hemispheral arteries and are due to amyloid angiopathy or hemorrhagic diatheses. In patients who survive, the hematoma is slowly resorbed over a period of months with some restitution of function.

MORPHOLOGY. Macroscopically, acute hemorrhages are characterized by extravasation of blood with compression of the adjacent parenchyma. Microscopically, resolution shows an area of cavitary destruction of brain with a rim of gliotic tissue containing pigment-laden macrophages.

Subarachnoid Hemorrhage (SAH)

Occurs most often with rupture of a *berry aneurysm* (*saccular aneurysm, congenital aneurysm*), the most frequent type of intracerebral aneurysm (fusiform atherosclerotic aneurysms and mycotic aneurysms also occur).

- Most berry aneurysms occur in the anterior circulation and are found near arterial branch points; multiplicity is found in 20 to 30% of patients.
- Most occur sporadically, but they also are associated with polycystic kidney disease.
- Hypertension and collagen disorders (Ehlers-Danlos syndrome, pseudoxanthoma elasticum, Marfan syndrome) also predispose to their development.

The probability of rupture increases with the size of the lesion; aneurysms greater than 10 mm have a roughly 50% risk of bleeding per year. Rupture often occurs with acute increases in intracranial pressure, such as with straining at stool or sexual orgasm. Between 25% and 50% of patients die with the first rupture. Rebleeding is common in the survivors, and with each episode of bleeding, the prognosis is more grave. Blood in the subarachnoid space can lead to arterial vasospasm. Eventually, blood resorption may lead to meningeal fibrosis and hydrocephalus.

MORPHOLOGY. At the neck of the aneurysm, the muscular wall and intimal elastic lamina are usually absent or fragmentary, and the wall of the sac is made up of thickened hyalinized intima. With acutely ruptured aneurysms, blood diffusely fills the subarachnoid spaces.

Vascular Malformations (p. 1313)

- *Arteriovenous malformations* (AVMs): Tangles of numerous, abnormally tortuous and misshapen vessels, and containing arteries and veins without an intervening capillary bed, most often in middle cerebral artery territory. Men are affected twice as frequently as women; the lesion is most often recognized clinically between the ages of 10 and 30 years, presenting as a seizure disorder, intracerebral and/or subarachnoid hemorrhage.

• *Cavernous hemangiomas:* Greatly distended, loosely organized vascular channels with thin, collagenized walls occurring most often in the cerebellum, pons, and subcortical regions.

• *Capillary telangiectasias:* Microscopic foci of dilated, thin-walled vascular channels separated by relatively normal brain parenchyma and occurring most frequently in the pons.

HYPERTENSIVE CEREBROVASCULAR DISEASE
(p. 1314)

In addition to hypertensive hemorrhage and arteriosclerosis, other pathologic processes include

• *Lacunes or lacunar state:* Small (<15 mm), often multiple cystic infarcts due to arteriolar occlusion, are most frequently seen in the lenticular nucleus, thalamus, internal capsule, deep white matter, caudate nucleus, and pons. Clinically, they can be silent or cause serious impairment. Because of the common involvement of basal ganglia, thalamus, and adjacent white matter, a number of stereotypic syndromes have been described.

• *Acute hypertensive encephalopathy:* A clinicopathologic syndrome characterized by diffuse cerebral dysfunction (headaches, confusion, vomiting, and convulsions, sometimes leading to coma), with increased intracranial pressure arising in a hypertensive patient. Rapid therapeutic intervention is required as the syndrome often does not remit on its own. Patients coming to postmortem examination may show an edematous brain with petechiae and necrosis of arterioles.

INFECTIONS (p. 1314)

Five categories based on the time course, etiologic agent, and site of involvement:

1. Acute bacterial (pyogenic) or viral (aseptic) infections that affect the leptomeninges and CSF (*meningitis*).
2. Acute bacterial infections of the subdural spaces (*subdural empyema*) or CNS parenchyma (*brain abscess*).
3. Chronic bacterial infections of the brain and meninges (*meningoencephalitis*).
4. Acute, subacute, or chronic viral infection of the brain (*encephalitis*).
5. Fungal and parasitic infections.

Four principal routes of entry of organisms into the nervous system:

1. *Hematogenous spread:* most common, usually arterial.
2. *Direct implantation:* usually traumatic.
3. *Local extension:* from an established infection in an air sinus.
4. *Axonal transport:* certain viruses (e.g., rabies, herpes simplex) travel along peripheral nerves.

MENINGITIS (p. 1315)

Bacterial

Include *Escherichia coli* and the group B streptococci in neonates; *Haemophilus influenzae* in infants and children; *Neisseria meningitidis* in adolescents and young adults; and *Streptococcus pneumoniae* and *Listeria monocytogenes* in elderly people.

CLINICAL FEATURES. Meningeal irritation with headache, photophobia, irritability, clouding of consciousness, and neck stiffness. Lumbar puncture: Cloudy or frankly purulent CSF under increased pressure, elevated protein, and a reduced glucose.

MORPHOLOGY. CSF is cloudy or purulent with neutrophils and organisms; meningeal vessels are engorged. Blood vessels become inflamed and occluded, and hemorrhagic infarction of the underlying brain ensues. In chronic or untreated cases, leptomeningeal fibrosis and consequent hydrocephalus may occur.

Viral

Enteroviruses (echovirus, coxsackie, and polioviruses) are the most commonly isolated pathogens; usually self-limited. Meningeal irritation and CSF with lymphocytic pleocytosis, moderate protein elevation, and nearly always normal sugar content. Often only a mild-to-moderate lymphocytic infiltration of leptomeninges.

BRAIN ABSCESS AND SUBDURAL EMPYEMA (p. 1316)

Predisposing conditions include acute bacterial endocarditis, cyanotic congenital heart disease, and chronic pulmonary sepsis. Streptococci and staphylococci are the principal organisms identified. With infection of the subdural space, thrombophlebitis may develop in the veins that cross the subdural space (bridging veins), resulting in venous occlusion and infarction of the brain.

CLINICAL FEATURES. Usually presents with progressive focal deficits and signs of raised intracranial pressure. CSF pressure, cell count, and protein are increased; glucose is normal. A systemic or local source of infection may be apparent. The increased intracranial pressure and progressive herniation can be fatal, and abscess rupture can lead to ventriculitis, meningitis, and sagittal sinus thrombosis.

MORPHOLOGY. Central region of liquefactive necrosis, a fibrous capsule surrounded by reactive gliosis, and often associated with marked cerebral edema.

CHRONIC MENINGOENCEPHALITIS (p. 1317)

Tuberculous Meningitis

Causes headache, malaise, mental confusion, and vomiting. Moderate CSF pleocytosis of mononuclear cells, sometimes with neutrophils, elevated protein, and moderately reduced or normal glucose. May cause arachnoid fibrosis, hydrocephalus, and obliterative endarteritis. Infection by *Mycobacterium avium-intracellulare* (MAI) in patients with AIDS may cause chronic meningitis, brain abscesses, and rarely diffuse encephalitis or cranial or peripheral neuropathy.

MORPHOLOGY. Subarachnoid space contains a gelatinous or fibrinous exudate of chronic inflammatory cells, with mixtures of lymphocytes, plasma cells, macrophages; rarely, well-formed granulomas, most often at the base of the brain, obliterating the cisterns and encasing cranial nerves. Arteries running through the subarachnoid space may show *obliterative endarteritis*, with inflammatory infiltrates in their walls and marked intimal thickening. Well-circumscribed intraparenchymal mass (*tuberculoma*) also may occur.

Neurosyphilis

A tertiary stage of syphilis; occurs in only about 10% of patients with untreated infections. *Meningovascular neurosyphilis*, chronic meningitis sometimes associated with an associated obliterative endarteritis. *Paretic neurosyphilis*, result of brain invasion by spirochetes; neuronal loss and proliferation of microglia (rod cells); insidious but progressive loss of mental and physical functions with mood alterations (including delusions of grandeur), terminating in severe dementia (general paresis of the insane). *Tabes dorsalis*, result of spirochete damage to the sensory nerves in the dorsal roots and loss of axons and myelin in the dorsal roots and dorsal columns; with impaired joint position sense, locomotor ataxia, loss of pain sensation leading to skin and joint damage (Charcot joints), and other sensory disturbances.

Lyme Disease

Caused by the spirochete *Borrelia burgdorferi* and transmitted by various species of *Ixodes* tick; may cause aseptic meningitis, encephalopathy, and polyneuropathies. Proliferation of microglial cells in the brain as well as scattered organisms.

VIRAL ENCEPHALITIS (p. 1318)

Parenchymal brain infections, almost invariably associated with meningeal inflammation, having a wide spectrum of clinical and pathologic expressions. Characteristic features: perivascular and parenchymal mononuclear cell infiltrate (lymphocytes, plasma cells, and macrophages), microglial nodules, and neuronophagia. The best characterized forms are

- *Arthropod-borne viral encephalitis:* Cause of most outbreaks of epidemic viral encephalitis; major types include Eastern Equine, Western Equine, Venezuelan, St. Louis, and California. All have animal hosts and mosquito or tick vectors. The typical clinical manifestations are seizures, confusion, delirium, and stupor or coma.
- *Herpes simplex virus type 1 (HSV-1, labialis):* Occurs in any age group but is most common in children and young adults; about 10% have a history of prior labial herpes. Common symptoms are alterations in affect, mood, memory, and behavior. Hemorrhagic, necrotizing encephalitis, most severe along the inferior and medial regions of the temporal lobes and the orbitofrontal gyri. Cowdry intranuclear viral inclusion bodies may be found in both neurons and glia.
- *Herpes simplex type 2 (HSV-2, genitalis):* Generalized, severe *encephalitis* in neonates; occurs in up to 50% of neonates born by vaginal delivery to women with primary HSV-2 infection.
- *Varicella-zoster virus (VZC, herpes zoster):* Reactivation of latent infection after chickenpox results in a painful vesicular skin eruption in the distribution of a dermatome ("shingles"). May cause a granulomatous arteritis or a necrotizing encephalitis in immunosuppressed patients.

- *Cytomegalovirus (CMV): In utero* infection leads to periventricular necrosis, microcephaly, and periventricular calcification. In patients with AIDS, CMV is the most common opportunistic viral pathogen, affecting the CNS in 15% to 20% of patients; causes a subacute encephalitis with microglial nodules or a periventricular necrotizing encephalitis with typical cytomegalic inclusions.
- *Poliomyelitis:* The virus attacks lower motor neurons and may cause flaccid paralysis with muscle wasting. Death can occur from paralysis of the respiratory muscles and myocarditis. Inflammatory reaction is usually confined to the anterior horns but may extend into the posterior horns. The postpolio syndrome typically develops 25 to 35 years after the resolution of the initial illness, is characterized by progressive weakness associated with decreased muscle bulk and occasional pain. There is no evidence to date for persistence of polio virus genomes.
- *Rabies:* Transmitted by the bite of a rabid animal, and virus ascends to the CNS along the peripheral nerves from the wound site. Causes extraordinary CNS excitability, hydrophobia, flaccid paralysis; death ensues from respiratory center failure. Widespread neuronal necrosis and inflammation, most severe in the basal ganglia, midbrain, and medulla. *Negri bodies* (intracytoplasmic eosinophilic inclusions) are found in hippocampal pyramidal cells and Purkinje cells, sites usually devoid of inflammation.
- *Human immunodeficiency virus 1 (HIV-1):* Up to 60% of patients with AIDS develop neurologic symptoms, and neuropathologic changes have been observed in 80% to 90%. These fall into three categories: *opportunistic infections* of the CNS (notably CMV, toxoplasmosis, polyoma virus, VZV, HSV, and cryptococcosis), *primary CNS lymphoma,* and *direct or indirect effects of HIV-1,* which comprise the following four syndromes.

  1. *HIV-1 aseptic meningitis,* occurs within 1 to 2 weeks of seroconversion in about 10% of patients; antibodies to HIV-1 can be demonstrated, and the virus can be isolated from the CSF. Microscopically, there is mild lymphocytic meningitis and some myelin loss in the hemispheres.
  2. *HIV-1 encephalitis,* manifest as HIV-related cognitive/motor complex, with insidious mental slowing, memory loss, and mood disturbances, later progressing to motor abnormalities, ataxia, bladder and bowel incontinence, and, rarely, seizures. Features are virus-containing microglial nodules with multinucleated giant cells, and myelin damage with gliosis.
  3. *Vacuolar myelopathy,* found in 20% to 30% of patients with AIDS at autopsy, consists of destruction of myelinated fibers and macrophages involving the posterior and lateral columns, resembling subacute combined degeneration, but vitamin B_{12} levels are normal. A disease with some similarities is *tropical spastic paraparesis,* an HTLV-1 related myelopathy.
  4. *Cranial and peripheral neuropathies and myopathies* include acute and chronic inflammatory demyelinating polyneuropathies, inflammatory myopathy, and a zidovudine (AZT)-related acute toxic reversible myopathy with "ragged red" fibers and myoglobulinuria.

In children with congenital AIDS, neurologic dysfunction, evident by the first years of life, includes microcephaly with mental retardation and motor developmental delay with long tract signs.

- *Progressive multifocal leukoencephalopathy (PML):* Infection of oligodendrocytes by a polyoma virus (JC virus) occurring in immunosuppressed patients. About 65% of normal asymptomatic people have serologic evidence of exposure to JC virus by the age of 14 years. Patients develop multifocal and progressive neurologic manifestations because of irregular regions of destruction of myelin. Lesions consist of patches of demyelination, greatly enlarged oligodendrocyte nuclei with viral inclusions, and astrocytes with greatly enlarged atypical nuclei.

FUNGAL AND PARASITIC INFECTIONS (pp. 1324, 1325)

Most frequently encountered in immunocompromised patients in the industrialized world. The brain is usually involved only late in the disease, when there is widespread hematogenous dissemination of the fungus, most often *Candida albicans,* mucor, *Aspergillus fumigatus,* and *Cryptococcus neoformans.* In endemic areas, pathogens such as *Histoplasma capsulatum, Coccidioides immitis,* and *Blastomyces dermatitides* may involve the CNS after a primary pulmonary or cutaneous infection. Three basic patterns of infection:

- *Chronic meningitis:* Most commonly by *Cryptococcus neoformans;* may occur in immunocompetent patients.
- *Vasculitis:* Most frequently seen with mucor and aspergillus, with invasion of blood vessel walls, thrombosis, and hemorrhagic infarction.
- *Parenchymal invasion* with granulomas or abscesses, most commonly encountered with candida and cryptococcus.

Other infectious agents that may involve the CNS include protozoa (malaria, toxoplasmosis, amebiasis, and trypanosomiasis); rickettsia (typhus, Rocky Mountain spotted fever), and metazoa (cysticercosis and echinococcosis).

- *Toxoplasma gondii:* One of the most common causes of neurologic symptoms and morbidity in patients with AIDS. Clinical symptoms are subacute and often focal; CT and MRI studies show multiple ring-enhancing lesions. Abscesses contain both free tachyzoites and encysted bradyzoites. Primary maternal infection with toxoplasmosis, particularly if it occurs early in pregnancy, may be followed by a cerebritis in the fetus and multifocal necrotizing cerebral lesions, which may calcify.
- Among amoeba species, *Naegleria* sp. causes a rapidly fatal necrotizing encephalitis. A chronic granulomatous meningoencephalitis has been associated with acanthamoeba.

SPONGIFORM ENCEPHALOPATHIES (p. 1323)

A group of diseases (including Creutzfeldt-Jakob disease [CJD] and kuru in humans, scrapie in sheep and goats, transmissible encephalopathy in mink and bovine spongiform encephalopathy) with a characteristic *spongiform change* in the gray matter, consisting of vacuolization of the gray matter neuropil and gliosis, but no inflammatory infiltrates. They are transmissible to experimental animals after a long latent period (usually about 18 months). They have been associated with a protein with unusual characteristics (*prion*), which is an abnormal form of a normal cellular protein.

- *Creutzfeldt-Jakob disease:* A rapidly progressive, fatal dementia that occurs sporadically and has a worldwide incidence of about one per million. Heritable forms exist, linked to specific point mutations in the prion protein; otherwise the mode of transmission is obscure, but there are a few cases of iatrogenic transmission (via corneal transplantation, deep implantation electrodes, and contaminated preparations of human growth hormone).

DEMYELINATING DISEASES (p. 1326)

Conditions characterized by a preferential damage to myelin with relative preservation of axons.

MULTIPLE SCLEROSIS (MS) (p. 1326)

Defined clinically as *distinct episodes of neurologic deficits, separated in time, attributable to demyelinating white matter lesions that are separated in space.* The natural course of MS is variable; often, it begins as a relapsing and remitting illness in which episodes of neurologic deficits develop over short periods of time (days to weeks) and show gradual partial remission. The frequency of relapses tends to decrease over time. In some patients, there is a steady neurologic deterioration. The cellular basis for recovery from symptoms is unknown.

Cellular immunity directed against myelin components is a strong candidate for the underlying mechanism of MS. The rate of MS increases with distance from the equator, and individuals take on the relative risk of the environment in which they spent their first 15 years. Risk is 15-fold higher when the disease is present in a first-degree relative, and the concordance rate for monozygotic twins is approximately 25%.

MORPHOLOGY. Lesions ("plaques") are sharply defined areas of gray discoloration of white matter occurring especially around the ventricles but potentially located anywhere in the central nervous system. *Active plaques* have evidence of myelin breakdown, lipid-laden macrophages, and relative preservation of axons. Lymphocytes and mononuclear cells are prominent at the edges of plaques and around venules in and around plaques. *Inactive plaques* lack the inflammatory cell infiltrate and show gliosis; most axons within the lesion remain unmyelinated.

- *Neuromyelitis optica (Devic's disease):* A variant of MS occurring especially in Asians, characterized by bilateral optic neuritis and especially destructive demyelinating lesions in the spinal cord.
- *Acute multiple sclerosis:* Occurs in younger individuals and has a rapid course; the plaques are large, with destruction of myelin and some axonal loss.

ACUTE DISSEMINATED ENCEPHALOMYELITIS (ADEM) (p. 1328)

- Monophasic disease that follows either a viral infection, or rarely, a viral immunization, characterized by headache, lethargy, and coma; findings include perivenous demyelination with accumulation of lipid-laden macrophages; some polymorphonuclear leukocytes in the early stages, which gradually give way to a mononuclear infiltrate.

- *Acute hemorrhagic leukoencephalitis (AHL)* shares the perivascular distribution of ADEM but is more fulminant and includes hemorrhagic necrosis of white and gray matter. These patients, typically young adults, may not have had a prior viral syndrome.
- ADEM may represent an acute autoimmune reaction to myelin and AHL, a hyperacute variant.

CENTRAL PONTINE MYELINOLYSIS (CPM) (p. 1329)

Selective damage to myelin in the basis pontis and portions of the pontine tegmentum, often leading to spastic paresis and associated with rapid correction of hyponatremia.

DEGENERATIVE DISEASES (p. 1329)

Characterized by

- Progressive and selective loss of functional systems of neurons.
- Onset without any clear inciting event in a patient without previous neurologic deficits.
- Empirically grouped according to regions of brain that are primarily affected.

DEGENERATIVE DISEASES AFFECTING THE CEREBRAL CORTEX (p. 1329)

Principal clinical manifestation is dementia.

Alzheimer's Disease (AD)

Usually begins after age 50 years, with insidious impairment of higher intellectual function, and progresses over 5 to 10 years. Most cases are sporadic, although at least 5% to 10% of cases are familial (loci on chromosomes 21, 14, and 19). Many patients with trisomy 21 who survive beyond 45 years develop a decline in cognition and the pathologic features of AD.

MORPHOLOGY. Gyri are narrowed and the sulci widened, especially in the frontal, temporal, and parietal lobes; hydrocephalus *ex vacuo* follows loss of tissue. Microscopic changes include

- *Neurofibrillary tangles (NFT)*: Bundles of argyrophilic paired helical filaments in neuronal cytoplasm, especially in entorhinal cortex, hippocampus, amygdala, basal forebrain, and the raphe nuclei. Contain hyperphosphorylated tau, MAP2, ubiquitin, and amyloid β-peptide (Aβ).
- *Neuritic plaques:* Spherical, 20- to 200-μm-diameter collections of dilated, tortuous, argyrophilic neuritic processes (dystrophic neurites), with a central amyloid core containing amyloid β-peptide (Aβ), a 40- to 43-amino acid peptide derived from a larger molecule, amyloid precursor protein (APP). Plaque is surrounded by microglia and reactive astrocytes. Occur most often in the hippocampus, amygdala, and neocortex.
- *Amyloid angiopathy:* Vascular wall deposition of Aβ, occurs in intracortical and subarachnoid vessels, and is an almost invariable accompaniment of AD.

These may also occur in the brains of elderly nondemented individuals, so the diagnosis of AD requires clinicopathologic correlation.

- *Pick's disease:* Much rarer; also causes dementia, often with prominent frontal signs. Brain shows atrophy of frontal and temporal lobes, with sparing of the posterior two-thirds of the superior temporal gyrus. Rather than plaques and tangles, there are large ballooned neurons (Pick cells) and smooth argyrophilic inclusions (Pick bodies).

DEGENERATIVE DISEASES OF THE BASAL GANGLIA AND BRAIN STEM (p. 1332)

Associated with movement disorders, tremor, and rigidity.

Parkinsonism

A clinical syndrome characterized by diminished facial expression, stooped posture, slowness of voluntary movement, festinating gait (progressively shortened, accelerated steps), rigidity, and a "pill-rolling" tremor, associated with decreased function of the nigrostriatal system.

- *Idiopathic Parkinson's disease (IPD):* A progressive parkinsonian syndrome that comes on in later life and in some is associated with dementia. Pallor of the substantia nigra and locus ceruleus with loss of their pigmented, catecholaminergic neurons and gliosis; *Lewy bodies* (intracytoplasmic, eosinophilic inclusions) occur in the remaining neurons.
- *Progressive supranuclear palsy:* A progressive striatal syndrome occurring after the fifth decade, characterized by loss of vertical gaze, truncal rigidity, dysequilibrium, loss of facial expression, and sometimes progressive dementia. There is widespread neuronal loss and neurofibrillary tangles in the globus pallidus, subthalamic nucleus, substantia nigra, colliculi, periaqueductal gray matter, and dentate nucleus of the cerebellum.
- *Multiple system atrophies:* Often overlapping group of disorders that include
  - *Striatonigral degeneration:* Similar to IPD but resistant to L-dopa therapy; widespread neuronal loss and gliosis of the caudate and putamen, as well as involvement of pigmented neurons of the zona compacta of the substantia nigra, without Lewy bodies.
  - *Shy-Drager syndrome:* Parkinsonism and autonomic system failure, with loss of the sympathetic neurons of the intermediolateral column of the spinal cord.

Huntington's Disease (HD)

Autosomal dominant movement disorder that becomes clinically manifest between 20 and 50 years of age. Affected patients develop chorea, characterized by jerky, hyperkinetic, sometimes dystonic movements affecting all parts of the body; they may later develop parkinsonism with bradykinesia, rigidity, and dementia. Striking atrophy of the caudate nucleus and, to a lesser extent, the putamen, with severe loss of medium-sized, spiny striatal neurons. Neurons that contain nitric oxide synthase and cholinesterase are spared. The disease is associated with expansion of a trinucleotide repeat in the HD gene on chromosome 4p, which encodes a protein of unknown function.

SPINOCEREBELLAR DEGENERATIONS (p. 1334)

Affect primarily, to a variable extent, the cerebellar cortex, spinal cord, and peripheral nerve.

- *Olivopontocerebellar atrophy:* Mostly autosomal dominant inheritance, with cerebellar ataxia, eye and somatic movement abnormalities, dysarthria, and rigidity. Findings are shrinkage of the basis pontis from loss of the pontine nuclei, widespread loss of Purkinje cells, especially in the lateral portions of the hemispheres, and retrograde degeneration in the inferior olives.
- *Friedreich's ataxia:* Autosomal recessive with a male preponderance. The disease comes on at around 11 years of age, and symptoms of gait ataxia, dysarthria, depressed tendon reflexes and Babinski signs, and sensory loss evolve progressively over about 20 years. Associated findings include pes cavus, kyphoscoliosis, diabetes, cardiac arrhythmias, and myocarditis. Changes include (1) fiber loss and gliosis in the posterior columns and distal corticospinal and spinocerebellar tracts; (2) neuronal loss in Clark column, the VIII, X, and XII cranial nerve nuclei, dentate nucleus, Purkinje cells of the superior vermis, and dorsal root ganglion cells; and (3) peripheral neuropathy.
- *Ataxia-telangiectasia:* Probable autosomal recessive disease; presents in childhood with evidence of cerebellar dysfunction and recurrent infections. Telangiectatic lesions are found especially in the conjunctiva. Findings include loss of Purkinje and granule cells, absence of a thymus, hypoplastic gonads, and lymphoid malignancy.

DEGENERATIVE DISEASES AFFECTING MOTOR NEURONS (p. 1336)

- *Amyotrophic lateral sclerosis:* Loss of lower motor neurons (muscular atrophy, fasciculations, weakness) and upper motor neurons (hyperreflexia, spasticity, and a Babinski reflex); may have predominantly bulbar manifestations (involvement of motor cranial nerves, sparing those that control the extraocular muscles). Degeneration of the upper motor neurons results in loss of myelinated fibers in the corticospinal tracts; occasionally there is atrophy of the precentral gyrus. The disease is more common in men, usually comes on after the fifth decade, and is relentlessly progressive, with death from respiratory complications.

  Approximately 10% of cases show autosomal dominant inheritance; a locus on chromosome 21 appears to be the Cu/Zn-binding superoxide dismutase gene.

- *Werdnig-Hoffmann disease (infantile progressive spinal muscular atrophy):* A severe autosomal recessive form of lower motor neuron disease, which presents in the neonatal period with hypotonia ("floppy infant"). Death ensues within a few months from respiratory failure or aspiration pneumonia. Spinal muscular atrophy has been linked to a locus on chromosome 5q.
- *X-linked spinal muscular atrophy:* Lower motor neuron loss associated with gynecomastia, testicular atrophy, and oligospermia. Has been linked to amplification of a trinucleotide repeat in the coding sequence of the androgen receptor gene, with severity of the disease related to the number of repeats present.

INBORN ERRORS OF METABOLISM (p. 1337)

Three main groups: neuronal storage diseases (*see p. 138 PBD*), leukodystrophies (white matter diseases), and mitochondrial encephalomyopathies.

LEUKODYSTROPHIES (p. 1337)

- *Krabbe's disease:* Autosomal recessive deficiency of galactocerebroside β-galactosidase, the enzyme required for the catabolism of galactocerebroside to ceramide and galactose, with diffuse myelin and oligodendrocyte loss and the aggregation of macrophages around blood vessels as multinucleated cells (*globoid cells*). These macrophages contain storage material (linear inclusions by EM).
- *Metachromatic leukodystrophy:* Autosomal recessive disease with several clinical subtypes (congenital, late infantile, juvenile, and adult), caused by deficiency of arylsulfatase A with an accumulation of sulfatides, especially cerebroside sulfate. Findings include myelin loss and gliosis, with macrophages containing metachromatic material.

Other leukodystrophies include adrenoleukodystrophy, Pelizaeus-Merzbacher disease, an X-linked leukodystrophy caused by a mutation in the gene for proteolipid protein (PLP), a major protein of central nervous system myelin; and Canavan's disease, a spongiform degeneration of white matter with Alzheimer type II cells associated with aspartoacylase deficiency.

MITOCHONDRIAL ENCEPHALOMYOPATHIES (p. 1338)

- *Leigh's disease:* Usually an autosomal recessive disorder, onset between 1 and 2 years of age as arrest of psychomotor development, feeding problems, seizures, extraocular palsies, weakness with hypotonia, and lactic acidemia. Various biochemical abnormalities have been found in the mitochondrial pathway for converting pyruvate to ATP. The brain reveals bilateral regions of destruction with a proliferation of blood vessels, usually symmetrically, involving the periventricular gray matter of the midbrain, tegmentum of the pons, and the periventricular regions of the thalamus and hypothalamus.
- *Myoclonic epilepsy and ragged red fibers* (*MERRF*): Associated with a mutation in a mtDNA gene for a mitochondrial-specific tRNA, resulting in altered function of several of the oxidative complexes. A similar tRNA mutation has been found in *mitochondrial encephalomyopathy, lactic acidosis, and strokelike episodes* (*MELAS*). *Leber hereditary optic neuropathy* is an example of a mtDNA-based disease associated with a point mutation in the gene for a single enzyme, although nuclear genes influence the expression of the disease. *Kearns-Sayre syndrome,* a mitochondrial disorder characterized by ophthalmoplegia associated with systemic defects, is associated with a deletion in the mitochondrial genome.

TOXIC AND ACQUIRED METABOLIC DISEASE (p. 1339)

VITAMIN DEFICIENCIES (p. 1339)

- *Thiamine (vitamin B_1) deficiency:* Beriberi has been discussed (*p. 420, PBD*); may also lead to sudden onset of psychosis (*Wernicke's encephalopathy*), which may be followed by a prolonged and largely irreversible disorder of memory (*Korsakoff's syndrome*). The disorder is particularly common with chronic alcoholism but also may follow thiamine deficiency from gastric disease (carcinoma, chronic gastritis, or persistent vomiting). Findings are foci of hemorrhage and necrosis, particularly in the mamillary bodies, but also adjacent to the third and fourth ventricles. Lesions in the medial dorsal nucleus of the thalamus appear to be the best correlate of memory disturbance.

- *Vitamin B₁₂ deficiency:* Causes nervous system symptoms as well as anemia. Usually begins with slight ataxia and numbness and tingling in the lower extremities and may progress rapidly to include spastic weakness of the lower extremities or paraplegia. Recovery from early symptoms may be expected with vitamin replacement; however, if complete paraplegia has developed, recovery is poor. Swelling of myelin layers producing vacuoles affects both ascending and descending tracts (subacute combined degeneration), beginning at the midthoracic spinal cord.

NEUROLOGIC SEQUELAE OF METABOLIC DISTURBANCES (p. 1340)

- *Hypoglycemia:* Cellular effects similar to those of oxygen deprivation, since the brain requires glucose and oxygen. Neurons that are relatively sensitive to hypoglycemia include large cerebral pyramidal cells, hippocampal pyramidal cells in area CA1, and Purkinje cells. If the level and duration of hypoglycemia are of sufficient severity, there may be a global insult to the neurons of the brain.
- *Hyperglycemia:* Most commonly found in the setting of inadequately controlled diabetes mellitus and can be associated with either ketoacidosis or hyperosmolar coma. The patient becomes dehydrated and develops confusion, stupor, and eventually coma. The fluid depletion must be corrected gradually, otherwise severe cerebral edema may follow.
- *Hepatic encephalopathy (hepatic coma):* Cellular response is predominantly glial, with Alzheimer type II cells in the cortex and basal ganglia and other subcortical gray matter regions.

TOXIC DISORDERS (p. 1340)

- *Carbon monoxide:* Pathology resembles hypoxia, with selective injury of the neurons of layers III and V of cerebral cortex, Sommer sector of the hippocampus, and Purkinje cells. Bilateral necrosis of the globus pallidus may also occur and is more common in carbon monoxide–induced hypoxia than in hypoxia from other causes.
- *Methanol poisoning:* May lead to blindness, with degeneration of retinal ganglion cells. Selective bilateral putamenal necrosis also occurs when the exposure is severe. Formate, a major metabolite of methanol, may play a role in the retinal toxicity.
- *Chronic ethanol abuse:* As many as 1% of patients with a history of long-term high intake of ethanol develop a clinical syndrome of truncal ataxia, unsteady gait, and nystagmus. The early changes are atrophy and loss of granule cells predominantly in the anterior cerebellar vermis. In advanced cases, there are loss of Purkinje cells and a proliferation of the adjacent astrocytes, *Bergmann gliosis*, as the layer between the depleted granule cell layer and the molecular layer of the cerebellum.
- Alcohol consumption during pregnancy, especially in high amounts, may result in the *fetal alcohol syndrome*, with growth retardation, facial abnormalities, cardiac septal defects, joint

abnormalities, microcephaly, delayed development with mental impairment that may range from mild to severe, and neuronal migration abnormalities.

- *Radiation-induced injury:* May develop months to years following irradiation; can be synergistic with methotrexate. Radionecrosis is composed of large areas of coagulative necrosis in the white matter with adjacent edema. Adjacent to these areas, proteinaceous spheroids may be identified, and blood vessels have thickened walls with intramural fibrin-like material.

TUMORS (p. 1342)

Important features of brain tumors include

1. *Consequences of location:* The ability to surgically remove the neoplasm may be restricted by functional anatomic considerations. Benign lesions can have lethal consequences because of their location.

2. *Patterns of growth:* Most glial tumors, including many with histologic features of a benign neoplasm, infiltrate entire regions of the brain leading to clinically malignant behavior.

3. *Patterns of spread:* Some types of tumor will spread through the CSF; however, even the most frankly malignant gliomas (glioblastoma multiforme) very rarely metastasize outside of the CNS.

Tumors of the central nervous system account for as much as 20% of all cancers of childhood. In childhood, 70% of primary tumors arise in the posterior fossa, whereas in adults a corresponding proportion arise above the tentorium. Among adults, there is a nearly equal incidence of primary and metastatic tumors.

GLIOMAS (p. 1342)

Astrocytomas

- *Fibrillary astrocytomas:* Represent about 80% of adult primary brain tumors, usually in cerebral hemispheres, but may also occur in the cerebellum, the brain stem, or spinal cord. All astrocytomas are composed of neoplastic astrocytic nuclei, distributed between astrocytic processes of varying density; grade is determined histologically.

  Low-grade tumors are poorly defined, gray-white, infiltrative tumors that expand and distort a region of the brain; they show hypercellularity and some nuclear pleomorphism. *Anaplastic astrocytoma:* Increased degree of nuclear anaplasia and the presence of mitoses and vascular cell proliferation. *Glioblastoma multiforme:* Most malignant astrocytoma, with a mixture of firm, white areas, softer, yellow foci of necrosis, cystic change, and hemorrhage. Increased nuclear density of the highly anaplastic tumor cells along the edges of the necrotic regions is termed *pseudopalisading.*

  Low-grade astrocytomas may remain static or progress only slowly for a number of years. Eventually, however, patients often enter a period of rapid clinical deterioration and rapid tumor growth, correlated with the appearance of anaplastic features. The prognosis for patients with glioblastoma is very poor: mean length of survival after diagnosis is only 8 to 10 months.

- *Brain stem gliomas:* Occur mostly in the first two decades of

life. By the time of autopsy, about 50% have progressed to glioblastomas. With radiotherapy, the 5-year survival rate is between 20% and 40%.
• *Pilocytic astrocytomas:* Occur in children and young adults, usually in the cerebellum, but also in the floor and walls of the third ventricle, the optic nerves, and, occasionally, the cerebral hemispheres. They are often cystic with a mural nodule in the wall of the cyst. The tumor is composed of bipolar cells with long, thin "hair-like" processes; Rosenthal fibers and microcysts are often present. These tumors are rarely infiltrative and grow very slowly.

Oligodendroglioma

These tumors constitute about 5 to 15% of gliomas and are most common in middle life in the cerebral white matter. In general, patients with oligodendrogliomas have a better prognosis than patients with astrocytomas. Current therapies have yielded an average survival of 5 to 10 years. Cases of poorly differentiated tumors with necrosis have a worse prognosis.

Oligodendrogliomas are well circumscribed, gelatinous, gray masses, often with cysts, focal hemorrhage, and calcification. Tumor is composed of sheets of regular cells with spherical nuclei containing finely granular chromatin, often surrounded by a clear halo of cytoplasm sitting in a delicate network of anastomosing capillaries. Calcification, present in up to 90% of cases, ranges from microscopic foci to massive deposits.

Ependymoma

These tumors arise from the ependymal lining of the ventricular system, including the central canal of the spinal cord. CSF dissemination is a common finding. In the first two decades of life, ependymomas typically occur in the fourth ventricle; in middle life, the spinal cord is the most common location.

The tumor cells have regular, round-to-oval nuclei with abundant granular chromatin; they may form ependymal rosettes, or, more frequently, perivascular pseudorosettes.

Myxopapillary ependymomas: Histologically benign lesions arising in the filum terminale of the spinal cord. Cuboidal cells, sometimes with clear cytoplasm, are arranged around papillary cores containing connective tissue and blood vessels. Myxoid areas contain neutral and acidic mucopolysaccharides.

Subependymomas: Solid, sometimes calcified, very slow-growing nodules attached to the ventricular lining and protruding into the ventricle. They have clumps of ependymal-appearing nuclei scattered in a very dense, finely fibrillar background.

Choroid Plexus Papillomas

These tumors almost exactly recapitulate the structure of the normal choroid plexus, with papillae of connective tissue stalks covered with a cuboidal or columnar ciliated epithelium. Hydrocephalus is common, due either to obstruction of the ventricular system or overproduction of CSF. The lateral ventricles of children are the most common site; in adults, fourth ventricle is more frequent.

Colloid Cysts of the Third Ventricle

Non-neoplastic lesion of young adults; location at the foramina of Monro, can result in noncommunicating hydrocephalus, sometimes rapidly fatal. The cyst has a thin, fibrous capsule and a lining of low-to-flat cuboidal epithelium; the cyst contents are gelatinous proteinaceous material.

NEURONAL TUMORS (p. 1346)
Ganglioglioma

Glial neoplasm with admixed ganglion cell component of irregularly clustered neurons with apparently random orientation of neurites and frequent binucleated forms. Most occur in the temporal lobe and are slow growing, but occasionally the glial component becomes frankly anaplastic and the tumor then assumes a much more rapid course. Mature-appearing neurons may constitute the entire population of a tumor, then termed *gangliocytoma*.

- *Cerebral neuroblastoma:* Rare, aggressive neoplasm that occurs in the hemispheres in children and resembles peripheral neuroblastomas, with small undifferentiated cells and Homer Wright rosettes (*p. 459, PBD*).
- *Neurocytoma:* Found adjacent to the foramen of Monro; evenly spaced, round, uniform nuclei resembling the oligodendroglioma, but ultrastructural and immunohistochemical studies reveal their neuronal origin.

POORLY DIFFERENTIATED NEOPLASMS (p. 1346)

Some tumors, although of neuroectodermal origin, express few, if any, of the phenotypic markers of mature cells of the nervous system and are described as poorly differentiated.

Medulloblastoma

Twenty per cent of childhood brain tumors; occurs exclusively in the cerebellum. Tumors are located in the midline in children, with lateral locations found more often in adults. Rapid growth may occlude the flow of CSF, leading to hydrocephalus. Often well-circumscribed, gray, and friable, they are usually extremely cellular, with sheets of anaplastic cells with hyperchromatic nuclei and abundant mitoses. The cells have little cytoplasm, and the cytoplasm is often devoid of specific markers of differentiation, although neuronal or glial features may be seen. Extension into the subarachnoid space may elicit a prominent desmoplastic response. Dissemination through the CSF is common.

The tumor is highly malignant, and the prognosis for untreated tumor is dismal; however, it is an exquisitely radiosensitive tumor. With total excision and radiation, the 5-year survival has been reported to be as high as 75%.

OTHER PARENCHYMAL TUMORS (p. 1348)
Primary Brain Lymphoma (PBL)

Approximately 2% of extranodal lymphomas. One or more dominant masses within brain parenchyma; nodal or bone marrow involvement or involvement outside of the CNS are extremely rare late complications. Within the immunosuppressed population, e.g., AIDS, all the neoplasms appear to be of B-cell origin and to contain Epstein-Barr virus genomes within the transformed B cells. Regardless of the clinical context in which they occur, PBL is an aggressive disease with relatively poor chemotherapeutic responses, compared with peripheral lymphomas, although it is initially responsive to radiotherapy and steroids. The morphology of the neoplastic lymphocytes is nearly always of a high-grade type. The malignant cells diffusely involve the parenchyma of the brain and accumulate around blood vessels, with some vessel walls expanded by multiple layers of malignant cells.

Germ Cell Tumors (GCT)

Occur along the midline in adolescents and young adults, with the pineal and suprasellar regions dominating the distribution. Tumors in the pineal region show a strong male predominance, not seen in suprasellar lesions. The histologic appearances of GCTs and their classification are the same as used for other extragonadal sites (see p. 1015).

MENINGIOMAS (p. 1349)

These are predominantly benign tumors of adults that arise from the meningothelial cell of the arachnoid. They show a moderate (3:2) female predominance within the cranial vault, but within the spinal canal a ratio of 10:1. Loss of heterozygosity of the long arm of chromosome 22 is a common finding.

They tend to be rounded masses with well-defined dural bases that compress underlying brain but are easily separated from it. Lesions are usually firm to fibrous and lack evidence of necrosis or extensive hemorrhage. Many histologic patterns exist with comparable prognosis:

- *Syncytial* (clusters of cells in tight groups without visible cell membranes).
- *Fibroblastic* (elongated cells and abundant collagen deposition).
- *Transitional* (features of the syncytial and fibroblastic types).
- *Psammomatous* (abundant psammoma bodies).
- *Papillary* tumors, with pleomorphic cells arranged around fibrovascular cores, have a worse prognosis.
- *Malignant meningiomas* are unusual tumors and may be difficult to recognize histologically. Features that support this diagnosis include single cell infiltration of underlying brain and abundant mitoses with atypical forms.
- *Sarcomas* of the meninges are uncommon but can include malignant fibrous histiocytomas and hemangiopericytomas.

METASTATIC LESIONS (p. 1349)

Among general hospital patients, metastatic lesions, mostly carcinomas, account for approximately half of intracranial tumors. Common primary sites are lung, breast, skin (melanoma), kidney, and gastrointestinal tract. The meninges are also a frequent site for involvement by metastatic disease.

Intraparenchymal metastases are sharply demarcated masses, often at the gray-white junction, usually surrounded by a zone of edema. Meningeal carcinomatosis, with tumor nodules studding the surface of the brain, spinal cord, and intradural nerve roots, is an occasional complication particularly associated with small cell carcinoma and adenocarcinoma of the lung and carcinoma of the breast.

Paraneoplastic syndromes: Functional and structural changes of the brain in response to malignancy elsewhere in the body, often small cell carcinoma of the lung. Syndromes may improve with plasmapheresis, immunosuppression, or treatment of the neoplasm.

- *Paraneoplastic cerebellar degeneration* is the most common pattern; loss of Purkinje cells, gliosis, and a mild inflammatory infiltrate associated with an antibody-mediated injury of Purkinje cells.
- *Limbic encephalitis* is a subacute dementia, usually with a prominent component of memory disturbance. Findings are most striking in the anterior and medial portions of the temporal lobe and resemble an infectious process with perivascular inflammatory cuffs, microglial nodules, some neuronal loss, and gliosis.

PERIPHERAL NERVE SHEATH TUMORS (p. 1351)

A large proportion of tumors occurring within the confines of the dura are derived from cells of peripheral nerve; comparable tumors arise along the peripheral course of nerves.

- *Schwannoma:* Benign tumors of neural crest–derived Schwann cells, most commonly associated with the vestibular branch of the eighth nerve at the cerebellopontine angle (vestibular schwannoma or acoustic neuroma). Spinal tumors mostly arise from dorsal roots; tumor may extend through the vertebral foramen, acquiring a dumb-bell configuration. When extra-dural, schwannomas are most commonly found in association with large nerve trunks. They are well circumscribed, encapsulated masses, attached to the nerve but separable from it. Axons are excluded from the tumor, although they may become entrapped in the capsule. Tumors show a mixture of two growth patterns: *Antoni A*, elongated cells with cytoplasmic processes arranged in fascicles in areas of moderate-to-high cellularity with little stromal matrix; and *Antoni B*, less densely cellular tissue with microcysts and myxoid changes. Electron microscopy shows basement membrane deposition encasing single cells and long-spacing collagen. Malignant change, rare.
- *Cutaneous neurofibroma and solitary neurofibroma:* Occur sporadically and in association with neurofibromatosis type 1 (NF1) (p. 148, PBD). The skin lesions are evident as nodules, sometimes with hyperpigmentation; these lesions may grow quite large and become pedunculated. The risk of malignant transformation from these tumors is extremely small. Present in the dermis and extending to the subcutaneous fat, these are well delineated but unencapsulated masses composed of spindle cells in a highly collagenized stroma. Lesions within peripheral nerves are histologically similar.
- *Plexiform neurofibroma:* Considered (by some) the defining lesion of NF1. Tumors irregularly expand a nerve as fascicles are infiltrated; unlike schwannomas, it is not possible to separate the lesion from the nerve. The lesion has a loose myxoid background with a low cellularity, including Schwann cells, fibroblasts, perineurial cells, and a sprinkling of inflammatory cells often including mast cells. Axons can be demonstrated within the tumor. A major concern in the care of NF1 patients is the difficulty of surgical removal of these tumors from major nerve trunks, combined with their potential for malignant transformation.
- *Malignant peripheral nerve sheath tumor (MPNST, malignant*

schwannoma): A highly malignant, locally invasive sarcoma. Do not arise from malignant degeneration of schwannomas; instead, they arise *de novo* or from transformation of a plexiform neurofibroma. The lesions are poorly defined tumor masses with frequent infiltration along the axis of the parent nerve as well as invasion of adjacent soft tissues. Tumor cells resemble Schwann cells with elongated nuclei and prominent bipolar processes; fascicle formation may be present. Mitoses, necrosis, and nuclear anaplasia are common. Patterns of other sarcoma types may be present.

NEUROCUTANEOUS SYNDROMES (PHACOMATOSES) (p. 1353)

A group of mostly autosomal dominant disorders characterized by hamartomas located throughout the body, often prominently involving the nervous system and skin. Neoplasms occur with a high incidence in most of the neurocutaneous disorders. These syndromes include

- *Neurofibromatosis Type 1 (NF1)*: Characterized by neurofibromas (plexiform and cutaneous), acoustic nerve schwannomas, optic nerve gliomas, meningiomas, pigmented nodules of the iris (*Lisch nodules*), and cutaneous hyperpigmented macules (*café au lait spots*). Even in the absence of malignant transformation of neurofibromas, have disfiguring potential and potential to create spinal deformity, most commonly kyphoscoliosis. Tumors arising in proximity to the spinal cord or brain stem may also have devastating consequences, independent of their histologic grade. The gene, located at 17q11.2, encodes a protein homologous to GTPase-activating proteins and may play a role in regulating signal transduction related to growth control.
- *Neurofibromatosis Type 2 (NF2)*: An entirely distinct autosomal dominant disorder (chromosome 22) with a propensity to develop bilateral eighth nerve schwannomas or multiple meningiomas. The gene encodes a member of a group of proteins that interact with both the membrane components and the cytoskeleton.
- *Tuberous sclerosis:* Characterized by angiofibromas, seizures, and mental retardation. Hamartomas within the central nervous system include *cortical tubers* (areas of haphazardly arranged neurons and large cells that express phenotypes intermediate between glia and neurons) and subependymal hamartomas (large astrocytic/neuronal cell clusters beneath the ventricular surface, which may give rise to a tumor unique to tuberous sclerosis—subependymal giant cell astrocytoma). In addition, may be renal angiomyolipomas; retinal glial phakomas; pulmonary and cardiac myomas; hepatic, renal, and pancreatic cysts; leathery cutaneous thickenings (shagreen patches); hypopigmented areas (ash leaf patches); and subungual fibromas. There is variable expressivity and penetrance, and at least two distinct loci are known, on chromosomes 9 and 16. The chromosome 16 gene codes for a GTPase-activating protein, distinct from the NF1 gene product.
- *von Hippel–Lindau disease:* Characterized by
  - Capillary hemangioblastomas in the cerebellar hemispheres, retina, and less commonly within the brain stem and spinal cord.

- Cysts involving the pancreas, liver, and kidney (with a strong propensity to develop renal cell carcinoma of the kidney).
- Paragangliomas.

The hemangioblastomas commonly are cystic lesions with a mural nodule and contain variable proportions of delicate capillary vessels with "stromal" cells of uncertain histogenesis and abundant vacuolated cytoplasm between them. Polycythemia is an associated finding in about 10% of cases, related to erythropoietin production by the tumor. The disease locus on chromosome 3 encodes a tumor suppressor gene that is also associated with renal cell carcinoma.

Index

Page numbers in *italics* refer to illustrations; numbers followed by t indicate tables.

A

Aβ_2 protein, 100
AA protein, 100
Abetalipoproteinemia, 328
abl gene, in cancer, 112, 113t
abl-bcr gene, in chronic myeloid leukemia, 114, 117, 279
ABO incompatibility, 189
Abortion, pelvic inflammatory disease after, 413
Abrasion, 165
Abscess(es), brain, 523
  breast, 427
  Brodie's, 484
  liver, 351
  lung, 299–300
  pancreatic, sterile, in pancreatitis, 368
Acantholysis, defined, 458
Acanthosis, defined, 458
Acanthosis nigricans, 462
  paraneoplastic, 126
Acetaldehyde, in pathogenesis of alcoholic liver disease, 353
Acetaminophen (Tylenol), adverse effects of, 158
  mechanism of cell injury in, 6
Acetylcholine receptors (AChRs), antibodies to, in myasthenia gravis, 512
Achalasia, 311–312
Achondroplasia, 478
AChRs (acetylcholine receptors), antibodies to, in myasthenia gravis, 512
Acne vulgaris, 471–472
Acquired immunodeficiency syndrome (AIDS), 95–99. See also *Human immunodeficiency virus (HIV-I)*.
  central nervous system infections in, 523, 525–526
  clinical features of, 97–98, 99t
  epidemiology of, 95
  fungal infections in, 135
  infections associated with, 143–146
  Kaposi's sarcoma in, 211
  major immune function abnormalities in, 97t
  modes of transmission of, 95
  mycobacterial infections in, 134–135, 523
Acrochordon, 462–463
Acromegaly, 434–435
Acrylamide, neuropathy due to, 509t
ACTH (adrenocorticotropic hormone), ectopic production of, 449
  pituitary hypersecretion of, 435, 449
Actin, 501
Actinic keratosis, 464
Acute phase protein(s), in inflammation, 39

M